Radical-Mediated Protein Oxidation

Radical-Mediated Protein Oxidation

From Chemistry to Medicine

Michael J. Davies

and

Roger T. Dean

The Heart Research Institute, Sydney

OXFORD • NEW YORK • TOKYO

OXFORD UNIVERSITY PRESS

1997

This book has been printed digitally in order to ensure its continuing availability

OXFORD
UNIVERSITY PRESS

Great Clarendon Street, Oxford OX2 6DP

Oxford University Press is a department of the University of Oxford.
It furthers the University's objective of excellence in research, scholarship,
and education by publishing worldwide in

Oxford New York

Auckland Bangkok Buenos Aires Cape Town Chennai
Dar es Salaam Delhi Hong Kong Istanbul Karachi Kolkata
Kuala Lumpur Madrid Melbourne Mexico City Mumbai Nairobi
São Paulo Shanghai Singapore Taipei Tokyo Toronto

with an associated company in Berlin

Oxford is a registered trade mark of Oxford University Press
in the UK and in certain other countries

Published in the United States
by Oxford University Press Inc., New York

© Michael J. Davies and Roger T. Dean, 1997

The moral rights of the author have been asserted
Database right Oxford University Press (maker)

Reprinted 2001

A catalogue record for this book is available from the British Library

Library of Congress Cataloging in Publication Data
Davies, M. J.
Radical-mediated protein oxidation : from chemistry to medicine /
Michael J. Davies and Roger T. Dean
Includes bibliographical references and index.
1. Proteins - Oxidation   2. Free radicals (Chemistry) –
Pathophysiology.   3. Free radicals (Chemistry) – Physiological
effect.   I. Dean R. T.   II. Title.
QP551.D355   1997   612'.01575—dc21   97–28433
ISBN 0-19-850097-1 (Hbk)

Preface

As far as we can discover, there has been no previous book solely devoted to radical-mediated protein oxidation. Yet there have been several books focused on adjacent issues, such as lipid peroxidation, photo-oxidation, atmospheric oxidation, radiation biology (e.g. von Sonntag 1987), and several excellent texts of free radical chemistry (e.g. Fossey *et al.* 1995) and free radical biochemistry and medicine (e.g. Halliwell and Gutteridge 1989). The introductory chapters of several of these (von Sonntag 1987; Halliwell and Gutteridge 1989; Bensasson *et al.* 1993) are appropriate background for a reader to appreciate the present book.

This immediately points to the fact that the delineation of the boundaries of any subject is inevitably fuzzy. Our emphasis is on the molecular mechanisms of protein oxidation, our understanding of which has developed significantly in the last decade. We place equal thrust upon the present and future application of these mechanisms to problems of biochemistry and medicine. We will refer much less to the extensive literature on oxidation in food, in which studies of protein oxidation have been only modest. Similarly, we will not be able to place as much emphasis on plants and lower organisms as on animals, particularly mammals and man, again mainly because the study of these topics has been more limited. In some aspects, notably the metabolism of oxidized proteins, bacteria have been studied quite extensively, but this literature is only mentioned briefly.

It is not possible even in a monograph such as this to refer to all publications with information on protein oxidation. For example, there are specialized series (such as *Methods in Enzymology*) and monographs (e.g. Punchard and Kelly 1996) on methodology including some relevant to protein oxidation. We do not provide practical details here, but rather discuss the interpretation of the various methods. We have only referenced a modest portion of the extensive literature from the 1920s–1950s, which was focused primarily on radiation biology, notably 'strahlentherapie', though we try to offer a judicious sampling. Another area which has been only briefly covered is photo-oxidation, and we have selected against studies which have little relevance to radical-intermediates in photo-oxidation, or which focus on photosensitizers; these areas have been extensively reviewed recently (Bensasson *et al.* 1993). Because our central concern is biological processes, in which proteins are endogenous, we have included studies on oxidation by hypohalous acids and other agents which give rise to radicals when these are endogenously generated in physiology. In general we concern ourselves with processes in which radicals formed on a protein lead, amongst other things, to oxidation of that protein. This occurs both in physiological and pathological circumstances, and can be either productive or non-functional and damaging. We cover only very briefly the literature on enzymes which use protein radicals as part of their mechanism for chemically transforming other molecules in a controlled way (e.g. ribonucleotide reductase). In the recent literature we have also had to be somewhat selective in our listings, though we aim to have fairly represented all the significant data and ideas in it.

Our literature searches were completed in November 1996, and have been based on Medline, Chemical Abstracts, and the Science Citation Index. This lead us to a compilation of more than 3000 references bearing on protein oxidation, of which only about half could be directly referenced in the text. We have concentrated on referencing journal articles rather than book chapters, for reasons of accessibility.

Most of the key contributors to the field have offered useful reviews of various aspects of its development, and many of these are listed here for convenience: (Arnow 1936; Swallow 1960, 1973; Augenstine 1962; Ebert et al. 1965; Garrison 1968, 1987; Tappel 1975; Gardner 1979; Davies 1986; Wolff et al. 1986; Dean 1987b; Pacifici and Davies 1990; Stadtman 1990a, b, 1992, 1993; Dean et al. 1992, 1993, 1994; Levine et al. 1994). We would like to thank the following colleagues who kindly reviewed all or part of this book in manuscript: Kelvin Davies, Shanlin Fu, Jan Gebicki, Jay Heinecke, Patrick Riley, and Roland Stocker.

Sydney   M. J. D.
February 1997   R. T. D.

Contents

Abbreviations

AAPH	2,2′-azobis(2-amidinopropane) dihydrochloride
ACAT	acyl-CoA acetyl transferase
AMA	2-aminomalonic acid
AMVN	2,2′-azobis(2,4-dimethylvaleronitrile)
BCA	bicinchoninic acid
BHA	*t*-butyl-4-hydroxyanisole; butylated hydroxyanisole
BHT	2,6-di-*t*-butyl-4-methylphenol; butylated hydroxy toluene
BPTI	bovine pancreatic trypsin inhibitor
BR	bilirubin
BSA	bovine serum albumin
CGD	chronic granulatomous disease
DEPC	diethyl pyrocarbonate
DMPO	5,5-dimethyl-1-pyrroline-*N*-oxide
DNPH	2,4-dinitrophenylhydrazine
DOPA	3,4-dihydroxyphenylalanine
EDTA	ethylenediaminetetraacetic acid
EGTA	ethylene glycol-bis(β-aminoethyl ether) N,N,N′,N′-tetraacetic acid
EPR	electron paramagnetic resonance
ESR	electron spin resonance
fMLP	formyl-Met-Leu-Phe
G	Radiation chemical yield. This used to be expressed in 'molecules per 100 eV' (electron volts); the (modern) SI unit is μmol per joule ($\mu mol\ J^{-1}$). The conversion between these is $(100\ eV)^{-1} \simeq 1.036 \times 10^{-7}\ mol\ J^{-1} = 0.1036\ mmol\ J^{-1}$. As nearly all the G values quoted in the literature are in the old units, we have not converted these, and all values in the text are in units of molecules $(100\ eV)^{-1}$.
GSH	reduced glutathione
GSSG	oxidized glutathione; glutathione disulfide
HDL	high density lipoprotein
4-HNE	4-hydroxynonenal
HPLC	high pressure liquid chromatography
HSA	human serum albumin
IGF1	insulin-like growth factor 1

LDL	low density lipoprotein
MDA	malondialdehyde
MP	metalloproteinase
MPO	myeloperoxidase
NF-κB	nuclear transcription factor-κB
NK	natural killer
NMR	nuclear magnetic resonance
PBN	α-phenyl-N-t-butylnitrone, N-t-butyl-α-phenylnitrone
RNI	generic term for all reactive nitrogen intermediates
ROS	generic term for all reactive oxygen species
TBA	thiobarbituric acid
TBARS	thiobarbituric acid reactive substances
TCA	trichloroacetic acid
TOPA	2,4,5-trihydroxyphenylalanine
TGFβ	transforming growth factor β

1 A historical survey of the study of radical-mediated protein oxidation

1.1 Early developments in the field and implications for current research

We will give here particular emphasis to the studies before 1970, since those published subsequently are more immediately pertinent to the discussions of later chapters, and are also reasonably well represented in the major review articles we have already listed in the Preface. The first publication we have located on radical-mediated amino acid oxidation without the addition of acid is that of Dakin (1906), and it is also the earliest of those referenced in the major reviews of Garrison (1968) and Stadtman (1993). It is worth summarizing the perceptive work it embodies, both as a taste of the openings of a field, and because of its entertaining contrasts with the styles of experiment and presentation we follow today. The paper is in the first volume of the *Journal of Biological Chemistry* (*JBC*), now by far the most extensive journal of biochemistry, publishing around 30 000 pages per volume, but then a modest, small-format single volume for the years 1905–6. It is also amusing and impressive to note that Dakin's follow-up publication 2 years later (Dakin 1908*a*) was accompanied by a large batch of other single-author publications of his own, taking up roughly half of the volume of *JBC*! Such relative occupancy would be impossible even for a large group to achieve today.

Dakin's 1906 paper is entitled 'The oxidation of amido-acids with the production of substances of biological importance'. As is often still the case, the title makes an assertive claim, whose latter part ('biological importance') is not truly investigated in the work presented. However, the important aspect of the work is that it set the standard and path for the proper and complete chemical characterization of specific products of amino acid oxidation, and protein oxidation, which may now be entering its terminal phases. Setting his work in the context of liver and organismal enzymatic conversion of amino acid into carbohydrate, Dakin points first to the importance of deamination and decarboxylation, and chooses what he describes as a Fenton system in order to investigate the non-enzymic basis of such reactions. As he says, 'this method of oxidation is due to Fenton and has led to most beautiful results in the chemistry of the carbohydrate group'. He then presents data on the oxidation of 'glycocoll' (glycine), alanine, and leucine, mentioning that the first member of a chemical series often shows idioscyncrasies, as he demonstrates for glycine, and as we will discuss later in the context of the particular stability of α-carbon backbone radicals from glycine as compared with other amino acids.

Dakin's experiments were undertaken at 'ordinary temperature' (room temperature). He gives experimental details of a 'typical' oxidation, in which he starts with 1 g of alanine, adds the 'calculated' amount of hydrogen peroxide (which seems to indicate a 1:1 molar stoichiometry as confirmed by the specific conditions defined in a later paper (Dakin 1908b)) and then a 'few milligrams of ferrous suphate'. The scale is impressive, and Dakin notes that after a 'couple of minutes the solution became warm and a slow evolution of carbon dioxide commenced, while the smell of acetaldehyde increased'. In our laboratories in the 1990s the smaller scale of such experiments often precludes the use of smell, with the exception of studies on human atherosclerotic plaque, where the smell of oxidation (mainly of lipids) is still clear-cut.

Dakin's products were thus carbon dioxide, ammonia and an aldehyde. He characterized the aldehyde by the formation of the β-hydrazone with phenyl hydrazine, and the acids by the formation of various salts, followed by elemental analysis. The characterized products from glycine were formic (methanoic) and glyoxylic (oxoethanoic) acids, plus formaldehyde (methanal). From alanine, acetic (ethanoic) acid and acetaldehyde (ethanal) were found, and from leucine, isovaleric (3-methylbutyric) acid and isovaleric aldehyde (3-methylbutanal). Dakin highlights the 'peculiar' oxidation of glycine by indicating the modest production of 'nitrogen-containing substances' .. 'probably oximido-acetic acid (HO–N=CH–COOH) and formaldoxime' (HO–N=C–CHO; structures added by us). Indeed, 'their isolation offers peculiar difficulties which need not be entered upon here'. A charming phrase, especially viewed from present density of publication strictures.

In a second paper in the same issue of *JBC*, Dakin described the oxidation of sarcosine, but his main follow up was in 1908, in which he studied leucine further, and also took on amino-valeric acids (Dakin 1908b). One of Dakin's purposes in the further studies of leucine was to counter claims (Breinl and Baudisch 1907) that leucine gave rise under the action of hydrogen peroxide largely to isobutyric aldehyde (2-methylpropanal), rather than isovaleric aldehyde (3-methylbutanal), which he did effectively and rigourously. Dakin refers to 'old observations' of Liebig discussed by Breinl in support of the claim, on acid/peroxide-induced leucine oxidation. Dakin points out that the elemental analysis published by Liebig showed 'somewhat too high percentages of carbon and hydrogen' to be isobutyric aldehyde (67.3 vs 66.7 per cent; 11.4 vs 11.1 per cent; observed vs calculated). He argues neatly that these impressively minor differences can be explained if isovaleric (3-methylbutanoic) acid were amongst the products. Mild controversy even after the earliest publications on non-enzymic amino acid oxidation! His summary states: 'Breinl and Baudisch's statement of the formation of isobutryic aldehyde by the oxidation of leucine is incorrect'.

The main purpose of Breinl and Baudsich's work was to demonstrate the oxidation by peroxide of keratin, or at least of the components of skin left after ether extraction. Theirs was one of the earliest papers on chemically-induced radical-oxidation of intact proteins, and it demonstrated formation of keto acids, ammonia, and acetaldehyde, together with the formation of peptides by protein fragmentation. This fragmentation was probably largely oxidative since most proteinases would be relatively well inactivated by the ether step. 30 per cent reagent hydrogen peroxide was used, and together with metals clearly constituted a 'Fenton' system. The authors commented (Breinl and Baudisch 1907) on the oxidation of glycine, alanine, and leucine, and on the relative lack of oxidation of tyrosine, an issue to which we will return later, since this was probably an interpretive problem. Probably the next important paper on oxidation of proteins per se by hydrogen peroxide is that of Edelbacher (1924). Edelbacher showed that oxidized protein suspensions contained soluble products, presumably on average smaller in size, which the author considered consequent on fragmentation, and these were positive in the Biuret reaction, and negative for Millon's (a test for phenols such as tyrosine), diazo (a method for detecting aromatic rings), PbS, and glyoxylic acid reactions.

After exposure of casein to peroxide, inflicting what we would consider very extensive oxidation, Edelbacher found that unlike the parent protein, 50 per cent of the resultant protein fracion (which he somewhat misleadingly termed 'apocasein') was resistant to the attack of pancreatin, a proteolytic enzyme mixture from the pancreas. This was perhaps the first demonstration that (strongly) oxidized proteins can be more resistant to proteolysis than their precursors, and anticipates the problem of enzymatic protein degradation and the mechanism by which oxidized proteins may accumulate in the body, which we will address later in the book.

Twenty years later it was found that proteolysis in a pancreatic extract shows a biphasic dependence on radiation exposure, increasing at low doses, and then decreasing again (Bevilotti 1945). This presumably involved initial increases in sensitivity of the substrates superimposed on the enzyme inactivation which would have been concurrent (see below). The enhanced sensitivity due to limited oxidation was more clearly shown with pseudo-globulins irradiated at pH 7.5 in phosphate buffer, and then exposed to trypsin (Haurowitz and Tumer 1949). In this study, various periods of irradiation were used, and after 30 minutes there was precipitation of the substrate. The combined precipitate and supernatant was exposed to trypsin as a suspension, and Kjeldahl nitrogen then measured in the protein-free filtrate, revealing increased release of such low molecular weight material from the oxidized protein. Similar increases in susceptibility of serum albumin to pepsin (Epshtein and Zabozlaeva 1955), and of casein and ovalbumin to trypsin after irradiation were reported, and it was shown in these cases that ascorbate could inhibit the effect (McArdle and Desrosier 1955). This protection may arise from both the repair of protein radicals formed during the irradiation, and simple competition for the primary irradiation products. The large doses of irradiation used in food preser-vation, when applied to insulin caused extensive oxidation, and resulted in decreased proteolytic susceptibility, consistent with the idea of a biphasic relationship between oxidation and proteolytic susceptibility (Drake *et al.* 1957).

Dakin continued his chemical investigations of amino acids by dem-onstrating a series of later reaction products from leucine, derived from the isovaleric acids, and including two hydroxylated derivatives, 'α- and β-oxyisovaleric acid' (2-hydroxy-3-methylbutyric acid and 3-hydroxy-3-methylbutyric acid, respectively (Dakin 1908*b*)). He also proposed an all-encompassing reaction scheme (Scheme 1.1). Subsequently, Dakin studied the Fenton oxidation of glutamate (which gave rise in ammoniacal conditions to succinate), and aspartate, which delivered acetic acid, acetaldehyde, and malonic acid, in agreement with the reaction scheme presented (Dakin 1908*a*). Later, Dakin resolved hydroxyaspartic (2-amino-3-hydroxybutane-1,4-dioic) acid into optically active forms, but he did not find any of it in a '5 months' tryptic digest of casein (Dakin 1922*b*). Other contemporaneous authors showed that the reactivity of different amino acids to peroxide (and also to 'blood charcoals', which seems to be a similar, insolubilized Fenton system), was greater for primary and secondary, than tertiary, amines (Negelein 1923). They also confirmed Dakin's product analyses for glycine, alanine, and leucine using both peroxide and electrolytic oxidation at the anode (Richter and Kuhn 1924). Formation of *p*-tyrosine from phenylalanine, and DOPA from tyrosine by a Fenton system was shown (Raper 1932). The latter was also soon shown to be formed on proteins during irradiation (Nurnberger 1937).

Dakin also performed much synthetic chemistry on amino acids, together with studies of their metabolism when administered to animals. Most interestingly he synthesized β-hydroxyglutamic (2-amino-3-hydroxy-

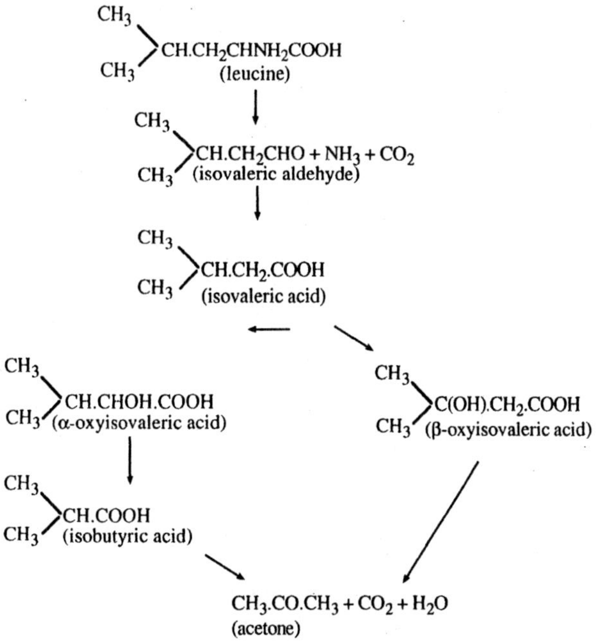

$$\begin{array}{c} CH_3 \\ \diagdown \\ CH_3 \diagup \end{array} CH.CH_2CHNH_2COOH$$
(leucine)

$$\downarrow$$

$$\begin{array}{c} CH_3 \\ \diagdown \\ CH_3 \diagup \end{array} CH.CH_2CHO + NH_3 + CO_2$$
(isovaleric aldehyde)

$$\downarrow$$

$$\begin{array}{c} CH_3 \\ \diagdown \\ CH_3 \diagup \end{array} CH.CH_2.COOH$$
(isovaleric acid)

$$\begin{array}{c} CH_3 \\ \diagdown \\ CH_3 \diagup \end{array} CH.CHOH.COOH$$
(α-oxyisovaleric acid)

$$\begin{array}{c} CH_3 \\ \diagdown \\ CH_3 \diagup \end{array} C(OH).CH_2.COOH$$
(β-oxyisovaleric acid)

$$\begin{array}{c} CH_3 \\ \diagdown \\ CH_3 \diagup \end{array} CH.COOH$$
(isobutyric acid)

$$CH_3.CO.CH_3 + CO_2 + H_2O$$
(acetone)

Scheme 1.1

pentane-1,5-dioic) acid (Dakin 1919), having found it in protein hydro-lysates, including those from gliadin and glutein. He did not undertake elaborate studies to preclude its generation as an artefact. Dakin also claimed, from indirect chemical evidence, that when this hydroxy amino acid was administered to dogs, it caused an enhanced glucose production, reflected in urinary glucose, and hence was catabolized like glutamate, proline or ornithine (Dakin 1919). In another metabolic study, Dakin administered tyrosine, and looked for its potential derivatives in urine. While he found tyrosine itself, he did not find homogentisic acid or other dihydroxyaromatic acids (Dakin 1909). As we discuss later, some di-hydroxyaromatic acids are generated in protein oxidation, and are found in urine (Dutton *et al.* 1993) though their quantities in urine are probably too low for detection by Dakin's methods. In 1944, Dakin synthesized γ–hydroxyleucine (4-hydroxyleucine: (Dakin 1944)), a moiety which we have very recently demonstrated definitively to be present in oxidized proteins *in vivo* (Fu *et al.* 1997). He published the synthesis of γ-methyl-proline subsequently (Dakin 1946).

The extent of oxidation illustrated in Dakin's Fenton systems is probably rather greater than achieved in most current radical-oxidation systems, and indeed in biological systems the emphasis seems to be appropriately placed on only limited oxidation. However, Dakin's work is inspiring in its approach and methodology, and it laid the foundation for further chemical characterization of oxidation products in the 1950s–1970s by Garrison and colleagues, and others such as Kopoldova, and then for contemporary developments. At the same time as Dakin was undertaking these studies, there were many publications on the oxidation of proteins induced by strong acid and alkaline conditions, which we will not review here (Whitaker and Feeney 1983).

Dakin, a chemist by training, was also interested in the application of chemistry to problems of medicine and hygiene, no doubt conditioned by the occurrence of the First World War. In 1916 he published a simple method for the electrolytic generation of hypochlorite from seawater, which could be used aboard ship for disinfection (Dakin and Carlisle 1916). He found that small quantities of the product could disinfect 'tons' of seawater. Dakin subsequently pursued interests in both disinfectants, and biological oxidations, and he wrote a book on each subject. The book on oxidations is a major effort, appearing first in 1912 with 135 pages, and then in a second, substantially enlarged edition (Dakin 1922a), which emphasizes the conversion of amino acids into sugars and fatty acids as potentially important metabolic features of micro-organisms, rather than non-enzymic oxidation, which it considers rather as an archetype for the enzymatic mechanisms.

Dakin's two major interests were by no means separate. Hypochlorite is fundamentally a two-electron, non-radical oxidant, yet it can also produce radicals in reactions with transition metals, and with nitrites and other species. We will generally include it in our considerations, particularly because it is a major product of stimulated neutrophils when chloride ion is present at physiological concentrations. Dakin's early work in this area was again remarkably prescient. He synthesized a germicidal organic chloroamine, given the name 'chloramine', with a view to its stability conferring advantages as an 'off the shelf' antiseptic and germicide, and in this publication he indicated also that protein chloroamines would be expected to possess the same action (Dakin et al. 1916a). In typical spirit, he then went on to show this activity directly with four different chlorinated proteins (Dakin et al. 1916b).

He also injected hypochlorite intravenously into rabbits, and demonstrated a fall in the 'anti-tryptic content' of blood, followed by a compensatory increase after 24 h (Dakin 1917). This may be the earliest example of oxidative inactivation of proteinase inhibitors, since both α-1-proteinase inhibitor and α-2-macroglobulin (to use current terminology) are important in the 'anti-tryptic' action of blood. Equally, it is one of the earliest examples of a biological compensatory response to an oxidative affront, in which the recovery of anti-tryptic activity presumably represented synthesis and/ or secretion of proteinase inhibitors. In order to explain the relative consumption of hypochlorite by various different quantities of serum, Dakin discussed the reactions in terms of selective action on proteins of blood, rather than lipids, again anticipating observations made much more recently on such selectivity during exposure of blood lipoproteins to hypochlorite, as will be discussed later.

Dakin (1880–1952) was an archetype of the 'brain drain': born and trained in the UK, but pursuing much of his career in the USA, he became both an academic and an industrialist (having a major role as a director with Merck and Co.). Similarly, protein oxidation was early to join the fields of industrial application: the products of peroxide oxidation were used in an early patent involving oxidized proteins, to stabilize and protect textiles (Lenssen and Wiegand 1942).

Some of the other early studies on hypochlorite oxidation of proteins were discussed by Engfeldt (1922), who used 'Dakin's hypochlorite', and demonstrated protein cleavage, deamination and carbon dioxide production, and effects on the biuret reactivity of the products. Wright (1926, 1936) distinguished the chlorination and oxidation paths, and demonstrated that the chlorinated derivatives of amino acids differed significantly in their stability, with those of glycine being relatively stable, and those of cystine relatively unstable. Hypobromite, which can also be formed biologically, was also studied by other groups (e.g. (Brigl et al. 1928). These studies together indicated that amino acids in proteins are attacked selectively (SH groups, ring structures with the apparent exception of phenylalanine, guanidino, and free amino groups being preferentially attacked). They also revealed that the reactions, and particularly the balance between oxidation and chlorination, are pH dependent. Later studies of Baker on sodium hypochlorite reacting with ovalbumin (Baker 1947) demonstrated the rapid fragmentation of the protein, using assays of phosphotungstic acid-precipitable Kjeldahl nitrogen to determine the remaining macromolecular portion. Baker deduced a reaction path for chlorination in which initially-formed RNCl groups are later hydrolysed to regenerate RNH functions. Baker estimated that about 2.9 molecules of hypochlorite are consumed for each chain breakage, on the basis of reasonable assumptions, except for taking the molecular weight of ovalbumin to be lower than is now known to be correct.

Probably the next major input of ideas to the field of protein oxidation after those generated by Dakin arose from the work of F. Gowland Hopkins in the 1920s which focused on the roles of glutathione. Again, it is worth considering in some detail the major publication of Hopkins in this area, though it is but one small aspect of his diverse overall contribution to biochemistry (Hopkins 1925). This included editing the series of books on Biochemistry in which that of Dakin on biological oxidations appeared. Matters of presentation in Hopkins' paper are again an instructive and amusing contrast to those of today. For example the article occupies 33 pages of the *Biochemical Journal*, which would currently be an astounding number. In his discussion of the potentially conficting observations of Meyerhof, Hopkins' phraseology also differs markedly from that of Dakin in relation to Breinl and Baudisch. Hopkins (p. 817): 'Nothing, I think, is now more sure than that both views may be correct'. What a subtle conglomerate of conviction and doubt!

The observations in Hopkins' article (Hopkins 1925) 'illustrate certain of the properties of glutathione as a promoter of oxidation', even though they are 'as yet quite insufficient to explain its precise function in living tissues'. Hopkins notes that contemporaneous studies of Warburg and colleagues (e.g. Warburg and Sakuma 1923) indicated that the autoxidation of glutathione requires both oxygen and 'minute traces of iron', as pure glutathione is stable (Dixon and Meldrum 1929). Hopkins comments that, as we still sometimes fail to appreciate now, the complete removal of such minute quantities of iron from biological samples is virtually impossible; it was soon recognized that the form in which iron is available is critical, and some may be inactive (Handovsky 1928). Hopkins' systems therefore contained transition metal, and he was careful to point to its importance in experimental results. He also explains that a statement of Szent-Gyorgi 'that the thiol group as it exists in the tissues .. is not oxidizable', is based only on observations over too short a time period (15 minutes) whereas the oxidation in tissue samples takes 5–6 hours.

Describing the data obtained from oxygen uptake measurements in the Barcroft manometer (the only type of data presented), Hopkins comments that the curves shown are 'quite unsmoothened' (sic), and indeed they are impressive. The experiments were undertaken at 37 °C, with shaking, and at neutral pH, though hardly buffered (in Ringer or distilled water). The paper first addresses oxidation of boiled water tissue extracts, and the stimulation of oxygen uptake by GSSG, and after focusing on fats, demonstrates clearly that the tissue extracts, at neutral pH, can reduce supplied GSSG, and that this remains the case in 'lipoid-free' extracts. This leads Hopkins to consider oxygen 'uptake of pure proteins' and to conclude that 'the establishment of the SH group in its molecule determines in every susceptible protein a capacity to take up oxygen..', far in excess of the quantity needed for direct oxidation of the SH, and particularly after denaturation. Hopkins thereby defines a reversible reduction-oxidation of glutathione and of protein-bound SH groups, and a catalytic action of GSH-GSSG on the oxidation of protein SH groups.

He concludes that the 'oxidation proceeds only when and while the protein itself displays (as shown by the nitroprusside reaction) an SH group'. This conclusion, of course, reflects the limits of sensitivity of the manometric technique, since we now know that modest oxygen uptake can occur during reductant- and metal-catalysed autoxidation of any protein (see Chapter 2). It is clearly implied from the comments about iron that transition metal reduction might be a component of the action of the protein SH, and indeed we confirmed this during our identification (Simpson *et al.* 1992) of (other) novel protein-bound reductants which may also contribute to the kinds of autoxidations studied by Hopkins. Similarly, a recent paper on oxidative events in Alzheimer's disease makes great play of observing the same SH-dependent phenomenon in the SH-rich amyloid precursor protein (Multhaup *et al.* 1996).

Hopkins does not concern himself much with the products of protein oxidation, in contrast to the studies of Dakin. However, he comments that 'Miss Thurlow (1925) has shown that the oxidation of the SH group when it occurs in the presence of a peroxidase may induce other oxidations (e.g. of nitrites) which do not occur in the absence of this latter factor' (Thurlow 1925), and attributes this to the formation of peroxide from the oxidation of the SH group. This phenomenon is an early example of the coupling of protein oxidation to damage to other species. The biological relevance of the autoxidative thiol chemistries is now quite well established, but Hopkins is duly cautious: 'I am well aware indeed that on first acquaintance the curious and at many points obscure phenomena described in this paper may seem to lack biological reality'. Hopkins later offered a stimulating review of his work in this area (Hopkins 1931).

Photochemistry and radiation chemistry provided major contributions in the 1920s onwards, for example particularly from the work of a substantial group of German radiation scientists, and in relation to enzyme inactivation. This impetus is reflected in the existence of the journals *Strahlentherapie* and *Am. J. Roentgenol.* It was also in the 1920s that the term 'free radical' appeared in *Chemical Abstracts*; and monographs on the subject were first published. The conclusions from this literature are reviewed by von Sonntag in his excellent book (von Sonntag 1987); though this early literature is sometimes poorly represented in English language articles. Recent reviews of the area of course suffer from the difficulty that the authors and sometimes the journals carrying the reviews desire contemporary coverage, to the exclusion of historical, and this may partly explain these omissions. For example, the important and lucid 1968 review by Garrison on radiation chemistry of organo-nitrogen compounds (Garrison 1968) lacks any references before 1949. The earlier major review of Augenstine (1962) on actions of ionizing radiation on enzymes covers the literature since 1940 well, but mentions only 10 articles before this (out of 270 references), and four of these are by the originator of current radiation dosimetry methods, Fricke.

One of the earliest substantial works on photo-oxidation of proteins and amino acids (Harris 1926) already demonstrates the selectivity of the emissions of a mercury arc lamp for aromatic amino acids, while also showing the photo-induced uptake of oxygen by several proteins. As noted in the Preface, we shall not consider photo-oxidation in detail, except where radical intermediacy is particularly important, or in the case of choloroplast function.

Even in 1915 it was appreciated that radium rays cause 'coagulation' of protein solutions, presumably reflecting primarily denaturation consequent on chemical modifications. Salt could protect against these changes (Fernau and Pauli 1915). The same authors subsequently showed that an aggregated protein preparation, gelatin, could conversely be induced to disaggregate, as judged by decreasing viscosity accompanied by liberation of protons, and presumably consequent on protein fragmentation (Fernau and Pauli 1922). Subsequently, the decomposition and inactivation of trypsin and pepsin solutions by radium radiations, and also by X-, β- and γ-rays was demonstrated (Hussey and Thompson 1923a,b). Inactivation of catalase solutions by X-rays (Maubert et $al.$ 1924) was also demonstrated. Structural changes consequent upon irradiation were demonstrated by several workers; for example Wels (1923) showed that the surface tension of serum and solution of albumins and globulins was decreased by Roentgen rays. This may have been a consequence of the increased hydrophobicity of the proteins, and their aggregation and loss from solution, though fragmentation might also have contributed. Wels also used an ultramicroscope method to demonstrate globulin aggregation by such radiation (Wels and Thiele 1925) and this was confirmed by others (Dessauer 1930). Others confirmed such structural changes by demonstrating characteristic differences in the absorption spectra of the irradiated proteins (Spiegel-Adolf and Krumpel 1927); these are often also affected by enhanced light scattering (Tyndall effect) due to unfolding. Such aggregation and structural alterations were also observed after ultraviolet irradiation (Rajewsky 1929, 1930; Gentner and Schwerin 1930; Spiegel-Adolf 1931) and high-frequency radiation (Fricke 1938). A particularly impressive early contribution by Arnow (1935) analysed the irradiation of egg albumin and compared acid/isoelectric pH conditions, with alkaline. In the acid conditions, an increase of UV absorbance was found, in association with coagulation and oxygen consumption. Arnow proposed that the increase in absorption was due to a hydroxylation of an aromatic ring, envisaging the formation of DOPA from tyrosine. At alkaline pH, a decrease in UV absorption, a decrease in viscosity, and no apparent 'coagulum' were found, and it was suggested that cleavage of the aromatic rings might be occurring. Later analyses of hydroxyl radical attack on free tyrosine demonstrated the selective formation of DOPA (3,4-dihydroxyphenyl-alanine), with little 2,4-DOPA, and apparent formation of p-hydroxy-phenylpyruvate through side chain reactions similar to those described by Dakin (Rowbottom 1955). This was also confirmed and extended in work which showed the additional formation of *p*-hydroxyphenylacetalde-hyde from phenylalanine, and the formation of the *p*-hydroxy analogues of both the keto acid and the aldehyde from tyrosine (Nosworthy and Allsop 1956).

In the 1930s further indications that protein chain cleavage might be caused by radicals were obtained, usually in the form of evidence that at certain doses, the viscosity of protein solutions decreased. Thus, biphasic effects were observed in studies on gelatin (Zhukov and Unkovskaya 1930; Woodward 1932), such that at low doses viscosity declined, and it rose again at higher doses, corresponding presumably to fragmentation and then superimposed cross-linking and aggregation (though neither fragmentation nor crosslinking were directly demonstrated in these studies). In a few studies, electrophoresis (usually on paper) was used to show that the originally relatively homogeneous electrophoretic pattern became more diffuse after irradiation (Crowther and Liebmann 1939; Dale and Russell 1956), though this was not apparent in all systems, especially with mixtures of proteins, such as serum (Kepp and Michel 1953). The precise causes of the electrophoretic changes were not defined until later, when size and charge heterogeneity could be analysed separately by electrophoretic and isoelectric focusing techniques.

Augenstine makes an excellent attempt to rationalize into a limited number of themes a large body of literature concerning the effects of radiation on enzymes (Augenstine 1962). He indicates that the action of ionizing radiation on solutes in solutions is due to the formation of solvent radicals and their subsequent action on the solute. He particularly focuses on enzyme inactivation, which of course is critically dependent only on a modest proportion of the radical attacks which occur; indeed he explains well that some enzymes possess functional groups critical for their action which are also particularly radiation-sensitive (e.g. cysteine), while others may be inactivated only when a range of different kinds of molecular damage has taken place.

Many of the inactivation studies reviewed by Augenstine concerned dried preparations, in which direct radiation effects are important; these will only be discussed briefly here, because of their very limited biological relevance. Generally, even in dried preparations, oxygen enhances the inactivation, but some disparities were noted, and probably depend mainly on the nature of co-solutes, and on the particular nature of the sensitive groups (or lack of any sensitive group) in the target enzyme. Protein inactivation was achieved when only small proportions of amino acids, except for the cyclic structures and for cysteine, were lost. EPR studies of proteins very shortly after irradiation (Combrisson and Uebersfield 1954) in the dried or solid state have led to the definition of α-carbon radicals as a primary site of radical formation on the proteins (reviewed: Box *et al*. 1961), and to the observation of sulfur radicals formed from cysteine groups (e.g. (Gordy and Miyagawa 1960)) which make many enzymes much more sensitive to inactivation than non-sulfydryl enzymes. Immediately after irradiation, proteins are also often chemiluminescent, or 'thermoluminescent' in the earlier terminology, due to decay of the excited state species they still contain.

Augenstine reviews well the studies on enzymes in aqueous solutions, indicating that the work of Dale and colleagues (to quote an early and a late example; Dale 1940; Dale and Russell 1956) was largely responsible for the realization that radicals, rather than direct primary radiation effects, were important. Dale also showed that with pancreatic carboxypeptidase, substrate dramatically protected against inactivation (Dale 1940). It was some time before the predominant importance of the hydroxyl radical was appreciated, but during the discussion of inactivation mechanisms, the idea of protein radicals, of lesser reactivity than the solute radicals, was put forward. It was also appreciated that solute competitors, and most notably, enzyme substrates, can significantly protect against inactivation. Augenstine tabulates 20 enzymes whose inactivation had been studied quantitatively, of which the most sensitive (glutamate dehydrogenase at pH 7.6, and pepsin at pH 5.4) showed G values of approx 5 (G = molecules inactivated per 100 eV absorbed; see von Sonntag 1987). The G value for radicals released in the γ-radiolysis of water, in the presence of an adequate supply of oxygen, is 5.4, of which half are hydroxyl and half superoxide (see Chapter 2). Thus, if hydroxyl radicals were solely responsible, one radical must inactivate more than one enzyme molecule in these particular cases. For most of the listed enzymes, G values are much lower, mostly around 0.2.

Augenstine's discussion does not assume that a certain minimum solute concentration is necessary for the maximum proportion of incident radicals to react with the solute, as we now appreciate is the case: below this solute concentration, inactivation is inevitably much less efficient. Several authors also argued that partial inactivation, due to partial denaturation, could take place, and was in some cases accompanied by changed substrate specificity. It was also noted that cytochrome *c* can be reduced during irradiation, and we now know this is often a function of superoxide and several organic radicals (though direct radiation effects can also play a role). The variable importance of superoxide, hydroperoxyl, and hydroxyl radicals in inactivation of different proteins was appreciated by Butler and colleagues (Butler and Robins 1960) from studies of the influence of oxygen (needed for superoxide radical formation) and pH (low pH results in the protonation of the superoxide radical to give hydroperoxyl radicals, pK_a 4.8). In some limited circumstances, irradiation can also cause activation of enzymes, as noted much earlier (Seitz 1938).

A few studies documented inactivation of a non-enzymic function, such as the clotting of fibrinogen by thrombin; this was defective after irradiation of fibrinogen (Rieser 1956; Rieser and Rutman 1957). Functional studies were combined with detailed chemical analyses in some particularly important papers, such as that on the oxidation of hormone insulin by irradiation (Drake *et al.* 1957). These authors found selective losses of cystine, tyrosine, phenylalanine, proline, and histidine, and lesser losses (detected at higher irradiation levels) of glycine, leucine, valine, and lysine. They also noted deamination of *N*-terminal glycine and phenylalanine. Drake used massive doses (up to 40 million roentgen equivalent physical, which corresponds to a very slightly smaller number of rads), even exceeding those used in the food industry. Insulin was used at 1 per cent, which from later knowledge would saturate the system in the sense of consuming the maximum proportion of incident radicals in reactions with the protein. Nevertheless, consumption of amino acids was considerably sub-stoichiometric with radical attack. Barron and colleagues (Barron *et al.* 1955) not only demonstrated inactivation of dye-binding during oxic irradiation of bovine serum albumin, but also changes in binding of copper, such that metal bound during equilibrium dialysis increased by approx 40 per cent. This has particular interest for later discussions of the roles of 'mis-localized' transition metals in pro-oxidant events in pathogenesis (see Chapter 5). Barron also presented detailed analyses of amino acid consumption, with results largely consonant with those of Drake. After exposure of sub-saturating concentrations (10 μM) of albumin to 75 000 roentgen (i.e. approx 70 kRad) they observed approx 20 per cent consumption of glycine, alanine, and glutamic acid; lesser consumption of lysine, threonine, tyrosine, and isoleucine (13–21 per cent), and approx 8 per cent loss of leucine, proline, and phenylalanine. They did not detect loss of valine, arginine, histidine, aspartic acid or serine (Barron *et al.* 1955). Though these experiments were conducted at sub-saturating protein concentrations, the amino acid consumption vastly exceeded the radical flux, a matter not discussed in the paper, but brought to the fore in much later studies by Stocker and colleagues demonstrating that in the presence of oxygen there is a chain reaction within protein oxidation (Neuzil *et al.* 1993; Neuzil and Stocker 1993).

There were several other studies of amino acid compositional changes in oxidized proteins in this period. For example, Okada and colleagues undertook studies of amino acid loss during DNAase I irradiation in the presence of oxygen, and interpreted these to indicate that one tryptophan was critical, and others less so: they observed loss of lysine, tryptophan (whose loss was biphasic with respect to radiation dose), isoleucine, histidine, and aspartic acid, in conditions in which other detectable amino acids seemed not to be lost (Okada 1957; Okada 1961; Okada and Gehrmann 1957). UV absorption at 250 nm was increased.

Careful studies were undertaken by Weiss and colleagues of the oxidative damage to histone in deoxyribonucleohistone solutions (Robinson *et al.* 1966*a*, *b*). These authors demonstrated that protein protected DNA from γ-irradiation in the presence of oxygen, in view of the lack of change of protein damage in the presence or absence of DNA, and consistent with relative rate constants for hydroxyl radical attack on important chemical constituents. The relative extent of loss of individual amino acids was also generally consistent with their relative rate constants for reaction with hydroxyl radicals. Thus the aromatic amino acids (tryptophan, tyrosine, phenylalanine and histidine) and methionine were particularly consumed, and the lower losses of aliphatic amino acids declined with decreasing side chain length, so that glycine was relatively poorly consumed; though it was selectively lacking from the polypeptides released from the intact histone as a consequence of the oxidation.

Selective losses of lysine, histidine, cystine, and proline were observed during anoxic radiolysis of RNAase, while other amino acids were not changed at radiation doses of up to 100 kRad (1000 Gray) with the enzyme at 100 μM (Levitzki and Anbar 1967). The loss of amino acids during irradiation in the presence of nitrous oxide (which efficiently converts e^-_{aq} into HO·) as measured by G values, was approx 5. This value is very similar to that for the production of hydroxyl radicals, and it was found to be unchanged by the addition of copper. In the presence of copper, which bound to the enzyme at histidine residues, the loss of histidine and proline was accentuated at the expense of the cystine and lysine, and at the same time, the inactivation of the enzyme (and of enolase) was increased. This was one of the earliest indications of the superimposition of site-specificity dictated by metal binding upon the selectivity of hydroxyl radical attack on proteins.

Similarly, it was found that during the cupric (Cu(II)) ion catalysis of γ-globulin cleavage by hydrogen peroxide (Phelps *et al.* 1961), histidine and proline (together with valine) were preferentially lost. These authors made an interesting comparison between consumption of free amino acids and protein-bound (γ-globulin) amino acids in their system. Unlike the situation with the protein, tryptophan, tyrosine, and phenylalanine were amongst the heavily damaged free amino acids, while histidine was highly susceptible in both circumstances. Their electrophoretic studies demonstrated fragmentation and aggregation, and confirmed this for bovine serum albumin also. The selective loss of tryptophan, but not tyrosine and histidine, during the oxidation of α-chymotrypsin by horse radish peroxidase and hydrogen peroxide was also noted (Wood and Balls 1955).

Interestingly, a surprisingly high G value (about 1) was reported for peptide chain breakage in pepsin and gelatin ((Jayko and Garrison 1958) and this is discussed later) though its bearing upon inactivation was not clear. Anaerobic fragmentation was also noted (Kumta and Tappel 1961) in terms of generation of TCA-soluble fragments. Fragmentation by copper and ascorbate was observed in early detailed studies of Orr, in which he detected small fragments by size-dependent gel filtration, and changes in paper electrophoresis behaviour of catalase (Orr 1967a, b). Some UV spectral changes occurred beyond those of the haem, consistent with aromatic amino acid oxidation, and it was also noted that radioactive ascorbate became incorporated into the protein, and that there was some formation of larger structures. Even without added copper, ascorbate could damage the protein, and one would now tend to interpret this as another indication of effects of low concentrations of metals endogenous to the buffers and the enzyme.

This area of radiation chemistry has been well reviewed by Swallow (Swallow 1960) and has been continued in studies by Adams, Land, Willson, and colleagues in the UK, Prutz, von Sonntag, and others in Germany, and Garrison in the USA, and encompasses both steady state radiolysis, and pulse radiolysis (Ebert et al. 1965); in the latter the transient spectra of reaction intermediates can be defined. For example, the early spectra of products during the reaction of lysozyme with hydroxyl radicals and the other primary radiolysis products of water can be largely explained by reactions at disulfides and tryptophan (Adams et al. 1969; Aldrich et al. 1969). These studies have developed the understanding of reaction routes, and of specific products which can be obtained largely from the radicals produced in water by radiation. Extensive studies of radiation damage to proteins in the solid phase (often at low temperatures) were started in the mid-1950s with the development of a technique which allowed the direct detection of paramagnetic species (i.e. free radicals and some metal ions)—electron paramagnetic (or spin) resonance (EPR or ESR) spectroscopy. Many of these early studies were reported in physics, or physical chemistry, journals despite their obvious biological relevance, emphasizing the early development of this methodology by physicists. These early EPR studies illustrated the importance of α-carbon radical formation and of SH dependent radicals (Gordy et al. 1955a, b; Gordy 1958). Secondary processes resulting from the warming (annealing), and oxygenation of protein samples irradiated dry at 77 °K, allowed the decay and interconversion of these initial species to be examined. Thus the formation of peroxyl radicals, and the interconversion of the thiyl (RS·) and the so-called 'glycylglycine' α-carbon radical signals were observed (Henriksen et al. 1963; Garrison et al. 1964; Patten and Gordy 1964; Henriksen 1967). The addition of SH compounds, such as cysteamine or cysteine, was found to lead to the formation of thiyl radicals, which subsequently gave rise to the glycyl α-carbon radical, presumably upon their further oxidation (Singh and Ormerod 1965). Seleno-amino acids are more protective than the corresponding sulfur-amino acids (Shimazu and Tappel 1964). These solid state and low temperature studies were subsequently extended to the reactions of hydroxyl radicals and related species with amino acids and small peptides in aqueous solution at room temperature, through irradiation (electron or UV) EPR methods in the 1960s and 1970s (see Chapter 2).

The pulse radiolysis approach also supported the realization in the 1960s–1970s that the initial site of radical formation in a peptide or protein is not necessarily the final site of reaction; radicals may be translocated to distal sites within the same molecule by various electron transfer processes. Even in di- and tri-peptides, the differential competition between tyrosine and amino acids such as cysteine, methionine, tryptophan (effective) and leucine, isoleucine, valine, glycine, alanine, or glutamate (ineffective) for radiation-induced radicals could be discerned, in terms of differential extents of production of DOPA (Fletcher and Okada 1961). Such studies emphasized the greater complexity of radical chemistry in proteins, with four levels of structure, than in free amino acids. At the same time, definition of oxidation of the free amino acids developed, using a variety of paper chromatography techniques to provide (provisional) identification of the products. For example, Nofre and colleagues studied solely the amino-group-containing products of Fenton oxidation of a range of amino acids, and qualitatively defined interesting conversions, such as histidine to asparagine, proline to glutamate, and many hydroxylation products of the aromatic amino acids (Nofre et al. 1961).

A complementary, more biological, approach was introduced by the extensive studies of Tappel and colleagues since the late 1950s. Tappel was particularly concerned with oxidation in membranes and organelles, and with relationships between lipid peroxidation and protein damage (reviewed: Tappel 1978). There was (and still is) considerable interest in these issues from the point of view of food science, since the development of toughness in stored foods often depends on lipid-protein interactions which result in the insolubilization of proteins (e.g. that of cod actomyosin by linoleic and linolenic acids (King et al. 1962)), and which usually involve oxidation. They also involve reactions between end products of lipid oxidation, such as the aldehydes, and protein. For example, MDA (malondialdehyde) could react by addition with free amino groups of bovine serum albumin; this seemed to involve reaction of each MDA with only a single amino group, as there was no significant cross-linking of gelatin induced (Crawford et al. 1967). Further characterization of the products followed (Chio and Tappel 1969b).

Tappel emphasized the interaction between lipid peroxidation products and protein as 'radiomimetic', discussing the quantities and to a lesser degree the qualities of products (Romani and Tappel 1959; Roubal and Tappel 1966a, b) and showing that peroxidizing lipid and peroxidation products such as MDA can inactivate ribonuclease and other enzymes (Chio and Tappel 1969a). For example, during the interaction of peroxidizing linolenic acid with cytochrome c, inactivation was associated with loss from the macromolecular fraction of 55–35 per cent of the initial content of the amino acids histidine, serine, proline, valine, arginine, methionine, and cystine (in descending order of loss) and 20–30 per cent of the other amino acids studied; the loss of tryptophan was not measured (Desai and Tappel 1963). Insolubilisation often results from the lipid-protein co-oxidation (Roubal and Tappel 1966b), and analyses of the amino acid constitution of the insolubilized portions of several proteins after reaction with arachidonate revealed the generally high susceptibility to loss of methionine, histidine, cystine, and lysine (Roubal and Tappel 1966a). In the insolubilized BSA and haemoglobin, glycine and the aromatic residues are also substantially lost. Tappel's work is discussed further in Chapter 3.

The interactions and competition between macromolecules may be such that one 'spares' another from damage, in that they may compete for radical fluxes. This is true of proteins in the presence of lipid, as had also been earlier pointed out for plasma proteins in the presence of bilirubin (Barae and Roseman 1946). This paper showed that bilirubin in alkaline solution autoxidizes rapidly, and this process can be inhibited by human or bovine serum albumin, though not by several other proteins. Current understanding is however that bilirubin is a significant antioxidant, one of whose functions may be to protect albumin from oxidation (Neuzil and Stocker 1993, 1994).

Studies in the 1970s were among the first to consider in detail how oxidation of a protein might influence its metabolism, emphasizing first the influence of S–S formation from SH groups. This thrust was vastly developed by Stadtman, who proposed that limited oxidation of proteins might be a signal for their accelerated degradation, a kind of biological garbage-munching machine. We have later elaborated this idea to accommodate the fact that oxidized proteins accumulate in a range of biological systems, during physiological ageing, and during several pathologies.

A recent development contributed by ourselves has been the idea that besides protein-radicals themselves, protein oxidation gives rise to several relatively stable, yet reactive intermediates, rather analogous to the lipid hydroperoxides of lipid peroxidation. Thus both oxidizing and reducing species have been defined, and their physiological and pathological roles are under investigation. As with many areas of research, in retrospect one can see this to have been foreshadowed in areas of the literature which subsequently were neglected. For example, the oxidizing species which we have defined, protein hydroperoxides, were observed from certain free amino acids (glycine, alanine, leucine, aspartic acid, and lysine) by Latarjet in the 1940s (Latarjet and Loiseleur 1942; Loiseleur *et al*. 1942), though no quantitation is given, and the positive observation on glycine, which actually yields little peroxide in these circumstances (Okada 1958) makes one suspect that hydrogen peroxide was a significant portion of what was measured. However, the occurrence of peroxides and TBA-reactive products on irradiated amino acids and proteins was subsequently suggested again (Alexander *et al*. 1956; Okada 1958; Ambe and Tappel 1961).

Indications of their presence on heavily irradiated proteins were sometimes incomplete, again because hydrogen peroxide was not always removed (Garrison *et al*. 1962). Garrison and colleagues themselves made detailed quantitative studies of carbonyl, ammonia, amide nitrogen, ketoacid, and organic peroxide formation during radiation of 1 per cent gelatin (Garrison *et al*. 1962). The organic peroxides ($G \simeq 0.4$) detected in this study were no doubt protein derived hydroperoxides, as distinct from the separately measured hydrogen peroxide ($G \simeq 1.24$).

However, the idea of their importance in reaction chains was also prefigured, and in some cases explicitly anticipated. It was observed (Anderson 1954; McDonald 1954) that the inactivation of trypsin and pepsin solutions, respectively, continued after irradiation. While this was probably largely due to reactions of metal ions and hydrogen peroxide, it may also have involved protein-bound reactive species such as hydroperoxides undergoing further reaction. More explicitly, Alexander and colleagues (Alexander *et al*. 1956) found that proteins irradiated in the presence of oxygen could induce polymerization of methacrylate, whereas samples irradiated in vacuo did not. This finds close parallels in the recent studies of protein peroxyl radicals on haem proteins inducing styrene oxidation (Ortiz de Montellano and Catalano 1985). Similarly, we have emphasized the possible importance of protein-bound catechols, such as DOPA, in autoxidation reactions. An important progenitor to this idea was the studies of the roles of catechols, be they exogenous or endogenous to protein, in hardening of insect cuticle, involving 'tanning' of the protein 'sclerotin' (Hackman 1953; Hackman and Todd 1953). Some of the reactions that occur during this process (e.g. those involving transition metal reduction, and radical additions), are in common with steps in melanogenesis, and are summarized by Horner (1961).

The various reactive species we have identified are probably, together with the protein-bound radicals, the main agents of the protein chain oxidation reaction, as we now appreciate it through the contribution of Stocker and colleagues; and our definition of a range of protein-bound radical species offers a plausible chemistry for the chain oxidation, and explains its essential features, differing from lipid oxidation, of slight oxygen consumption and modest chain length.

We are now at an exciting stage in the study of this field, in assessing the biological importance of the reactions and products discussed. It is our hope that this book will contribute to enhancing and accelerating that development.

1.2 The influence of technical advance on biochemical understanding of protein oxidation

From reviewing the earlier literature on protein oxidation above, it is quite apparent that there are repeated waves of publication on a particular area. Table 1.1 summarizes some of these. This is a well known phenomenon in bibliometrics, and it operates at levels of 'normal science' much more detailed and narrow than those associated with the 'paradigm shift' of a 'scientific revolution', as envisaged by Kuhn (1970). Subsequent authors have proposed substantial developments and modifications to Kuhn's views, and indicated that the sociological basis of such clusters may have some relevance to 'normal science' as well as to the revolutionary (Latour and Woolgar 1979; Charlesworth *et al.* 1989).

We are not here attempting a sociological analysis of the waves of Table 1.1, but rather providing an ethnographic synopsis which may be of use to future sociologists of science in considering this area. In doing so we point out the overlapping influences of new ideas, and of new kinds of technique and equipment. We shall refer for convenience to the latter as new 'technologies', while noting that the term is often used much more broadly and sociologically.

In assessing whether a development is the result of new analytical thoughts, or rather a secondary consequence of the availability of new technology, the simplest, default hypothesis is probably the cynical one, that developments are largely conditioned by technical change. This is well symbolized in a chapter title of Charlesworth and colleagues: 'The triumph of technique: from molecular biology to biotechnology' (Charlesworth *et al.* 1989). Note, however, that such technical developments themselves were more often probably the result of new analytical thought, but we will not discuss that here.

So what were the major advances in technique and equipment relevant to the field, during its parallel development? Most striking was the discovery at Kazan University in 1944 of the phenomenon of electron paramagnetic resonance (EPR) by Zavoisky; radio frequency absorption lines were detected from samples of Cu(II) and Mn(II) salts (Zavoisky 1944, 1945*a*, *b*, 1946). These fundamental studies laid the foundations for the subsequent rapid growth, and use, of EPR (or ESR) spectroscopy, first for detecting paramagnetic metal ions and later, organic radicals. The rapid exploitation

Table 1.1 A simplified chronology of the study of protein oxidation

Aspect	Periods	Comments and selected references
Characterization of oxidation products	1905–	Side chain Fenton oxidation products of amino acids, particularly aliphatic (Dakin 1906, 1922b)
	1960–	Stoichiometry and pathways for protein cleavage and modification (Garrison et al. 1962; Garrison 1968)
	1990–	Fenton oxidation revisited: role of bicarbonate (Stadtman and Berlett 1991)
Reactive non-radical products of protein oxidation	1942–	Amino acid hydroperoxides (Latarjet and Loiseleur 1942)
	1960–	Hydroperoxides on proteins (Ambe and Tappel 1961)
	1992–	Hydroperoxides and DOPA as oxidizing and reducing species, respectively (Simpson et al. 1992)
Radiation damage to proteins through free radical attack	1920–	'Coagulation' of protein
	1960–	Modification and fragmentation
	1980–	Selectivity of fragmentation and its effects on conformation (Schuessler and Herget 1980; Schuessler and Schilling 1984; Wolff and Dean 1986; Davies 1986; Davies and Delsignore 1987; Davies et al. 1987a, b)
Oxidation of proteins as an influence on enzymatic proteolysis	1975–	Limited oxidation as trigger (Francis and Ballard 1980; Levine et al. 1981; Goldberg and Boches 1982; Dean and Pollak 1985; Davies 1986) Substantial oxidation as limitation (Davies 1986; Dean et al. 1986a; Grant et al. 1992; Jessup et al. 1992b)
Protein bound radicals	1960–	Demonstration (Schaich 1980a, b, c; Floyd and Nagy 1984) Generated from protein-bound hydroperoxides (Davies, M.J. et al. 1995)
Protein oxidation as a chain reaction	1992–	Demonstration and determination of stoichiometry (Neuzil et al. 1993; Neuzil and Stocker 1993) Proposal of radical reaction scheme (Davies, M.J. et al. 1995)

of this technique, which preceded that of its more well known cousin nuclear magnetic resonance (NMR) spectroscopy, was undoubtedly aided by the Second World War due to the widespread availability of the microwave systems needed for the technique, which had originally been developed for radar. Thus many early machines, which were hand built, worked in the 9 GHz frequency region (X-band) partly due to the low cost of these components.

After the initial experiments in the USSR, EPR methods were rapidly developed both in the USA (Cummerow and Halliday 1946) the UK (Bagguley and Griffiths 1947), though the technique remained primarily the preserve of physicists, due to the requirement to hand-build the equipment, until machines became commercially available in the early 1960s. The steadily increasing sensitivity and ease of use of these machines catalysed their rapid spread in to both large numbers of chemical, and a few biological, departments. The first major reviews of the use of this technique in the biological sciences appeared in the late 1960s and early 1970s (Swartz et al. 1972).

Other spectrometers using the related technique of NMR have also proved very helpful in structural analyses, and became effective in the 1950s and 1960s, though their penetration into the biological field was slow due to the requirement for large quantities of pure materials (NMR being orders of magnitude less sensitive than EPR spectroscopy) and the enormous complexity of the spectra from most biological molecules. The subsequent development of multi-nuclear spectrometers and high-field machines has dramatically enhanced their use in biological systems.

Separation techniques also underwent a major development, from the paper and thin layer electrophoresis of the early part of the century, to column chromatography in the 1960s and 1970s, and then the development of high pressure liquid chromatography since then. These have been important for isolation of materials for structural definition, as well as for analytical procedures. Ancillary developments such as gel electrophoresis and, more recently, capillary electrophoresis, have primarily been useful in analytical separations, notably of proteins. Downstream of the separation and isolation, mass spectroscopy has vastly strengthened the researcher's armoury for structural determination, giving much more information than elemental analysis such as performed by Dakin, and working well in conjunction with NMR of small to moderately sized molecules. Mass spectroscopy has substantially accelerated the sequencing of peptides and proteins as well as oxidation products derived from them. Furthermore, recent techniques permit the direct sequencing of very small quantities eluted from HPLC columns or polyacrylamide gels.

These technological changes can explain several of the waves in the field. For example, the recurrence in the 1960s and then in the 1980s–1990s of structural definition of the kind initiated by Dakin, might largely reflect the availability, respectively of improved paper and column chromatography techniques, and improved HPLC and structural analysis techniques. This would also explain why the 1960s analyses were more a case of partial separation and hesitant (or confident) supposition of the associated structure (Kopoldova *et al.* 1963*a*, *b*, *c*), while the recent ones attempted more direct demonstrations of purity, and precise structural definition, including isomeric distinctions. The technological influences can also explain the progressive transfer of the radiation chemists' interest from small molecule studies, to enzyme inactivation, back to amino acid analysis within proteins, since the procedures for larger molecules became gradually available.

Which developments might reflect the input of novel ideas? And which of these ideas reflect the application of ideas from other fields? Again, the latter is simpler to divine as a possibility, though of course the realities of thought processes are beyond our space or capabilities here. A novel idea in the late 1970s and early 1980s, still under careful assessment, is that oxidized proteins, being unfolded are degraded by cells more rapidly than their parent native molecules. This could be seen to have arisen from the much earlier protein chemistry studies of protein unfolding and folding, in which a criterion of partial unfolding was often increased susceptibility *in vitro* to a proteolytic attack. Furthermore, there was a great thrust in the 1970s for the study of abnormal proteins, including error-containing proteins, resulting from incorrect protein synthesis. These latter proteins were often modelled by studies of proteins synthesized in the presence of amino acid analogues such as canavanine, 2-azetidine-carboxylic acid, and aliphatic amino acid hydroxides (related to arginine, proline, and the aliphatic amino acids repectively). These amino acids could be incorporated reasonably efficiently, when supplied to a variety of cells, and they lead to the production of classes of proteins which were much more unstable than average, in the sense of undergoing more rapid protein degradation in cells, and in lysates. The extent of incorporation of these analogues was always quite limited and, in a few cases, the degradation of individual proteins such as tyrosine amino transferase, was shown to be accelerated when they contained the analogues.

Thus it was a clear prediction from such studies that oxidized proteins, at least at modest levels of substitution of modified amino acids, might be more rapidly degraded than native ones. Such were the observations of Stadtman in lysate systems, ourselves using isolated mitochondria, and Goldberg, Davies and ourselves in intact cell systems, though the claimed magnitude of the effect varied very much from system to system (from a factor of around 1.5 to 50). Later studies have indicated that this simple interpretation may need to be modified in the face of more extensive oxidation, or perhaps in the face of certain specific modifications, such as some kinds of glycation (Fu *et al.* 1994; Dean *et al.* 1986; Wolff and Dean 1987) or oxidation (Grant *et al.* 1993) which are difficult for proteolytic enzymes to handle. Such changes may cause inefficiency of catabolism, which may be part of the mechanism of accumulation of oxidized proteins in ageing.

Thus the idea of oxidation as markers for proteolysis was an outgrowth of the more general idea of unfolding and chemical modification by other means functioning as such markers. Similarly, our more recent idea of protein oxidation as a route for the formation of relatively long-lived reactive species, which might transfer damage to other targets when eventually they react further, is an outgrowth of ideas from the much more heavily studied area of lipid peroxidation. If one searches Medline 1966–09/ 1996 one finds 12 387 hits for 'lipid peroxidation' (where the words have to be adjacent), which may be compared with the body of around 3000 references which we have gathered as relevant to protein oxidation, or with the lesser numbers found by similar Medline searches. To search Medline for literature on protein oxidation, it is necessary to exclude the significant literature on enzymatic amino acid oxidation, which also appears in metabolic studies of protein turnover as 'protein oxidation'. 'Protein peroxidation' (where the two words must be adjacent) is resistant to this problem as a search vehicle, but only finds 26 references (references from Medline 1966–09/1996), of which several have the words in the reverse order. Searching for the string radi* (where the asterisk indicates any termination) identifies words such as radical and radiation, and hence can usefully be used as a Boolean 'and' with 'protein oxidation' (as adjacent words). Articles concerned with protein turnover rarely contain the string radi*, and thus are quite well excluded by this approach. The combination search 'protein oxidation' (as adjacent terms), with the additional requirement of the presence of radi*, finds additional references, and the total of unique references from this and 'protein peroxidation' is only about 90. The frequency of such references does rise gradually towards the present, but clearly this change reflects terminology more than research activity.

This huge difference between the numbers of publications on lipid and protein oxidation is indicative of the disparity in effort applied to these fields: because of the breadth of the searches which has engendered 3000 protein oxidation references, the figure for lipid peroxidation is a substantial underestimate of the figure which would be similarly achieved. Conversely, if one searches 'lipid peroxidation' and 'lipid oxidation' (words adjacent in both cases), and adds the requirement for radi* as used in the protein oxidation searches, there are 4952 hits. The use of radi* is justifiable since lipid oxidation, like protein oxidation, gathers studies on metabolic turnover of lipids (through mitochondrial and peroxisomal fatty acid oxidation). From all these figures, it seems that a conservative estimate of the ratio of lipid:protein oxidation publications is at least 50 and so it is not surprising that the field of lipid oxidation is more advanced.

The protein enthusiast might also argue that lipids are easier to work with! Thus lipid peroxidation leads to the formation of hydroperoxides, which are intermediates in peroxidation, and first accumulate during peroxidation of a membrane or of lipoproteins, and then are removed. Removal may involve reduction to alcohols or further radical generation (Kenar *et al*. 1996). We rediscovered protein hydroperoxides while analysing total hydroperoxides in LDL, and comparing this with albumin (lipid free). We anticipated that at certain stages of protein oxidation, reactive species might be present, such as the hydroperoxides, which could damage secondary targets. These ideas led by analogy with lipid peroxidation to our search for both reducing and oxidizing reactive species, and to our subsequent demonstration of both radical products and alcohols from the reactions of protein hydroperoxides, as discussed later in this volume.

It is perhaps surprising that as yet, the recent increased public awareness of necessity for food quality control, has not led to much new data on protein oxidation in food. Particularly in the case of detection and quantification of food irradiation, which is a burning issue in many countries, some of the stable products of protein oxidation could be very useful. Furthermore, there may well be novel species among protein oxidation products in irradiated food, because of the special physical conditions which apply, and the coexistence of cell death without complete degradation by endogenous enzymes or spoilage by micro-organisms. Food science was amongst the earliest stimuli for the study of protein oxidation, particularly in relation to anoxic conditions (Garrison 1987) and it may become so again in the near future, and with reference to oxic as well as anoxic conditions, in view of changes in storage mechanisms.

Finally, the recent enhanced definition of radical species upon proteins, can be seen partially as an outgrowth of the development of ideas just discussed, and partly as a result of the discovery of proteins which use stable radicals within their enzymatic cycles. Changes in sensitivity of the equipment have been partly responsible for improved definition of protein-bound as opposed to free amino acid radicals. Awareness of the formation of radical species on proteins, and the relative importance of peroxyl and alkoxyl radicals, has, with the independent contribution of Stocker and colleagues, resulted in the realization that protein oxidation is a 'chain reaction' and is another example of the cross-over of ideas from lipid peroxidation to protein oxidation.

Most of the developments in the study of protein oxidation can thus be considered as examples of the influence of technical developments, and of analogous ideas from the fields of proteolysis and lipid oxidation, interacting with the novel inputs of the involved investigators. In saying this, we wish, of course, to strengthen appreciation of the major contributions of the key groups in the field, relatively well represented as authors of the list of major reviews given in the Preface to this book.

2 Formation and chemistry of radicals involved in amino acid, peptide, and protein oxidation

Radicals can be generated in both chemical and biological systems by a multitude of different pathways. In the first part of this chapter we will outline how radicals which may be important in protein oxidation can be formed, before discussing the types of reactions that each of these species can participate in. In neither case will the discussion and examples given be exhaustive, as the intention is to pick out what seem to be the key species, some of the mechanisms by which they can be formed, and examples of the major reaction processes which they undergo. These areas are covered in much greater detail in a number of books to which the reader is referred for further information (Pryor 1966; Huyser 1970; Kochi 1973; Nonhebel *et al.* 1977; Bensasson *et al.* 1983, 1993; Giese 1986; von Sonntag 1987; Halliwell and Gutteridge 1989; Motherwell and Crich 1992; Fossey *et al.* 1995). In the section following these, we will discuss in more detail the reactions of these different types of radicals with free amino acids, peptides and proteins.

In general the processes that give rise to radicals can be divided into two categories. First, those reactions which involve direct cleavage of bonds, and secondly, those that involve electron transfer processes; there are reactions which fit both categories.

In the first type of process the bond between two parts of a molecule is broken so that each part of the molecule ends up with an unpaired electron. Examples of such processes include the interaction of high energy radiation (e.g. γ-radiation, high energy electrons, neutrons, X-rays) with water, the action of high temperatures on molecules, and the action of UV and visible light (often in the latter case a sensitizer molecule is needed) (reactions 1 and 2).

$$H_2O_2 + UV \text{ light} \longrightarrow 2HO^\bullet \tag{1}$$

$$I_2 + \text{heat} / \text{light} \longrightarrow 2I^\bullet \tag{2}$$

In the second category are processes where an initial electron transfer to or from a molecule results in the generation of a species which very rapidly fragments. Examples of this type of process include metal-ion- (or enzyme-) mediated oxidation or reduction of peroxides, and the interaction of some forms of radiation with water.

$$H_2O_2 + e^- \longrightarrow (H_2O_2)^{\bullet -} \longrightarrow HO^- + HO^{\bullet} \tag{3}$$

$$H_2O_2 - e^- \longrightarrow (H_2O_2)^{\bullet +} \longrightarrow H^+ + HOO^{\bullet} \tag{4}$$

$$H_2O - e^- \longrightarrow (H_2O)^{\bullet +} \longrightarrow H^+ + HO^{\bullet} \tag{5}$$

In some of these cases the yield of the species generated can be readily quantitated. Thus, the yield of iodine atoms from the photolysis of iodine molecules (reaction 2) can be easily controlled by varying the intensity or exposure time to the illuminating source and the number of iodine atoms quantitated by knowing the quantity of energy supplied and the efficiency of the photochemical process (Bensasson *et al.* 1993). Radiation techniques, such as the irradiation of water outined above, can also be used to provide a defined quantity of a well characterized species. Here the species produced are calculated in terms of the number of atoms or molecules produced (G) per 100 eV (electron volts) of energy absorbed by the solution (Swallow 1960, 1973; Hart and Anbar 1970; von Sonntag 1987). Thus, in systems where a sparsely ionizing radiation source (e.g. electrons with energies below 3 MeV or ^{60}Co γ-rays) is employed, and the solutions are relatively dilute (i.e. most of the energy deposition is to the solvent, water, rather than with the solute), the initial radical species formed are the hydrated electron (e^-_{aq}), hydrogen atoms ($H^{\bullet}$), and the hydroxyl radical ($HO^{\bullet}$). Two major molecular products are also formed, hydrogen (H_2) and hydrogen peroxide (H_2O_2) (von Sonntag 1987). The yields of these different species under different experimental conditions are given in Table 2.1. These values alter somewhat if concentrated solutions, or densely ionizing radiation (such as α-particles) are employed. For further details of these effects and radiation techniques, refer to a number of other excellent texts (Swallow 1960, 1973; Hart and Anbar 1970; von Sonntag 1987).

Direct electron transfer reactions constitute oxidation and reduction reactions; in these cases the radicals generated can be neutral (reaction 6) or charged species: either radical-cations (positively charged species, reaction 7), or radical-anions (negatively charged species, reaction 8). Examples include the oxidation of anions by peroxidases and the reduction of some biologically important chemicals and drugs such as the herbicide methyl viologen (paraquat) and quinones (Mason 1982; Halliwell and Gutteridge 1989).

$$N_3^- - e^- \longrightarrow N_3^{\bullet} \tag{6}$$

Table 2.1 Radiation yields of reactive radicals from ^{60}Co γ-irradiation of water

Radical	N_2	N_2O^a	$N_2O/O_2{}^b$	$O_2{}^c$
HO$^\bullet$	2.7	5.4^d	5.4	2.7
H$^\bullet$	0.55	0.55	–	–
e$^-_{aq}$	2.65	–	–	–
HOO$^\bullet$/O$_2{}^{\bullet-}$	–	–	0.55	3.2

^{a} N$_2$O-saturated, 2.2×10^{-3} mol dm^{-3}
^{b} N$_2$O/O$_2$ 4:1 v/v
^{c} O$_2$-saturated, 2.2×10^{-3} mol dm^{-3}
^{d} Value dependent on the scavenger concentration; value increases at higher concentrations.

For further details see: Swallow 1960; Hart and Anbar 1970; von Sonntag 1987.

$$MV^{2+} + e^- \longrightarrow MV^{\bullet+} \text{ where } MV^{2+} \text{ is methyl viologen} \tag{7}$$

$$\text{Quinone} + e^- \longrightarrow \text{Quinone}^{\bullet-} \tag{8}$$

Once generated, such radicals can undergo an enormous variety of different types of reaction, but again these can be readily broken down in to a number of different categories. These include hydrogen abstraction, electron abstraction by the radical (oxidation of the substrate), electron donation by the radical (reduction of the substrate), addition, fragmentation, and substitution (addition followed by rapid elimination). Examples of these types of reaction are given below:

$$HO^\bullet + R\text{–}H \longrightarrow H_2O + R^\bullet \qquad \text{hydrogen abstraction} \tag{9}$$

$$HO^\bullet + Cl^- \longrightarrow HO^- + Cl^\bullet \quad \text{electron abstraction (oxidation)} \tag{10}$$

$$Q^{\bullet-} + O_2 \longrightarrow Q + O_2{}^{\bullet-} \quad \begin{array}{l}\text{electron donation (reduction),} \\ \text{where Q is a quinone}\end{array} \tag{11}$$

$$HO^\bullet + \begin{array}{c}\diagdown \\ \diagup\end{array}C=C\begin{array}{c}\diagup \\ \diagdown\end{array} \longrightarrow HO\text{-}\overset{|}{\underset{|}{C}}\text{-}\overset{|}{\underset{|}{C}}{}^\bullet \qquad \text{addition} \tag{12}$$

$$(CH_3)_3CO^\bullet \longrightarrow {}^\bullet CH_3 + CH_3C(O)CH_3 \qquad \text{fragmentation} \tag{13}$$

$$(CH_3)_3CO^\bullet + P(CH_2CH_3)_3 \longrightarrow (CH_3)_3CO\text{-}P(CH_2CH_3)_2 + {}^\bullet CH_2CH_3$$
$$\text{substitution (addition + rapid elimination)} \tag{14}$$

As can be discerned from the above examples, reaction of a radical with another molecule must give rise to either a further radical species or a species which is oxidized or reduced—good examples of the latter type of phenomenon are the reactions of radicals with certain metal ions (Bielski et al. 1985; Sukhov et al. 1986; Buxton et al. 1988). Thus:

$$O_2{}^{\bullet-} + Fe^{3+} \longrightarrow O_2 + Fe^{2+} \tag{15}$$

$$HO^\bullet + Cu^{1+} \longrightarrow HO^- + Cu^{2+} \tag{16}$$

Hence, in most biological situations reaction of a radical with a substrate generates a further radical which itself will undergo further reactions. This phenomenon underlies the common occurrence of chain processes in biological systems and is the reason for the importance of radical-scavenging antioxidants which, in the main, react with reactive radicals to give highly stabilized, unreactive radical species, thus limiting the further occurrence of radical-induced damage. Obviously, such chain reactions will only occur readily and rapidly when the overall energetics of the reaction are favourable: though many radicals are extremely reactive they can also show selectivity in their reactions. A good example of this phenomenon is the hydroxyl radical, HO·, which even though a very powerful oxidizing (and electrophilic) species, does show some selectivity in the types of bonds with which it will react. Thus, in the reaction of this radical with simple alcohols such as ethanol the majority of the hydroxyl radicals (approx 97.5 per cent) react with C–H bonds rather than the O–H bond (Asmus *et al.* 1973); this is a consequence of the much higher bond strength of the O–H bond compared with a typical C–H bond (about 495 kJ mol^{-1} compared to 385–410 kJ mol^{-1} (Fossey *et al.* 1995)) making reaction at the C–H bonds much more favourable (more exothermic). As might be expected from the above range of values for C–H bond strengths, there is also some degree of selectivity between different types of C–H bond, though this is often much less marked.

Reaction is preferred at sites where the radical will be stabilized by neighbouring functional groups such as double bonds, aromatic rings, electron-rich heteroatoms and, to a less significant extent, electron-releasing alkyl groups. There are two component stabilizing factors: firstly, delocalization of the electron on to other atoms through overlap of the orbital containing the unpaired electron with p or π orbitals; secondly, electron donation through a (σ) bond from an alkyl group to the electron deficient radical centre. In the case of the two possible types of C–H bonds in ethanol—those on the methyl group with those on the $-CH_2-$ group next to the -OH function—reaction is known to occur predominantly at the latter site (approx 84 per cent *vs* 13 per cent (Asmus *et al.* 1973)), despite the statistical weighting in favour of the three primary CH_3 hydrogens rather than the two secondary CH_2 hydrogens, as hydrogen abstraction at the latter site will give a radical which is stabilized by both the neighbouring methyl and hydroxyl functions.

With radicals such as HO· attention also has to be paid to their relative propensities to undergo the various types of radical reactions outlined above. Though HO· reacts rapidly with most C–H bonds by hydrogen abstraction, addition reactions with unsaturated systems (double bonds, aromatic rings etc.) are even more rapid and often predominate where there is a choice; this is particularly so where the unsaturated system is electron rich (a consequence of the oxidizing nature of this radical; see Table 2.2 for a list of the oxidation and reduction potentials of a number of radicals of biological importance). This preference for electron-rich sites (both between different molecules and between sites in the same molecule) arises from the electrophilic nature of this species and has important consequences in determining the selectivity of $HO^{\cdot}$ attack at certain positions on some amino acids (see later).

A consequence of these arguments is that the less reactive a species is, the more selective (in general) such a species will be. This has potentially very wide-reaching biological consequences, as the most reactive radicals may not necessarily be the most damaging, simply because they will react relatively indiscriminately at, or near, their site of formation, whereas less

Table 2.2 Reduction potentials of some free radicals of biological interest

Couple	Reduction potential (mV)	Couple	Reduction potential (mV)
aq/e^-_{aq}	-2870	$CH_3OO^{\cdot} / CCH_3OO^-$	$600-700$
$H^+ + e^-/ H^{\cdot}$	-2400	$RS^{\cdot} / RS^-$ (Cysteine)	$730-1100^a$
$(CH_3)_2CO + e^-/ (CH_3)_2CO^{\cdot -}$	-2100	$HOO^{\cdot} / HOO^-$	790
$CH_3CHO + e^-/ CH_3CHO^{\cdot -}$	-1930	Indole$^{\cdot}$ / Indole$^-$	970
$CO_2 + e^-/ CO_2^{\cdot -}$	-1900	$NO_2^{\cdot} / NO_2^-$	$\simeq 1000$
Cystine	$\simeq -1700$	$CCl_3OO^{\cdot} / CCl_3OO^-$	>1000
Oxidized lipoamide	-1600	$I_2^{\cdot -} / 2I^-$	$1000-1100$
β-mercaptoethanol	-1570	$RSSR^{\cdot +}/ RSSR$ (lipoic acid)	1130
$(CH_3)_2CO + e^- + H^+/$ $^{\cdot}C(CH_3)_2OH$	-1390	$(SCN)_2^{\cdot -} / 2SCN^-$	1330
$CH_3CHO + e^- + H^+/$ $^{\cdot}CH(OH)CH_3$	-1250	$N_3^{\cdot} / N_3^-$	1330
$CH_2O + e^- + H^+/ ^{\cdot}CH_2OH$	-1180	$RS^{\cdot} + e^- + H^+/ RSH$ (β-mercaptoethanol)	$\simeq 1330$
$O_2 + e^-/ O_2^{\cdot -}$	-330	$PhO^{\cdot} + e^- + H^+/ PhOH$ (phenoxy radical/phenol)	1340^a
Riboflavine	-318	$RSSR^{\cdot +}/ RSSR$ (dimethyl sulfide)	1391
Adriamycin	-341	$HOO^{\cdot} + e^- + H^+/ H_2O_2$	1480
$SO_2 + e^-/ SO_2^{\cdot -}$	$\simeq -280$	$Br_2^{\cdot -} / 2Br^-$	1660
1,4-Napthoquinone	-140	$HO^{\cdot} / HO^-$	1900
DOPA	14	$Cl_2^{\cdot -} / 2Cl^-$	$\simeq 2300$
1,4-Benzoquinone	78	$SO_4^{\cdot -} / SO_4^{2-}$	$\simeq 2430$
$SO_3^{\cdot -} / SO_3^{2-}$	630	$Cl^{\cdot} / Cl^-$	$\simeq 2550$
$RSSR^{\cdot -} / 2RS^-$ (Cysteine)	650		

^{a} For pH dependence of these reactions see Figure 2.1

Values at pH 7 *versus* the standard hydrogen electrode at room temperature using standard states of unit activity (i.e. approximately 1 mol dm^{-3} for solids and liquids and 1 atmosphere partial pressure for gases). Source: von Sonntag 1987; Wardman 1989.

reactive species will not only be more selective in the targets which they damage, but also are able to diffuse further before undergoing reaction.

2.1 Detection and identification of radical species and their reaction products

The examination of the reactions of radicals with amino acids, peptides, and proteins is inextricably linked with both the detection of these species and their reaction products. As we pointed out in Chapter 1, the development of analytical techniques has gone hand-in-hand with many of the major advances in this field. As methodology for detecting such species is not the major thrust of this work, and has been admirably covered elsewhere (e.g. the *Methods in Enzymology* series), we will only summarize briefly the major techniques which are of direct relevance to the studies discussed below.

Direct detection of radical species, particularly in biological systems, has always been a challenging area. Most of the readily available techniques rely on spectroscopic methods, and unfortunately few of these are specific for radical species. In most cases the observation of absorptions from low levels of a transient species has to be carried out against an intense background of other absorptions. An obvious corollary of this is that such measurements are easiest to make when the radical concentration is high and the rates of subsequent reaction of the radical are slow; thus most of the studies which have provided useful information on such radicals have tended to employ rapid generation and detection systems and/or techniques to slow down subsequent reactions (such as low temperatures). Each of these strategies brings with it complications (see below).

The major techniques which have given data on radical species are fast optical spectroscopy (plus occasionally fast infra-red), conductivity measurements (for charged radicals, or reactions which feature large changes in charge), and electron paramagnetic (or spin) resonance (EPR or ESR) spectroscopy. (The basis of this last technique is discussed in some detail in Swartz *et al.* 1972; Symons 1978; Carrington and McLauchlan 1979; Weil *et al.* 1994.) The former techniques are, of course, not specific for radicals and hence the assignment of the observed absorptions to particular species can be difficult, though they are extremely powerful techniques for examining the *kinetics* of reactions. The opposite is true of EPR spectroscopy; its specificity for species with unpaired electrons (i.e. free radicals and some metal ions, which are normally very readily discernible from each other) means that the assignment of the (often detailed) absorptions to particular species can be definitive, but obtaining kinetic information from this technique is more difficult. The information obtained from optical detection and EPR spectroscopy is therefore often complimentary.

It is also worth mentioning here some of the limitations of these techniques, which should be borne in mind when either examining literature data or planning experiments. Optical spectroscopy is, in general, limited to 'clean' or model systems due to the problems in obtaining well-resolved and characteristic absorption peaks from heterogenous solutions, and is therefore often limited to studies of decompartmentalized reaction mixtures; the influence of cellular localization and the role of membranes are difficult to probe. Though EPR spectroscopy can detect radical concentrations down to nM levels and is specific for radicals, it also has its minus points. The steady-state levels of most radicals in intact biological systems are below this level and hence other additional strategies must be employed to detect such species. These include the use of rapid freezing to slow the decay or further reaction of a radical species, and the use of spin trapping agents; the latter are compounds added to the reaction system at high concentration so as to react with the radicals present to give long-lived, and hence more readily detectable, adducts which will build up in concentration with time (reviewed: Janzen 1971; Perkins 1980; Janzen and Haire 1990; Davies and Timmins 1996). The freezing approach, though advantageous in some respects, suffers from the problem that the absorption lines become very much broader, indistinct, and often split into several components due to the freezing of the radical(s) in random orientations; this makes assignment of the peaks to particular radicals much more difficult and hence there are problems with identification. It also suffers from the problem that the species which are observed after freezing may not accurately reflect those present in the initial system, as the most reactive species may decay away during the finite period (often 10s to 100s of milliseconds) required to achieve freezing of the sample. The use of spin trapping agents also suffers from many problems (reviewed: Janzen 1971; Perkins 1980; Janzen and Haire 1990; Davies and Timmins 1996), not least of which are: i) the spectra from the adducts are much less informative than those of the parent radicals, and hence problems exist with their identification; ii) there are many artifactual reactions which give rise to similar signals which can be readily mistaken for spin-trapped radicals; iii) the spin traps, by trapping radical species, interfere with the process under study; and iv) the spin traps may cause toxicity due to their nature and the high concentrations that often need to be employed. Spin trapping data, though immensely useful, must therefore be treated with caution; the literature is unfortunately littered with misleading data.

The methods available for the detection and identification of the products of radical reactions are much more diverse and numerous than those available for the detection of radicals themselves, and a number of volumes (e.g. the *Methods in Enzymology* series) have covered such advances in technology very competently; the reader is referred to these for further information.

2.2 Reactivity and reactions of individual radical species

Having outlined briefly some of the mechanisms and processes by which radicals may be formed and detected/identified, we will now consider the individual characteristics of some of these reactive species. Particular emphasis is placed on the types of reactions which these entities may undergo in biological environments.

2.2.1 Hydroxyl radicals

As outlined above the hydroxyl radical can be generated in a multitude of different reactions including the interaction of high energy radiation with water (see above, where HO' is formed with $G \simeq 2.7$ in the absence of other added agents), via UV photolysis of hydrogen peroxide (reaction 1), and as a consequence of one-electron reduction of hydrogen peroxide (reaction 3). The last of these is most commonly brought about by low-valent transition metal ions; in the case of reaction with Fe^{2+} this process (reaction 17) is known as the Fenton reaction (Fenton 1894, 1899). Many of the properties of this powerful oxidizing species have been outlined (Swallow 1960, 1973; Pryor 1966; Huyser 1970; Kochi 1973; Nonhebel *et al.* 1977; von Sonntag 1987; Fossey *et al.* 1995) and will not be discussed further here.

$$Fe^{2+} + H_2O_2 \longrightarrow Fe^{3+} + HO^- + HO^{\cdot} \tag{17}$$

Considerable controversy exists in the literature as to the exact nature of the species generated during the reaction of some iron (and other transition metal ion complexes) with hydrogen peroxide. In some cases it has been suggested that other powerful oxidizing species are formed either in conjunction with or in place of HO' (reviewed: Barton 1992; Sawyer 1996). While it is clear that in some cases well-characterized high-oxidation-state iron species are formed, in other cases the evidence is less convincing and based on the lack of effects of scavengers, or altered product distributions. In a number of the latter cases, these variations can be explained in terms of either the formation of HO' in a site-specific manner, where scavengers may not have ready access, or the oxidizing or reducing activities of the metal ion complexes present (Croft *et al.* 1992). The reactions of some well characterized, high-oxidation-state species, including Fe^{4+}-oxo (ferryl) species, Cu^{3+} complexes, and metal ion-OOH complexes have been investigated (Aft and Mueller 1984; Tullius and Dombroski 1986; Tullius 1987; Balasubramanian *et al.* 1989; Rana and Meares 1990, 1991*a*, *b*). Whilst these are undoubtedly formed in at least some situations, they are relatively specialized cases and there is evidence, in at least some cases, for the reactions of these complexes being non-radical in nature (Tullius and Dombroski 1986; Tullius 1987).

2.2.2 Hydrogen atoms

Studies on the action of hydrogen atoms in biological systems have primarily employed the radiolysis of water as a generation method as this technique produces known, but relatively low, yields (at least at neutral pH) of this species (Table 2.1). This species is a relatively powerful reducing agent, though it is less powerful (by about 0.52 eV, see Table 2.2) than the hydrated electron which is also produced (in much higher yields) as a result of radiation exposure. Hydrogen atoms, like HO˙, readily add to double bonds and aromatic systems and can abstract hydrogen atoms from C–H bonds (Neta and Schuler 1972) to give molecular hydrogen and a new carbon-centred radical. The former type of reactions are very rapid (with rate constants in the range 10^8–10^9 $dm^3 mol^{-1} s^{-1}$ (Neta and Schuler 1972; Buxton 1988)) and also show some preference for electron-rich sites, as like HO˙ this radical is electrophilic in nature (Neta and Schuler 1972). It is, however, much less reactive than HO˙ in hydrogen atom abstraction (cf. data in Buxton *et al.* 1988), and is a much more selective radical, with the C–H bond strength of potential sites of attack being of major importance.

2.2.3 Solvated electrons

The third major reactive species generated as a result of the radiolysis of water is the solvated electron. This is the strongest reducing agent found in biological systems and the chemistry of this species is dominated by this property. Thus, unlike the other radicals discussed above, it shows little propensity for hydrogen atom abstraction, and its chemistry is dominated by addition reactions (Hart and Anbar 1970). This species also does not react readily with isolated carbon-carbon double bonds, but it does undergo ready reaction with conjugated systems and aromatic rings (cf. data in Buxton 1988). The addition species formed in these reactions are usually unstable radical-anions which undergo further reactions rapidly. Thus the radical-anion formed by addition of the solvated electron to an aromatic ring often undergoes rapid reaction with a proton from water to form a species which appears to be a hydrogen atom addition product (Gordon *et al.* 1977). This propensity for addition to electron-rich sites extends to the reactions of this species with other functional groups and electronegative heteroatoms. Thus it is known that this species will cause dehalogenation of halogen-containing species by dissociative electron capture (e.g. reaction 18 (Hayon and Allen 1961)). Analogous processes occur on reaction of this species with hydrogen peroxide (reaction 3, $k = 1.3 \times 10^{10}$ dm^3 mol^{-1} s^{-1} (Buxton 1988)) and N$_2$O (reaction 19, $k = 9.1 \times 10^9$ dm^3 mol^{-1} s^{-1} (Janata and Schuler 1982)); the latter process is often used by radiation chemists and biologists to convert the solvated electron into HO$^\cdot$ in order to generate high yields of this species and allow the selective study of this radical (Dainton 1962). A final example of the reactions of this species, which is of major importance in understanding the effect of the solvated electron on peptides and proteins, is the addition of this species to carbonyl ($-C=O$) bonds (Hart *et al.* 1967). This process, which can occur with free carbonyl functions as well as with amide and carboxyl groups, results in the formation of a radical-anion (reaction 20 (Hart *et al.* 1967)); this species when formed on amino acids, peptides and proteins can lead to deamination (loss of an amine group; see later).

$$e^-_{aq} + R\text{--}Cl \longrightarrow R^\cdot + Cl^- \tag{18}$$

$$e^-_{aq} + N_2O + H_2O \longrightarrow HO^\cdot + N_2 + HO^- \tag{19}$$

$$e^-_{aq} + RR'C=O \longrightarrow (RR'C=O)^{\cdot\,-} \tag{20}$$

2.2.4 Superoxide radicals

The superoxide radical-anion, $O_2^{\cdot\,-}$, can be generated readily in chemical systems as a result of electron attachment to oxygen (reaction 21, $k \simeq 2 \times 10^{10}$ dm^3 mol^{-1} s^{-1} (Gordon *et al.* 1963)) or by reduction of oxygen by powerful reducing agents such as semiquinones (reaction 22 (Patel and Willson 1973)) or the carbon dioxide radical-anion (formate radical, $CO_2^{\cdot\,-}$, reaction 23, $k = 2\text{--}4.2 \times 10^{10}$ dm^3 mol^{-1} s^{-1} (Adams 1972; Neta *et al.* 1988)). Semiquinone radical species can be readily generated by either reduction of a quinone (e.g. enzymatically) or by oxidation (catalysed or autoxidation) of a quinol (Yamazaki 1971; Mason 1982). $CO_2^{\cdot\,-}$ can be formed by the reaction of HO$^\cdot$ or H$^\cdot$ with a large excess of formic acid (methanoic acid, reaction 24). The latter process has been extensively used in radiation chemistry studies, as in the presence of excess oxygen it generates high yields of $O_2^{\cdot\,-}$ in a specific manner (Adams 1972); the solvated electrons produced by the initial radiation react with oxygen directly, while the hydrogen atoms and hydroxyl radicals react with excess formate to give rise, in the presence of excess oxygen, to more $O_2^{\cdot\,-}$ (reaction 24 followed by 23). Thus $O_2^{\cdot\,-}$ is both a product of the radiolysis of water in the presence of oxygen, and an almost ubiquitous species in aerobic organisms as a result of the use of molecular oxygen as the terminal acceptor of electrons in mitochondrial electron transport chains. Though the latter processes are very efficient, some leakage of electrons to oxygen appears to give rise to a continual flux of $O_2^{\cdot -}$ within aerobic cells.

$$e^-_{aq} + O_2 \longrightarrow O_2^{\cdot -} \tag{21}$$

$$Q^{\cdot -} + O_2 \longrightarrow O_2^{\cdot -} + Q \qquad \text{where } Q = \text{Quinone} \tag{22}$$

$$CO_2^{\cdot -} + O_2 \longrightarrow CO_2 + O_2^{\cdot -} \tag{23}$$

$$HO^{\cdot} / H^{\cdot} + HCO_2^- \longrightarrow H_2O / H_2 + CO_2^{\cdot -} \tag{24}$$

The superoxide radical is however a relatively unreactive species whose major type of reaction is reduction (i.e. donation of an electron); this occurs most commonly with high-oxidation-state metal ions. Thus this radical is capable of recycling higher valence metal ions to lower oxidation states. Examples of this type of behaviour include reduction of Fe^{3+} to Fe^{2+} (reaction 25), a key step in the metal-ion-catalysed Haber-Weiss reaction (Haber and Weiss 1932, 1934; Czapski and Ilan 1978), and reduction of Cu^{2+} to Cu^+ (reaction 26), a process which is of major importance in the removal of $O_2^{\cdot -}$ during the catalytic cycle of the Cu/Zn form of the protective enzyme superoxide dismutase (Klug-Roth and Rabani 1976). $O_2^{\cdot -}$ is also a weak oxidizing agent (i.e. electron acceptor) but these reactions only occur with easily oxidized materials (e.g. ascorbate) and are relatively slow (k for reaction with ascorbate $\simeq 1.5 \times 10^5$ $dm^3 mol^{-1} s^{-1}$ (Bielski and Richter 1977; Bielski et al. 1985)); the biological significance of these reactions is therefore open to question.

The only other major process undergone by this radical which is of great biological significance is its rapid dismutation to oxygen and hydrogen peroxide (reaction 27 (Bielski et al. 1985)); this reaction is probably a major source of cellular hydrogen peroxide. The superoxide radical is also capable of acting as a weak base; these reactions, however, do not usually involve radical species and hence are beyond the scope of this book. The ability of this radical to act as both a reducing agent and as a base is significantly enhanced in organic solvents, and these types of reaction may therefore play a role in some biological damage.

$$O_2^{\cdot -} + Fe^{3+} \longrightarrow Fe^{2+} + O_2 \tag{25}$$

$$O_2^{\cdot -} + Cu^{2+} \longrightarrow Cu^+ + O_2 \tag{26}$$

$$2O_2^{\cdot -} + 2H^+ \longrightarrow H_2O_2 + O_2 \tag{27}$$

The protonated form of this species, $HOO^{\cdot}$, which is formed at lower pH values (pK_a 4.8), does not undergo electron transfer reactions as readily as $O_2^{\cdot -}$ (e.g. with ascorbate) but is a much better hydrogen abstracting agent. Thus it will abstract hydrogen atoms from activated methylene $(-C=C-CH_2-C=C-)$ positions unlike $O_2^{\cdot -}$ (reaction 28, (Bielski et al.

1985)); the concentration of $HOO^\cdot$ in most biological systems, at neutral pH, will however only be a fraction of 1 per cent of the $O_2^{\cdot-}$ concentration. Its role in most biological protein oxidation reactions is therefore questionable and it is difficult to assess the contribution from this radical under most physiological conditions. There are, however, several specialized physiological and pathological environments in which low pH values may occur, and hence situations in which this radical may be important: examples of these sorts of environments include phagosomes, endosomes, lysosomes, and inflammatory foci.

$$HOO^\cdot \;+\; -C=C-CH_2-C=C- \;\longrightarrow\; H_2O_2 \;+\; -C=C-\overset{\cdot}{C}H-C=C- \qquad (28)$$

2.2.5 Carbon-centred radicals

Reaction of a large number of radicals with substrates containing C–H bonds results in the formation of carbon-centred radicals as a result of hydrogen-abstraction reactions. Carbon-centred radicals can also be readily generated by a number of other methods (reviewed: Fossey *et al.* 1995) including addition of an initiating radical to a double bond or aromatic system, decomposition of thermolabile azo ($R-N=N-R$) compounds in the absence of oxygen (reaction 29), by fragmentation reactions of alkoxyl and peroxyl species (see below), $HO^\cdot$-induced decomposition of sulfoxides (reaction 30), photolysis of alkyl chlorides, bromides, and iodides (reaction 31), metabolism of a number of drugs, and decarboxylation of carboxylate anions by strong oxidants (see section 2.2.10). Aryl radicals are less readily formed (often as a result of higher carbon-substituent bond strengths), though these can still be generated by a number of different methods; a convenient source is the metal-ion-mediated reduction of aromatic diazonium salts (reactions 32).

$$R-N=N-R + heat \longrightarrow 2R^\cdot + N_2 \qquad (29)$$

$$HO^\cdot \;+\; RR'S=O \;\longrightarrow\; R-\underset{\underset{O^\cdot}{|}}{\overset{\overset{OH}{|}}{S}}-R' \;\longrightarrow\; RSO_2H + R''^\cdot \qquad (30)$$

$$R-X + light \longrightarrow R^\cdot + X^\cdot \qquad X = Cl, Br, I \qquad (31)$$

$$R-N_2^+ + M^{n+} \longrightarrow R^\cdot + N_2 + M^{(n+1)+} \qquad (32)$$

The most common reaction of such species in biological systems is with oxygen to form peroxyl species (see below). This type of process is usually diffusion controlled, meaning that the reaction is controlled by how frequently the reactants collide, in turn determined by how fast they diffuse, and thus is the fastest category of reactions the species can undergo in solution (Neta 1990). Other biological reactions of these radicals are poorly understood, though these processes are much better characterized in chemical systems.

In the absence (or presence of only low concentrations) of oxygen, alkyl radicals will carry out hydrogen abstraction reactions, though these processes are slow, particularly with unactivated C–H sites; the nucleophilic nature of many of these species results in a different selectivity of damage when compared to most oxygen-, sulfur-, and nitrogen-centred species; thus they favour electron-poor rather than electron-rich sites. Reactions with thiols are usually faster and such processes are often classed as repair reactions in radiation chemistry (reviewed: Adams 1972; von Sonntag 1987). Addition of alkyl radicals to double bonds is a much faster process (Abell 1973), but these processes are of relatively little significance in protein and peptide chemistry.

Aryl radicals are in most cases considerably more reactive than their alkyl counterparts and there is some evidence that these nucleophilic species can play a role in protein damage in certain circumstances (Maples *et al.* 1988*a*, *b*).

With both alkyl and aryl species an additional important reaction is that with a further radical i.e. dimerization. These reactions are very fast and usually approach diffusion-controlled rates (i.e. $2k_t \simeq 10^9$ dm^{3}mol^{-1}s^{-1} (Fossey *et al.* 1995)), but are restricted by the presence of oxygen due to the very low concentrations of the radicals. In the absence of oxygen, dimerization is a very significant termination pathway and can give rise to multiple products (see later). In some specialized cases such dimerization reactions can also occur in the presence of oxygen, particularly when addition of oxygen to the initial carbon-centred radical is an unfavourable process; this is most commonly observed with some aromatic species, such as Tyr phenoxyl radicals where di-tyrosine is a major product (Karam *et al.* 1984; Simic and Dizdaroglu 1985; Jin *et al.* 1993).

2.2.6 Peroxyl radicals

The majority of carbon-centred species, as mentioned above, react rapidly with oxygen to give peroxyl, $ROO^{\cdot}$, species. These addition reactions of oxygen are in theory reversible, but the majority of $C–OO^{\cdot}$ bonds are stable (Slagle *et al.* 1985, 1986). The reverse process, loss of oxygen from a peroxyl radical, only appears to happen to any major extent (at room or physiological temperatures) in cases where the carbon-centred species is especially stable (e.g. the bisallyl radicals formed by hydrogen abstraction from polyunsaturated lipids (Morgan *et al.* 1982)); such reversal reactions can have a dramatic effect on the stereochemistry and distribution of the products formed, and can yield valuable mechanistic information (Porter *et al.* 1980, 1981).

Peroxyl radicals can be readily generated for experimental study from the thermal (or light-induced) decomposition of a number of azo compounds (R–N = N–R) in the presence of oxygen; this type of process can be used to generate *known* fluxes of peroxyl radicals in either aqueous or lipid environments as the rate of thermal decomposition of these species is often known (e.g. Dean *et al*. 1991; Fossey *et al*. 1995). It should, however, be noted that this is not a pure source of these species, as decay reactions of the peroxyl radicals (see below) can give rise to highly reactive alkoxyl radicals. Peroxyl radicals can also be generated, in the absence of oxygen, from the oxidation of hydroperoxides; this is usually achieved by use of high-valent transition metal ions (e.g. Ce^{4+}, Co^{3+}, Pb^{4+} (Kochi 1973)). The subsequent chemistry of these species is very structure dependent.

In the case of peroxyl radicals with heteroatoms attached to the carbon to which the oxygen is bound (i.e. an α-substituted species) a rapid unimolecular decay with loss of $HOO\cdot/O_2\cdot^-$ can occur (reaction 33 (Rabani *et al*. 1974; Ilan *et al*. 1976; Bothe and Schulte-Frohlinde 1978; Neta 1990)); a 5-membered transition state is likely to be involved in this reaction. This process can occur with both α-hydroxyl and α-amino groups (and hence can be important with the side chains of amino acids (Abramovitch and Rabani 1976; Neta 1990)) and α-amide functions (von Sonntag 1987); the latter type of reaction is of particular importance for peroxyl radicals formed at backbone α-carbon sites (Garrison *et al*. 1962, 1970; Mieden and von Sonntag 1989; Mieden *et al*. 1993), and appears to be a key reaction in peptide main chain degradation (see later). Similar elimination reactions are thought to occur when the peroxyl radical is formed on aromatic rings (e.g. on the phenol ring of Tyr) as a result of initial radical addition to the ring, formation of substituted cyclohexadienyl radicals, and addition of oxygen (reaction 34 (Pan *et al*. 1993)). Compared to the examples outlined above, most of these species have the heteroatom (oxygen) substituent at least one carbon removed from the site from which the HOO· is lost (i.e. these processes are not α-elimination reactions, but are β- or greater).

$$\text{—}\overset{|}{\underset{|}{\text{C}}}\text{—OH} \quad \longrightarrow \quad \text{—C=O} \quad + \quad HOO\cdot \qquad (33)$$
$$\overset{}{\underset{OO\cdot}{}}$$

(34)

Peroxyl radicals can also undergo a variety of bimolecular decay reactions, the primary step of which is believed to involve a short-lived tetroxide species (i.e. ROO–OOR, reaction 35 (Bartlett and Guaraldi 1967; Adamic *et al.* 1969; Bennett *et al.* 1970; Howard 1972)). These short-lived tetroxides can decompose by a number of pathways including homolysis back to two peroxyl species (i.e. the formation of the tetroxide is an equilibrium process, at least with secondary and tertiary peroxyl species). At room or physiological temperatures these tetroxides are very short lived and rapidly decompose by a number of different pathways, depending on the structure of the peroxyl radical. In the case of tertiary peroxyl species two major routes are possible (reactions 36 and 37); one of these gives rise to the dialkyl peroxide and oxygen (i.e. does not generate further radicals) whereas the second gives two alkoxyl radicals and a molecule of oxygen (Bennett 1990). The ratio of these two pathways is thought to be structure dependent; in the case of *t*-BuOO· the second, alkoxyl radical, pathway appears to dominate over the former by a ratio of approximately 6:1 in aqueous solution (Bennett 1990). In the case of secondary and primary peroxyl radicals, other reactions also play a very significant role; these are outlined in reactions 38–40 (reviewed: von Sonntag 1987). These processes are concerted reactions with one giving rise to further carbon-centred radicals; the others give rise to either alcohols and/or carbonyl-containing materials (aldehydes/ketones). The significance of each of these processes depends on the conditions and the radicals under study (Bothe *et al.* 1978; Schuchmann and von Sonntag 1979). Reaction 38 is the well characterized Russell mechanism which occurs via a 6-membered transition state (Russell 1957); this process must obey the spin conservation rule and hence at least one of the products must be generated in an excited state (either singlet oxygen or a triplet carbonyl species).

$$2ROO^\cdot \longrightarrow ROO\text{–}OOR \qquad (35)$$

$$ROO\text{–}OOR \longrightarrow RO\text{–}OR + O_2 \qquad (36)$$

$$ROO\text{–}OOR \longrightarrow 2RO^\cdot + O_2 \qquad (37)$$

$$(38)$$

$$(39)$$

$$R-\underset{\underset{R'}{|}}{\overset{\overset{H}{|}}{C}}-OO^\bullet \xrightarrow{\times 2} 2 \underset{\underset{R'}{|}}{\overset{\overset{H}{|}}{C}}=O + 2R^\bullet + O_2 \tag{40}$$

2.2.7 Alkoxyl radicals

Alkoxyl radicals can be generated either as a result of the above peroxyl radical reactions or via other more direct routes. The latter include direct generation as a result of the one-electron reduction of alkyl hydroperoxides (RO–OH) and dialkylperoxides (RO–OR), as well as a number of photochemical processes (e.g. photolysis of dialkylperoxides, alkyl nitrites (RO–NO) or hypochlorites (RO–Cl), and peresters (RC(O)O–OR); reviewed: Fossey et al. 1995). Alkoxyl radicals tend to have very short half-lives due to their high reactivity: in addition to undergoing standard addition and hydrogen-abstraction reactions, they also undergo a number of very facile unimolecular fragmentation and rearrangement reactions (Berdnikov et al. 1972; Gilbert et al. 1976, Gilbert 1981; von Sonntag 1987; Fossey et al. 1995). The latter processes are structure dependent. In the case of primary and secondary alkoxyl radicals, rapid hydrogen (formally 1,2) shift reactions (with $k \simeq 10^6 - 10^7 \, s^{-1}$) occur which result in the formation of α-hydroxyalkyl radicals (reaction 41 (Berdnikov et al. 1972; Gilbert et al. 1976, 1977)); these reactions compete with intramolecular hydrogen abstraction processes (usually via 6-membered transition states) if suitable labile hydrogens are available (reaction 42 (Gilbert et al. 1976, 1977)). In the case of tertiary alkoxyl radicals where 1,2-hydrogen shift reactions are not possible, β-fragmentation reactions occur (reaction 43) with formation of a carbon-centred radical and a ketone (Walling and Wagner 1964; Gilbert et al. 1981; Bors et al. 1984; Neta et al. 1984; Erben-Russ et al. 1987). The most stable pairing of these two species determines the mode of fragmentation in cases of multiple possible pathways. These processes can be very rapid ($k > 10^6 \, s^{-1}$) in aqueous solution (Gilbert et al. 1981; Bors et al. 1984; Neta et al. 1984; Erben-Russ et al. 1987). Both the 1,2-hydrogen shift reaction and these β-fragmentation reactions are very solvent dependent; in organic solvents these processes are very much slower, and can be uncompetitive compared to addition/hydrogen abstraction reactions (Walling and Wagner 1964). For these reasons, while there is a wealth of data on rate constants for alkoxyl radical addition/hydrogen abstraction reactions in organic solvents, the determination of similar data for aqueous systems is very difficult.

$$-\underset{|}{\overset{\overset{H}{|}}{C}}-O^\bullet \longrightarrow -\underset{|}{\overset{\bullet}{C}}-OH \tag{41}$$

$$CH_3-CH_2-CH_2-CH_2O^{\cdot} \longrightarrow {}^{\cdot}CH_2-CH_2-CH_2-CH_2OH \qquad (42)$$

$$R'-\overset{\overset{\displaystyle R}{|}}{\underset{\underset{\displaystyle R''}{|}}{C}}-O^{\cdot} \longrightarrow R'-\overset{O}{\underset{\underset{\displaystyle R''}{|}}{C}} + R^{\cdot} \qquad (43)$$

2.2.8 Thiyl radicals

Thiyl radicals can be readily generated in biological systems either by hydrogen abstraction from a thiol (reaction 44, $k = 1–2 \times 10^{10}$ dm^3 mol^{-1} s^{-1} (Neta and Fessenden 1971a)) or by cleavage of disulfide linkages (photolytically or as a result of electron transfer reactions, reactions 45 and 46, respectively (Davies, M. J. et $al.$ 1987)). They can also be formed as a result of some fragmentation reactions (e.g. reaction 47, reviewed: Davies and Gilbert 1991). The chemistry of these radicals is complex and has been the subject of extensive study (reviewed: von Sonntag 1987, 1990; Armstrong 1990; Prutz 1990). These radicals react readily by dimerization, with oxygen (in a reversible manner, reaction 48) and will also undergo both addition and hydrogen abstraction reactions; the latter type of process, which is the reverse of the well characterized thiol repair mechanism, only occurs at any appreciable rate with activated C–H bonds (e.g. bisallylic sites in polyunsaturated fatty acids, reaction 49, and sites adjacent to radical stabilizing functions such as α-hydroxy functions (Schoneich et $al.$ 1989a, b, 1992; Schoneich and Asmus 1990)). Further details of the complex chemistry of these species is given in the above mentioned reviews.

$$X^{\cdot} + RSH \longrightarrow XH + RS^{\cdot} \qquad (44)$$

$$RS–SR + light \longrightarrow 2RS^{\cdot} \qquad (45)$$

$$RS–SR + e^- \longrightarrow RS^{\cdot} + RS^- \qquad (46)$$

$$^{\cdot}CH(OH)CH_2SR \longrightarrow CH(OH)=CH_2 + RS^{\cdot} \qquad (47)$$

$$RS^{\cdot} + O_2 \longrightarrow RSOO^{\cdot} \qquad (48)$$

$$RS^{\cdot} + -C=C-CH_2-C=C- \longrightarrow RSH + -C=C-\overset{\cdot}{C}H-C=C- \qquad (49)$$

2.2.9 Nitrogen-centred radicals

The identification of nitric oxide (nitrogen monoxide, NO$^{\cdot}$) as an important biological signalling molecule has sparked considerable interest in the generation and reactions of nitrogen-centred radicals in biological systems. Though NO$^{\cdot}$ is, per se, a relatively unreactive radical (and may even be protective as it can react with a number of radicals to give non-radical products (Shelton and Kopczewski 1967; Eiserich et $al.$ 1995b)), there is now considerable evidence that reaction of this species with the superoxide radical, to form peroxynitrite (oxoperoxonitrate $(1-)$, reaction 50), may be an important route to biologically damaging agents. The exact nature of the species responsible for the observed damage is the subject of controversy, with various studies implicating a wide variety of radical and non-radical reactive species as well as intermediates formed on further reaction of the initial products with CO_2, HOCl and H_2O_2 (Scheme 2.1 (Moreno and Pryor 1992; Koppenol 1994; van der Vliet *et al.* 1994*a*, *b*, 1995; Goldstein and Czapski 1995; Denicola *et al.* 1996; Eiserich *et al.* 1996; Gow *et al.* 1996*b*; Lymar *et al.* 1996)). Some of these species appear capable of generating characteristic products (e.g. 3-nitrotyrosine) with amino acids and proteins, though there is no consensus as yet as to whether these are radical or non-radical processes (or a mixture of both) (Ischiropoulos *et al.* 1992; Haddad *et al.* 1993; Haddad *et al.* 1994*a*, *b*; Kaur and Halliwell 1994; van der Vliet *et al.* 1994*a*, *b*, 1995; Ischiropoulos and al-Mehdi 1995; Mirza *et al.* 1995; Oury *et al.* 1995; Eiserich *et al.* 1996). These reactive nitrogen species are also capable of oxidizing other amino acid residues in addition to tyrosine; these reactions are discussed in more detail later.

$$NO^{\cdot} + O_2^{\cdot -} \longrightarrow O{=}N{-}OO^- \tag{50}$$

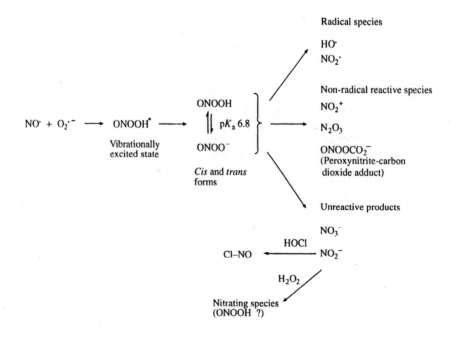

Scheme 2.1

Nitrogen dioxide ($NO_2{}^{\bullet}$), which is itself a radical, is an important atmospheric pollutant and may be responsible for damage to proteins in the lung and airways (Mustafa and Tierney 1978; Evans 1984; Frampton *et al.* 1991; Kikugawa *et al.* 1994). The chemistry of this species, unlike that of peroxynitrite and related species, is relatively well characterized (Pryor *et al.* 1982; Forni *et al.* 1986; Halliwell *et al.* 1992; Huie 1994).

2.2.10 Other inorganic radicals

The reactions of a number of other inorganic radicals such as the halogen radical anions ($Cl_2{}^{\bullet -}$, $Br_2{}^{\bullet -}$, $I_2{}^{\bullet -}$), $(SCN)_2{}^{\bullet -}$, $N_3{}^{\bullet}$, $CO_3{}^{\bullet -}$, $SO_3{}^{\bullet -}$, and $SO_4{}^{\bullet -}$ (amongst others) with amino acids and proteins have been examined. Many of these species can be readily generated by reaction of $HO^{\bullet}$ with a large excess of the parent anion (e.g. reaction 51), while $SO_4{}^{\bullet -}$ can be formed by the photochemical degradation, or one electron reduction, of peroxydisulfate (reactions 52 and 53) or peroxymonosulfate (von Sonntag 1987; Fossey *et al.* 1995). Most of these species show very marked selectivity in their reactions (Neta *et al.* 1988), when compared to $HO^{\bullet}$, and have been used to generate damage at specific sites on peptides and proteins and hence examine the role of specific residues. Though a number of these species are valuable tools in examining amino acid, peptide, and protein chemistry, it should be noted that most of them are unlikely to be formed to any significant extent in normal biological systems. Others have, however, been implicated in certain circumstances. Thus, $SO_3{}^{\bullet -}$, and $SO_4{}^{\bullet -}$ have been implicated in lung damage induced by atmospheric sulfur oxides (Rall 1974) and the chemistry of these species has been examined (reviewed: Neta and Huie 1985), whereas $CO_3{}^{\bullet -}$ may play a role in biological systems which contain hydrogencarbonate ($HCO_3{}^{-}$).

$$HO^{\bullet} + X^{-} \longrightarrow HO^{-} + X^{\bullet}, \qquad X^{\bullet} + X^{-} \longrightarrow X_2{}^{\bullet -} \tag{51}$$

$$S_2O_8{}^{2-} + UV\ light \longrightarrow 2\ SO_4{}^{\bullet -} \tag{52}$$

$$S_2O_8{}^{2-} + Fe^{2+} \longrightarrow Fe^{3+} + SO_4{}^{2-} + SO_4{}^{\bullet -} \tag{53}$$

The majority of the above radicals are selective oxidants of electron-rich sites (selected rate constants for these reactions are accumulated in Table 2.3, for further data see (Neta *et al.* 1988)), and hence generate damage primarily at aromatic and sulfur-containing amino acid side chains. Thus $N_3{}^{\bullet}$ shows great selectivity for Trp residues and has been employed to examine radical transfer (cascade) reactions of tryptophan-derived radicals in peptides and proteins (reviewed: Klapper and Faraggi 1979; von Sonntag 1987; Prutz 1990). $Cl_2{}^{\bullet -}$ and $CO_3{}^{\bullet -}$ also show considerable selectivity for Trp residues; $(SCN)_2{}^{\bullet -}$ favours Trp, the cysteine anion (pK_a (SH) 8.3) though this is environment dependent and the methionine monoanion;

Table 2.3   Rate constants for reaction of selected radicals with some amino acids, amino acid derivatives, peptides, and two proteins in aqueous solution

Substrate	Attacking radical	Rate constant $(dm^3\,mol^{-1}\,s^{-1})$	pH
Glycine	HO$^\bullet$	1.7×10^7	5.8–6
	HOO$^\bullet$	< 49	1.5
	O$_2^{\bullet-}$	< 0.42	8.8
	e$^-_{aq}$	8.8×10^6	6.2–7
	H$^\bullet$	7.7×10^4	$\simeq 7$
Alanine	HO$^\bullet$	7.7×10^7	5.5–6
	e$^-_{aq}$	9×10^6	6.4–7.4
Valine	HO$^\bullet$	7.6×10^8	6.6–6.9
	HOO$^\bullet$	< 10	1.5
	O$_2^{\bullet-}$	< 0.18	10.1
	e$^-_{aq}$	$< 5 \times 10^6$	6.4
	H$^\bullet$	1.2×10^7	$\simeq 7$
Leucine	HO$^\bullet$	1.7×10^9	5.5–6
	e$^-_{aq}$	$< 1 \times 10^7$	6.5
Serine	HO$^\bullet$	3.2×10^8	5.5–6
	e$^-_{aq}$	$< 3 \times 10^7$	6.1
Threonine	HO$^\bullet$	5.1×10^8	6.6
	e$^-_{aq}$	2×10^7	7
Cysteine[a]	HO$^\bullet$	3.4×10^{10}	5.8–7
	e$^-_{aq}$	1.2×10^{10}	5.8–7
	H$^\bullet$	1.8×10^9	6
	HOO$^\bullet$	$< 6 \times 10^2$	1.4
	O$_2^{\bullet-}$	< 15	10.9
	I$_2^{\bullet-}$	1.1×10^8	6.8
	I$_2^{\bullet-}$	1×10^9	10–11
	Br$_2^{\bullet-}$	1.8×10^8	6.6
	Br$_2^{\bullet-}$	2×10^9	10–11
Cystine	HO$^\bullet$	2.1×10^9	6.5
	e$^-_{aq}$	1.6×10^{10}	5.6–6.2
Methionine	HO$^\bullet$	8.3×10^9	5.5–7
	e$^-_{aq}$	4×10^7	6.0–7.3
	(SCN)$_2^{\bullet-}$	2×10^6	7.0
	(SCN)$_2^{\bullet-}$	3×10^8	> 9
	Br$_2^{\bullet-}$	1.7–2×10^9	5–11
Aspartic acid	HO$^\bullet$	7.5×10^7	6.8–7
	e$^-_{aq}$	1.8×10^7	7
Glutamic acid	HO$^\bullet$	2.3×10^8	6.5
	e$^-_{aq}$	1–2×10^7	5.7–7
Lysine	HO$^\bullet$	3.5×10^7	6.6
	e$^-_{aq}$	2×10^7	7–7.8
Arginine	HO$^\bullet$	3.5×10^9	6.5–7.5
	e$^-_{aq}$	1.5×10^8	6.1
Asparagine	HO$^\bullet$	4.9×10^7	6.6
	e$^-_{aq}$	1.5×10^8	7.3

Phenylalanine	$HO^{\bullet}$	6.5×10^9	5.5–8
	e^-_{aq}	1.4×10^8	5.5–7.5
Tyrosine	$HO^{\bullet}$	1.3×10^{10}	4–7
	e^-_{aq}	3.4×10^8	6.6–7.8
	$Cl_2^{\bullet-}$	2.7×108	1.8
	$Br_2^{\bullet-}$	2×10^{8b}	7
	$SO_4^{\bullet-}$	3.1×10^9	6.8–7
Histidine[c]	$HO^{\bullet}$	1.3×10^{10}	4–7
	e^-_{aq}	6.4×10^7	7–8
	e^-_{aq}	2.8×10^9	4.8
	$Cl_2^{\bullet-}$	1.4×107	1.8
	$Br_2^{\bullet-}$	1.7×10^7	7.6–9
	$HOO^{\bullet}$	< 95	1.8
	$O_2^{\bullet-}$	< 1	10
	$SO_4^{\bullet-}$	2.5×10^9	7
Tryptophan	$HO^{\bullet}$	1.3×10^{19}	6.1–8.5
	e^-_{aq}	2.9×10^8	5.9–7.8
	$H^{\bullet}$	2×10^9	$\simeq 6$
	$Cl_2^{\bullet-}$	2.6×10^9	1.8
	$Br_2^{\bullet-}$	7×10^8	6.2–13
	$N_3^{\bullet}$	4×10^9	6.1–12
	$O_2^{\bullet-}$	< 24	10.6
	$SO_4^{\bullet-}$	2×10^9	7
N-Ac–Gly	$HO^{\bullet}$	4×10^8	6.6–8.7
	e^-_{aq}	2×10^7	5.95
Gly–Gly	$HO^{\bullet}$	2.4×10^8	5.5–7
	e^-_{aq}	3×10^8	5.9–6.4
cyclo(Gly–Gly)	$HO^{\bullet}$	1.2×10^9	5
	e^-_{aq}	1.7×10^9	9.2
N-Ac–Gly–Gly	$HO^{\bullet}$	7.8×10^8	8.6
	e^-_{aq}	6.4×10^7	11.2
$(Gly)_3$	$HO^{\bullet}$	7.3×10^8	5.4
	e^-_{aq}	1.1×10^9	6.1
$(Gly)_4$	$HO^{\bullet}$	4.5×10^8	5.5
N-Ac–Ala	$HO^{\bullet}$	4.7×10^8	6.6–9.2
cyclo(Ala–Ala)	$HO^{\bullet}$	1.8×10^9	5.0
	e^-_{aq}	2×10^9	9.2
N-Ac–$(Ala)_3$	$HO^{\bullet}$	3.0×10^9	9.0
$(Ala)_5$	e^-_{aq}	1.9×10^9	6.0
$(Ala)_8$	e^-_{aq}	4.0×10^9	6.0
$(Ala)_{12}$	e^-_{aq}	6.1×10^9	6.0
$(Ala)_{20}$	e^-_{aq}	1.2×10^{10}	6.0
Lysozyme	$HO^{\bullet}$	$\simeq 5 \times 10^{10}$	5.6–7
Lysozyme	e^-_{aq}	$\simeq 5 \times 10^{10}$	4.3–8.4
Human serum albumin	$HO^{\bullet}$	7.8×10^{10}	7.0
Human serum albumin	e^-_{aq}	8.2×10^9	7.8

[a] pK_a for thiol group 8.3. Rate constants above pH 8.3 therefore involve reaction of the monoanion.
[b] This value rises to $\simeq 5 \times 10^8$ for reaction with the monoanion at pH > 10.1 (i.e. above the pK_a for the phenolic $-$ OH).
[c] pK_a for protonation of the imidazole ring approx. 6; values are pH dependent.
Source: Bielski *et al.* 1985; Buxton *et al.* 1988; Neta *et al.* 1988.

$Br_2^{\cdot -}$ reacts rapidly with Trp, the Tyr anion, Cys and the Cys anion, and the methionine monoanion. $SO_4^{\cdot -}$ behaves in a somewhat different manner as it is often much less selective than the above species and is a very powerful oxidant (see Table 2.2 above for oxidation potential); it is one of the few species capable of oxidizing HO^- to $HO^{\cdot}$ (reaction 54 (Roebke *et al.* 1969)), though this only occurs to a major extent in basic solution due to the low concentration of HO^- at most pH values. The chemistry of $SO_4^{\cdot -}$ is dominated by its very high electron affinity, and it is capable of oxidizing aromatic and Met side chains to the corresponding radical-cations which subsequently undergo either fragmentation or hydration reactions (see later (Davies *et al.* 1984*a*, *b*; Davies and Gilbert 1991)). This species is also capable of oxidizing carboxyl anions to acyloxyl radicals ($RCO_2^{\cdot}$) which subsequently rapidly decarboxylate to give carbon-centred species ($R^{\cdot}$) (reaction 55 (Davies 1985)). The analogous phosphate species $H_2PO_4^{\cdot}$ and $HPO_4^{\cdot -}$ (pK_a values 5.7 and 8.9, respectively) can be generated from reaction of $HO^{\cdot}$ with the corresponding anions, though the rate constant for these reactions are low ($< 3 \times 10^4$ $dm^3 mol^{-1} s^{-1}$ and 1.5×10^5 $dm^3 mol^{-1} s^{-1}$ for these two species, respectively (Maruthamuthu and Neta 1978; Buxton *et al.* 1988)) and hence are usually of little significance in biological systems where $HO^{\cdot}$ is generated in phosphate buffers. The corresponding dianion radical $PO_4^{\cdot 2-}$ is only formed at very high pH values. The reactions of these phosphate species are analogous to those of $SO_4^{\cdot -}$ in that they are also powerful one-electron oxidants (Maruthamuthu and Neta 1977, 1978).

$$SO_4^{\cdot -} + HO^- \longrightarrow SO_4^{2-} + HO^{\cdot} \tag{54}$$

$$SO_4^{\cdot -} + RCOO^- \longrightarrow SO_4^{2-} + RCOO^{\cdot} \longrightarrow R^{\cdot} + CO_2 \tag{55}$$

2.2.11 Singlet oxygen

Though not a radical, and hence outside the primary scope of this book, it is worth mentioning that singlet oxygen reacts rapidly with a number of amino acid side chains; the chemistry and actions of this species are reviewed (Bensasson *et al.* 1983, 1993; Frimer 1985). Such reactions can be of two forms; either a chemical reaction or a physical quenching of the excited state. In most cases, with the exception of tryptophan, reaction appears to occur mainly by chemical reaction. The chemical reaction rate constants for a number of amino acids are known; values of 3, 1.6, 0.8, and 0.7×10^7 $dm^3 mol^{-1} s^{-1}$ have been reported for Trp, Met, Tyr, and Ala, respectively (Wilkinson and Brummer 1981). In the case of histidine the rate constant is dependent on the pH of the solution with the values following the pK_a of the side chain; at pH > 8 the rate constant is 1×10^8 $dm^3 mol^{-1} s^{-1}$, whereas at low pH values it is about 0.5×10^7 $dm^3 mol^{-1} s^{-1}$. All of these values have, however, been suggested to be dependent on the experimental conditions and the sensitizer used (Gorman *et al.* 1979). In the case of Trp it is not always easy to distinguish the consequences of physical quenching from those of chemical reactivity; the end result, however, is not in doubt—the indolic ring is oxidized and *N*-formylkynurenine is formed as a major product (Creed 1984).

2.2.12 Other excited state species

The major excited state species formed during the photoexcitation of proteins are those of the three aromatic amino acids Trp, Tyr, and Phe and to a lesser extent cystine; the chemistry of these singlet and triplet excited states are reviewed in: (Bensasson *et al.* 1983, 1993). Such species are likely to play an important role in a number of biological situations including melanogenesis, induction of skin cancer, diseases such as porphyrias, and various phototreatments (e.g. photodynamic therapy of tumours) (Bensasson *et al.* 1993). Of major interest in the context of radical-induced oxidation processes is the observation that these excited states can undergo electron transfer reactions (and hence radical formation) as well as energy (usually triplet-triplet) transfer (Bensasson *et al.* 1983, 1993; Creed 1984*a*, *b*, *c*). Thus the triplet states of both Trp and Tyr (^{3}Trp and ^{3}Tyr, respectively) can oxidize disulfides via reactions 56 and 57. The reactions of the radicals generated as a result of these processes are covered later. Quenching of such triplet states by electron transfer can also occur readily with oxygen, with the concomitant formation of the $O_2^{\cdot-}$ and a corresponding amino acid-derived radical (e.g. reaction 58 (Bensasson *et al.* 1983)); some of these processes are very rapid ($k = 10^8$–10^9 $dm^3 mol^{-1} s^{-1}$ (Bensasson *et al.* 1983)). In some cases direct fragmentation of the excited state species can occur with formation of a pair of radicals; e.g. the fragmentation of the triplet state of phenylalanine which results in cleavage of the side chain to α-carbon bond (reaction 59 (Bent and Hayon 1975)).

$$^3\left[\underset{H}{\overset{}{\text{indole}}}\text{—CH}_2\text{CH(COO}^-\text{)NH}_3^+\right] + \text{RSSR} \longrightarrow \text{RSSR}^{\cdot-} + \left[\underset{H}{\overset{}{\text{indole}}}\text{—CH}_2\text{CH(COO}^-\text{)NH}_3^+\right]^{\cdot+}$$

$$\text{TrpN}^{\cdot+} \tag{56}$$

$$^3\left[\text{HO—}\langle\rangle\text{—CH}_2\text{CH(COO}^-\text{)NH}_3^+\right] + \text{RSSR} \longrightarrow \text{RSSR}^{\cdot-} + \left[\text{HO—}\langle\rangle\text{—CH}_2\text{CH(COO}^-\text{)NH}_3^+\right]^{\cdot+}$$

$$\tag{57}$$

$$3 \left[HO-\langle\!\!\bigcirc\!\!\rangle-CH_2CH(COO^-)NH_3^+ \right] + O_2 \longrightarrow O_2^{\cdot-} + H^+ + {}^\cdot O-\langle\!\!\bigcirc\!\!\rangle-CH_2CH(COO^-)NH_3^+$$

$$\text{TyrO}^\cdot \qquad (58)$$

$$3 \left[\langle\!\!\bigcirc\!\!\rangle-CH_2CH(COO^-)NH_3^+ \right] \longrightarrow \langle\!\!\bigcirc\!\!\rangle-CH_2^\cdot + {}^\cdot CH(COO^-)NH_3^+ \quad (59)$$

Direct photo-ionization of amino acids and peptides via one or two photon absorption has also been extensively examined, mainly with Trp-, Tyr-, and Phe-containing materials, with short wavelength excitation ($\lambda < 250$ nm) (e.g. reaction 60). These processes result, in many cases, in the same sort of radicals as mentioned above, though in some cases significant yields of main chain bond scission have been detected (Khoroshilova *et al.* 1990).

$$HO-\langle\!\!\bigcirc\!\!\rangle-CH_2CH(COO^-)NH_3^+ \xrightarrow{h\nu} H^+ + e^-_{aq} + {}^\cdot O-\langle\!\!\bigcirc\!\!\rangle-CH_2CH(COO^-)NH_3^+ \quad (60)$$

2.2.13 Hypochlorite and chloramines/chloramides

Reaction of hypochlorite with amino acids, peptides, and proteins does not appear in general to generate radicals directly on these targets, though there has been considerable interest in the processes by which both HOCl and the chloramines/chloramides, which are generated on reaction of this material with amines and amides (reactions 61 and 62), give rise to substrate oxidation. Previous studies have demonstrated that HOCl might give rise to radicals on reaction with reducing agents such as $O_2^{\cdot-}$ or low valence metal ions (reaction 63 (Candeias *et al.* 1993, 1994), but see also (Folkes *et al.* 1995)), whereas both light, heat, and reducing agents have been demonstrated to decompose chloramines and chloramides to reactive nitrogen-centred species such as aminyl (RNH$^\cdot$, or its protonated analogue RNH$_2^{\cdot+}$) and amidyl (RC(O)N(R')$^\cdot$) species (reactions 61 and 62, reviewed: Fossey *et al.* 1995). These species have been reported to carry out selective intra-molecular hydrogen abstraction reactions at suitable sites (particularly at low pH values, e.g. reaction 64), and/or rearrange to give α-aminoalkyl or α-amidyl species (e.g. reaction 65, Neale 1971; Michejda *et al.* 1978); the significance of these reactions in biological situations remains unclear.

$$RNH_2 + HOCl \longrightarrow H_2O + RNHCl \longrightarrow RNH^\cdot \qquad (61)$$

$$RC(O)NHR' + HOCl \longrightarrow H_2O + RC(O)NClR' \longrightarrow RC(O)N^\cdot R' \qquad (62)$$

$$HOCl + Fe^{2+} \longrightarrow HO^\cdot + Cl^- + Fe^{3+} \qquad (63)$$

$$--CH---NH^{\cdot} \longrightarrow --\overset{\cdot}{C}---NH_2 \tag{64}$$

$$-CH-NH^{\cdot} \longrightarrow -\overset{\cdot}{C}-NH_2 \tag{65}$$

Having discussed some of the chemistry of these specific species we will now turn to some of the more complex systems which are commonly encountered in biological systems, before outlining the chemistry of the radicals formed on amino acids, peptides, and proteins as a result of interaction with these initiating species. These more complex systems have been loosely collected together under the overall heading of 'mixed oxidation systems'.

2.2.14 Mixed oxidation systems

General observations

As should be obvious from the above discussion, it is extreme luxury to be able to study the reactions of known amounts of a single radical with a specific, well-defined, substrate. Thus, even systems which might initially appear to be 'clean' radical sources often are not. Even simple examples such as the reactions of peroxyl radicals clearly illustrate this point; even a clean source of $ROO^{\cdot}$ will need to take into account the reactions of alkoxyl and carbon-centred species generated via the dimerization and fragmentation reactions outlined in reactions 35–40 above. The situation with more physiologically relevant radical-generating systems can often be even more complex and hence result in data which, though of great interest in terms of the overall results and physiological relevance, can be difficult to decipher from a mechanistic view point. Two systems are of particular biological importance—the radicals generated during the process of lipid peroxidation, and those formed during sugar autoxidation. In each case the radicals formed during these processes are known to result in damage to neighbouring proteins.

Lipid peroxidation systems

During the peroxidation of lipids (reviewed: Chan 1987), the major species present are lipid-derived carbon-centred and peroxyl radicals. Under steady state conditions the concentrations of the latter species far exceed those of the former due to the rapid addition of oxygen to carbon-centred species and the relatively high oxygen content of most membrane/lipid systems. The absolute concentrations of these species have been estimated as being at maximum in the nM and μM ranges, respectively (Abuja and Esterbauer 1995; Waldeck and Stocker 1996). The levels of alkoxyl radicals generated via decomposition of the peroxyl radicals are also believed to be very low due to the rapid fragmentation and rearrangement reactions of this type of species (see above). Thus the major radical species believed to damage membrane proteins in systems undergoing lipid peroxidation is believed to be lipid-derived peroxyl radicals (Tappel 1973; Dean *et al.* 1991). Some of the products of lipid peroxidation reactions (e.g. aldehydes) are also known to be able to induce alterations; these are discussed in more detail later. The damage induced by such species has been, at least partly, characterized. These peroxyl radicals are believed to behave in a manner analogous to other peroxyl radicals (see above) though the rates of some of the dimerization reactions and subsequent fragmentation processes are affected by the altered polarity of the solvent and their mobility within the membrane/particle.

Autoxidation of sugars

The autoxidation of sugars is known to generate a variety of radical species. This process is particularly facile with sugars which can form vicinal dicarbonyls (e.g. glyceraldehyde). During the non-enzymic glycation of proteins, such as may occur during diabetes, there can be an 'autoxidative' glycation, in which radicals generated from the sugar subsequently damage proteins (Wolff and Dean 1987, 1988; Wolff *et al.* 1989). In addition, some of the protein-bound products of glycation can themselves autoxidize (Wolff and Dean 1987; McCance *et al.* 1993; Baynes 1996). Their rate of autoxidation is generally greater than that of the free sugars, and thus the relative importance of these two sites of autoxidation may vary according to the precise conditions (see Chapter 5). It is well established that such autoxidation processes can result in protein aggregation and fragmentation, though the exact nature of the species which cause the observed damage to the protein are poorly understood. It is likely that these include mixtures of carbon- and oxygen-centred (alkoxyl, peroxyl, hydroperoxyl/superoxide) radicals. Some of these radicals have been detected by EPR (Yim *et al.* 1995).

2.3 Sites of attack of radicals on amino acids, peptides and proteins

In this next section we will examine the chemistry of the radicals formed on amino acids, peptides and proteins that arise from reaction of these components with the above species. The diverse nature of the side chains of the 20 common amino acids means that there is a multitude of different possible sites of attack of an initiating radical on amino acids, peptides, and proteins. Though much data and considerable knowledge has been accrued on the rationale for the sites of attack of many radicals on free amino acids, the situation with more complex substrates is less well understood. Thus, we will examine first the situation with the most well understood systems—the free amino acids—before progressing to more complex systems.

2.3.1 Free amino acids

Glycine

For the majority of reactive radicals, the site of initial attack is decreed by the nature of the attacking species i.e. electrophilic versus nucleophilic. The simplest example is the case of glycine, though even with this material there is some discussion as to the relative yields of the different types of radicals which could be formed. In the majority of early studies it was assumed that the α-carbon position (i.e. C-2, numbering from the free carboxyl group) of Gly was the major site of attack by most radicals. Thus early EPR studies on the reaction of HO· with Gly resulted in the detection of signals from a radical arising from hydrogen abstraction from the methylene ($-CH_2-$) group (reaction 66 (Armstrong and Humphreys 1967; Taniguchi *et al.* 1968, 1970, 1972; Paul and Fischer 1969, 1971; Smith *et al.* 1970; Neta and Fessenden 1971*b*)). The rate constant for this process at neutral pH (i.e. reaction with the zwitterionic form) is low (see Table 2.3 for a compilation of rate constants for reaction of a variety of radicals with free amino acids and peptides (Buxton *et al.* 1988)). The reason for this low value is that this position is not an electron-rich site due to the presence of the neighbouring protonated amine function, and hence attack by electrophilic radicals such as HO· at this site is not favourable. Similar behaviour is observed with a number of other attacking radicals. The pK_a values of the Gly-derived radicals have been measured and, as expected, the radicals formed by hydrogen atom abstraction at the α-carbon position are more acidic than the parent compounds. Thus the pK_a value for protonation of the neutral/zwitterion ($·CH(NH_2)(COOH)/·CH(NH_3^+)(COO^-)$) species is < 1, the zwitterion species $·CH(NH_3^+)(COO^-)$ deprotonates to form $·CH(NH_2)(COO^-)$ with $pK_a \simeq 6.6$, and the last of these forms the dianion species $·CH(NH^-)(COO^-)$ with $pK_a > 12$ (Neta *et al.* 1970, 1972; Paul and Fischer 1971).

$$HO· + {}^+NH_3CH_2COO^- \longrightarrow H_2O + ·CH(NH_3^+)COO^- \tag{66}$$

The chemistry of this α-carbon radical, once formed, has been examined in some detail and it has been shown that there are a number of pathways which result in the loss of this species (Garrison 1968). These include dimerisation (chiefly in the absence of oxygen) to give α, α'-diaminosuccinic acid (reaction 67), disproportionation (reaction 68) to form one molecule of the parent compound and an imino acid (the latter can subsequently undergo hydrolysis in the presence of base or acid to form ammonium ions and the α-ketoacid, reaction 69; we are not aware of determinations of the rate constant for this reaction under physiological conditions), or reaction with oxygen to form a peroxyl radical at the α-carbon site (reaction 70) which then subsequently decomposes (via some, or all, of the pathways outlined in section 2.2.6) to give further imino acid and HO_2· (Garrison 1968, 1987). The formation of the latter species (or its de-protonated counterpart O_2·$^-$) has been directly observed by pulse radiolysis (Abramovitch and Rabani 1976). Steady state radiolysis experiments in the presence of high (non-limiting) concentrations of oxygen have been used to measure the yields (G) of the various products obtained from such reactions; these give $G(carbonyl) \simeq G(NH_4^+) \simeq 3$, which corresponds to the amount of HO· generated (Garrison 1968).

$$2 \cdot CH(NH_3^+)COO^- \longrightarrow {}^+NH_3CH(COO^-)CH(NH_3^+)COO^- \tag{67}$$

$$2 \cdot CH(NH_3^+)COO^- \longrightarrow {}^+NH_3CH_2COO^- + {}^+NH_2{=}CHCOO^- \tag{68}$$

$${}^+NH_2{=}CHCOO^- + H_2O \longrightarrow {}^+NH_4 + HCOCOO· \tag{69}$$

$$\cdot CH(NH_3^+)COO^- + O_2 \longrightarrow \cdot OOCH(NH_3^+)COO^- \tag{70}$$

More recently it has been suggested, on the basis of studies with model compounds such as trimethylamine, that the protonated amine group can be a major locus of attack (Das and von Sonntag 1986). Hydrogen abstraction from such a species would be expected to give rise to a nitrogen-centred radical-cation (reaction 71). This same sort of species has been suggested as a key intermediate in studies on the monoanion of Gly at high pH (reaction 72), and such a nitrogen-centred radical has been detected in studies with α-aminoisobutyric acid in basic solution (Neta and Fessenden 1971b). The intermediacy of this type of species may have eluded previous workers as a result of the rapid conversion of these nitrogen-centred radicals into carbon-centred radicals. This interconversion might occur by a number of different pathways including: i) direct decarboxylation (reaction 73, possibly via an electron transfer from the carboxyl group and rapid loss of CO_2 from the acyloxyl radical)—a process characterized for some amino acids (Monig et al. 1985), ii) deprotonation followed by reaction with another substrate (reactions 74 and 75 (Neale 1971; Michejda et al. 1978)), or iii) deprotonation followed by a rapid intramolecular 1,2-hydrogen atom shift reaction (reactions 74 and 76 (von Sonntag 1987)). The last of these processes is analogous to the 1,2-hydrogen shift reactions (reaction 41) which have been demonstrated to occur with alkoxyl radicals and which are known to be very rapid (Berdnikov et al. 1972; Gilbert 1976; Schuchmann and von Sonntag 1981); on this basis reaction 76 would also be expected to be rapid. The α-aminoalkyl radicals formed by such a reaction would be expected to undergo ready oxidation and hydration which will eventually result in the release of ammonium ions and the formation of a carbonyl group (Monig et al. 1985). The formation of such nitrogen-centred radicals has however been questioned on the basis of theoretical calculations (Armstrong et al. 1995).

$$HO^{\bullet} + {}^{+}NH_3CH_2COO^{-} \longrightarrow H_2O + {}^{+\bullet}NH_2CH_2COO^{-} \tag{71}$$

$$HO^{\bullet} + NH_2CH_2COO^{-} \longrightarrow HO^{-} + {}^{+\bullet}NH_2CH_2COO^{-} \tag{72}$$

$$^{+\bullet}NH_2CH_2COO^{-} \longrightarrow NH_2CH_2^{\bullet} + CO_2 \tag{73}$$

$$^{+\bullet}NH_2CH_2COO^{-} \longrightarrow {}^{\bullet}NHCH_2COO^{-} + H^{+} \tag{74}$$

$$^{\bullet}NHCH_2COO^{-} + {}^{+}NH_3CH_2COO^{-} \longrightarrow NH_2CH_2COO^{-} + {}^{\bullet}CH(NH_3^{+})COO^{-} \tag{75}$$

$$^{\bullet}NHCH_2COO^{-} \longrightarrow {}^{\bullet}CH(NH_2)COO^{-} \tag{76}$$

The reaction of the solvated electron with Gly in the absence of oxygen occurs via a somewhat different mechanism. Two reactions have been elucidated: electron attachment to the carboxyl function (the major site with Gly, reaction 77), and reaction at the protonated amine group (about 35 per cent of the e^{-}_{aq}, reaction 78). These reactions occur most rapidly, as expected, with the positively-charged species at low pH, and much less rapidly with the zwitterion and the monoanion at high pH (Peter and Neta 1972; Mittal and Hayon 1974). The radical-anion formed by addition at the carboxyl function rapidly eliminates ammonium ions to give an ethanoate radical (reaction 79). At low pH the yield of ammonium ions approaches the yield of the solvated electron, indicating that this is the predominant reaction under such conditions (Weeks and Garrison 1958) see also (Weeks *et al.* 1965). In the presence of oxygen these reactions occur only to a very limited extent as the solvated electron preferentially reacts with oxygen to give the superoxide radical (Hart and Anbar 1970).

$$e^{-}_{aq} + {}^{-}OOCCH_2NH_3^{+} \longrightarrow {}^{\bullet}C(O^{-})(O^{-})CH_2NH_3^{+} \tag{77}$$

$$e^{-}_{aq} + {}^{+}NH_3CH_2COO^{-} \longrightarrow H^{\bullet} + NH_2CH_2COO^{-} \tag{78}$$

$$^{\bullet}C(O^{-})(O^{-})CH_2NH_3^{+} \longrightarrow NH_3 + {}^{\bullet}CH_2COO^{-} \tag{79}$$

With other free amino acids, electrophilic radicals, such as HO$^{\bullet}$, can react with the side chain as well as at the backbone as outlined above. These side chain reactions become more significant: i) as the size of the side chain increases (particularly the number of C–H bonds), ii) where the side chain contains heteroatom substituents which can stabilize incipient radical centres, iii) where the side chain contains a sulfur atom, or iv) where the side chain is aromatic (reviewed: Garrison 1987; von Sonntag 1987).

Amino acids with aliphatic hydrocarbon side chains

On going from Gly and Ala, where attack is primarily at backbone sites, to other aliphatic side chains, the proportion of attack at side chain C–H bonds increases, with the larger the number of available bonds roughly determining the percentage attack at the side chain in contrast to the backbone. Thus the yields of material arising from attack at the backbone (e.g. keto acids, ammonium ions) decreases as the size of the side chain increases; with nor-leucine the percentage of attack at backbone sites has been estimated at about 10 per cent (Garrison *et al.* 1962; Kopoldova *et al.* 1963*a*, *b*, *c*; Garrison 1968; Rustgi *et al.* 1977*a*). Radical attack at such side chain sites is primarily by hydrogen atom abstraction to give a carbon-centred radical (Armstrong and Humphreys 1967; Taniguchi *et al.* 1968, 1970, 1972; Smith *et al.* 1970; Neta and Fessenden 1971*b*; Paul and Fischer 1971; Burgess and Easton 1987)), the subsequent reactions of which are very similar to other small carbon-centred radicals. Thus the major products in the absence of oxygen are dimers (Garrison 1968), whereas in the presence of oxygen, peroxyl radicals are formed. The latter undergo characteristic peroxyl radical reactions (reactions 35–40) and hence can give rise to hydroperoxides via hydrogen abstraction from further C–H bonds (reaction 80 (Simpson *et al.* 1992; Gebicki and Gebicki 1993; Fu *et al.* 1995*b*)), hydroxides, and carbonyl (aldehyde or ketone) groups (Kopoldova *et al.* 1963*a*, *b*, *c*). In the case of leucine the products formed as a result of exposure to a Fenton system with added bicarbonate ($Fe^{2+}/ADP/H_2O_2/$ bicarbonate) have both been characterized in some detail, and quantitated allowing a mass balance to be obtained (Stadtman and Berlett 1991). Reaction of proline (and proline-containing peptides) with radical-generating systems has been shown to give rise to a complex mixture of (*cis*- and *trans*-) 3- and 4-hydroxyprolines together with the corresponding keto materials (Trelstad *et al.* 1981). A list of some of the more well characterized products identified from such reactions, plus appropriate references, is given in Table 2.4. Further oxidation of some of these species (e.g. aldehydes to carboxylic acids) may also occur under certain experimental conditions; the detection of 2-aminomalonic acid ($^+H_3N–CH(COO^-)–COO^-$) under certain conditions (Wheelan *et al.* 1989; Copley *et al.* 1992), may arise from serine residues via a series of sequential oxidation reactions. Formation of dialkyl peroxide linkages, which would be expected from dimerisation of two peroxyl radicals via reactions 35 and 36 (see earlier), has not been characterized as yet, though such materials would be expected to be rare. Reactive nitrogen species are also believed to oxidize some aliphatic side chains as evidenced by a loss of such residues (Ischiropoulos and al-Mehdi 1995). The species formed in these reactions have not been characterized. If these reactions occur via hydrogen atom abstraction (as would be expected), the resulting radicals would be expected to undergo similar types of reactions to those outlined above; such processes may explain the observed increase in the level of carbonyl-containing compounds (Ischiropoulos and al-Mehdi 1995).

$$ROO^{\boldsymbol{\cdot}} + R'\!-\!H \longrightarrow ROOH + R''^{\boldsymbol{\cdot}} \tag{80}$$

Table 2.4 Selected stable, or semi-stable, products generated as a result of exposure of amino acids, peptides and proteins to radical species and their postulated mechanisms of formation

Parent amino acid	Product	Mechanisms of formation	Selected References
Tyrosine	DOPA[a] (3,4-dihydroxy-phenylalanine)	HO˙ attack or one-electron oxidation of aromatic ring. May also arise via reactions of reactive nitrogen species.	(Gieseg et al. 1993)
	Di-tyrosine	HO˙ attack or one-electron oxidation of tyrosine and subsequent radical-radical dimerization; HOCl.	(Heinecke et al. 1993a, c; Huggins et al. 1993)
	3-chlorotyrosine	Chlorination of tyrosine as a result of exposure to HOCl or other chlorinating agents.	(Kettle 1996)
	3-nitrotyrosine	Reaction of reactive nitrogen species with tyrosine.	(van der Vliet et al. 1995)
	Tyrosine hydroperoxide and subsequent cyclized materials[b]	Formation of tyrosine phenoxyl radical in presence of $O_2^{˙-}$.	(Jin et al. 1993; Pichorner et al. 1995)
Phenylalanine	o-, m-tyrosine	HO˙ attack or one-electron oxidation of aromatic ring. Possibly via reactive nitrogen species.	(Dizdaroglu and Simic 1980; Huggins et al. 1993)
	Dimers of hydroxylated aromatic amino acids	HO˙ attack or one-electron oxidation before or after dimerization.	(Marquez and Dunford 1995)
Tryptophan	N-formylkynurenine, kynurenine, 5-hydroxytryptophan, 7-hydroxytryptophan	HO˙ attack or one-electron oxidation of ring.	(Armstrong and Swallow 1969; Guptasarma et al. 1992; Maskos et al. 1992; Neuzil and Stocker 1993)
Histidine	2-oxo-histidine	HO˙ attack or one-electron oxidation.	(Uchida and Kawakishi 1993; Winter and Butler 1996)

Table 2.4   (*cont.*)

Parent amino acid	Product	Mechanisms of formation	Selected References
	aspartate	HO⁺ attack followed by ring opening; mechanistic details unclear.	(Amici *et al.* 1989; Dean *et al.* 1989*a*; Stadtman 1990*a*)
Glutamic acid	Glutamic acid hydroperoxide	Hydrogen atom abstraction from side chain in presence of O_2.	(Simpson *et al.* 1992; Gebicki and Gebicki 1993)
Lysine	Lysine hydroperoxide, 5-hydroxylysine,[c] other hydroxylysines, aldehydes/ketones.	Hydrogen atom abstraction from side chain in presence of O_2	(Trelstad *et al.* 1981; Simpson *et al.* 1992; Gebicki and Gebicki 1993; Morin *et al.*, unpublished data)
Leucine	Leucine hydroperoxides, hydroxy-leucines, α-ketoisocaproic acid, isovaleric acid, isovaleraldehyde, isovaleraldehyde oxime, other carbonyl compounds.	Hydrogen atom abstraction from side chain in presence of O_2.	(Stadtman and Berlett 1991; Simpson *et al.* 1992; Gebicki and Gebicki 1993; Fu *et al.* 1995*a*; Dean *et al.* 1996; Fu and Dean 1997)
Valine	Valine hydroperoxides, hydroxyvalines, aldehydes/ketones.	Hydrogen atom abstraction from side chain in presence of O_2.	(Simpson *et al.* 1992; Gebicki and Gebicki 1993; Fu *et al.* 1995; Fu *et al.* 1995)
Proline	Proline hydroperoxides, 3- or 4-oxo (keto)prolines, 3- or 4-hydroxyprolines,[d]	Hydrogen atom abstraction from side chain in presence of O_2.	(Trelstad *et al.* 1981; Simpson *et al.* 1992; Gebicki and Gebicki 1993)
	5-hydroxy-2-aminovaleric acid, glutamic acid.	Hydrogen atom abstraction from side chain in presence of O_2, and subsequent ring opening.	(Dean *et al.* 1989*a*; Ayala and Cutler 1996; Ayala and Cutler 1996)
Isoleucine	Isoleucine hydroperoxides	Hydrogen atom abstraction from side chain in presence of O_2.	(Simpson *et al.* 1992; Gebicki and Gebicki 1993)
Methionine	Methionine sulfoxide	Variety of routes including both radical and non-radical reactions.	(Li *et al.* 1995; Li *et al.* 1995; Vogt 1995); Garner *et al.*, unpublished data)

Cysteine	Cystine	Hydrogen abstraction from SH group and subsequent radical dimerization.	(Armstrong 1990; von Sonntag 1990)
	Oxy acids	Hydrogen abstraction from SH group, subsequent reaction with oxygen, and isomerization.	(Armstrong 1990; von Sonntag 1990)
Glycine	2-aminomalonic acid	Originally suggested to be formed via reaction of Gly α-carbon radical and $CO_2^{\cdot-}$. May also be formed via successive oxidations of other amino acids (eg. serine).	(Wheelan et al. 1989; Copley et al. 1992)
Arginine	5-hydroxy-2-aminovaleric acid	Hydrogen atom abstraction from side chain in presence of O_2, and subsequent loss of guanidine group.	(Ayala and Cutler 1996a,b)
All non-aromatic side chains?	Protein carbonyls	Hydrogen atom abstraction from side chains in presence of O_2.	(Levine et al. 1994)
All amino acids?	RCHO species (e.g. 4-hydroxyphenyl acetaldehyde from Tyr) formed by decarboxylation and deamination.	By a wide variety of processes including: the conventional Dakin hydroxyl radical mechanism, photodecarboxylation, reaction with powerful one-electron oxidants, and HOCl.	(Rowbottom 1955; Nosworthy and Allsop 1956; Zgliczynski et al. 1968, 1971; Pereira et al. 1973; Hazen et al. 1996)

[a] Can undergo further reaction to give rise to: a) the trihydroxy compound TOPA and b) ring-closed indolic materials.
[b] Cyclized materials are only generated in significant amounts if a free amine group is present; these materials are therefore probably only significant with the free amino acid.
[c] A natural amino acid, and hence not a useful marker for oxidative damage in most situations.
[d] Constituents of some natural products and hence unlikely to be a useful marker for oxidative damage in most situations.

Recent studies have shown that hydroperoxides can be major products of some free amino acids when exposed to a variety of initiating radicals in the presence of oxygen (Simpson *et al.* 1992; Gebicki and Gebicki 1993); these materials had been detected, but not quantified in earlier studies (Latarjet and Loiseleur 1942; Loiseleur *et al.* 1942). Thus it has been shown that aliphatic hydrocarbon side chain amino acids such as Val, Leu, Ile, and Pro can give high yields of side chain hydroperoxides; these can account for up to 40 per cent of the initiating radical flux (Simpson *et al.* 1992; Gebicki and Gebicki 1993). These materials appear to be formed solely on the side chain of free amino acids, with little evidence for formation at the α-carbon. This presumably reflects the low extent of attack at this site with these substrates, together with the fact that the presumed precursor of the hydroperoxide— the corresponding peroxyl radical (which would be an α-aminoperoxyl species)—would be expected to be highly unstable (cf. the ready elimination of HOO˙ from the corresponding α-hydroxyperoxyl species, reaction 33). The situation with amino acid derivatives and peptides is somewhat different (see below). Other amino acids such as Ala give very much lower yields (Gebicki and Gebicki 1993); this may reflect the lower reactivity of this amino acid compared with the former species, though the stability of the carbon-centred radical initially generated, the rates of reaction of the corresponding peroxyl radical, and the stability of the hydroperoxide itself, may all play a role in determining the overall yield of hydroperoxide (Mieden and von Sonntag 1989; Mieden *et al.* 1993).

Subsequent 2-electron reduction of these hydroperoxides (e.g. with NaBH$_4$) gives rise to the corresponding hydroxides; a number of these have been characterized in some detail (Fu *et al.* 1995*b*). One-electron reduction of the hydroperoxides (e.g. by reaction with low-valent metal ion complexes) has been shown to give rise to the formation of further radicals (Davies, M. J. *et al.* 1995). The initial species formed in each case is believed to be an alkoxyl radical. These can undergo a number of subsequent rearrangement and fragmentation reactions to give carbon-centred species, including 1,2-hydrogen atom shifts for primary and secondary alkoxyl species (e.g. reaction 41) and β-scission reactions for the tertiary alkoxyl radicals (reaction 43) (Davies, M. J. *et al.* 1995).

The formation of these hydroxide, hydroperoxide and carbonyl products would be expected to occur almost randomly with highly reactive radicals such as HO˙. This has been shown to be the case with a number of side chains either by use of EPR spectroscopy or product analysis (Armstrong and Humphreys 1967; Taniguchi *et al.* 1968, 1970, 1972; Paul and Fischer 1969, 1971; Garrison *et al.* 1970; Smith *et al.* 1970; Neta and Fessenden 1971*b*; Rustgi *et al.* 1977*a*; Stadtman and Berlett 1991; Fu *et al.* 1995*b*). With less reactive radicals however a degree of selectivity would be expected to occur, with formation of the most stable carbon-centred radicals (i.e.

tertiary favoured over secondary over primary, $R^1R^2R^3C^\cdot > R^1R^2CH^\cdot > R^1CH_2^\cdot$). This would particularly be the case with species, such as $Br^\cdot$, where the abstraction of a hydrogen atom can be endothermic (rather than exothermic) in nature, thereby resulting in very late transition states where the radical stability is of great importance (Pryor 1966). Few studies to date have investigated this phenomenon in aqueous solution in any detail, though some work has been carried out in organic solvents.

In contrast to the situation with $HO^\cdot$, $H^\cdot$, and other electrophilic radicals, attack at backbone sites is still preferred with some species. Thus, reaction of the hydrated electron with free aliphatic amino acids in the absence of oxygen (in its presence reaction occurs primarily with O_2) takes place mainly at the ionized carboxyl group (reaction 77 above) with a small percentage of addition at the protonated amine function (reaction 78 (Weeks et al. 1965; Willix and Garrison 1967, 1968)). These are rapid processes with rate constants in the range 10^8–10^9 $dm^3 mol^{-1} s^{-1}$, with the former process resulting in deamination as outlined above. Reaction of the solvated electron with some of the products of oxidation of the side chains may, however, be important under conditions where extensive conversion of starting material into products occurs. Thus the observation that the yield of hydroperoxides obtained with these amino acids in the presence of oxygen does not continually increase with increasing radiation dose (Simpson et al. 1992; Gebicki and Gebicki 1993), even in conditions where the substrate and oxygen are not limiting, suggests that subsequent decomposition of the hydroperoxide group is occurring during the radiolysis. This may be due to electron attachment and subsequent reductive fragmentation of the hydroperoxide functions; this would be expected to be a fast process (cf. $k \simeq 1.1 \times 10^{10}$ $dm^3 mol^{-1} s^{-1}$ for hydrogen peroxide and 1.6×10^{10} $dm^3 mol^{-1} s^{-1}$ for t-butyl hydroperoxide (Buxton et al. 1988)). This type of process would only be expected to compete with electron attachment to molecular oxygen (which occurs with $k = 1.9 \times 10^{10}$ $dm^3 mol^{-1} s^{-1}$, (Buxton et al. 1988)) when the hydroperoxide yield approaches the steady state concentration of oxygen in the samples; this appears to be the case, with maximal hydroperoxide concentrations in the 100–200 μM range detected (Simpson et al. 1992; Gebicki and Gebicki 1993). Thus, some of the products detected as a result of radiolysis may arise from the subsequent breakdown of initially generated hydroperoxides.

Reaction of HOCl with simple aliphatic amino acids has been extensively studied; the damage induced by this agent is of a dramatically different nature to those outlined above, and hence is worthy of mention. Though the side chains of some other amino acids (such as Cys, Met, Trp, Lys, His) are much more reactive than the aliphatic amino acids (Winterbourn 1985), reaction can still occur with excess HOCl. This involves initial reaction at the free amino group to form a semi-stable chloramine species; these species can have considerable lifetimes, can be isolated in some cases, and are potent bactericidal agents (Wright 1926; Van Tamelen *et al.* 1968; Zgliczynski *et al.* 1968, 1971; Pereira *et al.* 1973; Zgliczynski and Stelmaszynska 1975; Hazen *et al.* 1996). It is well established that these materials can undergo decomposition to form aldehydic materials which have lost both the amine group (as ammonia) and the carboxyl function (as CO_2); i.e. an amino acid of structure $^+H_3NCH(R)COO^-$, gives the aldehyde RCH(O) (Van Tamelen *et al.* 1968; Zgliczynski *et al.* 1968, 1971; Pereira *et al.* 1973; Zgliczynski and Stelmaszynska 1975). Early studies did not investigate the mechanism(s) of these interconversions in great detail; recent studies suggest that these reactions may involve decomposition of the chloramine to a nitrogen-centred radical (see earlier) which subsequently undergoes a series of rearrangement and fragmentation reactions (Hawkins and Davies, unpublished data). The formation of radicals from these chloramine species may be the reason for both their cytotoxicity, and their ability to promote damage to proteins (see Chapter 1 for historical precedents; also (Thomas 1979a, b; Weiss *et al.* 1983; Grisham *et al.* 1984; Katrantzis *et al.* 1991; Davies, J. M. *et al.* 1993).

Amino acids with aliphatic heteroatom-containing side chains

The presence of a functional group containing heteroatoms on the side chain of a free amino acid can have a dramatic effect on the selectivity of radical attack. Thus while hydrocarbon side chains are attacked with little selectivity by species such as HO·, much greater selectivity is observed with other side chains.

With the hydroxylated side chains Ser and Thr (and the less common amino acids 4-hydroxyproline and 5-hydroxylysine), attack by electrophilic radicals such as HO· occurs preferentially, by hydrogen atom abstraction, at the C–H bond(s) α to the hydroxyl group due to stabilization of the incipient radical by the electron-delocalising hydroxyl group (e.g. reaction 81 (Armstrong and Humphreys 1967; Rustgi *et al.* 1977a; Behrens and Koltzenburg 1985)). Reactive nitrogen radicals would be expected to behave in a similar manner, though such reactions have not been well characterized, apart from a gross loss of the amino acid (Ischiropoulos and al-Mehdi 1995). In the absence of oxygen, α-hydroxyalkyl radicals which have a β-amine group (e.g. those formed with Ser and Thr (Behrens and Koltzenburg 1985)) can undergo a rapid unimolecular elimination reaction which results in the loss of ammonium ions (e.g. reaction 82). The mechanism of these reactions has been elucidated in some detail, and is analogous to the β-elimination reactions seen with a large number of other α-,β- diheteroatom-substituted radicals (e.g. 1,2 diols, β-amino alcohols, and related compounds (Buley *et al.* 1966; Livingstone and Zeldes 1966; Foster and West 1973, 1974; Steenken *et al.* 1986; reviewed: Davies and Gilbert

1991). Similar reactions may occur with the analogous radicals from 4-hydroxyproline and 5-hydroxylysine. In the presence of oxygen, the peroxyl radicals formed from these initial radicals would be expected to undergo a rapid elimination reaction which results in the formation of a carbonyl function and the release of a hydroperoxyl (HOO·) radical (e.g. reaction 83 (Bothe *et al.* 1977, 1978)). This may explain the low yield of hydroperoxides obtained on radiolysis of these amino acids (Gebicki and Gebicki 1993).

$$HO^{\cdot} + HOCH_2\text{-}CH(NHR)C(O)R'' \longrightarrow H_2O + {}^{\cdot}CH(OH)\text{-}CH(NHR)C(O)R'' \qquad (81)$$

$$^{\cdot}CH(OH)\text{-}CH({}^{+}NH_3)R \longrightarrow O{=}CH\text{-}CH(R)^{\cdot} + NH_3 \qquad (82)$$

$$^{\cdot}CH(OH)R + O_2 \longrightarrow {}^{\cdot}OOCH(OH)R \longrightarrow HOO^{\cdot} + O{=}CHR \qquad (83)$$

The presence of an ionized carboxyl group on the side chain (e.g. Asp, Glu) also results in greater selectivity, with the radical delocalizing effect of the carboxyl group favouring hydrogen abstraction at C–H bonds next to such groups (Sokol *et al.* 1965; Armstrong and Humphreys 1967; Taniguchi *et al.* 1968, 1970, 1972; Smith *et al.* 1970; Neta and Fessenden 1971*b*; Paul and Fischer 1971; Rustgi *et al.* 1977*a*). Thus the C-4 position is the major site of hydrogen abstraction with Glu (reaction 84). This is also probably the site of reaction of reactive nitrogen radicals, though this has not been well characterized (Ischiropoulos and al-Mehdi 1995). A similar selectivity argument applies to the reaction of electrophilic radicals with amide-containing side chains.

In contrast to the above positive effects of substituents, the presence of a protonated side chain substituent can disfavour attack at particular sites. Thus with Lys, positions away from the amine group are somewhat favoured, and the C–H bonds of C-4 and C-5 appear to be the major sites of hydrogen abstraction (Hawkins and Davies 1997). In the absence of oxygen these carbon-centred radicals mainly undergo dimerization reactions, whereas in the presence of oxygen typical peroxyl radical chemistry (see above) is observed in most cases. 5-Hydroxylysine has been identified, with both free lysine and lysine-containing peptides, as a product of such reactions (Trelstad *et al.* 1981; Morin *et al.*, unpublished data). A number of other oxygenated products are also generated from Lys (Morin *et al.*, unpublished data); these are probably other isomeric alcohols, carbonyl-containing materials, and hydroperoxides. The (relatively low yield of) carbon-centred radicals formed at C-6 on Lys (i.e. α- to the side chain amine function) react rapidly with oxygen, then readily eliminate ammonium ions and HOO· in a reaction analogous to that seen with α-hydroxyalkylperoxyl species (reaction 85 (Garrison 1987)). Further oxidation of the Lys-derived aldehydes formed in such reactions may be the source of the α–aminoadipic–δ–semialdehyde generated from proteins such as elastin and collagen by Cu^{2+}/pyrroloquinoline quinone complexes (Shah *et al.* 1992).

$$HO^{\bullet} + {}^{-}OOCCH_2CH_2CH(NHR)C(O)R' \longrightarrow H_2O + {}^{\bullet}CH(COO^-)CH_2CH(NHR)C(O)R' \quad (84)$$

$$\sim CH_2\overset{\bullet}{C}HNH_3^+ + O_2 \longrightarrow \sim CH_2\underset{OO^{\bullet}}{CHNH_3^+} \longrightarrow \sim CH_2CHO + NH_3 + HOO^{\bullet} \quad (85)$$

A similar type of reaction, though in this case involving loss of the guanidine group, occurs with radicals formed at C-5 on Arg (i.e. α- to the guanidinium function, reaction 86 (Garrison 1987)); this type of process may explain the formation of 5-hydroxy-2-aminovaleric acid, which has been recently postulated as a marker of radical-induced damage to proteins and peptides (Ayala and Cutler 1996*a*, *b*). Table 2.4 lists some of the more well characterized products of these reactions.

$$\sim CH_2\overset{\bullet}{C}HNH\underset{\parallel}{C}NH_3^+ + O_2 \longrightarrow \sim CH_2CHNH\underset{\parallel}{C}NH_3^+ + O_2$$

Reduction and hydrolysis

$$^{-}OOCCCH_2CH_2CH_2OH \longleftarrow \longleftarrow \sim CH_2CHO + NH_2\underset{NH}{\overset{\parallel}{C}}NH_2 + HOO^{\bullet} \quad (86)$$

5-hydroxy-2-aminovaleric acid (HAVA)

When such rapid elimination reactions cannot occur, significant amounts of hydroperoxides can be formed on the side chain, particularly when this is a major site of initial attack (i.e. has a large number of C–H bonds); Glu and Lys give particularly high yields (see Table 2.4 above) (Gebicki and Gebicki 1993). Subsequent decomposition of the hydroperoxides formed on Lys, by metal ion complexes, gives further radical species as outlined above for aliphatic side chains (Davies *et al.* 1995). The situation with Glu, however, is slightly different. Decomposition of hydroperoxide groups on Glu, which appear to be primarily located on the C-4 carbon (i.e. α to the carboxyl group), by Fe^{2+} complexes to alkoxyl radicals has been shown to result in the loss of the side chain carboxyl group as $CO_2^{\bullet -}$ (Davies, M. J. *et al.* 1995). This appears to be a novel, and very rapid, β-scission reaction (reaction 87). The observation that the well characterized 1,2 -hydrogen shift reaction does not compete successfully with this new reaction, suggests that the rate of this fragmentation must occur with a unimolecular rate constant of $> 10^7 \text{ s}^{-1}$.

Some of the side chain functional groups present in the parent amino acids are targets for the attachment of the solvated electron, in addition to the

$$
\begin{array}{c}
\text{-NH} \\
\diagdown \\
\text{CHCH}_2\text{CH} - \text{COO}^- \\
\diagup \quad\quad | \\
\text{-C(O)} \quad\quad \text{OOH}
\end{array}
\xrightarrow[-\text{ HO}^-]{\text{Fe(II)-EDTA}}
\begin{array}{c}
\text{-NH} \\
\diagdown \\
\text{CHCH}_2\text{CH} \quad\text{C}-\text{COO}^- \\
\diagup \quad\quad | \\
\text{-C(O)} \quad\quad \text{O}^\cdot
\end{array}
\longrightarrow
$$

$$
\begin{array}{c}
\text{-NH} \quad\quad\quad \text{O} \\
\diagdown \quad\quad\quad\quad || \\
\text{CHCH}_2\text{CH} \quad + \; \text{CO}_2^{-\cdot} \\
\diagup \\
\text{-C(O)}
\end{array}
\tag{87}
$$

already mentioned backbone carboxyl function. Thus, it would be expected that electron attachment would also occur, though to a limited extent, to the ionized carboxyl side chains of Glu and Asp, as well as the protonated amine group of Lys, etc. These reactions would only be expected to be of any significance, however, in the absence of molecular oxygen.

The side chain amine group of Lys is a major site of reaction of HOCl, and this results in the formation of a chloramine species (Hazell and Stocker 1993; Hazell *et al.* 1994). This species, when present on a protein, can promote aggregation either via subsequent hydrolysis to form an aldehyde, which can react with another free amine function to form a Schiff base (Hazell *et al.* 1994), or possibly via further radical generation as outlined earlier.

Amino acids with aromatic side chains

The presence of an aromatic ring on the side chain of an amino acid almost invariably results in attack at that site by addition, though in many cases the initial radical often undergoes rapid subsequent reactions. Direct hydrogen abstraction, unlike the case of the aliphatic side chains, appears to be only a very minor process. Thus HO· adds rapidly to the aromatic ring of phenylalanine with little positional selectivity (i.e. the ring substituent has little directing effect) which result in the formation of a mixture of positional isomers with the ratio of *o*-:*m*-:*p*-tyrosine being 2:1:1.5 or 2.3:1:2.1 depending on the report consulted (Brodskaya and Sharpatyi 1967; Wheeler and Montalvo 1969; Lynn and Purdie 1976; Dizdaroglu and Simic 1980). Peroxynitrite has also been reported to bring about hydroxylation (van der Vliet *et al.* 1994*a*). The mechanism of formation of these species appears to be dependent on whether oxygen is present or not. In the presence of oxygen these materials appear to be formed via reaction 88 with release of HOO·. However the exact nature of these reactions is poorly understood, as the yield of HOO· formed is only about 50 per cent of what would be expected if all the four positional isomers of the hydroxycyclohexadienylperoxyl radical were reacting via this route (Brodskaya and Sharpatyi 1967; Dizdaroglu and Simic 1980; von Sonntag 1987). On the basis of model studies with benzene, some of the peroxyl radicals formed in the former process would be expected to undergo other side reactions which result in cleavage of the aromatic ring (cf. the detection of β-hydroxymuconaldehyde from benzene (Balakrishnan and Reddy 1970)). In the absence of O_2, reaction 89 is thought to occur (Eberhart 1974; Gordon *et al.* 1977; Simic *et al.* 1985). The overall yield of these tyrosines formed is, however, low, as the major fate of the intermediate hydroxycyclohexadienyl radicals is dimerization to give a number of biphenyls (Yamamoto 1973; Eberhart 1974; Gordon *et al.* 1977; Kim *et al.* 1984*a, b*; Simic *et al.* 1985). These subsequent reactions are pH dependent and at low pH radical-cation species formed by acid-catalysed loss of water from the initial adduct can occur; the subsequent reactions of these radical-cations have been investigated and it has been demonstrated that these can lead to damage transfer to other intramolecular sites (oxidation at the – CH_2– (benzylic) group next to the ring (reaction 90) or loss of the carboxyl group (reaction 91 (Davies *et al.* 1984*a*; Davies and Gilbert 1991)).

$$C_6H_5{-}CH_2CH(COO^-)NH_3^+ \;+\; HO^{\bullet} \;\longrightarrow\; HO{-}C_6H_6{-}CH_2CH(COO^-)NH_3^+ \qquad \downarrow O_2 \qquad (88)$$

$$HOO^{\bullet} \;+\; HO{-}C_6H_4{-}CH_2CH(COO^-)NH_3^+ \;\longleftarrow\; {}^{\bullet}OO{-}HO{-}C_6H_6{-}CH_2CH(COO^-)NH_3^+$$

$$C_6H_5{-}CH_2CH(COO^-)NH_3^+ \;+\; HO^{\bullet} \;\longrightarrow\; HO{-}C_6H_6{-}CH_2CH(COO^-)NH_3^+ \qquad \downarrow 2\text{x} \qquad (89)$$

$$HO{-}C_6H_4{-}CH_2CH(COO^-)NH_3^+ \;+\; C_6H_5{-}CH_2CH(COO^-)NH_3^+$$

$$C_6H_5{-}CH_2CH(COO^-)NH_3^+ \;+\; HO^{\bullet} \;\longrightarrow\; HO{-}C_6H_6{-}CH_2CH(COO^-)NH_3^+ \qquad \downarrow H^+ \qquad (90)$$

$$C_6H_5{-}\overset{\bullet}{C}HCH(COO^-)NH_3^+ \;\overset{-H^+}{\longleftarrow}\; [C_6H_6]^{+\bullet}{-}CH_2CH(COO^-)NH_3^+ \;+\; H_2O$$

$$C_6H_5{-}CH_2CH(COO^-)NH_3^+ \;+\; HO^{\bullet} \;\longrightarrow\; HO{-}C_6H_6{-}CH_2CH(COO^-)NH_3^+ \qquad \downarrow H^+ \qquad (91)$$

$$C_6H_5{-}CH_2\overset{\bullet}{C}HNH_3^+ \;\overset{-CO_2}{\longleftarrow}\; [C_6H_6]^{+\bullet}{-}CH_2CH(COO^-)NH_3^+ \;+\; H_2O$$

In contrast to the above, HO· addition to Tyr is much more selective due to the strong directing effect of the hydroxyl substituent (Steenken 1977), though still very rapid (Buxton *et al.* 1988). The major product, at most pH values, in the absence of oxygen is DOPA (3,4-dihydroxyphenylalanine) formed via the disproportionation of two of the initial adduct species (reaction 92) (Rowbottom 1955; Lynn and Purdie 1976; Boguta and Dancewicz 1981, 1982). Low yields of the 2,4-dihydroxy isomer are also formed. In the presence of oxygen, addition of oxygen is believed to be followed by rapid elimination of HOO·, as would be expected of α-hydroxy-alkylperoxyl radicals (reaction 93, cf. reaction 33 above (Fletcher and Okada 1961; Lynn and Purdie 1976)). As the latter process generates one DOPA per initial adduct, whereas the former requires two initial adducts per DOPA, the yield of DOPA is much higher in the presence of oxygen. In accordance with this, DOPA has been detected as a product of protein oxidation in both the presence and absence of oxygen (Gieseg *et al.* 1993). Multiple hydroxylations may infrequently convert phenylalanine to DOPA and tyrosine to TOPA (6-hydroxyDOPA; 2,4,5-trihydroxyphenylalanine), though this has not been studied carefully. The initial adduct radicals can also rapidly lose water, in both acid- and base-catalysed reactions, to give phenoxyl radicals (reaction 94).

(92)

(93)

$$HO-\bigcirc-CH_2CH(COO^-)NH_3^+ \ + \ HO^\bullet \longrightarrow \quad \begin{array}{c} HO \\ HO-\bigcirc-CH_2CH(COO^-)NH_3^+ \end{array}$$

$$\downarrow H^+/HO^- \qquad\qquad (94)$$

$$H_2O \ + \ \dot{O}-\bigcirc-CH_2CH(COO^-)NH_3^+$$

$$TyrO^\bullet$$

Phenoxyl species are also generated very efficiently and rapidly from Tyr by a number of other more selective oxidants (e.g. $N_3^\bullet$) with such reactions usually proceeeding via initial one-electron oxidation of the phenolic ring, to form a radical-cation, and subsequent very rapid loss of the phenolic proton. The formation of the neutral phenoxyl radical can be monitored readily either by the strong optical absorbances of such species or by their EPR signals (Land and Ebert 1967; Chrysochoos 1968; O'Neill *et al.* 1977; Prutz *et al.* 1983). These radicals undergo very ready dimerisation to yield hydroxylated biphenyls (di- or bi-Tyr) via reaction through the o- positions to give a dicyclohexadienone which rapidly rearranges to the phenolic tautomer (reaction 95) (Lehrer and Fasman 1967; Boguta and Dancewicz 1981, 1982; Butler *et al.* 1984; Jin *et al.* 1993). The rate constant for such dimerization has been measured as $\simeq 5 \times 10^8 \ dm^3 \ mol^{-1} \ s^{-1}$ (Cudina and Josimovic 1987; Hunter *et al.* 1989; Jin *et al.* 1993). Cross-links between the o- site and the oxygen have also been characterized (reaction 95 (Karam *et al.* 1984)). As might be expected from the delocalized nature of this radical, reaction with oxygen is slow (k estimated as $< 1 \times 10^3$ dm^3 mol^{-1} s^{-1}), and hence the yield of di-tyrosine is not affected by the presence of oxygen (Hunter *et al.* 1989; Jin *et al.* 1993).

The situation when tyrosine phenoxyl radicals and $O_2^{\cdot -}$ are generated simultaneously is however somewhat different, as it has been shown that a rapid addition reaction between the superoxide radical and the phenoxyl radical can occur with $k = 1.5 \times 10^9$ dm^3 mol^{-1} s^{-1} (Jin *et al.* 1993); this results in a dramatic suppression of di-tyrosine formation. Previous suggestions that the reaction between these two radicals occurs via electron transfer (Prutz *et al.* 1983; Cudina and Josimovic 1987; Hunter *et al.* 1989) appear to be incorrect. The addition of the superoxide radical on to the phenoxyl radical at the *o*- and *p*- positions results in the generation of short-lived ring hydroperoxide species which have a half life of about 4.2 hours at pH 8 (Jin *et al.* 1993). These hydroperoxides decay to give stable products which have been characterized; these are believed to arise via a ring closure reaction of the free amino group on to the ring (reaction 96). Similar tyrosine-derived peroxides have been detected as a result of the enzymatic generation of tyrosine phenoxyl radicals by a horse-radish peroxidase/H$_2$O$_2$/tyrosine system in the presence of glutathione (Pichorner *et al.* 1995). Scavenging of the initial tyrosine phenoxyl radicals by GSH gives rise to GS$^{\cdot}$ which, in the presence of oxygen, gives rise to superoxide radicals via the reactions outlined earlier. Subsequent reaction of the $O_2^{\cdot -}$ with excess phenoxyl radicals gives rise to the observed peroxide. It should be noted that the formation of these peroxides requires a free amine function, and hence these reactions are unlikely to be of any major significance in the chemistry of peptides or proteins unless the tyrosine is in the proximity of a free amine group. This may occur if Tyr is present at the N-terminus, or if there is a another amine present (e.g. a Lys side chain), but this is unlikely to be a common occurrence.

As mentioned earlier, reactive nitrogen species are also known to react readily with the activated aromatic ring of Tyr (in both the free amino acid,

peptides, and intact proteins) with the consequent formation of 3-nitro-
tyrosine (i.e. the nitro group *o*- to the hydroxyl substituent) and di-tyrosine
(Ischiropoulos and al-Mehdi 1995; van der Vliet *et al.* 1995; Denicola *et al.*
1996; Eiserich *et al.* 1996; Gow *et al.* 1996*b*; Lymar *et al.* 1996; Zhu *et al.*
1996)). These reactions can also result in the production of chemiluminescence, suggesting the formation of excited state species (Watts *et al.* 1995).
The positional selectivity of nitration (i.e. the predominance of the 3-isomer
over the alternative 2-isomer) is diagnostic of attack by an electron-deficient
species, but as both cations and radicals fulfill this criteria, this observation
cannot be used as a method of distinguishing between radical *versus* non-
radical attack. The product of nitration, 3-nitrotyrosine, may not be an inert
product and has been suggested to promote further radical damage particularly to DNA (Prutz 1986). The tyrosine phenoxyl radical, which has
been suggested as an intermediate in nitration reactions, may also initiate
further damage. Thus it has been shown that nitration of hen-egg white
lysozyme with tetranitromethane can result in cleavage of the protein backbone at a neighbouring Gly residue (Gly-104), with this process thought to
be mediated by the phenoxyl radical intermediate (Yamada, H. *et al.* 1990).
The detection of di-tyrosine in other studies (see references above), which
presumably arises from dimerization of tyrosine phenoxyl radicals, suggests
there is at least some radical contribution to the observed reactions; these
phenoxyl radicals, as outlined above, could arise from reaction of HO˙ with
the ring via an addition/elimination process, or one-electron oxidation of the
ring and rapid deprotonation of the radical-cation at the hydroxyl group.

The reaction of HOCl with the aromatic ring of tyrosine has also been
the subject of considerable study (Pereira *et al.* 1973; Rudie *et al.* 1980;
Domigan *et al.* 1995; Kettle 1996). This process is rapid and can result in the
chlorination of the ring to give 3-chlorotyrosine; this material has been
suggested to be a potential marker for *in vivo* exposure of proteins to HOCl
from neutrophils (Domigan *et al.* 1995; Kettle 1996). The formation of this
material appears to involve initial formation of a chloramine/chloramide
species which subsequently decomposes to give the chlorinating species
(Domigan *et al.* 1995); these reactions may involve Cl_2 (Heineck *et al.*, in
press).

Rapid addition reactions to the aromatic rings are also observed with both
Trp and His, though the products of these reactions are much less well
characterized. In the case of Trp, HO˙ is known to add to both the benzene
ring and the pyrrole moiety at the C-2 – C-3 double bond (e.g. reactions 97
and 98 (Armstrong and Swallow 1969; Winchester and Lynn 1970; Moan
and Kaalhaus 1974; Josimovic *et al.* 1993)). The former process results in
the formation of relatively low yields of phenolic materials such as 5- and
7-hydroxytryptophan (Armstrong and Swallow 1969; Maskos *et al.* 1992)
in the absence of oxygen. The relative ratios of attack at the two different

rings have been estimated as 40:60 (Solar 1985). Recent studies have demonstrated that in the presence of oxygen 27 per cent of the initial HO$^{\cdot}$ adducts lose water to give the neutral indolyl radical, TrpN$^{\cdot}$; this species reacts slowly with molecular oxygen (Jovanovic and Simic 1985). When the indolyl radical is generated simultaneously with super-oxide radicals a rapid reaction between these two species occurs with $k = 4.5 \times 10^9$ dm^3 mol^{-1} s^{-1} (Josimovic et al. 1993). The remaining initial HO$^{\cdot}$ adducts are believed to react with oxygen to form peroxyl radicals. Of these peroxyl species, about 30 per cent are believed to eliminate HOO$^{\cdot}$/O$_2$$^{\cdot}$$^{-}$ to give hydroxylated products such as 5- and 7-hydroxy-tryptophan. The peroxyl species formed at C-3 on the pyrrole ring as a result of initial addition of HO$^{\cdot}$ at the C-2 position, gives rise to N-formyl-kynurenine, a well characterized degradation product in oxygenated solution, via a ring opening reaction (reaction 99 (Dale et al. 1949; Jayson et al. 1954; Winchester and Lynn 1970; Josimovic et al. 1993)). The formation of this material, together with the loss of fluorescence from the parent amino acid, have often been used as markers of the oxidation of Trp residues in proteins (Giessauf et al. 1995, 1996). In contrast, the peroxyl radical formed at C-2 (as a result of initial HO$^{\cdot}$ addition at C-3) is believed to undergo typical alkyl peroxyl chemistry in that it gives rise to organic peroxides via dimerization reactions and the tetroxide (see earlier); these peroxides, which have not been completely characterized, account for about 25 per cent of the initial HO$^{\cdot}$ adducts (Josimovic et al. 1993). The effect of substituents on the chemistry of neutral indolyl radicals (and the corresponding cation radicals) together with their redox properties and kinetics of one-electron transfer reactions, have been examined in some detail by pulse radiolysis and steady-state radiolysis (Jovanovic and Simic 1985; Jovanovic et al. 1991; Jovanovic and Steenken 1992). Both reactive nitrogen species and HOCl are also known to react with the indole ring of Trp (usually monitored by loss of the characteristic fluorescence bands) but neither the nature of the species formed, nor the mechanism(s) of reaction have been fully characterized (Van Tamelen et al. 1968; Hazell and Stocker 1993; Hazell et al. 1994; Ischiropoulos and al-Mehdi 1995); either radical or electrophilic (non-radical) reactions could bring about such a loss of fluorescence. Autoxidation of sulfite ions, SO$_3$$^{2-}$, which generates SO$_3$$^{\cdot}$$^{-}$, has also been shown to result in the destruction of Trp; this is almost certainly a radical process, but the exact site of attack and the products formed have not been characterized (Yang 1973).

(97)

$$\text{(98)}$$

$$\text{(99)}$$

N-formylkynureine

HO$^•$ is known to add to the imidazole ring of histidine mainly at C-2, C-4, and C-5; these reactions result in the formation of stabilized allyl-type radicals (reaction 100 (Samuni and Neta 1973; Mittal and Hayon 1974; Bansal and Sellers 1975; Rao *et al.* 1975; Kopoldova and Hrneir 1977)). Subsequent addition of oxygen to these species results in the formation of a mixture of products (Kopoldova and Hrneir 1977). The initial allyl radicals can also undergo base-catalysed loss of water to give a highly stabilized bisallylic radical (reaction 101 (Samuni and Neta 1973; Bansal and Sellers 1975)). The products of these reactions are complex and remain incompletely characterized, though they include 2-oxo-histidine (Uchida and Kawakishi 1986, 1993), asparagine, and aspartic acid (Dean *et al.* 1989*a*). 2-Oxo-histidine has also been detected in the inactivated form of the enzyme vanadium bromoperoxidase, and has been suggested to be the cause of inactivation; this species may arise via suicidal oxidation of a histidine residue in the protein (possibly the fifth ligand of the vanadium atom) by reaction of hydrogen peroxide with the catalytic metal ion in the absence of the enzyme substrate (Winter and Butler 1996). Reactive nitrogen species and HOCl also give rise to damage at the imidazole ring but these processes are poorly understood (Winterbourn 1985; Ischiropoulos and al-Mehdi 1995).

The presence of the aromatic ring on these side chains offers an alternative site for electron attachment for the solvated electron in competition with the protonated amine group (a minor site) and the ionized carboxyl function. Addition of the electron to the ring results in the formation of a transient radical-anion, which subsequently rapidly picks up a proton to give a cyclohexadienyl radical (e.g. reaction 102), which behaves as outlined above. For phenylalanine the ratio of attachment at the ring relative to attachment

$$\text{(reaction scheme 100)}$$

(100)

2-oxohistidine

$$\text{(reaction scheme 101)}$$

Adducts to ring
(cf. reaction 100)

HO⁻

(101)

at the carboxyl group appears to be about 1:1 as judged from spectroscopic data (Mittal and Hayon 1974). With His the major site of attachment appears to be at the imidazole ring at pH values where this is protonated (reaction 103); the non-protonated ring is much less reactive and the carboxyl group is then the major site of attachment (Rao *et al.* 1975; Klapper and Faraggi 1979).

$$\text{(reaction scheme 102)}$$

(102)

$$\text{(reaction scheme 103)}$$

(103)

A large number of other (electrophilic and oxidizing) radicals, such as $N_3\cdot$, $SO_4\cdot{}^-$, and the halogen and pseudo-halogen radical anions, are also known to undergo rapid reaction with the aromatic side chains of Phe, Tyr,

Trp, and His (see section 2.2.10 above) (Adams 1972; von Sonntag 1987). Unlike species such as $HO^\cdot$, $H^\cdot$, and $CO_3^{\cdot -}$, which are believed to add to the aromatic ring of Trp (Adams 1972), species such as the pseudo halogen radical anions, $N_3^\cdot$ and $SO_4^{\cdot -}$ are thought to oxidize the ring via electron transfer to give initially a radical-cation species (reaction 104); this species has a pK_a of 4.3, and hence at neutral pH exists in the deprotonated form (Posener et al. 1976; Land and Prutz 1977). This neutral form has a much shorter wavelength optical absorption than the radical-cation species formed, for example, from the N-1 methyl-substituted indole (Redpath et al. 1975b). A similar radical-cation, and hence neutral radical, is believed to be formed as a result of photoionization (Evans et al. 1976). The selective formation of such neutral Trp radicals has been employed in a large number of studies on electron transfer within peptides and proteins as such radicals can selectively oxidize Tyr side chains to the phenoxyl radical (reaction 105 reviewed: (Klapper and Faraggi 1979; von Sonntag 1987; Prutz 1990), see also (Faraggi et al. 1989; DeFelippis et al. 1990)). Such transfer processes can be easily studied as both radical species have intense and highly characteristic optical absorption spectra; for further details of the information obtained from such studies see page 96).

TrpN$^\cdot$ (104)

$$TrpN^\cdot + TyrOH \longrightarrow TrpNH + TyrO^\cdot \qquad (105)$$

Radical-cation species are also believed to be formed during the oxidation of other aromatic residues.

In each case the radical-cation species is short lived and the charge lost rapidly by a number of processes including hydration (e.g. reaction 106 for the Phe radical-cation formed on reaction with $SO_4^{\cdot -}$), loss of a proton from an adjacent C–H bond (a reaction observed with Phe at low pH, reaction 107), and loss of an N–H as observed with Trp, see above, or His (reaction 108) or O–H proton (as seen on oxidation of Tyr, reaction 109, see above) (Davies et al. 1984a; Davies and Gilbert 1991).

$$C_6H_5-CH_2CH(COO^-)NH_3^+ + SO_4^{\cdot-} \longrightarrow SO_4^{2-} + [C_6H_6]^{\cdot+}-CH_2CH(COO^-)NH_3^+$$

$$\downarrow H_2O/-H^+ \tag{106}$$

$$HO-\overset{\cdot}{\underset{H}{C_6H_5}}-CH_2CH(COO^-)NH_3^+$$

$$[C_6H_6]^{\cdot+}-CH_2CH(COO^-)NH_3^+ \longrightarrow H^+ + C_6H_5-\overset{\cdot}{C}HCH(COO^-)NH_3^+ \tag{107}$$

$$\text{(imidazole)}-CH_2CH(COO^-)NH_3^+ + SO_4^{\cdot-} \longrightarrow SO_4^{2-} + \left[\text{(imidazole)}-CH_2CH(COO^-)NH_3^+\right]^{\cdot+}$$

$$\downarrow -H^+ \tag{108}$$

$$\text{(imidazolyl radical)}-CH_2CH(COO^-)NH_3^+$$

$$HO-C_6H_4-CH_2CH(COO^-)NH_3^+ + SO_4^{\cdot-} \longrightarrow SO_4^{2-} + HO-[C_6H_4]^{\cdot+}-CH_2CH(COO^-)NH_3^+$$

$$\downarrow -H^+ \tag{109}$$

$$^{\cdot}O-C_6H_4-CH_2CH(COO^-)NH_3^+$$

Sulfur-containing amino acids

Reaction of cysteine with radicals such as HO$^{\cdot}$ occurs very rapidly, and almost exclusively, at the sulfur centre to give a thiyl radical (RS$^{\cdot}$) by hydrogen abstraction (reviewed in: (von Sonntag 1987, 1990; Armstrong 1990; Wardman and von Sonntag 1995)). In the presence of oxygen these species react rapidly, though reversibly, with oxygen to form a peroxy species RSOO$^{\cdot}$ (reaction 48 above). In acidic conditions these radicals have been shown to be able to consume another thiol molecule, in a short chain reaction, which gives RSOOH (and hence disulfides from reaction of RSOOH with more RSH) and oxyacids as products. At physiological pH values, reactions of the thiol anion (RS$^-$) become much more important, and different behaviour is observed. Competition between reaction of the thiyl radical with oxygen and a further thiol anion, to give a disulfide radical anion, appears to become important (reaction 110 (von Sonntag 1987, 1990; Armstrong 1990; Wardman and von Sonntag 1995)). The resulting radical-anion reacts readily with oxygen in an electron transfer process to form the disulfide and the superoxide radical-anion (reaction 111). The release of the latter radical was originally postulated (in order to account for the observed

chain lengths of up to 30) to be a chain-propagating process, with this
radical undergoing further reaction with another RSH molecule. This
reaction has, however, been shown to be very slow. Dimerization of thiyl
radicals can also occur relatively readily, and such processes can result in
cross-linking either within a peptide or protein structure, or between
molecules. The overall chemistry of these systems is complex and the reader
is referred to specialized reviews of this area (von Sonntag 1987, 1990;
Armstrong 1990; Wardman and von Sonntag 1995).

$$RS^{\cdot} + RS^{-} \longrightarrow (RSSR)^{\cdot \, -} \tag{110}$$

$$(RSSR)^{\cdot \, -} + O_2 \longrightarrow RSSR + O_2^{\cdot \, -} \tag{111}$$

The thiol group and the corresponding anion react rapidly with the
solvated electron. Two major reactions appear to occur (reactions 112 and
113) which result in the formation of a carbon-centred radical (which
will behave in a manner similar to that outlined above for aliphatic hydrocarbon side chains), via R–S bond cleavage, and hydrogen atoms via S–H
cleavage; the subsequent reactions of the latter radical are covered above
(Jayson 1971). For cysteine the former process is believed to dominate
(Armstrong and Wilkening 1964), with alanine (from 'repair' by H-atom
donation, reaction 114) being a major product. Reactive nitrogen species
also readily oxidize free cysteine or these residues when present in peptides
or proteins (Gatti *et al.* 1994; van der Vliet *et al.* 1994*b*; Ischiropoulos and
al-Mehdi 1995). HOCl reacts very rapidly with the thiol group of cysteine
to give a mixture of products including short-lived sulfenyl chlorides,
disulfides, and oxy-acids (Pereira *et al.* 1973; Winterbourn 1985). These
reactions are believed, in general, not to involve radical (one-electron)
reactions, but two-electron (nucleophilic) processes, though some evidence
has been obtained to the contrary (Hawkins and Davies, unpublished
data).

$$e^{-}_{aq} + RSH \longrightarrow R^{\cdot} + HS^{-} \tag{112}$$

$$e^{-}_{aq} + RSH \longrightarrow RS^{-} + H^{\cdot} \tag{113}$$

$$e^{-}_{aq} + HSCH_2CH(NH_3^{+})COO^{-} \longrightarrow HS^{-} + {}^{\cdot}CH_2CH(NH_3^{+})COO^{-}$$
$${}^{\cdot}CH_2CH(NH_3^{+})COO^{-} + R{-}H \longrightarrow R^{\cdot} + CH_3CH(NH_3^{+})COO^{-} \tag{114}$$

Reaction of HO$^{\cdot}$ with cystine is also known to be extremely rapid (Buxton
et al. 1988) and proceeds via two pathways resulting in formation of either a
radical-cation or RSOH and RS$^{\cdot}$ species (reactions 115 and 116 (Bonifacic
et al. 1975; Elliot *et al.* 1981)). Subsequent reactions of these species in the
presence of oxygen results in the formation of RSO$_2$H and RSO$_3$H as the
principal products, with the former predominating (Purdie 1967).

$$HO^{\cdot} + RSSR \longrightarrow HO^- + (RSSR)^{\cdot +} \tag{115}$$

$$HO^{\cdot} + RSSR \longrightarrow RS^{\cdot} + RSOH \tag{116}$$

Cystine reacts rapidly (at diffusion-controlled rates) with the solvated electron (and other strongly reducing radicals such as $CO_2^{\cdot -}$) by electron attachment (or electron transfer in the case of $CO_2^{\cdot -}$) to give the corresponding radical-anion (reaction 117), which can be identified readily by optical (at 410 nm) or EPR spectroscopy (Willson 1970; Gilbert et al. 1975; Elliot et al. 1984). This species undergoes a number of further reactions depending on the conditions employed. In the absence of oxygen, cleavage of the S–S link occurs to yield a thiyl radical and a thiol anion (i.e. the reverse of the reaction 110); this process is reversible and the equilibrium favours the radical-anion at moderate thiol anion concentrations, though this is substrate dependent (Adams et al. 1967). The equilibrium can however be readily perturbed if there are other routes out for the species concerned. In the presence of oxygen, electron transfer from the radical-anion to oxygen regenerates the disulfide and forms the superoxide radical (reaction 111 (Barton and Packer 1970; Chan and Bielski 1973)).

$$e^-_{aq} \, / \, CO_2^{\cdot -} + RSSR \longrightarrow (RSSR)^{\cdot -} \tag{117}$$

The thioether side chain of methionine is readily damaged by radicals, and current evidence suggests that the majority of radicals react at the sulfur centre (Asmus 1979). In the presence or absence of oxygen, the subsequent chemistry is complex and results in multiple products (see Scheme 2.2) including decarboxylated materials (from damage transfer to the amino or carboxyl functions (Hiller et al. 1981; Bobrowski et al. 1991)), low yields of materials arising from cleavage of the C–S–C linkage and, in the presence of oxygen, methionine sulfoxide ($RS(O)CH_3$) and methionine sulfone ($RS(O)_2CH_3$) (Kopoldova et al. 1967; Asmus 1979). The decarboxylated radical formed with the free amino acid is, by virtue of being an α-aminoalkyl radical, a powerful reducing species which can react to give thiyl radicals ($k = 2.7 \times 10^8 \ dm^3 \, mol^{-1} \, s^{-1}$ (Prutz 1990)), and reduce disulfides to the corresponding radical anion ($k = 7 \times 10^6 \, dm^3 \, mol^{-1} \, s^{-1}$ (Prutz 1990)). Decarboxylation can also be observed in some small Met-containing peptides (Bobrowski et al. 1991), with the yield of CO_2 dependent on the peptide sequence, the overall charge, and the distance between the reacting groups; these reactions appear to involve electron transfer from the carboxyl function to the oxidized thioether centre, either via an intramolecular 'outer-sphere' electron-transfer reaction, or via the intermediacy of a three-electron cation species formed by reaction of the sulfur radical-cation and a suitably positioned amine group. The ring-closed, three-electron species Met–S–N$^{\cdot +}$ formed when the decarboxylation pathway is blocked, is a powerful oxidant and can transfer damage to other readily oxidized species. Thus it can oxidize Trp to the corresponding nitrogen-centred radical ($k = 4 \times 10^7$ dm^3 mol^{-1}s^{-1} (Prutz 1990)), thiols to the corresponding thiyl radicals ($k \simeq 8 \times 10^7$ dm^3 mol^{-1}s^{-1} for Cys (Prutz 1990)), and Tyr residues to the corresponding phenoxyl radicals. Reaction with other oxidizing radicals (and also photo-oxidation) occurs primarily at the sulfur centre. Thus, reaction with Br$_2^{\cdot-}$ occurs to give an adduct species (Met$\therefore$Br) which contains a two-centre, three-electron bond (reaction 118). This species is capable of undergoing a number of subsequent reactions, as it is a powerfully oxidizing species (e.g. it will readily oxidizes Tyr residues to the corresponding phenoxyl radical, reaction 119, $k = 4 \times 10^4$ dm^3 mol^{-1}s^{-1} (Prutz 1990)).

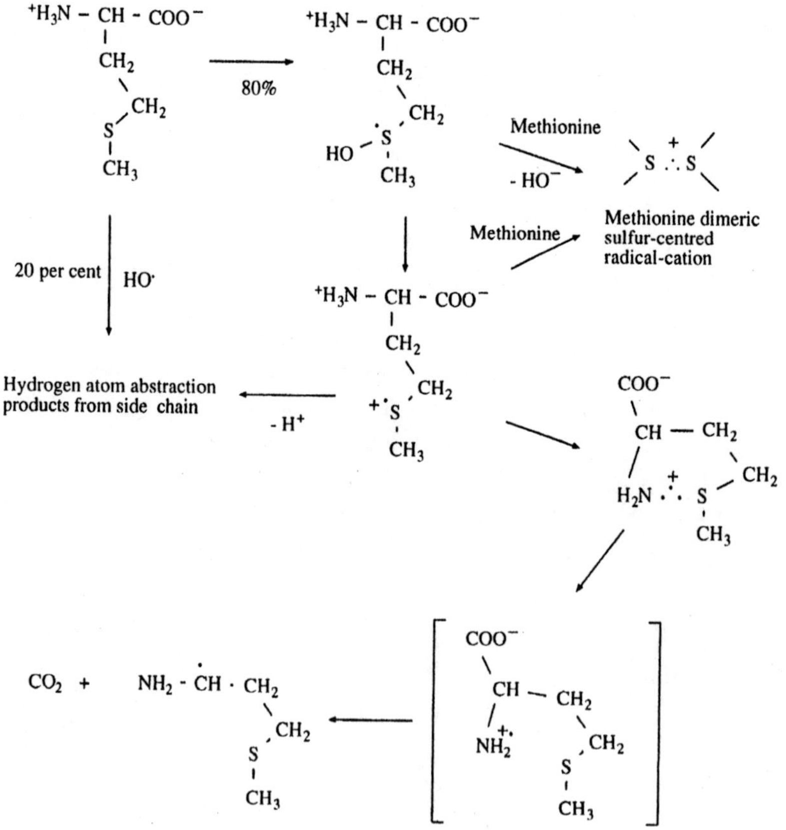

Scheme 2.2

$$Br_2^{\cdot-} + CH_3SCH_2CH_2CH(NH_3^+)COO^- \longrightarrow Br^- + {}^{\cdot}S(Br)(CH_3)CH_2CH_2CH(NH_3^+)COO^-$$
$$Met {\therefore} Br \qquad (118)$$

$$Met {\therefore} Br + Tyr-OH \longrightarrow Met + TyrO^{\cdot} + H^+ + Br^- \qquad (119)$$

$$e^-_{aq} + CH_3SCH_2CH_2CH(NH_3^+)COO^- \longrightarrow CH_3^{\cdot} + {}^-SCH_2CH_2CH(NH_3^+)COO^- \qquad (120)$$

$$e^-_{aq} + CH_3SCH_2CH_2CH(NH_3^+)COO^- \longrightarrow CH_3S^- + {}^{\cdot}CH_2CH_2CH(NH_3^+)COO^- \qquad (121)$$

Reaction of the thioether group with the solvated electron is believed to fragment either C–S bond to give a carbon-centred radical and a thiol anion (reactions 120 and 121 (Shimazu and Tappel 1964). These reactions are slow (Buxton *et al.* 1988) and do not compete well with attachment at the ionized carboxyl group in the free amino acid. Both peroxynitrite and HOCl have also been reported to react rapidly with the thioether group to give methionine sulfoxide (Pereira *et al.* 1973; Winterbourn 1985; Moreno and Pryor 1992). There is some doubt, particularly with HOCl, as to whether these reactions involve radical species (Pereira *et al.* 1973; Winterbourn 1985).

It should also be noted that molecular reaction of thioether groups, such as the methionine side chain, with hydrogen peroxide and other hydroperoxides is well known; this results in the formation of methionine sulfoxide via a nucleophilic (non-radical) reaction (reaction 122; reviewed: (Vogt 1995)).

$$ROOH / H_2O_2 + CH_3SCH_2R \longrightarrow ROH / H_2O + CH_3S(O)CH_2R \qquad (122)$$

2.3.2 Peptides and proteins

Backbone chemistry

Incorporation of an amino acid into a derivative (such as an *N*-acetyl amino acid) or peptide can have a profound influence on both the radicals formed and the products detected. Removal of the deactivating influence of the protonated amine function by formation of an amide bond is known to increase the rate of hydrogen abstraction at the α-carbon position and hence yield of species derived from such attack. Thus the rate constant for hydrogen abstraction from *N*-Ac-Gly ($CH_3C(O)NHCH_2COO^-$) is markedly greater ($\simeq 4 \times 10^8$ $dm^3 mol^{-1} s^{-1}$) than that for Gly itself (1.7×10^7 $dm^3 mol^{-1} s^{-1}$) at neutral pH (Buxton *et al.* 1988). This value for *N*-Ac–Gly is still less than that for the corresponding monoanion of Gly ($H_2NCH_2COO^-$, $k = 1.9$–5.3×10^9 $dm^3 mol^{-1} s^{-1}$ (Buxton *et al.* 1988)), suggesting that the stabilizing influence of the amide function, as a result of delocalization of the unpaired electron, is less than that of the free amine lone pair. This is as would be expected given the electron withdrawing effect of the neighbouring carbonyl function in the amide. A similar (though slightly less marked) enhancement in the magnitude of the rate constant is observed on going from Ala to N-Ac–Ala (see Table 2.3). Further increases in the magnitude of the rate constant for hydrogen abstraction are observed on lengthening the peptide chain (cf. reported values of 2.4×10^8 dm^3 mol^{-1} s^{-1} for the zwitterion Gly–Gly, and $\simeq 7 \times 10^8$ dm^3 mol^{-1} s^{-1} for N-Ac–Gly–Gly and Gly–Gly–Gly (Buxton et al. 1988)).

Attack at the α-C–H bonds of N-acetyl amino acids appears to be preferred over attack at the methyl group of the acetyl function (Paul and Fischer 1969); this is probably because the radical formed at the α-carbon can be stabilized by the 'capto-dative' effect of the amide nitrogen and ionized carboxyl group (Viehe et al. 1985)), whereas the methyl group of the N-acetyl group is not activated due to the neighbouring carbonyl function. The capto-dative effect arises from stabilization of the radical centre by the lone pair of the amide nitrogen and the electron withdrawing (delocalization) effect of the carbonyl function.

In dipeptides, the α-C–H bond(s) next to the amide nitrogen are preferred as sites of hydrogen abstraction over those next to the free amine. This preference for attack at the C-terminal site in dipeptides can again be removed by derivatization of the N-terminal free amine group. In situations where two alternative types of such α-C–H bond(s) next to the amide nitrogens are present, attack appears to be preferred at Gly residues over other amino acids, at least in some solvents and with particular attacking radicals (Sperling and Elad 1971a; Schwarzberg et al. 1973; Easton 1991). Thus for the peptide N-trifluoroacetyl–Gly–Ala methyl ester attack at the Gly α-C–H bonds is favoured (as judged by product analysis) over attack at the Ala α-C–H bond by a factor of 7:1 (Sperling and Elad 1971a). A similar effect is observed when the same pair of amino acids are present in the reverse order (i.e. N-trifluoroacetyl–Ala–Gly methyl ester) where the ratio for attack at Gly over Ala is 20:1 (Sperling and Elad 1971a). This selectivity is the opposite to that expected from the relative stabilities of these two types of α-carbon radical, as the radical formed from Ala should be more stable than that from Gly, being a tertiary radical whereas the latter is a secondary species (see also: Rauk et al. 1997). This behaviour has been rationalized in terms of the steric effects of the side chain (in this case the methyl side chain of Ala) on the ability of the α-carbon radical to adopt the planar conformation which would maximize stabilization by the neighbouring nitrogen and carbonyl groups (Easton and Hay 1986; Burgess et al. 1989; Easton 1991); this effect is discussed in greater detail later. Thus, not all sets of α-C–H bonds appear to be equally susceptible to radical attack, at least under certain circumstances. Obviously the *overall* extent of attack at the backbone is also dependent on the nature of the side chains, with these offering a competing locus for attack; this is particularly true when these contain sulfur or aromatic sites.

In the absence of oxygen, α-carbon radicals appear to decay mainly by dimerization ($G \simeq 3$ in N_2O-saturated solution (Dizdaroglu and Simic 1983)). A number of the products arising from such reactions with small peptides have been characterized (e.g. Ala–Ala and to a lesser extent tetra Ala (Dizdaroglu and Simic 1983)). Given that racemization can occur at the radical centres, the analytical problems associated with the exact analysis of the yields of these materials are not trivial; there are ten possible species with Ala–Ala alone. These have been resolved in to four separate fractions by HPLC, and it appears that all possible types of cross-link can be formed (carboxyl α-carbon to carboxyl α-carbon, carboxyl α-carbon to N-terminal α-carbon, *vice-versa*, and N-terminal α-carbon to N-terminal α-carbon, see Scheme 2.3 (Dizdaroglu and Simic 1983)). Analysis of all of the cross-links from tetra-Ala has not proved possible, so it is not possible to comment on the selectivity of attack at different sites within this peptide. With more complex peptides (i.e. those where significant reaction also occurs at side chain sites) significant levels of cross-links between side chain-derived radicals has also been observed. Thus experiments with Phe-containing peptides have provided evidence for both biphenyl linkages (Dizdaroglu *et al.* 1984; Simic *et al.* 1985) and other types of cross-links (Kim *et al.* 1984*a*). With large peptides, e.g. glucagon (a 29-mer), cross-links between aromatic, sulfur and basic residues have been identified, but the exact nature of all of the observed materials remains to be established (Kim *et al.* 1984*b*).

Reaction of the solvated electron with small linear peptides of amino acids with unreactive side chains (such as small Gly and Ala peptides) occurs primarily by attachment at the carbonyl function of the N-terminal residue; these radical-anions rapidly protonate (reaction 123). The α-hydroxy, α-amino radicals so formed undergo deamination at the N-terminus via reaction 124 (Willix and Garrison 1967; Garrison *et al.* 1973). The carbon-centred species formed by this type of process can subsequently hydrogen

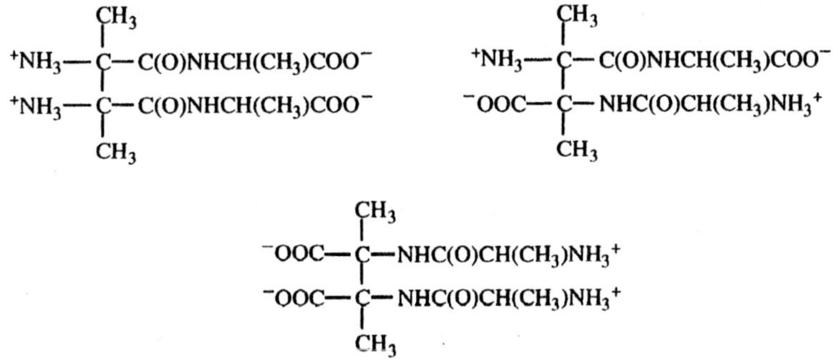

Scheme 2.3

abstract from another parent molecule (e.g. at a non-deactivated α-carbon position) or dimerize (Garrison et al. 1973; Dizdaroglu and Simic 1983). The yields of ammonium ions formed via reaction 124 approximate to the initial yield of solvated electrons (G $\simeq$ 3) for small peptides such as $(Gly)_2$ and $(Gly)_3$.

$$e^-_{aq} + {}^+NH_3CH_2C(O)NHCH_2COO^- + H^+ \longrightarrow {}^\cdot C(OH)(CH_2NH_3{}^+)NHCH_2COO^- \qquad (123)$$

$${}^\cdot C(OH)(CH_2NH_3{}^+)NHCH_2COO^- \longrightarrow {}^+NH_4 + {}^\cdot CH_2C(O)NHCH_2COO^- \qquad (124)$$

As the chain length is increased, however, the extent of electron attachment at the N-terminal carbonyl function decreases, with attachment at carbonyl groups of mid-chain peptide bonds observed to increase (reaction 125); the latter process occurs with $k \simeq 1 \times 10^9$ $dm^3 mol^{-1} s^{-1}$ (Rustgi and Riesz 1978b, c; Simic 1978; D'Arcy and Sevilla 1979; Klapper and Faraggi 1979). Thus, the yield of ammonium ions from tetra Gly is about 2.4 and from poly Ala about 0.3. With more complex side chains (i.e. those containing reactive functional groups such as aromatic, sulfur, protonated amine, and ionized carboxyl groups) reaction at the side chain (as outlined above for free amino acids) can also become significant. The reactions of the mid-chain α-hydroxy,α-amino radicals generated via reaction 125 have been studied in some detail. It has been suggested that the major decay route for these species is reaction with a further radical, with the favoured partner being an α-carbon radical formed by hydrogen abstraction; this results in the repair of both lesions (reaction 126 (Rodgers et al. 1970)). The initial electron adduct to the carbonyl group can also undergo electron transfer reactions with suitable electron acceptors. Thus, this species can be repaired by electron transfer to either disulfide groups (reaction 127) or histidine residues (Faraggi et al. 1975). Electron transfer to the former gives a disulfide radical-anion which can then give rise to thiyl radicals via dissociative reduction (reaction 46) or the formation of superoxide radicals via a further electron transfer to oxygen (reaction 111). Little main chain-cleavage (G < 0.3) appears to occur via reaction 128 for species such as N-Ac–Ala; this is consistent with pulse radiolysis data (Simic 1978; Klapper and Faraggi 1979), but not with some EPR studies where carbon-centred radicals appear to be formed via reaction 128 (Sevilla 1970; Sevilla and Brooks 1973; D'Arcy and Sevilla 1979). This difference in behaviour may be due to the experimental conditions employed. In cases where relatively high radical fluxes are employed and the radicals are free to diffuse (e.g. at room temperature in solution in the above mentioned pulse radiolysis studies), the bimolecular process (reaction 126) may predominate. In contrast, with the low-temperature EPR studies, where the radicals are formed in low yields in a rigid matrix and cannot diffuse freely, the unimolecular process shown in reaction 128 may predominate. In the presence of oxygen these processes may be much less important as a result of the scavenging of the solvated electron by oxygen.

$$e^-_{aq} + \sim C(O)NH \sim \longrightarrow \sim {}^{\cdot}C(O^-)NH \sim \longrightarrow \sim {}^{\cdot}C(OH)NH \sim \qquad (125)$$

$$\sim {}^{\cdot}C(OH)NH \sim + \sim NH{}^{\cdot}C(R)C(O) \sim \longrightarrow 2 \sim NHCH(R)C(O) \sim \qquad (126)$$

$$\sim {}^{\cdot}C(O^-)NH \sim + RSSR \longrightarrow \sim C(O)NH \sim + (RSSR)^{\cdot -} \qquad (127)$$

$$e^-_{aq} + CH_3C(O)NHCH(CH_3)COO^- \longrightarrow {}^{\cdot}C(O^-)(CH_3)NHCH(CH_3)COO^-$$
$$\longrightarrow CH_3C(O)NH_2 + {}^{\cdot}CH(CH_3)COO^- \qquad (128)$$

Some of the products arising from reaction of HOCl with small peptides which do not contain reactive side chains have been characterized (Pereira *et al.* 1973; Stelmaszynska and Zgliczynski 1978). The observed products, which are mainly N-(2-oxacyl)amino acids and nitriles (i.e. Ala–Ala gives CH_3-$C(O)$-$C(O)$-NH-$CH(CH_3)$-COO^-, and CH_3-CN plus free Ala), are believed to arise via initial reaction of HOCl at the free amine group at the N-terminus, and subsequent decomposition of the chloramine species so formed; this may involve radical species, or it may involve non-radical hydrolysis and dehydrochlorination reactions. With longer peptides, analogous species are likely to be formed via a similar route. The aldehyde and nitrile products generated as a result of such reactions would be expected to undergo further reactions (e.g. Schiff base formation) if formed in more complex biological systems, and may generate significant toxicity. These reactions may however only be of major significance in situations where HOCl is in large excess, as HOCl preferentially reacts at other, more reactive side chain sites (see above).

In the presence of oxygen the reaction of peptides with electrophilic radicals such as HO$^{\cdot}$ is much more complex than that observed in the absence of oxygen. In early studies it was postulated that the overall stoichiometry of main chain degradation could be formulated in terms of reaction 129, with the individual steps giving rise to this overall picture being given in Scheme 2.4 (Garrison *et al.* 1962, 1970; reviewed: Garrison 1987). Thus, radiolysis of simple peptide derivatives such as N-Ac–Gly and N-Ac–Ala was demonstrated to give rise to labile peptide derivatives which could be readily degraded under mild hydrolytic conditions to give ammonia (a material which is not an initial product) and carbonyl-containing materials (keto acids and aldehyde). If such reactions were the only reactions occurring it would be expected that the overall stoichiometry for ammonia formation should equal that of carbonyl group formation, and these in turn should account for all the HO$^{\cdot}$ consumed. However it has been determined that while the yields of ammonia are indeed what would be expected (G $\simeq$ 3, which equals that for HO$^{\cdot}$ consumption), the yield of carbonyl-containing materials is always much lower than that which would be expected ($G \simeq 1$ instead of 3) (Atkins *et al.* 1967; Garrison *et al.* 1970). Thus there must be other pathways which also play a role, in addition to those outlined above.

$$\sim C(O)NHCH(R)C(O)\sim \ + O_2 + H_2O \longrightarrow \ \sim C(O)NH_2 + O{=}C(R)C(O)\sim \ + H_2O_2 \quad (129)$$

In more recent studies (reviewed: Garrison 1987) it has been shown that there are other carbon-containing products in addition to the keto acids and aldehydes originally postulated. Thus, it has been determined that reaction of *N*-Ac–Ala with HO· also gives rise to pyruvic acid, acetaldehyde (ethanal), acetic (ethanoic) acid, and carbon dioxide; these materials were postulated to arise from further reactions of the initial α-carbon peroxyl radical as outlined in reactions 130–132 (Garrison *et al.* 1970). The di-acetamide product $CH_3CONHCOCH_3$ generated via reactions 131 and 132 can be further decomposed in the presence of base to give acetamide (ethanamide) and acetic (ethanoic) acid (reaction 133). The overall yields of material resulting from the radiolysis of *N*-Ac–Ala are summarized in Table 2.5, though it should be noted that these are the materials formed after subsequent base hydrolysis of the reaction mixture and do not reflect the initial products of radiolysis.

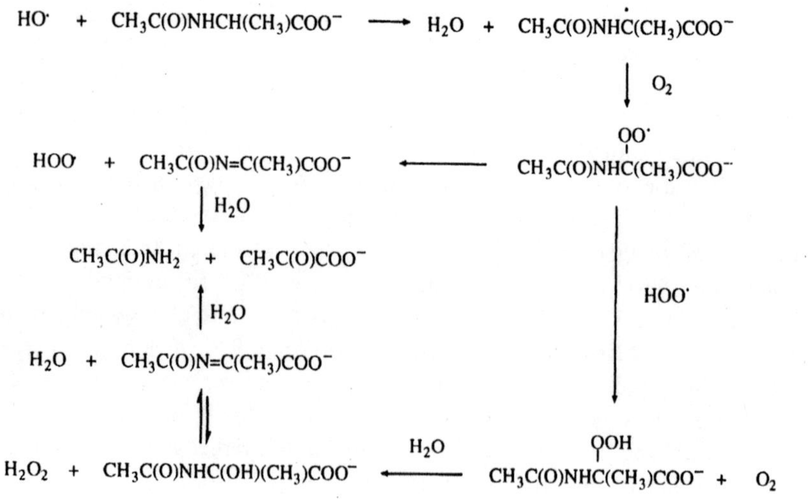

HO· + $CH_3C(O)NHCH(CH_3)COO^-$ ⟶ H_2O + $CH_3C(O)NH\overset{\cdot}{C}(CH_3)COO^-$

$\downarrow O_2$

$\overset{OO^{\cdot}}{\underset{|}{}}$
$CH_3C(O)NH\overset{|}{C}(CH_3)COO^-$

HOO· + $CH_3C(O)N{=}C(CH_3)COO^-$ ⟵

$\downarrow H_2O$

$CH_3C(O)NH_2$ + $CH_3C(O)COO^-$

$\uparrow H_2O$

H_2O + $CH_3C(O)N{=}C(CH_3)COO^-$ HOO·

$\Updownarrow$

H_2O_2 + $CH_3C(O)NHC(OH)(CH_3)COO^-$ ⟵ $\overset{H_2O}{\quad}$ $CH_3C(O)NH\overset{OOH}{\underset{|}{C}}(CH_3)COO^-$ + O_2

Scheme 2.4

$2CH_3C(O)NH\overset{OO^{\cdot}}{\underset{\underset{CH_3}{|}}{\overset{|}{C}}}{-}COO^- \longrightarrow 2CH_3C(O)NH\overset{O^{\cdot}}{\underset{\underset{CH_3}{|}}{\overset{|}{C}}}{-}COO^- + O_2 \qquad (130)$

$$2CH_3C(O)NH - \underset{\underset{CH_3}{|}}{\overset{\overset{OO\cdot}{|}}{C}} - COO^- \longrightarrow CH_3C(O)NH - \underset{\underset{CH_3}{|}}{\overset{\overset{OH}{|}}{C}} - COO^- + CH_3C(O)NH - \overset{\overset{O}{\parallel}}{C} - CH_3$$

$$+ O_2 + CO_2 \qquad (131)$$

$$CH_3C(O)NH - \underset{\underset{CH_3}{|}}{\overset{\overset{O\cdot}{|}}{C}} - COO^- + O_2 \longrightarrow CH_3C(O)NH - \overset{\overset{O}{\parallel}}{C} - CH_3 + CO_2 + O_2^{\cdot -} \qquad (132)$$

$$CH_3CONHCOCH_3 + HO^- \longrightarrow CH_3CONH_2 + CH_3COO^- \qquad (133)$$

It has been shown recently that significant yields of hydroperoxides can be formed on the backbone of N-Ac amino acids at the α-carbon (Davies 1996), in addition to those which are known to be formed on certain side chains (see earlier). These are semi-stable products, and do not all undergo immediate reaction as outlined above in Scheme 2.4. These materials would not be expected to survive the subsequent work-up procedure for product analysis used in earlier studies. Examination of the modes of decomposition of these materials has allowed some of the fragmentation pathways of these hydroperoxide species to be examined. Thus, it has been shown in studies on a range of γ-irradiated N-Ac amino acids, that a β-scission (fragmentation) reaction of the backbone alkoxyl radical can occur which gives rise to a carbonyl species and $CO_2^{\cdot -}$ (reaction 134) (Davies 1996). This process

Table 2.5 Product yields arising from the γ-radiolysis of N-acetylalanine and poly Ala in aqueous solution in the presence of oxygen

Product[a]	Yield	
	N-acetylalanine[b]	Poly Ala[c]
NH$_3$	2.9	3.9
CH$_3$COOH	3.0	≃ 3.9
CO$_2$	2.0	2.4
H$_2$O$_2$	2.2	2.2
ROOH[d]	0.5	–
CH$_3$C(O)COOH	≃ 0.2	1.2
CH$_3$CHO	≃ 0.2	0.4

[a] After hydrolysis of amide products to ammonia (Garrison et al. 1970).
[b] 0.05 mol dm^{-3}
[c] 0.5 per cent
[d] R group unspecified. See text for further discussion of this product and its potential further reactions.

Source: Garrison et al. 1970.

appears, on the basis of competition kinetics, to be a very rapid process with $k \simeq 10^7 \text{ s}^{-1}$ (Davies 1996). The formation of such intermediates is still consistent with the above overall product stoichiometry, as the former species is a diacetamide (which in the presence of base would hydrolyse as above, reaction 133). This type of material is, however, relatively stable at neutral pH, and analysis of the yield of these species may give important indications of the percentage of backbone cleavage occurring via the imine pathway shown in Scheme 2.4 and those arising from the alkoxyl radical pathway outlined above. The $CO_2 \cdot^-$ formed in this process would be expected to react with excess oxygen to give carbon dioxide (as observed) and superoxide radicals (reaction 23). The latter radical would give rise, on disproportionation, to some of the hydrogen peroxide detected. Similar hydroperoxide groups are generated with certain dipeptides (Davies 1996; see also Mieden and von Sonntag 1987; Mieden *et al.* 1993), as the major site of initial attack on the backbone is at the α-carbon adjacent to the carboxyl group. These undergo similar degradation reactions.

$$CH_3C(O)NH - \underset{\underset{CH_3}{|}}{\overset{\overset{OOH}{|}}{C}} - COO^- + Fe^{2+} \longrightarrow Fe^{3+} + HO^- + CH_3C(O)NH - \underset{\underset{CH_3}{|}}{\overset{\overset{O \cdot}{|}}{C}} - COO^-$$

$$\downarrow$$

$$(134)$$

$$CH_3C(O)NH - \overset{\overset{O}{\|}}{C} - CH_3 + CO_2 \cdot^-$$

Studies on *N*-Ac amino acid amides have shown that hydroperoxide formation at the α-carbon also occurs with these materials, and that analogous fragmentation reactions result in the loss of the C-terminal amide function as the $\cdot C(O)NH_2$ radical (reaction 135). Analogous reactions occur with larger peptides; in such cases backbone cleavage occurs as a result of formation of a mid-chain hydroperoxide and subsequent loss of a $\cdot C(O)NHR$ radical from the initial alkoxyl radical ((Davies 1996), see also later).

$$CH_3C(O)NH - \underset{\underset{CH_3}{|}}{\overset{\overset{OOH}{|}}{C}} - C(O)NH_2 + Fe^{2+} \longrightarrow Fe^{3+} + HO^- + CH_3C(O)NH - \underset{\underset{CH_3}{|}}{\overset{\overset{O \cdot}{|}}{C}} - C(O)NH_2$$

$$\downarrow$$

$$(135)$$

$$CH_3C(O)NH - \overset{\overset{O}{\|}}{C} - CH_3 + \cdot C(O)NH_2$$

Pulse radiolysis and EPR studies on larger peptides have shown that attack by species such as HO˙ occurs rapidly at α-carbon sites away from the charged termini (Hayon and Simic 1971; Makada and Garrison 1972; Rao and Hayon 1975; Simic 1978; Davies, M.J. *et al.* 1991, 1993). Thus, with tri, tetra, and poly Ala and Gly derivatives, reaction at such sites accounts for > 90 per cent of the initial radicals (Makada and Garrison 1972), with $k \simeq 10^9$ dm^3 mol^{-1}s^{-1} (Buxton *et al.* 1988). Thus reaction at backbone sites, unlike the situation with the free amino acids, often competes very successfully with reaction at reactive side chain sites.

We now return to the subject of selectivity between various different backbone (α-carbon) sites. Studies on the abstraction of hydrogen atoms from the α-carbon sites of a number of mixed peptides (and analogues with blocked termini) in organic solvents by relatively selective radicals, such as *t*-BuO˙, *N*-bromosuccinamidyl radicals, and Br˙, have suggested that not all α-carbon radicals are of equal stability. Thus, it has been shown that reaction with the peptides A and B results in the selective formation of products from radicals C and D in preference to those from the alternative species E and F (reactions 136 and 137, reviewed in: (Easton 1991)). This type of behaviour, as discussed earlier, might not have been expected, since the α-carbon radical from Gly is a *secondary* species compared to the *tertiary* radicals formed at other α-carbon sites. This apparent selectivity has been rationalized in terms of a destabilization of the tertiary radicals as a result of steric interactions between the side chain substituent and carbonyl function; such interactions would be expected to force the radical from a planar conformation with a resultant loss of stabilization from delocalization of the unpaired electron on to the carbonyl function (Easton 1991). Thus, the (secondary) Gly α-carbon radical appears to be more stable than other (tertiary) α-carbon species; this conclusion has however been disputed in theoretical studies (Rauk *et al.* 1997). A similar argument has been expounded to explain the selectivity of attack at Pro residues, as in this case the products formed from radical G predominate over those generated from radical H when the peptide I is reacted with *N*-bromosuccinimide (reaction 138, (Easton and Hay 1986; Burgess *et al.* 1989; Easton 1991)). In this case the secondary radical formed at the C-5 site of Pro is thought to be more stable than the tertiary α-carbon species as a result of steric interactions between the two carbonyl groups when radical H tries to adopt the planar conformation required for significant delocalization of the radical on to the neighbouring atoms. This would suggest that attack will occur at other α-carbon sites in preference to the α-carbon of Pro. Radical H would be expected to behave as outlined previously, which in a peptide could also lead to backbone breakage. Such a reaction has been observed during HO˙-induced damage to small peptides (Uchida *et al.* 1990). It should also be noted, however, that the subsequent reactions of radicals such as G can lead

to backbone cleavage via pathway (a) shown in reaction (139) (Dean *et al.*
1989*a*) as a result of the hydrolysis of the diketocompound J. Pathway (b) in
reaction (139) would be expected to give rise to the replacement of the Pro
residue with a Glu, and hence an increased Glu content of the peptide under
study; such increases have been observed experimentally in some cases, but
not all (Gruber and Mellon 1975; Cooper *et al.* 1985; Dean *et al.* 1989*a*).

$$(139)$$

It should, however, be borne in mind that it can be dangerous to extrapolate from data obtained on the reactions of small peptides with relatively selective attacking radicals in organic solvents to, for example, the situation with $HO^{\cdot}$ attack on proteins in aqueous conditions at physiological temperatures. In the latter type of reaction, current data suggests that there is less selectivity, if any, for particular sites as judged from the destruction of individual amino acids (Davies, K. J. *et al.* 1987*b*; Neuzil *et al.* 1993). The situation with systems where radicals may be generated at particular sites on, or near, a peptide or protein (for example, as a result of metal ion binding) is however dramatically different. This topic is discussed in more detail both below, and in Chapter 3.

From the discussion above it should be obvious that there are at least two major pathways which can give rise to backbone cleavage, starting from backbone radicals (as will be shown later there are other minor reactions which start from side chain radicals). Both of these major pathways involve the formation of peroxyl radicals on the α-carbon as obligatory intermediates, thus explaining the observed requirement for oxygen in order to obtain significant yields of peptide fragments; low yields may arise in the absence of oxygen via the solvated electron reactions shown in reaction 128, though this may not play a significant role in solution chemistry. One of these fragmentation pathways involves the formation of a peroxyl radical, loss of $HO_2^{\cdot}$, and subsequent hydrolysis of the imine species. The other process involves the formation of an alkoxyl radical at the α-carbon which then undergoes further fragmentation to cleave the backbone. It should be noted that each reaction gives a different spectrum of products (for example isocyanates, and hence CO_2, are only formed via the second pathway), and it should therefore be possible to determine the relative importance of these different pathways. Work is currently underway to achieve this goal.

Side-chain chemistry

The other major site of initial radical attack is the side chains. The exact ratio of attack at side chain *versus* backbone with mixed peptides will obviously depend crucially on the nature of the amino acids present. Little data on such selectivity is available, and the analysis of such complex systems is complicated by the possibility of transfer reactions between various sites (see below). In general, however, the chemistry of the side-chain-derived radicals is believed to be very similar to that outlined above for the free amino acids in both the absence and presence of oxygen, and many of the products detected on the side chains of free amino acids are also observed with peptide or protein side chains; a list of well characterized side chain oxidation products detected on peptide and protein side chains is given in Table 2.4.

Transfer between sites: backbone to backbone

Measurement of the yield of amides released in the radiolysis of some oligopeptides gives higher values than might be expected from the arguments outlined above. Thus, the yield (G) of amide, measured as ammonia, approaches 5, which is considerably more than the expected equivalence of ammonium ion production (from the base-catalysed hydrolysis of the amides generated via reaction 133) and hydroxyl radical consumption of $G \simeq 3$ observed with the *N*-Ac amino acids (Garrison 1987). This strongly suggests that there must be transfer of damage to other sites, and hence short chain reactions. This higher than expected yield has been suggested to occur via the involvement of a backbone alkoxyl radical (arising from the corresponding peroxyl radical, reactions 35 and 37) in an *intramolecular* process (reaction 140 (Garrison 1987)); direct spectroscopic evidence for the occurrence of such reactions is however lacking. Similar processes might be expected to occur with alkoxyl radicals on other substrates (e.g. *N*-Ac amino acids) but these reactions would have to be *intermolecular* in nature (e.g. reaction 141), and hence would be expected to be less efficient. Thus, the increasing yield on going from the *N*-Ac amino acid system to the larger peptides could be accounted for on the basis of changing from a relatively inefficient intermolecular process to a very efficient intramolecular reaction involving a relatively strain-free 6-membered ring. This is borne out by analysis of the product yields from small peptides: thus, on going from *N*-Ac–Gly to di-Gly, the yields change from $G(NH_3) \simeq G(\text{carbonyl}) \simeq G(HO^{\cdot})$ to $G(NH_3) \simeq 4.8$, $G(HCOOH) \simeq 1.7$, and $G(CHOCOOH) \simeq 1.9$ respectively (Makada and Garrison 1972). Furthermore, with the mixed dipeptide Gly–Ala both glyoxylic and pyruvic acids are formed with $G(\text{carbonyl}) \simeq 2$ and $G(NH_3) \simeq 4.8$ (Makada and Garrison 1972). The same type of process may also occur with homo polypeptides. Thus, poly-Ala gives yields of $G(NH_3) \simeq 4$, $G(RCOCOOH) \simeq 1.2$, $G(RCOOH) \simeq 3.0$, and $G(CO_2) \simeq 2.4$ (Garrison *et al.* 1970). These product yields were assumed to arise from random attack along the chain, formation of peroxyl radicals, and subsequent backbone cleavage via both the formation of imines (Scheme 2.4) and alkoxyl radicals (reactions analogous to 130–132).

$$\underset{\sim NH-CH(R)-C(O)-NH-\overset{\displaystyle |}{\underset{\displaystyle }{C}}(R)\sim}{\overset{\displaystyle \overset{\displaystyle O^\cdot}{|}}{}} \quad ----> \quad \underset{\sim NH-\overset{\displaystyle \cdot}{C}(R)-C(O)-NH-\overset{\displaystyle |}{\underset{\displaystyle }{C}}(R)\sim}{\overset{\displaystyle \overset{\displaystyle OH}{|}}{}} \tag{140}$$

$$\underset{CH_3-C(O)-NH-\overset{\displaystyle }{\underset{\displaystyle }{C}}(CH_3)COO^-}{\overset{\displaystyle \overset{\displaystyle O^\cdot}{|}}{}} + \quad CH_3-C(O)-NH-CH(CH_3)-COO^- \; ----> \tag{141}$$

$$\underset{CH_3-C(O)-NH-\overset{\displaystyle }{\underset{\displaystyle }{C}}(CH_3)COO^-}{\overset{\displaystyle \overset{\displaystyle OH}{|}}{}} + \quad CH_3-C(O)-NH-\overset{\displaystyle \cdot}{C}(CH_3)-COO^-$$

More recent studies have, however, suggested that this product distribution may arise in a slightly different manner. Thus it has been shown that hydroperoxide formation at α-carbon sites also occurs with cyclic dipeptides and larger acyclic peptides (Davies 1996). It has been suggested that the β-scission process of the alkoxyl radicals outlined above (reactions 134 and 135), arising from both these materials and from peroxyl radical dimerization (reaction 35 followed by 37), is a general phenomenon, and that this type of fragmentation reaction can give rise to backbone scission and release of a further radical via the general mechanism outlined in reaction 142 (Davies 1996). This pathway is in accord with the observed products, though the individual steps of the overall process are somewhat different.

$$\sim C(O)-NH-C(O^\cdot)(R)-C(O)-NHR \sim \quad \longrightarrow \quad \sim C(O)-NH-C(R)=O + \; ^\cdot C(O)-NHR \sim \tag{142}$$

Transfer between sites: backbone to side chain and vice-versa

Much of the side chain chemistry of peptides and proteins is exactly analogous to that discussed earlier for the free amino acids, though the extent of attack at the side chain is often reduced in a peptide compared to a free amino acid due to a greater extent of reaction at the α-carbon site. The ratio of attack at various sites will also, obviously, depend on their accessibility. There are however a few exceptions where the presence of the peptide function can affect the chemistry of side-chain-derived radicals, and of particular importance are those processes which result in transfer of damage either to or from the α-carbon site. Such processes can obviously enhance or diminish the extent of backbone cleavage or side chain alterations. Of these theoretical possibilities, evidence has been obtained for transfer to α-carbon sites, but little from α-carbon sites; this is as would be expected on the grounds that α-carbon radicals are relatively stable when compared to most carbon-centred radicals on side chains. Transfer from an α-carbon site to a side chain probably only occurs to any great extent with very good hydrogen atom donors such as thiols (e.g. reactions such as 143); this repair of carbon-centred radicals by thiols has been much studied in radiation chemistry ((Adams *et al.* 1968; Adams *et al.* 1969*a*; Baker *et al.* 1982), reviewed in: (Adams 1972)) and has also been suggested to occur in some proteins (Davies, M. J. *et al.* 1993). A large number of examples of side chain to side chain reactions are known; these are outlined below after a discussion of the more limited data on transfer to an α-carbon site.

$$\sim NH - {}^{\bullet}C(R)-C(O) \sim \; + \; \sim SH \longrightarrow \; \sim NH-CH(R)-C(O) \sim \; + \; \sim S^{\bullet} \tag{143}$$

Hydrogen abstraction at γ-carbon sites on the side chain of certain peptides amino acids has been suggested to yield dehydropeptides, in the presence of oxygen, via the formation of peroxyl radicals (Scheme 2.5 (Garrison 1987)). This type of process, which has precedent with other peroxyl radicals (Howard 1972), could have important consequences, as these dehydropeptides are equivalent to the corresponding oxygenated enol species which undergo ready tautomerism to the keto form (reaction 144). In this case the analogue of the keto form is an imine species; such compounds can be hydrolysed in the presence of base to give a new amide function and a keto acid (reaction 145).

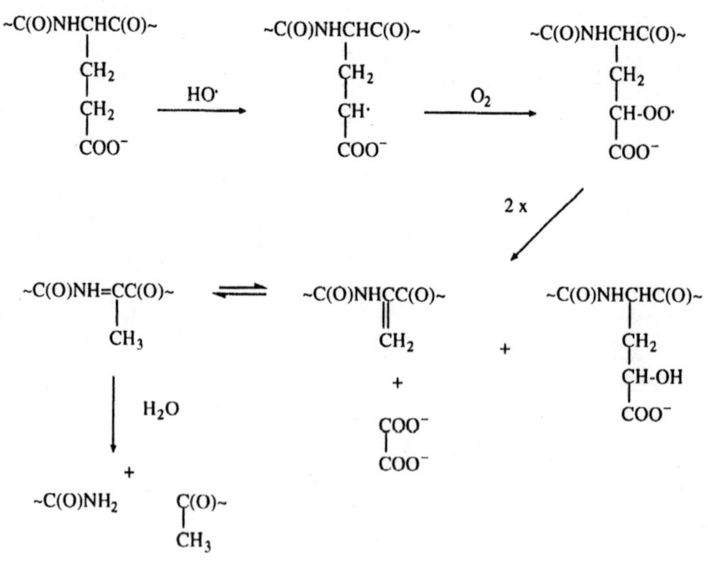

Scheme 2.5

Such reactions, for which there is limited direct evidence, could be very important processes in peptide and protein decomposition as they provide a mechanism by which attack at the side chain can result in cleavage of the peptide backbone (Garrison 1987).

$$\sim C(O)\text{–}NH\text{–}C(=CH_2)\text{–}C(O) \sim \; \rightleftharpoons \; \sim C(O)\text{-}N=C(CH_3)\text{–}C(O) \sim \qquad (144)$$

$$\sim C(O)\text{-}N=C(CH_3)\text{–}C(O) \sim \; + \; HO^- \; \longrightarrow \; \sim C(O)NH_2 + CH_3C(O)\text{–}C(O) \sim \qquad (145)$$

It is also possible that the formation of suitably positioned side chain alkoxyl radicals, via initial hydrogen atom abstraction to give a carbon-centred radical, formation of a peroxyl species, and subsequent reaction as outlined in reactions 35 and 37, may transfer damage from the side chain to the α-carbon site. Thus the formation of alkoxyl radicals at C-5 on Lys (a known site of hydrogen abstraction, see earlier) might result in an intramolecular 1,5-hydrogen abstraction reaction (reaction 146) to form an α-carbon radical. Similar reactions may occur with alkoxyl radicals formed at the C-5 sites on the side chains of Arg, Ile, and Leu. 1,4 shifts, such as those that might occur with an alkoxyl radical at the C-4 sites of Val, Leu, Ile, Gln, Glu, Lys, Arg, and Met, are less favourable, and hence much slower, than the analogous 1,5 (and 1,6) reactions (Gilbert et al. 1976, 1977); nevertheless they may occur to a minor extent. In many of these cases these sites are known to be major sites of initial hydrogen atom abstraction. Further reaction of these α-carbon radicals may then result in backbone cleavage via formation of peroxyl radicals and the series of reactions outlined above. Such intramolecular reactions are known to occur very readily with simple model compounds (e.g. reaction 147, with $k \simeq 8 \times 10^6 \text{s}^{-1}$ (Gilbert 1976)) and therefore may be possible candidates for side chain to backbone damage transfer reactions.

$$^+H_3NCH_2CH_2CH_2CH(COO^-)NH_3^+ \; \longrightarrow \; \longrightarrow \; ^+H_3NCH_2\text{—}\overset{|}{\underset{O^\bullet}{C}}H\text{—}CH_2CH_2CH(COO^-)NH_3^+$$

$$(146)$$

$$\downarrow$$

$$^+H_3NCH_2\text{—}\overset{|}{\underset{OH}{C}}H\text{—}CH_2CH_2\overset{\bullet}{C}(COO^-)NH_3^+$$

$$^\bullet OCH_2CH_2CH_2CH_3 \; \longrightarrow \; HOCH_2CH_2CH_2CH_2{}^\bullet \qquad (147)$$

Sulfur-centred radicals, such as those formed from hydrogen abstraction at Cys side chains, may also play a role in such transfer processes. Thus it has been shown that the thiyl radical formed on oxidation of the Cys residue in glutathione can hydrogen abstract from suitably placed backbone α-carbon sites (reaction 148 (Grierson *et al.* 1992; Zhao *et al.* 1994; Zhao, in press)). It has been suggested that this process occurs readily in this case, unlike normal hydrogen abstraction reactions of thiyl radicals (the reverse process repair of a carbon-centred radical by a thiol is usually favoured, e.g. reaction 143), due to the relatively weak nature of the α-carbon C–H bond arising from the stabilization provided by the neighbouring (capto-dative)–NH– and carbonyl functions. This is in accord with previous studies on the reaction of thiyl radicals with other activated C–H bonds (e.g. those in polyunsaturated fatty acids and alcohols (Schoneich *et al.* 1989*a*, *b*; Schoneich and Asmus 1990, 1992)). This reaction might be envisaged as occurring either intermolecularly, a process which might not compete successfully with either reaction of the thiyl radical with oxygen or dimerization, due to its slow nature, or intramolecularly with a neighbouring α-carbon site. The latter type of reaction has been demonstrated to occur with glutathione at pH values where the γ-glutamyl amine function is deprotonated, even though this involves a 9-membered transition state (reaction 149 (Zhao *et al.* 1994)). A similar process might also be expected to occur with the glutathione C-terminal (Gly) α-carbon site. An analogous transfer process has been shown to occur (i.e. thiyl to α-carbon transfer) with the thiyl radical from the free amino acid analogue, homocysteine (reaction 150), when the amino group is deprotonated (Zhao *et al.* 1994). This process does not appear to occur rapidly with the α-carbon site of the Cys residue itself (either in GSH or the free amino acid), as this would involve a highly strained 4-membered transition state (Zhao *et al.* 1994). Such transfer reactions may play a role in peptides and proteins, particularly when other reactions of the thiyl radical are disfavoured (steric constraints to dimerization, low oxygen tensions).

$$RS^{\bullet} + \sim NH–CHR–C(O) \longrightarrow RSH + \sim NH–{}^{\bullet}C(R)–C(O) \sim \qquad (148)$$

$$(149)$$

$$H_2NCH(CH_2CH_2S^{\bullet})COO^- \longrightarrow {}^{\bullet}C(NH_2)(CH_2CH_2SH)COO^- \qquad (150)$$

Evidence has been obtained for the repair of side chain carbon-centred radicals by thiols (i.e. transfer of damage) in some specific cases. Thus it has been demonstrated that electron addition to the thiol groups of GSH and Cys leads to efficient cleavage of the C–S bond with elimination of HS^- (see reaction 112 above). The carbon-centred radicals formed by this process, which are primary alkyl radicals, can rapidly oxidize ($k = 5 \times 10^6$ $dm^3 mol^{-1} s^{-1}$ for the Cys radical, and $k = 7.2 \times 10^6 dm^3 mol^{-1} s^{-1}$ for the corresponding GSH species (Prutz et al. 1989; Prutz 1990)) further molecules of the parent thiol (reaction 151). The species formed with Cys is, of course, the same species that would be formed as a result of hydrogen abstraction from the side chain of Ala, suggesting that similar repair processes should occur with the vast majority of side chain carbon-centred radicals. The rates of these processes would be expected to be slower with more stable carbon-centred species, i.e. the rates of repair of these carbon-centred species would decrease in the order primary > secondary > tertiary. The significance of these reactions in complex peptides and proteins remains to be established, though they have been suggested to occur (Davies, M. J. et al. 1993); such processes would appear to require the close approach of the two reactants, a situation which will be affected by the local environment and their freedom of motion, and will also be dependent on the extent of competition from other reactions, such as (the diffusion-controlled) reaction of the carbon-centred species with oxygen. Thus, these repair/ transfer reactions may only be of major significance under low oxygen tensions.

$$\sim HNCH(CH_2^{\bullet})C(O) \sim + RSH \longrightarrow \sim HNCH(CH_3)C(O) \sim + RS^{\bullet} \qquad (151)$$

Evidence has been presented for transfer of damage from the various oxidized sulfur species that can be generated on reaction of a number of radicals with the sulfur atom of methionine residues; in some cases these involve transfer to neighbouring amino acids in peptides (Bobrowski et al. 1991; Schoneich et al. 1993). This type of process occurs when the decarboxylation process outlined in Scheme 2.2 for the free amino acid (Hiller et al. 1981) is blocked by the incorporation of the free amino acid in to a peptide. In these studies it has been shown that a neighbouring Thr or Ser residue on the N-terminal side of Met can undergo fragmentation (and formation of formaldehyde and acetaldehyde, respectively) after initial oxidation at the sulfur atom of Met (e.g. by $HO^{\bullet}$) (Schoneich et al. 1994). This process is believed to occur via the mechanism outlined in Scheme 2.6. Though mechanistically interesting, this type of reaction can however only occur under very special circumstances, and its more general relevance to peptide and protein degradation is probably limited, and hence will not be discussed further here.

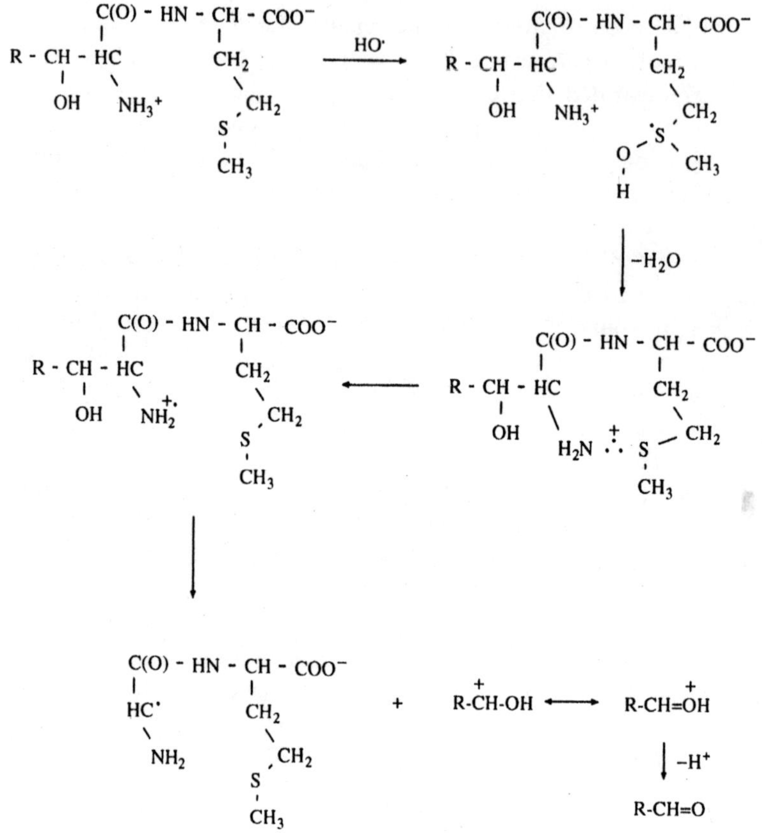

Scheme 2.6

A more subtle change exerted by the presence of a peptide or protein structure on the chemistry of side chain radicals has been outlined in studies where the product yields obtained from poly Glu were compared with those from smaller model systems (Sokol *et al.* 1965; Garrison 1972). Thus, with N-Ac–Glu the yield of products obtained (G(amide) $\simeq$ 2.3, G(α-keto-glutaric acid) $\simeq$ 0.8, and G(pyruvic acid) $\simeq$ 0.9) was found to be relatively constant over the pH range 3–8. In contrast, while similar yields were obtained with poly Glu over the pH range 6–8, the yield of amide and pyruvic acids decreased abruptly as the pH was lowered from 6 to 4; the yield of α-ketoglutaric acid, however, remained constant. This change in product yield with varying pH has been interpreted in terms of a change in structure of the polypeptide. At pH values > 6, poly Glu adopts a random coil conformation which allows various sections of the macro-molecule to interact freely, both intra- and intermolecularly, thus giving rise to behaviour analogous to that seen with the small model compounds. However, at lower pH values this polypeptide adopts a helix conformation; this type of structure would be expected to severely hinder intramolecular radical reactions and also possibly limit intermolecular processes. This is thought to affect the decay routes of the peroxyl radicals formed on the side chains, and hence the ratio of the observed products, as it will limit peroxyl radical self-dimerization reactions (such as formation of tetroxides via reaction 35 above) and thereby favour other routes such as reaction of ROO˙ with HOO˙ or reaction of ROO˙ with other R–H (Sokol *et al.* 1965; Garrison 1972, 1987). Such conformation-dependent effects on radical yields and reactions are poorly understood, but may play an important role in protein radical chemistry, and the relative yields of end products.

Transfer between side chain sites

By far the most well characterized examples of radical transfer reactions are those which involve transfer of damage from one side chain to another. These have been extensively studied for many years and have provided important information about the mechanisms and pathways of transfer of both electrons and oxidizing equivalents through proteins. This area has been reviewed extensively and only the most salient points are discussed here. For further information the reader is referred to the following reviews and recent papers (Klapper and Faraggi 1979; von Sonntag 1987; Faraggi and Klapper 1988; Faraggi *et al.* 1989; DeFelippis *et al.* 1990; Prutz 1990; Gray and Winkler 1996). The case of electron transfer from, and to, metal ion prosthetic groups within haem proteins and related species is covered separately below.

The extensive studies referred to above have allowed some general rules to be determined for the transfer of oxidizing equivalents through proteins and peptides. Examination of the reduction potentials of a number of peptide radicals at different pH values has resulted in the plot shown in Figure 2.1 (adapted from (Prutz 1990)). This diagram suggests that the ultimate sink for oxidizing equivalents in proteins should be Tyr residues, via the formation of the ring radical-cation and subsequent rapid de-protonation to give a phenoxyl radical (reaction 94), as the other radicals shown in this diagram are all capable of oxidizing this residue. It should, however, be noted that the reverse of some of these reactions can also occur, for example repair of a Tyr phenoxyl radical by a thiol to give a thiyl radical (reaction 152 (Prutz *et al.* 1983; Prutz 1990)), as such reactions are equilibria, which can be moved to one side or the other by manipulation of the concentrations of the species concerned. Thus the above repair re-action can be forced to the thiyl radical side by the presence of excess thiol anion, which removes the thiyl radicals by formation of the disulfide radical anion.

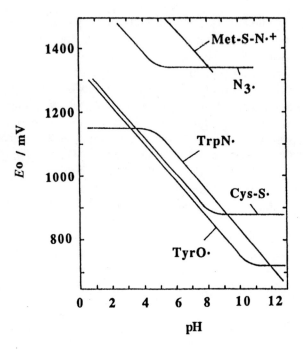

Figure 2.1

$$TyrO^\bullet + RSH \longrightarrow TyrOH + RS^\bullet \qquad (152)$$

By use of selective radical generation techniques, the factors which control the rates, and hence possible biological significance, of these reactions have been elucidated. Thus, reaction of peptides and proteins containing both Tyr and Trp residues with the azide radical ($N_3^\bullet$) gives rise, as mentioned earlier, to the selective formation of the nitrogen-centred indolyl radical. This species, as predicted from the reduction potentials in Figure 2.1, can oxidize the Tyr moiety to give the phenoxyl radical (Land and Prutz 1979; Prutz et al. 1982). Such transitions, which usually occur on the millisecond timescale, have been observed in many proteins and peptides (Land and Prutz 1977; Prutz and Land 1979; Prutz et al. 1980, 1981, 1982; Butler et al. 1982; Faraggi et al. 1989; DeFelippis et al. 1990). In a large number of these cases the pathways and specific residues involved are poorly characterized due to the presence of multiple Tyr and Trp units.

In model peptides the pathways and factors that control the rate of this transfer can be more readily investigated. Thus it has been shown that in the (62 amino acid) neurotoxin erabutoxin *b*, which has only a single Trp (residue 25) and a single Tyr (residue 29), little transfer occurs in the native protein, even though these two residues are only about 1.3 nm apart (Prutz *et al.* 1982). This has been attributed to the rigid nature of this material, which is held in a relatively inflexible conformation by four disulfide bonds, and the environment of the Tyr residue which is unable to rotate. However, reduction of the disulfide links and subsequent blocking of these sulfur residues (to prevent re-oxidation), results in efficient Trp → Tyr radical transfer (Prutz *et al.* 1982). This study also demonstrates that such transfers require direct contact of the residues (or contact with suitable intervening residues), and that the peptide backbone does not provide a conduit for the transfer of such oxidizing equivalents. The case with reducing equivalents or free electrons is however different (see below). As would be expected from these results the rates of transfer in model Trp/Tyr peptides have been found to be dependent on the distance (i.e. number of separating amino acids) between these residues (see Table 2.6). As can be seen from this data, inclusion of further residues does not always result in a further decrease in rate (Prutz *et al.* 1982; Faraggi *et al.* 1989; Prutz 1990). In contrast, when rigid spacers are employed (e.g. Pro residues) a decrease in rate has been observed with increasing number of spacers; this has been rationalized in terms of the ability of the flexible peptides to adopt a conformation where the reactive groups are in close contact, and the inability of rigid peptides to do this (Faraggi *et al.* 1989; DeFelippis *et al.* 1990; Prutz 1990). Furthermore, the absolute conformation of the peptide is also important—thus alteration of the stereochemistry (use of D- rather than L-amino acids) affects the rates. Similar transfer pathways have been observed with other residues, and examples of some of these interconversions are given in Scheme 2.7 (adapted from Prutz 1990).

The situation with reducing species is somewhat similar, though the pathways involved and the constraints on these are somewhat different. Thus, it is generally accepted that solvated electrons, if they do not react with oxygen, can react relatively randomly with sites on the surface of proteins, with addition occurring primarily at the carbonyl groups of peptide bonds; some addition also probably occurs at side chain sites (see above) (Holian and Garrison 1968; Adams *et al.* 1973; Rao and Hayon 1974; Rustgi and Riesz 1978*b*, *c*). These electron adducts are often not the ultimate site of these reducing moieties, and it has been shown that electron transfer can occur within the protein sufficiently rapidly to compete with reaction with molecular oxygen; disulfide bonds, if present, are major electron sinks (cf. reaction 127 (Klapper and Faraggi 1979)).

EPR studies on irradiated proteins at low temperatures have confirmed that electron transfer between peptide units can be rapid (Symons and Petersen 1978). Thus with lysozyme, approximately 65 per cent of the initial electron yield ends up at disulfide sites (Faraggi *et al.* 1985). In the case of RNAase A, the percentage is lower (about 20 per cent), but the observation

Table 2.6 Rate constants for inter- and intramolecular radical reactions of L-amino acid and peptide radicals.

Intramolecular reactions

Substrate	Process	Rate constant (s^{-1})
TyrOH–TrpNH	TrpN$^{\bullet}$ $\longrightarrow$ TyrO$^{\bullet}$	5.4–6.7×10^4
TyrOH–Pro–TrpNH	TrpN$^{\bullet}$ $\longrightarrow$ TyrO$^{\bullet}$	7.2×10^3
TyrOH–(Pro)$_2$–TrpNH	TrpN$^{\bullet}$ $\longrightarrow$ TyrO$^{\bullet}$	3.2×10^3
TyrOH–(Pro)$_3$–TrpNH	TrpN$^{\bullet}$ $\longrightarrow$ TyrO$^{\bullet}$	2.0×10^3
TrpNH–TyrOH	TrpN$^{\bullet}$ $\longrightarrow$ TyrO$^{\bullet}$	7.3–7.7×10^4
TrpNH–TyrOD (in D$_2$O)	TrpN$^{\bullet}$ $\longrightarrow$ TyrO$^{\bullet}$	2.3×10^4
D–TrpNH–L–TyrOH	TrpN$^{\bullet}$ $\longrightarrow$ TyrO$^{\bullet}$	1.5×10^5
TrpNH–Gly–TyrOH	TrpN$^{\bullet}$ $\longrightarrow$ TyrO$^{\bullet}$	5.1×10^5
TrpNH–(Gly)$_2$–TyrOH	TrpN$^{\bullet}$ $\longrightarrow$ TyrO$^{\bullet}$	2.4×10^4
TrpNH–(Gly)$_3$–TyrOH	TrpN$^{\bullet}$ $\longrightarrow$ TyrO$^{\bullet}$	3.5×10^4
TrpNH–Val–TyrOH	TrpN$^{\bullet}$ $\longrightarrow$ TyrO$^{\bullet}$	6.6×10^4
TrpNH–Pro–TyrOH	TrpN$^{\bullet}$ $\longrightarrow$ TyrO$^{\bullet}$	2.6×10^4
TrpNH–(Pro)$_2$–TyrOH	TrpN$^{\bullet}$ $\longrightarrow$ TyrO$^{\bullet}$	4.9×10^4
TrpNH–(Pro)$_3$–TyrOH	TrpN$^{\bullet}$ $\longrightarrow$ TyrO$^{\bullet}$	1.5×10^3
Erabutoxin b (denatured)	TrpN$^{\bullet}$ $\longrightarrow$ TyrO$^{\bullet}$	1.2×10^4
Met–TyrOH	Met(S$\therefore$Br) $\longrightarrow$ TyrO$^{\bullet}$	5.1×10^4
Met–TrpNH	Met(S$\therefore$Br) $\longrightarrow$ TrpN$^{\bullet}$	$> 10^6$
Cysteine-SH	RS$^{\bullet}$ $\longrightarrow$ α-carbon radical	2.5×10^4
Homocysteine-SH	RS$^{\bullet}$ $\longrightarrow$ α-carbon radical	2.2×10^5
Glutathione-SH	RS$^{\bullet}$ $\longrightarrow$ α-carbon radical	1.8×10^5

Intermolecular reactions

Process[a]	Rate constant ($dm^3\ mol^{-1}\ s^{-1}$)	pH
Met α-carbon$^{\bullet}$ + Cys-SH $\longrightarrow$ Cys-S$^{\bullet}$	2.7×10^8	8.2
Met α-carbon$^{\bullet}$ + (Gly–Cys-)$_2$ $\longrightarrow$ (Gly–Cys)$_2$SS$^{\bullet -}$	$\simeq 7 \times 10^6$	8.1
(Met–Gly)SN$^{\bullet +}$ + Cys-SH $\longrightarrow$ Cys-S$^{\bullet}$	$\simeq 8 \times 10^7$	8.0
(Met–Gly)SN$^{\bullet +}$ + Trp–Gly $\longrightarrow$ Trp(N$^{\bullet}$)–Gly	4×10^7	6.8
(Gly–Met)$_2$SS$^{\bullet +}$ + Cys-SH $\longrightarrow$ Cys-S$^{\bullet}$	3.5×10^8	8.3
(Gly–Met)$_2$SS$^{\bullet +}$ $\longrightarrow$ (Met–Gly)SN$^{\bullet}$	6.0×10^7	8.2
(Gly–Met-Gly)$_2$SS$^{\bullet +}$ + Cys-SH $\longrightarrow$ Cys-S$^{\bullet}$	1.7×10^8	8.2
(Gly–Met)$_2$SS$^{\bullet +}$ + Gly–Tyr-OH — Gly–Tyr-O$^{\bullet}$	9.0×10^7	8.9
(Gly–Met)$_2$SS$^{\bullet +}$ + Gly–Tyr-OH $\longrightarrow$ Gly–Tyr-O$^{\bullet}$	2.3×10^7	7.5
(Gly–Met)$_2$SS$^{\bullet +}$ + Trp–Gly $\longrightarrow$ Trp(N$^{\bullet}$)–Gly	4.8×10^8	7.0
(Met)$_2$SS$^{\bullet +}$ + Tyr-OH	3.8×10^7	1
(Met)$_2$SS$^{\bullet +}$ + Trp-NH	3.8×10^8	1
(Cys-Gly)S$^{\bullet}$ + Gly–Tyr-OH $\longrightarrow$ Gly–Tyr-O$^{\bullet}$	6.3×10^6	6.8
$^{\bullet}$CH$_2$-R (Ala side chain) + Cys-SH $\longrightarrow$ Cys-S$^{\bullet}$	5.0×10^6	8.2
Glutathione-S$^{\bullet}$ + Gly–Tyr-OH $\longrightarrow$ Gly–Tyr-O$^{\bullet}$	5.8×10^6	8.1
$^{\bullet}$CH$_2$-R (GSH side chain) + GSH $\longrightarrow$ Glutathione-S$^{\bullet}$	7.2×10^6	8.0

[a] Radical species involved: Met α-carbon$^{\bullet}$, α-carbon radical from Met; Cys-S$^{\bullet}$, thiyl radical from Cys; (Gly–Cys)$_2$SS$^{\bullet -}$, disulfide radical-anion of disulfide-linked peptide (Gly–Cys)$_2$; (Met–Gly)SN$^{\bullet +}$, three-electron species formed by oxidation of thioether group of Met and subsequent reaction with amine group (see also Scheme 2.2); Trp(N$^{\bullet}$)–Gly, nitrogen-centred indolyl radical from Trp side chain; (Gly–Met)$_2$SS$^{\bullet +}$, dimeric sulfur-centred radical-cation of peptide Gly–Met; (Gly–Met-Gly)$_2$SS$^{\bullet +}$, dimeric sulfur-centred radical-cation Gly–Met-Gly;

Gly–Tyr-O·, tyrosine phenoxyl radical from peptide Gly–Tyr; (Met)$_2$SS·$^+$, dimeric sulfur-centred radical-cation derived form Met; (Cys–Gly)S·, thiyl radical from peptide Cys–Gly; ·CH$_2$-R (Ala side chain), primary carbon-centred radical formed on side chain of Ala (or from loss of SH group from Cys radical anion); Glutathione-S·, glutathione thiyl radical; ·CH$_2$-R (GSH side chain), primary carbon-centred radical formed from loss of SH group from Cys residue of GSH radical anion.

Source: Faraggi *et al.* 1989; Prutz *et al.* 1989; Prutz 1990; Zhao *et al.* 1994.

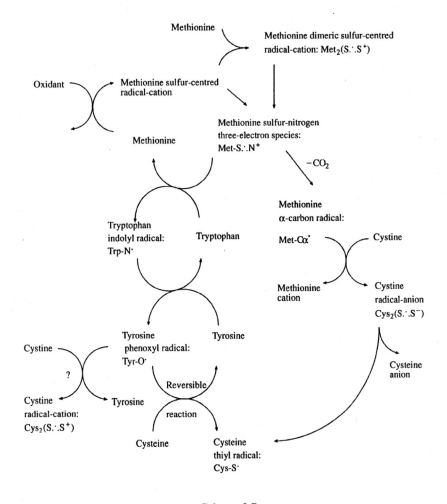

Scheme 2.7

of disulfide radical-anions in this case (these can be readily monitored by optical spectroscopy as they give rise to a broad band at about 410 nm) demonstrates that transfer can occur readily, as the disulfide groups in this protein are internal to the protein structure and not believed to be accessible to species in bulk solution (Faraggi *et al.* 1985). The formation of disulfide radical-anions can subsequently give rise to the formation of thiyl radicals, via reductive dissociation (reaction 46), and these thiyl radicals can then oxidize tyrosine residues to phenoxyl radicals (the reverse of reaction 152). Thus, both the oxidative pathways and the reductive routes finally converge at Tyr residues.

Transfer of electrons within peptides and proteins therefore appears to be both rapid and efficient. The transfer pathway in such cases is believed to be via the hydrogen bond network; i.e. the backbone can act as an efficient conduit, unlike the situation with positive holes (Faraggi et al. 1985; Gray and Winkler 1996). Unfortunately, as the initial attachment sites of the solvated electron are relatively random, exact information about the rates and pathways is difficult to obtain. Such information has, however, been obtained from pulse radiolysis (and other) techniques using chemically modified metalloproteins which have a very reactive metal ion attached to the surface, which subsequently reduces an internal metal site (Christensen et al. 1990; Liu, R.Q. et al. 1995; Quinkal et al. 1996). Knowledge of the distance between these sites and the structure of the intervening protein structure has allowed considerable information to be obtained about the mechanism and control of such electron transfer reactions (for further details see: Marcus 1956; Marcus and Smith 1985). These reactions, though intrinsically very interesting, do not result in oxidation of the protein per se, and hence are omitted from further discussion.

The carbon dioxide radical-anion $CO_2^{\cdot-}$ is a less powerful reductant than the solvated electron, and has been shown not to undergo rapid electron transfer to main chain carbonyl groups. However, reaction of this reductant with RNAase A also results in the formation of disulfide radical-anion species, despite the fact that these groups are inaccessible to $CO_2^{\cdot-}$ in the bulk solution (Faraggi et al. 1985). The observation of disulfide radical-anions therefore raises the possibility that there are other electron transfer routes through the protein which do not involve the initial addition of an electron to the carbonyl function. As expected, these reactions are slower than those seen with the solvated electron; the pathways through which this transfer occurs have not been further elucidated (Faraggi et al. 1985).

Interestingly it has also been shown (Simic and Taub 1978) that reaction of (oxidizing) $HO^{\cdot}$ can lead to reduction of a metal centre in a metallo protein such as ferric cytochrome c. This has been suggested to occur via initial reaction at the outer surface of the protein and subsequent formation of reducing moieties; these may be on the surface or buried within the structure, and ultimately result in reduction of the Fe^{3+} ion to Fe^{2+}. It has been estimated that approximately 50 per cent of the initial $HO^{\cdot}$ ultimately gives rise to reduction of the metal centre (Simic and Taub 1978), making this a remarkably efficient process for such a reactive radical. The processes by which this occurs and the residues involved are poorly understood; the formation and subsequent reactions of species such as DOPA are one possible source of some of this reducing activity.

Transfer reactions involving high-oxidation state prosthetic groups within haem proteins and related reactions

Damage transfer reactions have also been observed in haem proteins where the initial radical generation occurs at the haem moiety. Thus it has been known, for a number of years, that reaction of hydrogen peroxide, alkyl hydroperoxides, and a number of other two-electron oxidants, with the ferric (met) form of a number of haem proteins (e.g. haemoglobin, myoglobin, leghaemoglobin) gives rise to the formation of protein (globin) radicals (Gibson and Ingram 1956, 1958; King and Winfield 1963; King *et al.* 1967; Ortiz de Montellano 1987; Davies and Puppo 1992; McArthur and Davies 1993). These species are believed to be formed via initial two-electron oxidation of the Fe^{3+} protoporphyrin IX moiety to give a species which is formally Fe^{5+} and analogous to the Compound I species of peroxidases; this species is probably better formulated as an Fe^{4+}-oxo (ferryl) species and a porphyrin radical-cation (reaction 153). The latter species is a good oxidant, and is believed to undergo electron transfer with the surrounding protein, resulting in the repair of the porphyrin moiety and the formation of an oxidized protein via a one-electron transfer process (reaction 154). Similar ferryl species have also been proposed as reactive intermediates during the reaction of some iron complexes with hydrogen peroxide, and thus these reactions may have an intermolecular counterpart. As with the haemprotein versions, these 'free' ferryl species would be expected to readily oxidize amino acid residues.

$$Fe^{3+}(porphyrin)(protein) + H_2O_2 \,/\, ROOH \longrightarrow Fe^{4+}\text{-}OH(porphyrin^{\cdot\,+})(protein) + H_2O \,/\, ROH \tag{153}$$

$$Fe^{4+}\text{-}OH(porphyrin^{\cdot\,+})(protein) \longrightarrow Fe^{4+}\text{-}OH(porphyrin)(protein^{\cdot}) + H^{+} \tag{154}$$

Though the formation of such globin radicals has been known since the late 1950s (Gibson and Ingram 1958), the exact site(s) of the protein radicals have remained elusive and are still not fully characterized. Early workers postulated, on the basis of the arguments outlined in the above sections, that the aromatic residues in these proteins ought to be the sites of the radical species (Gibson and Ingram 1958; King and Winfield 1963)—this is particularly the case with myoglobin and leghaemoglobins as the forms of the proteins employed do not contain any sulfur-containing amino acids (Cys or Met). More recent studies, both on the radicals themselves by EPR spectroscopy and the products of the reactions using a variety of analytical techniques, have suggested that there might be multiple sites for these globin radicals with both tyrosine-derived phenoxyl radicals (Davies,

M. J. 1990*a*; Davies and Puppo 1992, 1993; Kelman and Mason 1992; McArthur and Davies 1993), tryptophan species (Kelman *et al.* 1994; Gunther *et al.* 1995), and other carbon-centred radicals (Moreau *et al.* 1996) having been identified in various studies. In the case of the Tyr- and Trp-derived radicals, these species probably arise via initial oxidation of the side chain to a radical-cation species, which subsequently rapidly deprotonates to give a phenoxyl radical in the case of Tyr, or an indolyl species in the case of Trp (i.e. reactions analogous to 109 and 104). In the case of the Trp-derived species, this radical has been detected by EPR spin trapping through the C-3 site of this stabilized allyl-type species (reaction 155 (Gunther *et al.* 1995)).

It is not clear at present whether these species are sequential sites on a single oxidation pathway, or whether such species arise from the occurrence of various alternative transfer pathways. The latter process appears to be the more likely, at least in the case of leghaemoglobin, where several different protein-derived radicals have been detected under identical reaction conditions. Attempts to determine the site(s) of the radicals in the case of myoglobin by use of site-directed mutagenesis have met with some success (Wilks and Ortiz de Montellano 1992; Rao *et al.* 1993; Kelman *et al.* 1994; Gunther *et al.* 1995). Removal of certain key residues, particularly the Tyr residues, alters the observed EPR signals, suggesting that some of these residues are either the site(s) of these species or are important conduits to their formation. However in nearly all the mutants examined, radical signals were still observed, suggesting that removal of a particular site, or key transfer pathway, merely switches the site of the oxidizing equivalent to another readily oxidized residue such as Trp or His (Wilks and Ortiz de Montellano 1992; Rao *et al.* 1993; Kelman *et al.* 1994; Gunther *et al.* 1995).

The formation of these globin-derived species has deleterious effects on the protein. In the case of myoglobin and soybean leghaemoglobin, these species can lead to the formation of cross-links between protein molecules; in the former case as a result of di-Tyr formation, in the latter by some process which does not involve this type of species (Tew and Ortiz de

(155)

Montellano 1988; Catalano *et al.* 1989; Wilks and Ortiz de Montellano 1992; Moreau *et al.* 1995*b*). Globin-derived species also appear, in the case of myoglobin and leghaemoglobin, to be able to back react with the porphyrin group to form haem-protein cross-links, which cannot act as efficient oxygen carriers (i.e. the process causes functional deactivation) (Catalano *et al.* 1989; Moreau *et al.* 1995*b*). These species are also capable of reacting with other species in bulk solution. This can be a repair process, when the reacting molecule is a low-molecular-weight antioxidant (such reactions have been characterized with a large number of such species including thiols, ascorbic acid, phenols, and a vitamin E analogue (Davies 1990, 1991; Davies and Puppo 1992; McArthur and Davies 1993)), or deleterious; thus in the case of leghaemoglobin, evidence has been presented for the reaction of the globin radical with biological membranes and the initiation of lipid peroxidation (Moreau *et al.* 1996).

There are also a number of examples where metal ion hydroperoxide complexes (M^{n+}–OOH) have been proposed as damaging species. These can be very selective agents, and a number of these complexes have been developed to carry out site-specific cleavage reactions with proteins (Tullius and Dombroski 1986; Rana and Meares 1990, 1991*a*, *b*; Platis *et al.* 1993), in a manner analagous to those developed earlier to selectively 'foot-print' DNA (Tullius and Dombroski 1985; Tullius 1987). By selectively locating the metal ion complex at a particular site, for example by use of thiol exchange or thiol oxidation to a disulfide, it has proved to be possible to dictate where the protein is cleaved and hence generate specific fragments. The mechanism of some of these reactions appears however to be hydrolysis, rather than oxidation, and involve nucleophilic attack of the metal ion-peroxide complex on the peptide carbonyl bond, rather than radical reactions. In other cases site-specific formation of HO˙ may be involved (Platis *et al.* 1993).

2.4 Random *versus* site-specific damage in proteins and peptides

2.4.1 As a result of random radical generation

From the above discussion it should be obvious that reaction of highly reactive radicals with peptides and proteins can occur at a large number of different sites, and hence that the damage observed on a peptide or protein ought to be at least semi-random, if not completely random. Thus with the most reactive radicals, such as HO˙, the difference in rate constants for attack at different side chains, and also at α-carbon sites on the backbone, is relatively small (Buxton *et al.* 1988) and hence damage to most, if not all, amino acids should be observed (Garrison 1987). This assumption is borne out by most reports in the literature (see, for example, (Drake *et al.* 1957; Robinson *et al.* 1966*a, b*; Duda 1981; Davies, K. J. *et al.* 1987*b*; Neuzil *et al.* 1993)), especially when the initial damaging radical is generated in a homogeneous manner in the reaction mixture (e.g. by radiolysis). Loss of all amino acids does not occur to a similar extent with, as expected, the most reactive amino acids, Cys, Met, Trp, Tyr, His and Phe, decreasing at a faster rate than many of the aliphatic amino acids with hydrocarbon side chains.

Nonetheless, there have been a number of studies which have shown that even random generation of radicals, such as HO˙, in free solution by radiolysis can result in *selective* cleavage at certain sites within a protein. Thus it has been shown that reaction of HO˙ with BSA gives non-random breaks, as evidenced by the observation of discrete bands rather than a smearing on SDS PAGE gels (Schuessler and Schilling 1984); similar behaviour has been observed with the haem proteins haemoglobin and myoglobin (Puchala and Schuessler 1993, 1995) and other systems (Wolff and Dean 1986; Davies, K. J. 1987). This selective cleavage has been suggested to be due to specific cleavage at proline residues, though the rationale behind such selective damage has not been fully explored in these studies. This selectivity would seem surprising as the studies outlined earlier, on the reaction of various radicals with Pro-containing peptides, suggested that attack at the α-carbon site of Pro was disfavoured relative to attack at C-5 (i.e. next to the nitrogen on the opposite side of the ring due to stabilization by the nitrogen lone pair). As pointed out in the Chapter 3, the molecular weights of observed fragments are also consistent with selective cleavage at Gly residues. Such selective fragmentation may arise as a result of the greater stability of the α-carbon radicals generated from Gly residues, compared to those from other amino acids, due to the lack of unfavourable steric interactions between the side chain and the carbonyl function as the radical adopts a planar conformation (see earlier). Such an explanation would require either initial attack to be selective for this residue (which is unlikely for radicals such as HO˙ even though there are often significant numbers of exposed Gly residues on the surface of proteins), or rapid and specific transfer of damage through the protein structure to these particular sites, by pathways which may involve the processes outlined in the previous sections. In the former case an increased loss of Gly residues relative to other amino acids would be expected, and this is not observed with irradiated proteins (see references above). With regard to the latter possibility, it should be noted that specific transfer solely to Gly residues would *not* be expected, as some of the side chain-derived radicals, such as those derived from Tyr and Trp residues, are more stable than these α-carbon species. Radical generation at Tyr and Trp residues is, however, not likely to lead to backbone cleavage and hence might not be observed using the techniques employed in these studies. Thus though the observation of these discrete SDS PAGE bands could be interpreted as being due to highly selective attack at certain key residues, it may not be nearly as selective as these gels would indicate, as much of the initiating radical flux may end up damaging side chain sites which would not lead to dramatic changes in molecular weight and hence would not be observed by this method.

2.4.2 As a result of selective radical attack

As might be expected, the difference between the extent of damage at different sites appears to become more marked as the attacking radical becomes less reactive and hence more selective. Thus selective damage has been observed with some small peptides as a result of attack by t-BuO˙, Br˙, N-bromosuccinamidyl, and triplet ketones in organic solvents (Elad and Sperling 1969; Sperling and Elad 1971a, b; Schwarzberg *et al.* 1973; Easton and Hay 1986; Burgess *et al.* 1989; Easton 1991). Unfortunately, too few studies have been carried out to determine whether there is a definite correlation between the rate constants for reaction with, for example, amino acid side chains, and the percentage decrease in their content under well-defined conditions. Attempts to carry out such correlations may, however, be misguided, in the light of the above discussion on radical transfer processes, as the initial site of attack may not reflect the final location of the radical, and hence the products observed or the extent of amino acid loss. This is particularly the case in well-defined and organized structures such as globular proteins, where the presence of defined structures, such as the hydrogen-bonding network, can aid damage transfer processes (cf. the transfer of reducing and oxidizing equivalents referred to above). Though the extent of such transfer reactions under particular conditions can only be guessed at, at present, it is likely that they play a major role in the majority of situations. The occurrence of such reactions would help explain the relatively rapid loss of Trp, Tyr, and Phe residues in many proteins when subject to γ-radiolysis; such residues would be expected, and are often known to be, buried in the hydrophobic cores of many proteins, and hence not immediately accessible to the reactive radicals generated in the aqueous phase, yet they are often the most rapidly lost.

Further evidence that such transfer reactions play a very significant role in peptide and protein damage, by radicals generated in a homogenous way in solution, has been obtained in recent studies on the consumption of amino acid residues in proteins when exposed to fixed fluxes of attacking radicals generated by γ-radiolysis in the presence of oxygen. Thus the studies of Stocker and colleagues (Neuzil *et al.* 1993) have shown that this does not occur in a stoichiometric manner, and that far larger numbers of amino acids are consumed than initiating radicals generated. This strongly implicates the presence of chain reactions under these conditions. These chains are relatively short, with approximately 15 amino acids being damaged per initiating HO$^{\cdot}$. Furthermore, under such conditions the oxygen consumption per attacking radical is of the order of two, implicating a number of non-oxygen-consuming reactions in these transfer and damaging processes. This study is supported by previous studies which also measured amino acid consumption in proteins exposed to γ-radiation in the presence of oxygen (e.g. (Davies, K. J. et al. 1987) and see Chapter 1), though the authors of these studies did not mention these yields. The nature of the chain-carrying species in such reactions is as yet poorly defined. The low consumption of oxygen requires that a number of these reactions be non-oxygen dependent; some of the processes outlined in the preceding sections fulfil this criteria and may therefore play a significant role. A summary of the reactions which we envisage play a role in this chain process, in the presence of oxygen, is given in Scheme 2.8. The main basis for this proposed reaction scheme is the identification of specific radicals during the reaction of oxidized proteins with metal ions (Davies, M.J. et al. 1995; Davies 1996) in conjunction with the earlier work of Garrison and colleagues (Garrison 1987). In addition, evidence such as that obtained by Traverso et al. (1996) supports specific parts of the pathway, in this case the formation of carbonyl functions as a result of decay of hydroperoxides.

2.4.3 As a result of metal-ion binding

A number of other cases are also known where radical formation occurs (or is believed to occur) at specific sites within a peptide or protein even though the attacking radical is not highly selective, as is the case with Br$_2^{\cdot -}$ or N$_3^{\cdot}$, or the site thermodynamically favoured (e.g. in the case of transfer to Tyr or Cys residues). In these cases selective attack is believed to arise from the binding of a metal ion, or other initiating species, at a particular site on, or within, the protein (Stadtman 1993). Thus evidence has been presented for the formation of specific, rather than random, radical formation on proteins during studies of Cu^{2+} and ascorbate damage to catalase (Orr 1967a, b), BSA (Marx and Chevion 1986), and some small peptides such as thyrotropin-releasing hormone (Bateman et al. 1985). In each case selective cleavage to give discrete fragments was detected, and this has been ascribed to the selective complexation/binding of the metal ion at particular sites on the protein, with the copper ions, once bound, still redox active and able to generate HO$^{\cdot}$ at the site of copper binding. These radicals, once formed, would be expected, on account of their high reactivity, to react in the immediate vicinity of the copper ion, thus inducing site-selective damage

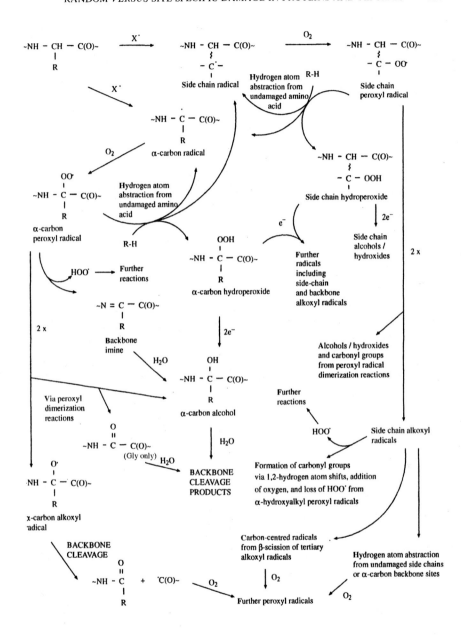

Scheme 2.8

(see also Hawkins and Davies 1997). Thus in the case of thyrotropin-releasing hormone, copper ion complexation to the His residue in the sequence ~Glu–His–Pro–amino acid, and subsequent reduction of the

Cu^{2+} to Cu^{+} by ascorbate, is believed to give rise (on reaction with H_2O_2) to site-specific $HO^{\cdot}$ (Bateman *et al.* 1985). This species abstracts a hydrogen atom from the α-carbon site between Pro and the neighbouring amino acid. Reaction with oxygen gives a peroxyl radical and subsequent strand breakage, with formation of an aldehyde and a new N-terminal amide (i.e. ∼ Glu-His-Pro-NH$_2$ from the above sequence) as would be predicted from the pathways discussed earlier. Several cases of (apparently) site-specific oxidation of particular amino acids have been reported. For example, selective histidine modification has been observed with glutamine synthetase ((Levine 1983*a*, *b*; Rivett and Levine 1990); this particular system is discussed in more detail in the following Chapter), selective methionine modification during treatment of peptides with Fe^{3+}/O_2/ascorbate (Li, S. *et al.* 1993, 1995), selective oxidation of both histidine and methionine in human relaxin treated with mixtures of either Fe^{3+} or Cu^{2+} and ascorbate in the presence of oxygen (Li *et al.* 1995), and selective oxidation of Trp residues in peptides exposed to $Fe^{3+}/O_2^{\cdot-}$ (Itakura *et al.* 1994). A similar rationale has been advanced to explain the greater extent of loss of certain amino acids in metal ion-catalysed damage by $HO^{\cdot}$ compared to that seen with the same radical generated homogeneously in solution by radiolysis (reviewed: Stadtman 1993)). Most of the amino acids which have been observed to be rapidly lost in such systems are those (e.g. His, Cys, Met, Lys, Arg, Trp) which are most likely to be involved in the binding of metal ions, and hence at, or very near, the site of radical formation. In some of these cases it has been suggested, on the basis that radical scavengers or protective enzymes have limited or no effect, that oxidants other than radicals may be involved (e.g. metal ion-peroxy complexes or hydrogen peroxide itself (Itakura *et al.* 1994; Li, S. *et al.* 1995*a*)). While this is a distinct possibility in some situations, for example in cases where oxidation of methionine to the sulfoxide occurs (Li, S. *et al.* 1995*a*, *b*), as this can be achieved readily by hydrogen peroxide alone via a molecular reaction (see earlier), in other cases the lack of effect of radical scavengers may merely be due to the putative protective agent being unable to approach the site of radical formation for steric or electronic reasons.

Selective oxidation of particular residues via site-specific oxidation may also be occuring in a large number of other systems where, for example, a metal ion is employed to generate radical species and the metal ion concerned is not strongly ligated to particular ligands which will keep the metal ion in solution and not bound to the protein. There are also a number of cases where what may inititially appear to be selective oxidation of particular amino acids is not, with the selectivity arising from the formation of alternative reactive species to those presumed to be present. An example of this effect is the observation that the presence of bicarbonate stimulates the oxidation of Trp residues in proteins when they are exposed to radiation

(Davies, K. J. *et al.* 1987); this stimulation is probably due to the partial scavenging of HO$^{\cdot}$ by the bicarbonate to form the CO$_3^{\cdot-}$ radical which is a highly selective oxidant and reacts with Trp at least 15 times faster than with any other amino acid residue (Neta *et al.* 1988). A similar situation may arise in other cases where bicarbonate has a dramatic stimulatory effect (e.g. oxidation of glutamine synthetase by ascorbate/Fe^{2+}/O$_2$ (Stadtman 1993)). In other cases, however, the effect of bicarbonate on the oxidation of amino acids, peptides, and proteins is more likely to be due to the action of this material as a ligand for metal ions present in the reaction mixture. The dramatic effect of bicarbonate on Mn^{2+}-catalysed oxidation of amino acids by H$_2$O$_2$ has been suggested ((Berlett *et al.* 1990; Stadtman *et al.* 1990), reviewed in (Stadtman 1993)) to be due to the formation of complexes which may also involve an amino acid. In the latter case the amino acid ligand may be oxidized at a more rapid rate and to a greater extent (relatively low levels of aldehydes/ketones are observed compared to the corresponding Fe^{3+}-catalysed system (Berlett *et al.* 1990; Stadtman and Berlett 1991)) than normal, via a 'site-selective' process due to the proximity of the amino acid to the site of radical formation. Alternatively, the intermediate amino acid radicals (or products) may react with the (oxidized) manganese ion resulting in further (or more rapid) oxidation; an enhanced rate may also arise from the effect of the amino acid and/or bicarbonate on the redox properties of Mn^{2+}. The effect of bicarbonate on corresponding Fe^{3+}-catalysed amino acid oxidation reactions (Stadtman and Berlett 1991; Stadtman 1993) may be due to the solubilizing effect that this species can have on the otherwise relatively insoluble Fe^{3+} complexes, and/or an effect on the redox properties of the metal ion.

2.4.4 As a result of lipid oxidation

Site-specific damage can also be a characteristic of the protein damage induced by both lipid peroxidation and sugar autoxidation reactions. In the former case, attack on membrane proteins is thought to occur mainly at residues which are at the interface between the lipid and protein regions within the membrane. Originally such damage was described as 'radiomimetic' (i.e. showing a degree of commonality of mechanism with radiation systems (Tappel 1973)), but this is probably an incorrect characterization, as it would be expected that both the initial sites of attack, the species involved (see earlier), and the subsequent mechanisms of damage, are dramatically different, though the end products (at least in terms of the generation of fragments, aggregates etc. and the conditions under which they occur) may be similar, as once radicals are formed on the protein, the subsequent chemistry of these species are probably reasonably similar, if not identical.

2.4.5 As a result of sugar autoxidation

In the case of sugar autoxidation two different categories of site-specific damage can be defined. First, site-specific damage in terms of where the sugar molecule initially attaches to the protein, and hence the damage that might be induced in this vicinity. Secondly, damage which arises from the autoxidation of a sugar molecule once it has been chemically linked (either by a radical process or enzymatically) to the protein. As with the systems outlined above, such systems may give rise merely to local damage, though there is also the possibility of remote oxidation in such systems as a result of long-range damage transfer. The exact nature of these reactions and the lesions which they generate, and hence the relative importance of local *versus* remote damage, remains to be elucidated. It is, however, clear from a number of studies that both types of damage can occur, and that such reactions do lead to extensive protein alterations (Wolff and Dean 1987a, b, 1988; Wolff et al. 1989, 1991; Hunt et al. 1990; Jiang et al. 1990; Hunt and Wolff 1991a, b).

It should, however, be noted that site-specific generation of oxidizing species at a particular site on the surface of, or within, a protein does not always result in localized damage. It has been demonstrated both in the special cases of the haem protein reactions outlined above, and other studies such as those carried out using BSA with photosensitizing porphyrins bound at particular sites on the protein surface (Timmins and Davies 1993a, 1994; Silvester et al. 1995), that damage can be readily transferred fom the initial site to remote residues. Thus it should be obvious, from the examples discussed in the above paragraphs, that a system which might be expected to give rise to random damage (e.g. γ-radiolysis) can give rise to selective fragmentation under particular circumstances, whereas systems which might be expected to give solely site-specific damage can also result in damage at sites far removed from the site of generation.

2.5 Secondary modification reactions

2.5.1 Modification of proteins by other biological components

It is now well established that a number of the products arising from cellular and other chemical reactions can result in further protein oxidation and alteration, and that protein oxidation reactions can in turn result in modification of other, previously undamaged, molecules. The initiation of further damage by radicals derived from hydroperoxides formed from lipids, carbohydrates, DNA, and proteins will occur in a similar manner to that outlined above for other small hydroperoxides. Some of these reactions are believed to have important biological consequences (e.g. transfer of damage from DNA to the histone proteins); these areas are discussed in more detail in later chapters. Further details of such reactions will only be covered below where the chemistry of these reactions results in different behaviour to that outlined above.

It has been known for a number of years that reactive aldehyde groups formed from lipid molecules as a result of lipid peroxidation can react with amino groups on protein molecules to form Schiff bases (Chio and Tappel 1969a, b; Kautiainen 1992; Szweda et al. 1993; Cohn et al. 1996). The initial formation of some of these materials can be reversed (Hazell et al. 1994; Yim et al. 1995), but after further rearrangement reactions this process becomes irreversible. This process results in the loss of surface charge on a protein and may be responsible for the increased electrophoretic mobility of proteins which have been oxidized in the presence of lipids (e.g. low density lipoproteins). Similar reactions are possible with aldehydes and carbonyl functions generated during the autoxidation of sugar and carbohydrate molecules; this process may be a key reaction in protein glycation (Riley and Harding 1993; Wells-Knecht, M. C. et al. 1995; Yim et al. 1995). In the latter case, the adduct species may undergo further autoxidation reactions, as outlined above, with resulting site-specific radical generation. In both cases the resulting adducts may also act as metal ion binding sites, which may allow metal ion-catalysed site-specific radical generation.

The reaction of amine groups on proteins with carbonyl functions is not limited to those generated from lipid or sugar/carbohydrate moieties. Thus it is possible that the formation of aldehydes on one part of a protein molecule can react with an amine function, such as on a Lys side chain, on either another part of the same molecule or another, damaged or un-damaged, protein (Hazell et al. 1994). This will result in the formation of either intra- or intermolecular cross-links, which would not be easily repaired. Though such reactions might be expected to occur readily, direct evidence for the occurrence of this type of cross-link is scarce.

2.5.2 Modification of other biological molecules by protein oxidation products

Evidence for a direct transfer of a radical from a protein to previously undamaged lipid molecules (either free fatty aids or more complex membrane or particle systems) has been sought by a number of different investigators. These studies have often been limited in nature, and are difficult to interpret in a number of cases as it is often not clear whether the observed damage arises via mediation of a protein-derived radical or via direct reaction of the initiating species with the target lipid (i.e. by-passing the protein). Such studies are still in their infancy.

The most clear cut examples of this type of phenomenon have come from systems where the radical is generated on the protein via a process which does not involve the formation of radicals in bulk solution where they could react directly with the target lipid system. Thus a number of groups have investigated the transfer of damage from haem proteins which have been treated with hydrogen peroxide (or other two electron oxidants) under conditions where little release of iron from the haem protein would be expected to occur (and hence little radical generation in free solution). These reactions are known (see earlier) to give rise to high-oxidation-state iron (Fe^{4+}-oxo, ferryl) species and globin-derived radicals, both of which might then be expected to oxidize lipid molecules. This has been shown to be the case in a number of systems using a variety of different techniques including EPR spectroscopy of both the precursor and product radicals, and the analysis of lipid oxidation products (Kanner and Harel 1985; Fantone *et al.* 1989; Galaris *et al.* 1990; Dee *et al.* 1991; Newman *et al.* 1991; Turner *et al.* 1991; Rao *et al.* 1994; Moreau *et al.* 1996). The nature of the oxidizing species (i.e. Fe^{4+}-oxo *versus* protein radical) is unclear in many of these cases. In some situations (Rao *et al.* 1994) the Fe^{4+}-oxo species has been shown to be the oxidant, whereas in other cases, where protein radicals have been shown to be involved (Newman *et al.* 1991; Moreau *et al.* 1996), the nature of the reactive haem-protein-derived radical(s) is still the subject of controversy. Hence the exact mechanism of initiation of these lipid oxidation reactions, e.g. the nature of the radical which adds or abstracts a hydrogen atom from these lipid molecules, is poorly understood. It is, however, clear that such haem protein-derived radicals can initiate oxidation of free fatty acids, phospholipids, micelles, membrane fractions, and lipoproteins. In some of these situations the reaction may involve the formation of an α-tocopherol radical (as a result of repair of a protein-derived radical by this antioxidant) and subsequent initiation of lipid peroxidation by this species (Witting *et al.*, in press).

Evidence has also been presented recently to show that the chloramine/chloramide species generated on the apoB protein molecule of low density lipoprotein (LDL), may initiate damage to the lipid fraction of the particle. Thus treatment of LDL with low excesses of hypochlorite (< 500 HOCl molecules per LDL particle), at low temperatures (4 °C), has been shown to result in complete consumption of the HOCl, oxidation of protein residues (chiefly Lys, Trp, Cys, and Met), but little or no lipid oxidation (Hazell and Stocker 1993; Hazell *et al.* 1994). Subsequent incubation of such treated LDL at 37 °C results in a dramatic increase in lipid oxidation products (LOOH or LOH) and consumption of lipid-soluble antioxidants, in a process which can be inhibited by radical scavengers and methionine (which destroys chloramines/chloramides). These results have been interpreted in terms of the formation of radical species (probably nitrogen-centred radicals, see earlier) from chloramines/chloramides on the protein and subsequent hydrogen atom abstraction from lipid molecules by these radicals or other radicals that arise from them (Hazell and Stocker 1993; Hazell, Davies and Stocker, unpublished data).

Transfer of radical damage from proteins to DNA and *vice versa* has been the subject of considerable study as a result of its possible relevance to radiation damage. As such the majority of studies have been carried out with histone proteins, as these materials are the most likely to participate in such reactions due to their proximity to DNA (Mee and Adelstein 1981). It has been demonstrated that a number of radicals derived from both proteins and peptides can cross-link to DNA (see Table 2.7) (Kornhauser 1976; Hartman *et al.* 1979; Summerfield and Tappel 1984*c*; Dizdaroglu and Simic 1985; Peak *et al.* 1985; Simic and Dizdaroglu 1985; Gajewski *et al.* 1988; Margolis *et al.* 1988; Dizdaroglu and Gajewski 1989; Dizdaroglu *et al.* 1989; Gajewski and Dizdaroglu 1990; Nackerdien *et al.* 1991; Olinski *et al.* 1992; Misra *et al.* 1993; Zhuang *et al.* 1994; Altman *et al.* 1995). In some cases the nature of these cross-links has been characterized, while in others evidence for cross-linking has been obtained purely on the basis of retention of protein by isolated DNA or *vice versa*. Evidence has been presented in some of these studies for the majority of these links arising from the addition of a protein or peptide radical to the C5–C6 double bond of the pyrimidine

Table 2.7   DNA-amino acid and DNA-protein cross-links

Amino acid	DNA base
Tyrosine	Thymine
Tyrosine	Cytosine
Glycine	Thymine
Alanine	Thymine
Valine	Thymine
Leucine	Thymine
Isoleucine	Thymine
Threonine	Thymine
Lysine	Thymine

These selected examples are of well characterized (primarily by gas chromatography-mass spectroscopy with selected ion monitoring) cross-links formed by exposure to γ-irradiation, transition metal ions (such as copper and iron species), and a number of carcinogenic metal ion salts.

Source: (Dizdaroglu and Simic 1985; Simic and Dizdaroglu 1985; Gajewski *et al.* 1988; Margolis *et al.* 1988; Dizdaroglu and Gajewski 1989; Dizdaroglu *et al.* 1989; Gajewski and Dizdaroglu 1990; Dizdaroglu 1991, 1992; Nackerdien *et al.* 1991; Olinski *et al.* 1992; Misra *et al.* 1993; Zhuang *et al.* 1994; Altman *et al.* 1995; Toyokuni *et al.* 1995). Other studies have examined cross-links induced by UV and visible light (e.g. Kornhauser 1976; Shetlar *et al.* 1984; J. G. Peak *et al.* 1985; M. J. Peak *et al.* 1985) and reported other, less-well-defined DNA-protein cross-links (e.g. Mee and Adelstein 1981; Schuessler *et al.* 1987; Schuessler and Hartmann 1987; Schuessler and Jung 1989*a*, *b*); such data is not included.

bases. Such selectivity is in line with studies with a number of other electrophilic and nucelophilic radicals, which have demonstrated that this position is the major reactive site on these substrates (von Sonntag 1987; Catterall *et al.* 1992, 1993; Hazlewood and Davies 1995). Addition of protein-derived radicals at the C8 position of the purines might also be expected to occur, but such materials are poorly characterized. In all cases, the yield of cross-links would be expected to be oxygen dependent as the majority of the attacking radicals would be expected to undergo competing reactions with oxygen to give peroxyl radicals. The major type of cross-link observed in the presence of oxygen has been characterized as arising from addition of a tyrosine phenoxyl radical to the base thymine. Such a product is not unexpected, as this species is one of the very few protein-derived species which has a long lifetime in the presence of oxygen and does not readily form a peroxyl radical.

Recent studies have shown that radicals derived from histone, and other protein, hydroperoxides may react with DNA molecules (Luxford and Davies, unpublished data). Similarly, protein-bound DOPA, specifically generated by tyrosinase (Simpson *et al.* 1993), can lead to metal-ion-dependent formation of oxidized DNA bases (Morin *et al.*, unpublished). The exact nature of the radicals involved in these reactions, both on the protein and the DNA, have yet to be characterized, though it is believed that such transfer can occur. For the hydroperoxides, it is likely that the addition of protein alkoxyl or carbon-centred species to the DNA bases is involved. The reverse process, reaction of DNA hydroperoxide-derived radicals with histone proteins, has also been shown to occur (Ho *et al.*, unpublished data).

Peroxyl-radical-induced cross-links are unlikely to survive the analytical procedures required for their characterization, as the cross-link would involve a relatively weak peroxide linkage. Addition to the sugar moieties of DNA cannot occur directly, but protein or peptide peroxyl radicals would be expected to readily abstract hydrogen atoms from sites on the sugar moiety. The occurrence of such damage is difficult to discern from that generated by other low-molecular-weight initiating radicals, as outlined above in the case of the corresponding protein radical reactions with lipids. Such reactions may however occur, and would be of considerable biological consequence, as sugar radicals are known precursors of DNA strand breaks.

Damage transfer from carbohydrates to proteins has been suggested to occur. It has been demonstrated that proteoglycans exposed to controlled doses of radiation undergo fragmentation of the protein moiety preferentially over the carbohydrate fraction (Dean *et al.* 1984*a*; Hawkins and Davies 1997). With the attacking radical in question (HO$^{\cdot}$) such selectivity may partly result from the greater rate constants for reactions with protein than polysaccharide, but may also involve damage transfer reactions.

Transfer of damage from one damaged protein to another undamaged molecule is also a distinct proposition. This may occur either via an indirect process, where a damaged protein could catalyse further radical formation which then initiates damage to other protein molecules, or via a direct reaction of a radical on one protein with another protein. We will discuss the former, indirect, case first.

It is now well established (see earlier) that modification of Tyr residues on proteins, in the presence of oxygen, gives rise to DOPA, and that the presence of this material can give rise to further oxidation reactions. Thus it has been shown that this species can reduce metal ions such as Cu^{2+} and Fe^{3+} (Simpson et al. 1992, 1993; Gieseg et al. 1993); this type of reaction (reaction 156) would be expected to result in redox cycling of the metal and an increased flux of radicals. The semiquinone species generated in this type of reaction would be expected to also undergo further reaction. This might occur either by disproportionation with another semiquinone species, a reaction which may be sterically very unfavourable when the semiquinone is present on a protein, or via electron transfer reactions with oxygen to form superoxide radicals (e.g. reaction 22), or another metal ion. In each case the corresponding DOPA quinone would be formed. This species can in turn undergo further reactions which result in the overall release of six electrons (starting from DOPA itself) and the formation of an indole derivative (reaction 157 (Gieseg et al. 1993)).

$$(156)$$

$$(157)$$

It has also been shown that DOPA can react with free thiol groups (such as free Cys) to form cysteinyl-DOPA species via Michael addition (reaction 158 (Ito et al. 1984, 1988)). Though no evidence for such adducts of protein-bound DOPA with protein thiols (on either the same or a different protein) has been obtained (Dean et al. 1996), such reactions could in theory contribute to the formation of protein-protein cross-links. Thus there are a number of routes to the formation of protein cross-links in addition to the direct radical processes outlined in earlier sections (e.g. thiyl dimerization, carbon-centred radical dimerization, di-Tyr and di-phenyl formation etc.) with only a few of these readily repairable (e.g. disulfide links).

$$O= \!\!\!\!\!\bigcirc\!\!\!\!\!-CH_2\!\sim \quad + \quad RSH \quad \longrightarrow \quad HO\!-\!\!\!\!\!\bigcirc\!\!\!\!\!-CH_2\!\sim \qquad (158)$$

Direct evidence for the transfer of damage, i.e. radical transfer, from one protein molecule to another, is relatively scarce except in a few very well characterized cases where the radical species is deliberately generated as part of an enzymatic, or other protein-mediated, process. Thus it is known that rapid transfer of reducing equivalents can occur from protein to protein as part of electron transport chains, such as those in mitochondria, chloroplasts, and haem protein systems such as the cytochrome P450 family. Similar rapid electron transfer reactions occur during the photo cycles of photosystems (PSI and PSII) where photo excitation is used to form both an oxidized (radical-cation) and reduced (radical-anion) species (Innes and Brudvig 1989; Hoganson and Babcock 1992; Pedersen and Finazzi 1993; Szalai and Brudvig 1996). Transfer of these oxidizing and reducing species away from the reaction centre is required to prevent rapid back reaction (repair). It is known that the protein matrix plays a key role in all of these processes. However as such reactions only result, under normal circumstances, in a transient oxidation or reduction of the protein, and specific repair processes are present to return these proteins to their resting states, these reactions will not be discussed further here. There is also a growing family of enzymes which are known to form transient protein radicals as part of their enzymatic cycles, and these radical species play an important role in carrying out the chemical transformations brought about on the substrate (reviewed: Pedersen and Finazzi 1993). These species are discussed further in Chapter 3.

Unlike the above processes, inadvertent transfer of a radical from one protein to another, other than via the formation of protein dimers, has been investigated only to a minor extent. Thus it is has been shown, by EPR spectroscopy, that radicals generated on myoglobin molecules as a result of the interaction of hydrogen peroxide with the haem centre can oxidize other proteins with the formation of a further protein radical on the target species (Miller et al. 1996; Ostdal et al. 1996; Irwin and Davies, unpublished data). As yet the site(s) of the radical on the target proteins (BSA, apoB, lactoglobulin) have not been characterized, but it would be expected that these would be surface species and readily oxidizable residues. Further studies on similar protein radical to protein systems are in progress.

2.6 Prevention of protein oxidation and antioxidants

The reactions of protein and peptide-derived radicals with antioxidants and scavengers have been studied in some detail on a number of occasions, as such reactions might be expected to protect the protein against either or both fragmentation and aggregation. Though such reactions are of immense potential importance, detailed mechanistic studies of the reaction of potential antioxidants have only been carried out on a limited number of occasions. There is, however, a wealth of data on the prevention of fragmentation or aggregation per se, with such changes usually assessed by either SDS PAGE or HPLC. Such studies, though they give information about the overall effect of the added agent, give little information on the nature of the chemical reactions that are occurring. This facet of antioxidant protection is covered in more detail in Chapters 3 and 6.

Mechanistic studies of protein antioxidation are again limited both by the problem of selectively generating a particular radical species on a protein, such that its reactions can be characterized, and by the fact that the kinetics of such reactions will almost certainly be highly dependent on the exact position and accessibility of the residue on which the radical is situated to the added scavenger. Thus kinetic data obtained for a particular radical on one protein may be completely erroneous for the same radical on a different protein. That said, some information has been obtained with a number of potential scavengers particularly through the use of either EPR spectroscopy or pulse radiolysis. The former has allowed information to be obtained about the identity/nature of the species reacting, but little on the kinetics of such reactions, whereas the opposite is true, in general, for the pulse radiolysis studies. It is also true that the most frequently (and readily) studied species are the more stable protein-derived radicals, which may be the least important with regard to fragmentation of the protein; this may not however be true about cross-linking where radicals such as Tyr-derived phenoxyl radicals are thought to be important (see earlier).

Pulse radiolysis with optical detection has been employed to measure the rate constants for the repair of radicals derived from some free amino acids at neutral pH by the vitamin E analogue Trolox C. Thus rate constants have been measured for the radicals from Trp ($k \simeq 5 \times 10^7$ $dm^3 mol^{-1} s^{-1}$), Tyr ($k \simeq 4 \times 10^8$ $dm^3 mol^{-1} s^{-1}$), Met ($k \simeq 7 \times 10^8$ $dm^3 mol^{-1} s^{-1}$), and His ($k \simeq 8 \times 10^8$ $dm^3 mol^{-1} s^{-1}$) (Bisby et al. 1984). These reactions result in the formation of the corresponding phenoxyl radical from the Trolox C (e.g. reactions 159 and 160), though it is likely that these reactions occur via electron transfer and subsequent rapid deprotonation of the Trolox C radical-cation. This is supported by the observation that the Trp radical-cation reacts more rapidly ($k \simeq 2 \times 10^9$ $dm^3 mol^{-1} s^{-1}$) than the neutral indolyl radical (Bisby et al. 1984). Repair of Trp-derived radicals has also been observed in the protein lysozyme ($k = 2$–5×10^7 $dm^3 mol^{-1} s^{-1}$ (Bisby et al. 1984)). The occurrence of this type of reaction with an intact protein molecule, where the residue is not completely exposed on the surface of the protein, supports the hypothesis that damage transfer, or repair in this case, can occur over quite large distances and that this process is very efficient. Thus the rate constant for repair of the free Trp radical is very similar to that for the same species in the intact protein. Attempts to extend these studies to vitamin E itself have proved to be complex due to the poor solubility of vitamin E in aqueous solutions. Use of vitamin E dissolved in 20 mM SDS did give positive results with free Trp-derived radicals ($k \simeq 1 \times 10^8$ $dm^3 mol^{-1} s^{-1}$ (Hoey and Butler 1984)), but no evidence was found for this reaction with lysozyme itself (i.e. $k < 1 \times 10^7$ $dm^3 mol^{-1} s^{-1}$ (Hoey and Butler 1984)) even though the lysozyme was partially unfolded under these conditions due to the presence of the SDS. Trolox C has also been shown to react rapidly with Tyr phenoxyl radicals in a number of proteins (Davies 1991; Davies and Puppo 1992; Giulivi et al. 1992; Giulivi and Cadenas 1993; McArthur and Davies 1993), though little kinetic data on these reactions is available, and α-tocopherol has been shown to slowly repair Tyr phenoxyl radicals in lysozyme (in the presence of 20 mM SDS, i.e. with partially unfolded protein (Hoey and Butler 1984)).

These observations suggest that vitamin E molecules present in membranes may act as antioxidants for membrane-bound proteins and transfer damage from the protein in to the lipid phase (Dean and Cheeseman 1987; Dean et al. 1991). In certain circumstances, particularly where the radical flux is low, the vitamin E phenoxyl radical can then initiate further lipid oxidation (tocopherol-mediated lipid peroxidation (Bowry et al. 1992b, 1995; Ingold et al. 1993; Stocker 1994)). Thus such reactions may repair proteins at the expense of generating further lipid damage.

$$\text{TrpN}^{\bullet} + \text{Trolox-OH} \longrightarrow \text{TrpNH} + \text{Trolox-O}^{\bullet} \tag{159}$$

$$\text{TyrO}^{\bullet} + \text{Trolox–OH} \longrightarrow \text{TyrOH} + \text{Trolox–O}^{\bullet} \tag{160}$$

Reaction of Trolox C with the protein peroxyl radical derived from myoglobin has also been observed, though the kinetics of this reaction were not determined (Davies, M. J. 1990a). Reaction of Trolox C with a number of radicals (alkoxyl and/or carbon-centred species) derived from protein hydroperoxides has also been demonstrated (Davies, unpublished data). In these cases, however, the reactions are not strictly repair reactions, as the products of the reaction on the protein are altered amino acids. Thus protein hydroperoxides would arise as a result of 'repair' of peroxyl radicals (reaction 161) (which may go on to generate further radicals: see earlier), and the products of 'repair' of protein alkoxyl radicals would be alcohols (hydroxides) (reaction 162).

$$\text{Protein–OO}^\bullet + \text{Trolox–OH} \longrightarrow \text{Protein–OOH} + \text{Trolox–O}^\bullet \tag{161}$$

$$\text{Protein–O}^\bullet + \text{Trolox–OH} \longrightarrow \text{Protein–OH} + \text{Trolox–O}^\bullet \tag{162}$$

As would be expected from the occurrence of the above reactions, a number of other phenolic compounds would also be expected to be protein antioxidants. This has been demonstrated in a number of cases with free Tyr, and other phenolic compounds such as n-propyl gallate and sesamol (3,4-methylenedioxyphenol), with these materials able to repair free Trp- and Tyr-derived radicals both in free solution and in lysozyme (though in some cases these reactions were carried out in the presence of SDS) (Hoey and Butler 1984). In some cases it should be noted, however, that formation of a free phenoxyl radicals via such 'repair' reactions may not be wholly advantageous, as such free phenoxyl radicals may then react with a further protein Tyr radical and hence generate di-tyrosine (Heinecke et al. 1993a). Such reactions are less likely to occur with sterically hindered phenols.

A number of studies have demonstrated that, as expected from the discussion earlier, thiols are good protective agents, and can repair a number of well-defined protein radical species. Thus it has been shown that both free cysteine and cysteine derivatives, such as N-acetylcysteine and glutathione, can readily repair Tyr phenoxyl radicals on proteins, with the concomitant generation of a free thiyl radical (reactions analogous to reaction 152 (Davies 1991; Davies and Puppo 1992; McArthur and Davies 1993; Puppo et al. 1993)). The rate constants for reaction of free Tyr phenoxyl radicals with a number of thiols have been determined, though it should be noted (as outlined earlier) that this process is a reversible reaction and repair will only be a viable process when there are routes out for the thiyl species (e.g. reaction with O_2 or thiol anions) (Prutz et al. 1986). The rate constants for reaction with protein Tyr phenoxyl radicals have been shown to be both protein and thiol dependent, with steric effects playing a major role. Thus repair of the Tyr phenoxyl radical in the haem protein leghaemoglobin is much more rapid with Cys than GSH, presumably for steric reasons (Davies and Puppo 1992).

Thiols have also been shown to react with the protein peroxyl radical formed on myoglobin (Davies, M. J. 1990a; Gunther et al. 1995; Irwin and Davies, unpublished data), and radicals formed from a number of protein hydroperoxides (Davies, unpublished data). It should again be noted that the protein peroxyl and alkoxyl radical reactions are not, strictly speaking, repair processes, in that altered amino acids are formed on the protein as a result of this process.

Vitamin C (ascorbate) has been shown to be a very efficient antioxidant for protein-derived radicals. It has been demonstrated that reaction with both free Tyr phenoxyl and Trp indolyl radicals is very rapid ($k = 6.9 \times 10^8$ $dm^3 mol^{-1} s^{-1}$ for reaction with TyrO· and $9 \times 10^7 dm^3 mol^{-1} s^{-1}$ for Trp· (Schuler 1977; Packer et al. 1981; Hoey and Butler 1984)), and that such reactions can also occur with lysozyme-derived Tyr and Trp radicals (Hoey and Butler 1984). The rate constants for the latter processes are similar to those for the free amino acid radicals. This antioxidant would also be expected to react rapidly with a number of other protein-derived radicals, and evidence has been obtained for repair of protein thiyl radicals, protein alkoxyl, and protein peroxyl radicals (Davies, unpublished data). The last two of these processes are again reactions which, though exporting the radical centre from the protein and hence limiting further protein damage, do not repair the initial lesion.

Uric acid has also been shown to repair Trp-derived radicals in free solution, and to repair both this species and Tyr phenoxyl radicals (in the presence of SDS) in lysozyme (Hoey and Butler 1984). Again there is little difference between the kinetics of repair of the free Trp indolyl radical and that of the same radical in lysozyme. The urate radical, in the presence of oxygen, can also inflict selective damage on alcohol dehydrogenase, and possibly other proteins with appropriate key functional amino acids (Kittridge and Willson 1984; Willson et al. 1985).

There are a number of other protective reactions which are limited to certain proteins. Thus it has been shown that bilirubin bound to HSA or BSA protects the protein from damage induced either by aqueous peroxyl radicals (from AAPH) or from radicals generated from γ-radiolysis (Stocker et al. 1987a, b; Neuzil and Stocker 1993). Whether such protection arises from the bilirubin acting as a sacrificial target and hence protecting a section of the protein surface from radical attack, or whether this protection results from the repair of radicals formed on the protein as a result of radical attack remains to be determined. It should, however, be noted that this reaction can also be looked at from an alternative viewpoint; i.e. that the protein is protecting the bilirubin from damage, and hence that it is the protein that is the antioxidant (Adhikari and Gopinathan 1996). Similar 'protection' might be expected with other carrier molecules, though whether these are true antioxidant functions is a matter of conjecture.

3 The biochemistry of protein oxidation in cells and cell-free systems

Here we deal primarily with protein oxidation in cells in culture and in cell-free systems derived from them, leaving consideration of its relevance to organismal function to later chapters. Note that we also defer consideration of markers for protein oxidation which can be used reliably in cellular studies until the next chapter, since the critical issues are similar for cellular and organismal systems, and there are currently more data available on the latter.

3.1 Functional inactivation of proteins by radicals: reversible and irreversible mechanisms

Even in the early studies of radical attack upon proteins, particularly those of Gowland-Hopkins, it was appreciated that functional inactivation was a common consequence. The very large literature in the 1920s and 1930s concerned with radiation damage to proteins also established this fact for a range of enzymes (see Chapter 1). However it was only since about 1960 that the chemical mechanisms for inactivation, and the selectivity of inactivation by certain radicals were studied closely. Here we discuss first mechanisms which lead to limited modification, some of which may be reversible, especially during the radical reactions themselves. Later we consider more extensive modifications which may eventually be associated with gross unfolding of the protein structure.

Adams and his colleagues studied lysozyme (Adams *et al.* 1969*b*; Aldrich *et al.* 1969), ribonuclease (Adams *et al.* 1972*b*), papain (Adams and Redpath 1974), chymotrypsin (Adams and Redpath 1974; Baverstock *et al.* 1974), pepsin (Adams *et al.* 1979), and bovine carbonic anhydrase B (Hoe *et al.* 1981) in some detail. Most of their studies concerned radiolysis in deoxygenated conditions, in which the hydroxyl radical was the most effective inactivator. Radicals which can result in selective modifications (see

Chapter 2), such as $(CNS)_2^{\cdot-}$, $Br_2^{\cdot-}$, $Cl_2^{\cdot-}$, $I_2^{\cdot-}$, and $SCN_2^{\cdot-}$, were also studied. $SCN_2^{\cdot-}$ effected a reaction with an important tryptophan in pepsin which, though the damage can be reversed by the same radical, was effective in inactivating the enzyme. In the case of carbonic anhydrase these radicals modified tryptophan and histidine particularly, but these alterations were not so relevant to the maintenance of active enzyme as in pepsin. In studies on D-amino acid oxidase, the same group showed that near neutral pH, the removal of the coenzyme, FAD, enhanced such selective free radical attack, illustrating again the influence of conformation (Anderson et al. 1977), as previously noted for the effects of the presence of substrate (Chapter 1).

Later studies have further analysed the selectivity of the $Br_2^{\cdot-}$ and $SCN_2^{\cdot-}$ systems, for example in the case of radiolytic inactivation of dehydrorotate dehydrogenase, which depends on modification of cysteine and aromatic residues, without requiring significant fragmentation or aggregation of the protein (Saha et al. 1992). Inactivation by the hydrated electron, generated by radiolysis under deoxygenated conditions (Chapter 2), has also been studied extensively, a recent examples being studies on the inactivation of tyrosinase (Terato and Yamamoto 1994). As noted already, the significance of these selective radical and hydrated electron conditions to biological systems may be limited, though these studies have given useful mechanistic information. Many early studies on enzyme inactivation using radiolytic conditions have been reviewed (Augenstine 1962 also reviewed in von Sonntag 1987).

As we have noted in the Preface, several enzymes contain an intrinsic radical species while in their active form (reviewed: Stubbe 1989; Pedersen and Finazzi 1993), and they have this in common with photosystems of the chloroplast, and electron transport chains of the mitochondrion. In some circumstances, the reactions of these radicals may lead to functional inactivation. In order to discuss this possibility, we first provide a little background on protein-radical enzymes. In recent years, however, primarily as a result of the advent of more sophisticated spectroscopic techniques and the advances made in site-directed mutagenesis, there has been explosive growth in this area and there are now recognizable sub-families of enzymes which use radicals as a means of bringing about specific chemical transformations. There have been several attempts to classify this diverse group of enzymes; the most sensible, in the light of the topic of this volume, is that based on the nature of the radical species involved.

Many of the radicals formed in enzymes are relatively stable species. As might be expected from the link between the reactivity of a radical and the selectivity of its reactions, such radicals would be expected to be the most discriminatory in terms of the reactions they carry out. Thus it has ben demonstrated that there are enzyme systems which involve tyrosine-derived radicals—chiefly phenoxyl species, though there are also enzymes which employ modified species derived from Tyr, tryptophan-derived radicals (and some derivatives), a couple which involve glycine-derived radicals, and a few where the species are not fully categorized. Though the mechanisms of action of these enzymes are very diverse, there appear to be two major roles for radicals in these enzymes. In the major grouping the radical acts as a sink, or store, for a single oxidizing equivalent either as a means of inducing a further transformation or arising from such a process. As expected on the basis of the chemistry discussed in Chapter 2 these enzymes employ the most readily oxidized residues in these reactions (Tyr and Trp and their derivatives). Ultimately, this oxidized species is repaired by an electron or hydrogen atom transfer reaction (i.e. reduction). In the second, much smaller, grouping, which chiefly involves those enzymes employing Gly radicals, the radical appears to be generated as a means of carrying out a hydrogen atom abstraction reaction. There have also been suggestions that thiyl radicals maybe generated in some enzyme systems and that these species also act as hydrogen atom abstracting agents; these processes would again be expected to be very specific, in the light of the known chemistry of such systems, with only the most reactive C–H bonds susceptible to hydrogen atom abstraction by this type of radical.

Though many of these enzymes have been the subject of extensive study over a number of years, the exact details of many of these processes are still poorly understood. For further details the reader is directed to a recent review of this area (Pedersen and Finazzi 1993) and some key papers (Booker *et al.* 1994; Licht *et al.* 1996).

The reaction of these protein radicals with oxygen or other components may sometimes lead to enzyme inactivation, and in some cases this involves protein chain cleavage. For example, the reduction of the intrinsic tyrosyl radical on the R2 subunit of ribonucleotide reductase, which is part of the catalytic mechanism, can be accompanied by cleavage of the R1 subunit into 26 and 61 kDa fragments, respectively, from the N- and C-terminals of R2, and the new N-terminal of the latter is blocked. The precise site of cleavage is not clear (Mao *et al.* 1992*a*, *b*). Similarly, inactivation of *E. coli* pyruvate formate lyase by oxygen or hypophosphite appears to involve reactions with the intrinsic glycyl radical, and is initially reversible (possibly via loss of oxygen from the peroxyl radical species), since the damage is both very localized and limited in extent (Brush *et al.* 1988). This enzyme is found in anaerobically grown bacteria, and inactivation is believed to arise via reaction of oxygen with the glycyl α-carbon radical present at position 734 in the sequence R–Ser–Gly–Tyr–R2. This process results in chain cleavage and formation of an N-terminal oxalyl residue from the glycine (Wagner *et al.* 1992). Serine 733, which would have been expected to form the new C-terminus of the N-terminally derived fragment from the parent protein, was not recovered, suggesting that this species is also altered in some way.

These products are consistent with the Garrison α-amidation mechanism of fragmentation discussed in Chapter 2.

In addition, many oxidative enzymes may generate radical species during their interaction with certain substrates, such that a gradual 'self-inactivation' occurs. Lipoxygenases show such self-inactivation by a modest proportion of enzyme turnovers, and oxygen sensitizes this process with some substrates (Hartel et al. 1982; Cucurou et al. 1991b). For example, the hydroperoxides of linoleic acid generated during the action of the reticulocyte enzyme can inactivate it when iron is available, be it supplied by the enzyme active site or in other forms, and this process is accentuated by the presence of oxygen; indeed the enzyme presents 'hydroperoxidase' activity (Hartel et al. 1982). With lipoxygenases, only limited oxidation of the enzyme polypeptide seems to be necessary, though this has not been fully characterized.

Many different radical species of biological relevance can inactivate proteins, sometimes including those derived from antioxidants such as urate by reactions with superoxide (Kittridge and Willson 1984; Aruoma and Halliwell 1989), and peroxyl radicals (Willson et al. 1985). For example, radicals produced during lipid autoxidation, like those produced during lipoxygenase action, can inactivate. Thus, α-1-PI (α-1-proteinase inhibitor) can be inactivated by reactions involving oxidation of its Met 358, caused by peroxidizing lipids (Mohsenin and Gee 1989). In addition, some of the aldehyde end-products of lipid oxidation have been shown to be potent inactivating agents, as in the cases of malondialdehyde (Chio and Tappel 1969a) and 4-hydroxynonenal (Szweda et al. 1993). Similarly, both singlet oxygen and free radical species can participate in photosensitizer-induced inactivation of enzymes, as studied with purified catalase or within erythrocyte ghosts or K562 cells (Gantchev and van Liet 1995). The photosensitized inactivation of protein kinase C due to calphostin (Gopalakrishna et al. 1992) is dependent on oxygen, suggesting the mediation of peroxyl radicals, and is reversible in solution. However, within cells this process becomes irreversible, and is focused on the membrane bound portions of the enzyme complex, rather than the cytosolic portions. This implies a change in the site and/or mechanism of inactivation under these different conditions. Oxidative events are clearly involved, but require further study.

Stadtman and colleagues have emphasized inactivation in cell-free systems by 'metal catalysed oxidations', usually meaning metal-dependent auto-xidations with ascorbate, reduced nucleotides and P450, non-haem iron-sulfur proteins, or low molecular weight metal chelates, usually with the addition of peroxide or autoxidizable thiols. They introduced this terminology to clarify some of their earlier usage of the term 'mixed function oxidation', which could be confused with 'mixed function oxidases'. Such mechanisms are probably a major part of previously described cell-free oxidative inactivation systems, such as that of *B. subtilis* active on its glutamine phosphoribosyl-pyrophosphate amidotransferase (Turnbough and Switzer 1975*a*, *b*). This early system showed strong dependence on oxygen, and was perturbed by metal chelators, but its chemistry was not defined in detail. It was noted that inactivation proceeded normally in a mutant strain double minus for important proteinases, and that oxidation of a (4Fe-4S) centre was apparently important.

Although metal-catalysed oxidations are highly diverse mechanistically, they all produce radicals akin to Fenton systems because of their metal content, involve the intermediacy of hydrogen peroxide (and hence can be blocked by catalase) and can inactivate a wide range of proteins and enzymes as shown in the seventies by several authors. For example, the carbamyl phosphate synthetase of *E. coli* seems to be inhibited by dithiothreitol by such an oxidative mehcanism, duplicated by model experiments with hydrogen peroxide. Oxidation of chymotrypsinogen, cyctochrome *c*, and several other proteins by ferrous ion and air, due to peroxide reactions, was well defined, and it was noted that the buffer ions have a major impact, such that reactions on proteins proceed more in the presence of phosphate than Tris (Taborsky 1973). Taborsky also noted the formation of multiple species of protein carbonyls, and their labelling by tritiated borohydride. Major loss of aromatic residues and histidine from collagen or from free amino acid solutions, due to reactions with hydrogen peroxide and copper, were described (Gruber and Mellon 1975). Some proline was retained in the collagens, but free proline was converted to 3-hydroxyproline and to β-alanine; losses of aliphatic residues were modest.

Metal-catalysed oxidations were subsequently formalized by Stadtman and colleagues (Levine *et al.* 1981; Stadtman 1991; Fucci *et al.* 1983; Nakamura and Stadtman 1984; Nakamura *et al.* 1985; Stadtman and Wittenberger 1985). Stadtman and colleagues have suggested that this is important for their proteolytic turnover (Levine *et al.* 1981), and for the accumulation of such modified forms in ageing (Fucci *et al.* 1983), as we will discuss later. The inactivation of glutamine synthetase in vitro depends on the adenylation state of the enzyme (Levine *et al.* 1981), a factor which has been previously shown to be an important regulator of both this enzyme, and some multi-enzyme regulatory cascades (Stadtman *et al.* 1968; Ginsburg and Stadtman 1970; Stadtman and Chock 1978; Shacter *et al.* 1988; Stadtman 1990*b*). The inactivated enzyme can comprise hybrid polymers containing both active and inactive subunits (Nakamura and Stadtman 1984).

The experimental systems used by Stadtman and colleagues, like many others, involve generation of a complex mixture of radical species, and while specific damage can be demonstrated in some cases, such as to histidines in glutamate synthetase (Nakamura *et al.* 1985; Farber and Levine 1986;

reviewed: Rivett *et al.* 1985), it is likely that such changes are accompanied by a wide range of other alterations, as indicated in this case by both protein fragmentation (Kim *et al.* 1985), and by complex changes in hydrophobicity. Limited oxidation increases hydrophilicity of the enzyme, while further oxidation increases hydrophobicity (Cervera and Levine 1988). It was initially suggested that modification of a single histidine was sufficient for both inactivation and increased proteolytic susceptibility (Levine 1983*b*), but later, more detailed, studies have shown that while inactivation does occur concomitant upon modification of a single histidine, the enhanced proteolytic susceptibility requires the modification of two histidines per subunit (Rivett and Levine 1990). The latter takes place at a stage by which several other modifications have already occurred, such as that later defined for Arg 344 (Climent and Levine 1991).

The most detailed study of this issue of the extent, or type, of amino acid changes which are necessary for either inactivation or changed proteolytic sensitivity, is discussed below (Rivett and Levine 1990). Using an ascorbate/metal/oxygen system, this work confirms that inactivation occurs when only one of the 16 histidines mol^{-1} has been lost. On the other hand, even when 2 histidines mol^{-1} have been lost, and there is a changed proteolytic susceptibility, carbonyl formation only reaches 0.7 mol mol^{-1}, so that the majority of the altered histidine residues are not present as carbonyl derivatives, strongly suggesting that other products are generated. More importantly, tritiated borohydride incorporation in to the enzyme at various stages of oxidation was studied, by the separation of (unidentified) radioactive peaks using a conventional amino acid HPLC separation method, after protein hydrolysis. Some of these peaks might represent derivatized carbonyls. Eight peaks were partially separated using this procedure, and the authors concluded, as the chromatographic pattern was relatively constant at different times, that the spectrum of products is constant. This interpretation is not very strong, but it is clear that all but two or three of these materials are generated within the first hour of the experiment, which corresponds to the period in which the first histidine is oxidized. After two hours little further histidine oxidation takes place (at least for several hours) under the conditions used. Unfortunately, an un-incubated control is not shown, with the earliest time point displayed being after 20 minutes. It cannot therefore be definitively concluded that the critical event for inactivation, or proteolytic susceptibility, is the histidine oxidation, since it is clear that many modifications are occurring simultaneously. The proportional consumption of any other individual amino acid is clearly smaller than that of histidine, and cannot be detected by the several amino acid analyses performed, but the aggregate of all amino acids consumed could not be quantitated, and so could be rather significant.

Related processes seem to be involved in the hemin-mediated oxidative degradation of proteins, and oxygen-dependent fragmenting process (Aft and Mueller 1984). This is readily observed with myoglobin and haemopexin, though not very effective with albumin. The authors could not detect carbonyl formation or loss of amino acids other than cysteine. Similarly, the ascorbate/iron-catalysed loss of phosphoglucomutase activity can be a subtle process, involving loss of covalently bound phosphate, and enhanced proteolytic susceptibility, but the precise chemistry of accompanying events has not been defined (Deshpande and Joshi 1985).

The glutamine synthetase of the fungus *N. crassa* is also susceptible to metal-catalysed oxidative inactivation, and inactivated enzyme has been detected *in vivo* (Aguirre and Hansberg 1986). Similarly, a careful study has been made of oxidative inactivation of enzymes in living *Klebsiella pneumoniae* (Chevalier *et al.* 1990). Concomitant with changing metabolic pathway expression, several enzymes in this organism are lost during the switch from anaerobic to aerobic conditions. Glycerol dehydrogenase has been the most extensively studied, and it has been shown that this enzyme is inactivated *in vivo* after either a switch to oxygen, or after exposure to hydrogen peroxide. The enzyme purified from cells exposed to peroxide was compared with the native enzyme. Although the preparation was 90 per cent inactivated, there were no detectable differences in either subunit molecular size or amino acid composition (including levels of reduced sulfydryl groups). The lack of gross changes in the amino acid composition is not surprising, as very limited modification appears to be necessary for inactivation. The intact oligomer migrated in gel filtration as if slightly larger than the native, and there was a significantly enhanced hydrophobicity expressed by the inactivated enzyme. This careful and interesing study points to one of the extreme difficulties in studying the role of metal-catalysed oxidation *in vivo*: even the detailed characterization of this isolated inactivated enzyme gave no direct evidence that the inactivation was due to direct oxidation of the protein, though it was clearly initiated by an oxidative affront to the cells. We will return to this issue later in this chapter.

Enzyme and protein inactivation in cells may also involve interactions with species generated during lipid peroxidation. These changes may also be metal-catalysed. For example, Tappel and his colleagues have recently demonstrated hemichrome formation during ferrous ion induced oxidation of liver slices (Andersen *et al.* 1993). In later studies using liver homogenates, they also demonstrated slower glutathione peroxidase inactivation (Andersen *et al.* 1994). In both systems these reactions were accompanied by lipid peroxidation.

Proteins other than enzymes, for example proteinase inhibitors, are equally well inactivated by radical generating systems. The inactivation of α-1-proteinase inhibitor (formerly known inappropriately as α-1-antitrypsin) has been studied extensively, as a result of the dependence of the inhibitor on an active methionine residue which, as discussed earlier, is particularly susceptible to oxidation. A neutrophil cytosolic serine-proteinase inhibitor (serpin), susceptible to inactivation by hydrogen peroxide, has been identified (Thomas *et al.* 1991). Peroxynitrite has been shown to react with a peptide model of the active site of α-1-PI without significant hydroxyl radical formation, and by selective attack on the methionine (Moreno and Pryor 1992). In contrast, Fenton systems inactivate this inhibitor by generating a wide range of lesions (Kwon *et al.* 1990). It has been shown that such systems, which generate a complex mixture of radicals and oxidants, including some with reactivity comparable to the hydroxyl radical, inactivate other proteinase inhibitors, not dependent on methionine with comparable efficiency (Dean *et al.* 1989*a*). Thus, methionine containing inhibitors are not automatically vulnerable, with their susceptibility appearing to depend very much upon the radical or oxidizing conditions which pertain *in vivo*.

As expected from the discussion above intermediates and products of lipid peroxidation, such as the terminal aldehydes, may also modify non-enzyme proteins. Thus the binding of the apoB protein of low density lipoprotein to its cellular receptor is perturbed by reaction with 4-hydroxynonenal at modest levels (Jessup *et al.* 1986), and is grossly altered when suprapathological levels are provided (Hoff *et al.* 1989); the latter conditions lead to protein aggregation.

We need to consider the nature of the reactions involved most commonly in the limited modifications included in the preceding survey, especially in terms of those which are at least transiently reversible, since such reversal might be expected to cause reactivation. Direct enzyme *activation* by radical processes is discussed at the end of this chapter. One of the earliest events during radical oxidation of proteins is believed to be conversion of sulfydryl groups to disulfides and other oxidized species, with the ratio depending on the chemical environment. For example, with lens crystallins *in vitro*, hydrogen peroxide (presumably via a metal-catalysed reaction) causes preferential thiol and subsequently methionine consumption, with most other amino acids hardly altered (McNamara and Augusteyn 1984). Higher sulfides and persulfides may also be produced (Prutz 1992). Conformational changes in these proteins can also be detected (Leader and Mosson 1980; McNamara and Augusteyn 1984). The inactivation of some enzymes by limited sulfydryl oxidation has also been studied, for example in the case of aldose reductase (Cappiello *et al.* 1994); such work has usually involved oxidized thiols such as GSSG as oxidants, to restrict the range of other reactions. Aldose reductase is inactivated by GSSG, upon the formation of a mixed disulfide with the enzyme, and may be reactivated by GSH. In the mixed-disulfide form, the enzyme exists in an altered conformation.

Such S-thiolation has also been observed with cytosolic proteins in hepato-cytes exposed to radical-generating oxidants (Rokutan *et al.* 1989), and reversibly with glyceraldehyde-3-phosphate dehydrogenase in endothelial cells (Schuppe *et al.* 1994*a, b*). Furthermore, during the respiratory burst of human monocytes (but not of chronic granulomatous disease monocytes, which generate virtually no radical flux), rapid and reversible S-thiolation of a group of cytosolic proteins has been observed. As discussed below, it is apparent, therefore, that biological thiols such as GSH and cysteine can influence these processes, either directly by reacting with the radical fluxes, or indirectly by forming reversible bonds with normally free thiols on proteins, such that the protein activity may be regenerated (Cappiello *et al.* 1994; Seres *et al.* 1996). Controlled disulfide formation is of course essential for appropriate *de novo* folding and maintenance of conformation of many proteins (States *et al.* 1980; Jeppesen and Morten 1985).

We focus next on the oxidation of methionine residues, which can be a feature of limited protein oxidation contributing to inactivation, and also one which is reversible in the early stages. Methionine oxidation has already been mentioned with regard to α-1PI, but it is equally relevant to some other proteinase inhibitors (Smith *et al.* 1987; Boudier and Bieth 1994). Furthermore, the proteinase subtilisin depends on a methionine residue for its activity, and also for its susceptibility to hydrogen peroxide *in vitro*; replacement of this residue by a range of others by genetic engineering is effective in decreasing its inactivation by peroxide (Estell *et al.* 1985). Determination of methionine residues in proteins can be based on the cleavage reaction with cyanogen bromide, which is unreactive with the oxidized methionine sulfoxide (Asquith and Carthew 1972), or on mass spectroscopy (Wagner and Fraser 1987; Chowdhury *et al.* 1995). Such approaches have shown that limited methionine oxidation can occur during chemical synthesis or preparative processing of proteins (Milton *et al.* 1988). Selective oxidation with chloramine T or N-chlorosuccinimide may be achieved (Shechter *et al.* 1975), though under some conditions the latter may also cleave tryptophanyl peptide bonds (Shechter *et al.* 1975). Con-versely, a selective chemical reduction procedure for methionine sulfoxide, the first oxidation product, has been developed using $TiCl_4$ (Pennington and Byrnes 1995).

t-Butyl hydroperoxide reacts selectively with exposed methionines in isolated proteins, while hydrogen peroxide is also selective for methionines, but reats with the less exposed methionines also (Keck 1996). These reactions may be molecular reactions rather than radical-mediated pro-cesses. Similarly, isolated human erythrocyte glycophorin, when exposed to a 10-fold molar excess of ozone, undergoes loss of both methionines, and becomes resistant to cleavage by cyanogen bromide, while other amino acids are retained (Banerjee and Mudd 1992). Ferrate can selectively oxidize a methionine in *E. coli* DNA polymerase 1 (Basu *et al.* 1987), though it is less discriminating with free amino acids and attacks the amino group rather than the thioether (Rush and Bielski 1995). Isolated glyceraldehyde-3-phosphate dehydrogenase also undergoes selective methione oxidation by ozone, but in this case cysteine and aromatic residues are also oxidized (Knight and Mudd 1984). Several inhibitors of neutrophil neutral proteinases show significant oxidation of methionine, with lesser oxidation of histidine and aromatics when exposed to ozone (Smith *et al.* 1987); analogous results have between obtained with isolated *E. coli* glutamine synthetase and bovine serum albumin during oxidation by ozone (Berlett *et al.* 1996). During the respiratory burst of neutrophils, triggered by fMLP, the peptide is itself inactivated through methionine oxidation (Rossi *et al.* 1983).

The oxidation of protein methionines may be reversible at two stages. Firstly, the initial radical species derived from methionine by one-electron oxidation may be reduced by the water-soluble tocopherol analogue, Trolox, as discussed in Chapter 2 (Bisby *et al.* 1984). Secondly, the first stable oxidation product of the methionine thioether moiety, methionine sulfoxide, can be reduced by a specialised reductase present in a wide variety of mammalian cells (Brot *et al.* 1995; Moskovitz *et al.* 1995; Moskovitz *et al.* 1996). This process may reactivate α-1-PI (Mohsenin and Gee 1989). The enzyme shows stereospecificity with artificial substrates, but the significance of this for protein substrates remains to be established (Minetti *et al.* 1994). Once methionine sulfoxide has been oxidized further to the sulfone (e.g. in the case of whey proteins (Nielsen *et al.* 1985)) the reductase is no longer able to reverse the process. The field of methionine oxidation and reduction has been reviewed (Vogt 1995) and the argument is presented there that the process may be a biological control mechanism, analogous to the reversible thiolation discussed above. Other repair mechanisms exist for damaged protein functions such as cis-prolines and iso-aspartyl residues (reviewed: Visick and Clarke 1995) but these are of limited relevance to radical damage.

Schiff bases, the transient products of reactions between carbonyl functions and amino groups, are formed during exposure of proteins to lipid aldehydes (such as malondialdehyde and 4-hydroxynonenal (Kautiainen 1992)), to autoxidizing sugars (which form vicinal dicarbonyl compounds), and to amino acid aldehydes (see Chapter 2). Since the initial adducts formed in these reactions are unstable (Yim *et al.* 1995), they too may play a role in reversible inactivation, as reversal of Schiff base formation can occur. However, Schiff base formation is often very rapidly followed by Amadori rearrangements (in the case of sugars (Wells-Knecht, M. C. *et al.* 1995)) and so this reversal route may be of limited importance. Furthermore, recent studies have indicated that with certain carbonyls, Schiff base formation may be subsidiary to Michael addition reactions in the case of lipids (Bruenner *et al.* 1995; Nadkarni and Sayre 1995). In insulin (which contains no cysteine) histidines are selecively modified by 4-HNE (4-hydroxynonenal) by Michael addition (Uchida and Stadtman 1992*a*). The thioether linkage of SH-proteins with 4-HNE may be somewhat selectively cleaved with Raney nickel (Uchida and Stadtman 1992*b*), but the applicability of this approach to complex biological samples is not clear. In the case of dialdehydes, Schiff base formation and Michael addition appear to be simultaneous, forming cross-links between two lysines (Riley and Harding 1993; Cohn *et al.* 1996). 4-HNE can inactivate glucose-6-phosphate dehydrogenase and glyceraldehyde-3-phosphate dehydrogenase, and in the latter case both intra- and intermolecular cross linking may be important (Szweda *et al.* 1993; Uchida and Stadtman 1993). During hypochlorite oxidation of LDL, in which protein is the preferential target, amino acid aldehydes derived from lysine are believed to be responsible for the formation of protein cross-links; this reaction is initially reversible (Hazell *et al.* 1994).

3.2 Protein unfolding after radical attack

Some of the examples of limited chemical modification of proteins mentioned above appear to involve very little unfolding, as judged by a number of techniques including intrinsic fluorescence, fluorescence probes such as aniline naphthalene sulfonate (ANS), hydrophobic chromatography, and circular dichroism. In the case of the multi-subunit enzyme, glutamine synthetase, limited oxidation by a metal/ascorbate system can, as mentioned above, give rise to hybrids containing both fully active and damaged subunits, as judged by interactions with substrate molecules (Nakamura and Stadtman 1984). The observation that the adenylation state of the subunits also affects this process is interesting, as this involves only limited conformational change; and it parallels the observations of Adams and colleagues on the protection of proteins by FAD during pulse radiolysis with selective radicals. *In vivo*, changes in glycerol dehydrogenase during exposure of *Klebsiella pneumoniae* to hydrogen peroxide (Chevalier *et al.* 1990) similarly involve little change in size and only slight hydrophobicity increases. In agreement with this, only small free energy changes (0.25–0.5 kJ mol^{-1}) seem to be involved in the inactivation of glutamine synthetase *in vitro* (Fisher and Stadtman 1992).

Several other *in vitro* studies have noted that under physiological conditions the formation of species of changed size from the parent protein is quite limited. For example, when bovine serum albumin is exposed to radiolytic attack by hydroxyl radicals in the presence of oxygen, dose-dependent generation of smaller fragments is apparent by SDS gel electrophoresis; yet when the protein is subjected to non-denaturing size separation by HPLC, only small proportions of molecules of reduced size are observed (Dean *et al.* 1986*b*; Wolff *et al.* 1986). Under non-aerated conditions, the hydroxyl radical causes substantial cross-linking, which can be observed with both techniques to result in larger moieties than the initial protein. Similar observations have been made with lens crystallins exposed to prolonged autoxidation *in vitro* (Dean *et al.* 1986b; Wolff *et al.* 1986), and have been extended in the work of Spector and his colleagues (Wang and Spector 1995) who have identified aggregates by both light scattering and size-exclusion chromatography.

While protein modifications which cause aggregation will necessarily alter the protein size, those which cause breakage of the main chain may not initially do so, since the fragments may remain associated with the parent molecule in a conformation which is sometimes only minimally altered. This is true of certain membrane proteins: for example, (non-oxidatively) fragmented band 3 of bovine erythrocyte membranes generated by chymotrypsin, and solubilized in detergent. The two fragments remain associated, and only partly unfolded unless denaturants are supplied (Makino and Nakashima 1982). Similarly, it is found that large protein fragments resulting from recombinant technology often form complexes approximating to the conformation of the native parent protein, and this can facilitate peptide bond synthesis by the reverse reaction of proteinases to form the parent molecule (Proudfoot *et al.* 1989).

Such conclusions are consonant with a recent study of damage to acetylcholinesterase by iron/edta/ascorbate/hydrogen peroxide (Weiner *et al.* 1994), in which UV and fluorescence changes were observed, together with fragmentation and increased ANS binding, while the molecule yet retained its (native) dimeric form. In this case, however, tertiary structure was largely lost, to form a 'molten globule'. Protein fragmentation is discussed in more detail in the following section.

In the case of glutamine synthetase, and several other enzymes, it has been shown that the changes needed to cause inactivation are sufficiently limited as to not bring about drastic conformational change. On the other hand, limited oxidation of glyceraldehyde-3-phosphate dehydrogenase and alcohol dehydrogenase by singlet oxygen or hydroxyl radicals causes intrinsic fluorescence changes (Prinsze *et al.* 1990). This raises the issues of whether a limited conformational change can be functionally reversible, independent of repair of the chemical lesions which were responsible for it; and similarly, whether large-scale unfolding can be reversed. Limited unfolding can clearly be reversed (Prinsze *et al.* 1990). Unfortunately, there seem to have been no systematic studies to date on the possibility of refolding proteins which have been extensively damaged by radicals.

The importance of correct SH -----> S–S oxidation during refolding of expressed proteins, or those which have been oxidatively 'jumbled' at their cysteines, is well known (States *et al.* 1980; Bolewska *et al.* 1995). The roles and redox mechanisms of protein disulfide isomerase in achieving this are partly understood (Ostermeier *et al.* 1996; Walker *et al.* 1996), and will not be discussed in detail here. Similarly, the importance of chaperonins for correct (non-radical) oxidation of SH groups to S–S functions shortly after synthesis, within the endoplasmic reticulum, has been widely studied (Yamashita *et al.* 1996). The conformations of a given polypeptide sequence are, in theory, exchangeable with each other, but the energy barriers involved in such refolding may often be too great for the exchange to occur at a detectable rate under physiological conditions. Furthermore, recent studies of folding of newly-synthesised proteins indicate the possible importance of 'nucleation' steps in the pathway, making it unlikely that all conformational paths are explored (Flanagan *et al.* 1993; Walker *et al.* 1996). One can conclude from these studies that the likelihood of refolding of a substantially damaged, oxidized protein is extremely limited, even when it is recognized by chaperonins.

However, *during* oxidative stress, at which time partially unfolded proteins may exist, chaperonins may protect against irreversible denaturation. This, at present, can only be inferred from correlations between the induction of oxidative stress, unfolded proteins, and heat shock proteins (HSPs), including a range of chaperonins. For example, macrophage colony stimulating factor (M-CSF) enhances superoxide radical output by the cells, and also induces synthesis of a number of HSPs (HSP60, 70, and 90), concomitantly conferring enhanced resistance to hydrogen peroxide on the cells. Such HSP induction may be a protection against autoxidative damage during the respiratory burst, and the chaperonins amongst the HSPs may participate is providing such protection (Teshima *et al.* 1996). A parallel induction of chaperones is caused in the intracellular facultative bacterium *Francisella tularensis LVS* exposed to hydrogen peroxide, presumably as part of its defence against oxidative stress produced by the host macrophages (Ericsson *et al.* 1994). Similarly, human umbilical vein endothelial cells (HUVECs) respond to oxidative stress, initiated by xanthine oxidase plus hypoxanthine, with induction of several HSPs, including at least some present in both endoplasmic reticulum and cytosol (Dreher *et al.* 1995). In each of these systems, a component of the oxidative stress response may be a signal from the complexes of partially unfolded proteins with chaperones, which can trigger further responses.

The lens of the eye is a special case in relation to oxidative damage to proteins, since the crystallins are exceptionally long lived molecules. Thus it is not surprising that α-crystallin has been found to be a chaperonin, restricting the aggregation of other proteins (which might otherwise lead to opacity and cataract). Such a chaperone function operates not only in relation to thermal denaturation of lens crystallins, but also with oxidatively-damaged crystallins generated by an iron/ascorbate/hydrogen peroxide system (Wang and Spector 1995). Exposing cultured rat lenses to oxidative stress leads to enhanced phosphorylation of both chains of this crystallin, yet with little effect on their chaperone activity (Wang *et al.* 1995). On the other hand oxidation of this crystallin *in vitro* diminishes its chaperone capacity, and α-crystallin from senile human lenses also shows decreased chaperonin activity together with enhanced post-translational modification (Cherian and Abraham 1995). Oxidation of crystallins by hydroxyl or peroxyl radicals (generated radiolytically) enhances the susceptibility of the substrates to enzymatic transglutamination, for example, leading to incorporation of putrescine (Seccia *et al.* 1991). This is mainly due to enhanced availability of the intrinsic acceptor sites, rather than to the generation of new sites (Groenen *et al.* 1993).

Oxidation of isolated phosphoglycerate kinase by iron/ascorbate causes unfolding, as evidenced by the susceptibility of the protein to thermal denaturation (Zhou and Gafni 1991). These changes were, at best, poorly reversible by chemical reduction of the oxidized protein. This study is one example, of many, in which proteolytic senstitivity to trypsin (or other proteinases) has been used as a criterion of unfolding, sensitivity being enhanced as a result. However, this classical criterion of unfolding is not always fulfilled when proteins which have been subject to oxidation are studied: for example, Prinsze *et al.* (1990) found ADH relatively more resistant to elastase and proteinase K than several other proteins after limited oxidation by singlet oxygen or hydroxyl radicals. It is also clear that more extensively oxidized proteins may be denatured and aggregated to such an extent that proteolytic access is restricted rather than enhanced, though the distinction between limited and extensive oxidation is, of course, an arbitrary division of a continuum. We return to these issues in more detail later in this chapter. An important component of irreversible oxidation of proteins is protein fragmentation, and when this is extensive it seems inevitably to lead to loss of conformation.

3.3 Protein fragmentation and polymerization

As discussed in Chapter 2 on the chemistry of protein oxidation, oxidative main chain cleavage, unlike enzymatic proteolysis, does not necessarily involve hydrolysis or cleavage of the peptide (amide) bond. Enzymatic proteolysis is effectively irreversible in biological systems, since the energetics of the reverse reaction are highly unfavourable. Only in model systems, and under non-physiological conditions, can this reaction be readily reversed. The other main-chain cleavage reactions of protein oxidation are at least as difficult to reverse, and being somewhat more diverse, it is hardly surprising that no enzymatic machinery for achieving this is known. Thus, oxidative fragmentation can be considered one of the key irreversible steps in protein oxidation. It is for this reason that this area has been concentrated on, and is routinely investigated whenever it is technically possible (Dean *et al.* 1985)

The measurement of protein fragmentation which is not accompanied by the generation of new amino termini is not straightforward, and deserves separate discussion. In most literature it is demonstrated qualitatively, and some of the claims of quantitative measurement are misleading. As noted already, protein fragmentation can be difficult to observe when oxidized proteins are subjected to non-denaturing size-filtration chromatography, because the fragments tend to remain associated. However, denaturing conditions, such as the addition of SDS and reductants, allows ready visualisation of fragments in gel filtration, or more commonly gel electrophoresis, as extensively studied by Schuessler (Puchala and Schuessler 1993). It is difficult to use gel electrophoresis for quantitation of fragmentation for several reasons; and no-one has claimed great precision in doing so. In many cases the fragments are small, and are difficult to retain on the gel, either during the electrophoresis, or during the staining process. Secondly, individual fragments will give different staining intensities depending on their composition and their degree of oxidation, and this is true of both gel staining techniques (e.g. Coommassie Blue or the more sensitive silver staining), and protein assays such as those of Lowry and Bradford (Davies and Delsignore 1987). Comparisons between proteins are also difficult for the same reasons. Since under most conditions fragmentation and formation of reductant-resistant cross-links occur simultaneously, it is difficult to use the extent of disappearance of the parent monomer band from the gel as a precise index of the extent of fragmentation.

What of chemical measures of protein fragmentation? As discussed already, oxidative fragmentation does not always involve peptide (amide) bond hydrolysis, and a number of other main chain cleavage mechanisms have been characterized. Thus determination of the release of new amino groups is not sufficient to quantify the overall extent of such reactions. In early studies, as clearly discussed by Garrison (1987), it was noted that in the γ-radiolysis of gelatin, and several model peptides, in the presence of oxygen, the G value for release of amino groups, representing the new C-terminal of the original N-terminal portion of the polypeptide, was similar to that for the keto acid generated on the other side of the cleavage, according to Chapter 2. Other reactions generating free RCOOH were also noted. The generation of carbonyl functions also cannot be simply equated with fragmentation, since these functions are known to be readily formed on amino acid side chains. G values for fragmentation, estimated by separation of reduced products in SDS, varies between proteins as might be expected, as the extent of competing side chain reactions varies. It is not clear from these experiments to what degree fragmentation is accompanied by the generation of terminal amide functions. Garrison has also pointed out that the extent to which the putative imino-peptide intermediate in his scheme would hydrolyse spontaneously is not clear; it may well be facilitated at acid pH, such as is often used in protein precipitations (e.g. by trichloracetic acid).

What is the relationship between extent of fragmentation and terminal amino group generation? While Davies and colleagues (Davies and Delsignore 1987) found vast losses of albumin monomers after hydroxyl/ superoxide radical attack in the presence of oxygen at 25 nmol radicals per nmol BSA, they only found small quantities of low-molecular-weight (TCA-soluble) amino groups which were reactive with fluorescamine (less than 6 per cent of the initial precipitable amino reactivity). On the other hand, the total amino group reactivity declined by 20 per cent, as measured without denaturants. When measuring amino groups after unfolding by guanidine hydrochloride, we found modest *increments* in total amino groups after low dose hydroxyl/superoxide radical attack in the presence of oxygen and losses at higher doses (Dean et al. 1985). We also found very small quantities of TCA-soluble amino groups. Similarly, during exposure of lysozyme to copper and hydrogen peroxide, there is an initial loss of ε-amino groups of lysine, and a subsequent increase in amino groups, detected on oxidized samples unfolded by SDS; if the lysine groups are blocked by succinylation prior to oxidation, then only the modest increase in amino groups is observed (Kang et al. 1985). Therefore, until there are precise means of quantitating the several fragmentation pathways, the observations on release of TCA-soluble amino groups cannot be used as a quantitative index of fragmentation.

The difficulty with TCA precipitation (or any of its congeners) is that it requires absolute measurement of the materials, and unless one determines Kjeldahl nitrogen or total amino acids after hydrolysis, this is difficult with native proteins, let alone with oxidized fragments. With native proteins the Lowry assay, which is the basis also of the BCA assay, is most commonly used. This methodology depends on copper reduction under alkaline conditions, and gives responses per unit weight of protein which vary by a factor of more than five. Since alkaline autoxidation of aromatic residues, particularly tyrosine, is important in this assay, responses depend significantly on the content of these amino acids in the substrate and the extent of their loss during oxidation (alkaline protein modification is reviewed generally and thoroughly in (Whitaker and Feeney 1983)). Thus, even with protein fragments of moderate size, tyrosines may be absent, or vary significantly in their abundance between fragments. Thus the quantitative response of individual peptides may vary substantially, and an aggregate quantitation may be very inaccurate. Similarly, if the low-molecular-weight (TCA-soluble) peptide-carbonyls are measured using DNPH (Marx 1991), one is faced with the same risk that peptides may vary significantly in their content of amino acids appropriate for carbonyl formation. This may be less of a problem than that outlined above with tyrosine residues, as a larger number of amino acid side chains are believed to give rise to such materials, and hence variations may be less extensive. The extent of further reaction of such carbonyl functions could, however, compound such measurements. In measuring fragmentation of an *individual* protein, it may be found that the release of measured material in the low-molecular-weight fraction is linear with time during radical attack at a constant radical flux per unit time: this at least gives some comfort in such data interpretation. However, in experiments with BSA under hydroxyl radical attack (oxic), it is found that most DNPH-reactive materials are formed in the fraction soluble in 5 per cent TCA, so that their distribution between TCA-soluble and insoluble fractions is not a good index of fragmentation (Dean *et al.* 1985).

Several of the above difficulties are even more extreme with oxidized proteins than with native, since tyrosines may already have been converted into DOPA and subsequent indoles, such that their electron donating (reductant) capacity has been changed or lost, and hence their activity in several of the assays (such as the Lowry assay) decreased (Davies and Delsignore 1987). For this reason it is difficult to interpret studies which compare fragmentation of *different* proteins on the basis of such assays. Thus in a comparison between non-lenticular proteins (such as albumin, ovalbumin, ADH etc.) and lenticular crystallins it was suggested that the non-lenticular proteins were highly susceptible to fragmentation by copper and hydrogen peroxide, while the lenticular crystallin proteins were hardly susceptible at all, unless cleaved beforehand with cyanogen bromide (Carmichael and Hipkiss 1991). While the latter observation suggests that conformation of the native crystallins may be limiting their accessibility to fragmentation, and thus supports the basic observation, it is difficult to be sure of more than qualitative differences. This in turn may be due to the efficiency and sites of binding of the transition metal to the different substrates, rather than to differential 'susceptibility' to cleavage. In other words, no such differential susceptibility might be observed with radicals generated by, for example, radiolysis or decomposition of azo compounds where metal ions are not involved.

A more secure approach to measuring oxidative protein fragmentation is to use proteins which are radioactively labelled at main chain carbon sites (by biosynthesis) or on the side chains, for example by use of reductive methylation (Davies and Delsignore 1987). Iodination of tyrosines has also been used for this purpose, but the generation of free iodide, as well as iodotyrosine, during fragmentation makes this approach quite difficult. Iodination is routinely used in studies of cellular metabolism of proteins and lipoproteins, and in these circumstances, de-iodination is substantial, and a separate analytical step with silver nitrate is used to remove free iodide, in addition to the TCA precipitation step. However, providing removal of the labelling moiety itself can be distinguished from fragmentation, the radioactive approach is probably the most quantitative and reliable.

What has been learnt of the biochemistry of oxidative protein fragmentation using these approaches? The important series of studies of Schuessler and colleagues on the 'oxygen effect in the radiolysis of proteins' stemmed from the radiation biology literature on oxygen sensitization of organisms to radiation damage (Schuessler and Herget 1980; Puchala and Schuessler 1993, 1995; Schuessler and Schilling 1984). It showed that even during radiolytic attack of hydroxyl radicals on albumin, fragmentation is extensive, but selective. With such metal-free proteins, fragmentation is highly dependent on the availability of oxygen. Under anoxic conditions, cross-linking, involving both reductant sensitive and resistant cross-links, becomes predominant, though it is also detectable under oxic conditions; and furthermore, formation of fragments is also detectable during anoxic irradiation, as with LDH in the earliest studies (Schuessler et al. 1975). These observations have been confirmed and extended (Wolff and Dean 1986; K. J. A. Davies 1987; Davies and Delsignore 1987; M. J. Davies et al. 1987a, b). It has been shown that there is also a synergy in radiolytic fragmentation between hydroxyl and superoxide radicals (Wolff and Dean 1986). This has been demonstrated by quantitative comparison of the materials formed by radiolysis in the presence of oxygen under conditions which generate only hydroxyl radicals with those where both hydroxyl and superoxide radicals are formed. A possible explanation for this observation lies in the additional decay pathways available for α-carbon peroxyl radicals in the latter set of conditions via reaction with the hydroperoxyl/superoxide radicals (see section 2.3.2 in Chapter 2).

The site specificity of cleavage is dependent on the nature of the radical-generating system. Thus, metal-catalysed oxidation can induce selective fragmentation as a consequence of the localization of the metal ions at particular binding sites on the target protein, as demonstrated first in elegant model studies by Levitzki and colleagues using $IrCl_6^{2-}$ as oxidant (Levitzki and Anbar 1967; Levitzki et al. 1967; Pecht et al. 1967; Levitzki and Berger 1971; Levitzki et al. 1972), and in the work of Orr on catalase fragmentation by copper and ascorbate (Orr 1967a, b). Subsequently it was shown that there are parallel effects during copper-catalysed fragmentation of BSA (Marx and Chevion 1986), where fragments of 50, 47, 22, 18, and 3 kDa are prominent. However, even during radiolytic hydroxyl radical attack, fragmentation can be selective. The reasons for this selectivity are not entirely clear, but they may include the accessibility of certain sites to the attacking species, the stability of the radicals generated on the protein, and the occurrence of radical transfer reactions, as discussed in Chapter 2. Schuessler has pointed out that the sizes of the fragments generated from BSA by radiolytic HO· attack are compatible with an important role for proline in this fragmentation, which can be rationalized in terms of the stability of the backbone α-carbon radical formed from this amino acid (see Chapter 2). Thus the released fragments have sizes (around 62, 58, 54, 51, 48, 42, 39, 34, 31, and 27 kDa) which could be generated by single cleavages at proline residues, within the admittedly significant ranges of precision of the gel electrophoretic determinations. She also noted that the same is true of fragmentation of haemoglobin (Puchala and Schuessler 1993) and myoglobin (Puchala and Schuessler 1995). In accordance with this, we have shown that proline, together with histidine, is an important site of radical attack on BSA (Dean *et al.* 1989*b*), but were unable to find the predicted product(s) from cleavage at this site, though we could demonstrate new products from radioactive proline in proteins. In other simpler peptide systems, this putative pathway has been demonstrated (Uchida *et al.* 1990). We have now re-assessed the data on the sizes of fragments obtained by Schuessler from BSA and haemoglobin, and considered whether they can be explained alternatively by single cleavages at glycine, whose α-carbon radical is especially stable (as discussed in Chapter 2). In bovine serum albumin, which has more glycines than prolines, and human haemoglobin α-chain, which has six glycines and seven prolines amongst its 141 residues, the observed fragments can be just as readily rationalized by cleavage at glycine. With myoglobin, there are only four prolines, yet seven major fragments (Puchala and Schuessler 1995), and the authors describe two as 'not expected' and indicative of 'another radiosensitive site'. With 14 glycines, even granted that two are terminal, it is easy to envisage the formation of all the fragments by single cleavages at glycines. Glycine also seemed important in the radical-mediated fragmentation of calf skin collagen by a xanthine oxidase system (Monboisse *et al.* 1983), which probably produced hydroxyl radicals by metal-catalysed processes, since it is clear that the primary superoxide produced is inactive in chain breakage. Here 90 per cent of the N-terminal amino acids generated by fragmentation were glycine, even though the parent molecule only contains roughly one-third of its residues as glycine. Other studies of proline/glycine model peptides show complementary results with increasing glycine N-terminal generation from oligopeptides which initially contain proline N-termini, but these results can be explained by selective fragmentation at the proline (Kato *et al.* 1992). Comparison of the data from several papers suggests that the fragments from metal/peroxide and radiolytic systems are distinct; this has been confirmed by direct comparison (Hunt et al. 1988a, b).

It is notable that in a series of papers with peptides, synthetic poly-peptides, and a few proteins, studied in largely organic (denaturing) solvents, Elad and colleagues have described selective UV-photochemically induced alkylation of glycine residues by agents such as toluene or 1-butene (Sperling and Elad 1971a, b). The limited studies with proteins (Sperling and Elad 1971a) presented data on photoalkylation of lysozyme in largely organic solution, and while demonstrating alkylation of glycines by 1-butene, also showed proportionally greater destruction of histidine, cysteine, methionine, tyrosine, and tryptophan, which was independent of the alkylating agent, and only slightly inhibited by phenol. The mechanism of the alkylation was not closely defined (though it was proposed to involve a glycyl α-carbon radical reacting with a radical derived from the alkylating agent), and indeed there was only a limited attempt to assess alkylation of other residues. Thus the relevance of these studies to the selectivity of radiation or radical attack on proteins is quite restricted. The importance of glycine during radical attack on proteins in aqueous physiological environments will only be resolved by protein sequencing of the fragments from such systems.

With haemoglobin, the extent of fragmentation induced by radiolysis is very similar when carried out in both the presence and absence of oxygen (unlike the situation with albumin). This presumably arises because of the iron atom present in the protoporphyrin IX prosthetic group. This transition metal may generate sufficient oxygen from the hydrogen peroxide generated during radiolysis to permit fragmentation and restrict cross-linking. A similar type of process may also explain why cross-linking in the copper/hydrogen peroxide system with albumin is negligible (Marx and Chevion 1986). Both aggregation and fragmentation can be observed in a similar system with lysozyme (Kang et al. 1985), but the aggregation is coincident in time with the loss of lysine amino groups, and was probably largely non-covalent. Selective protein fragmentation has also been observed with the apoB protein of LDL during either radiolysis or metal-ion-catalysed damage (Bedwell et al. 1989). In this last case, however, it is difficult to assess the relevance of cleavage at proline or glycine residues, due to the difficulty is measuring the sizes of the (large) fragments with sufficient precision.

The mechanisms of protein covalent cross-linking in the presence of oxygen, have been particularly well studied by Guptasarma and colleagues (Guptasarma et al. 1992). Using several proteins, chosen so as to lack one of either tyrosine, tryptophan, or histidine, they indicated the importance of histidine in such cross-linking, confirming the comparative approach by studies in which the residue was blocked with DEPC. As observed in other systems, they also found that lysine was involved, again by blocking studies.

In the tyrosine containing proteins, BPTI (bovine pancreatic trypsin inhibitor), RNAase A, and the crystallins, di-tyrosine cross-links were not observed, but oxygen was present, and thus would have inhibited radical-radical recombination.

Guptasarma et al. (1992) point out that in the tyrosine lacking protein, melittin, hydroxyl radicals can induce changes in protein fluorescence spectra (e.g. ex c. 320 em c. 405) characteristic of di-tyrosine in proteins, yet clearly due to other products, such as tryptophan derivatives. Thus they caution against the identifcation of di-tyrosine on this basis, and comment on the likelihood that there is an additional requirement, beyond limitation of oxygen, for structural proximity of the tyrosines to permit cross-linking, as can occur in calmodulin. However, in some cases it has also been claimed that anoxic, and to a lesser extent oxic, irradiation of insulin, RNAase, and other proteins generated di-tyrosine, detectable in protein hydrolysates by Bio-gel P2 chromatography and fluorescence detection (Boguta and Dancewicz 1983). Unfortunately, the inconsistencies in chromatographic profiles, and the possible conflation with pyridinoline derivatives, undermine this interpretation. For definitive definition, it is necessary to use contemporary HPLC separations, verified by mass spectral criteria, as well as fluorescence, diode array spectra (Eiserich et al. 1996), and co-elution. This has been done for exampe in MPO catalysed oxidation of proteins, and also incorporation of exogenous tyrosine in di-tyrosines with endogenous tyrosines (Francis et al. 1993; Heinecke et al. 1993a). Unfortunately, experiments continue to be published with inadequate verification of di-tyrosine formation in complex systems, such as intact cells, in which it has been claimed as a marker of oxidized proteins and their metabolism (Giulivi and Davies 1993).

Aggregation of fibrinogen due to oxidative attack catalysed by copper and ascorbate is probably a rather special case, since peptide chain cleavage, involving release of some small peptides, may lead to the subsequent unfolding and aggregation (Marx and Chevion 1985; Karpel et al. 1991; Marx 1991), as it does during proteolytic conversion of fibrinogen to fibrin. Fibrinogen appears to be the protein most sensitive to in vitro metal-catalysed carbonyl formation during plasma oxidation (Shacter et al. 1994), and this susceptibility does not appear to be substantially influenced by its carbohydrate moiety (Lee and Shacter 1995). These authors also noted that while oxidized purified fibrinogen is normally cleaved by thrombin, the resulting products do not aggregate properly to form clots (Shacter et al. 1995), in essential agreement with earlier studies on deficiencies in clotting after exposure of fibrinogen to irradiation (Rieser 1956; Rieser and Rutman 1957). It is not entirely clear how this can be reconciled with the earlier results of Marx and colleagues, as both studies were done with isolated fibrinogen.

3.4 Protein oxidation and antioxidation in soluble, membrane-bound, and lipoproteins

In this section we will first compare the features of radical damage to proteins in solution, be it in isolation, or in protein mixtures, with those of membrane proteins and lipoproteins. Building on this, we will then consider the mechanisms which may be used intra- or extracellularly to protect against such reactions.

3.4.1 Protein oxidation in solution, in membranes and in lipoproteins

Our purpose here is not to reiterate the features of oxidation of soluble proteins discussed in Chapter 2, nor the discussion of functional inactivation and protein fragmentation in the section preceding this. Rather, we wish to reveal how the immediate environment of polypeptides influences the nature and extent of their reactions with radicals. In this subsection we will consider these reactions without regard to the possible presence of specialized, mainly non-protein antioxidants, to which we will turn in Section 3.4.3.

With protein solutions, the key factors influencing radical interactions are the concentration of protein present, the nature and relative concentrations of the different proteins (and other potential scavengers), and the nature, extent, and location of the radical flux. Thus the yield of protein oxidation products for a given radiolytic radical flux increases with protein concentration until the system is saturated, in the sense that all incident radicals react with the protein rather than with other components such as buffer ions, or with each other. This principle is the same as is used in the manipulation of radiolytic systems described in Chapter 2, such that all hydroxyl radicals can be converted to superoxide radicals in the presence of sufficiently high concentrations of formate and oxygen. It is also applicable to radicals generated by means of the decomposition of thermolabile azo-compounds, such as AAPH. In such saturating conditions, different proteins in a mixture can be expected to interact with a proportion of the incident radicals, dependent on their relative volume occupancy and their relative rate constants for reaction; though the latter are often similar for proteins. Whether this then locates the damage to the proteins in the same proportion depends on two major factors: first, whether the conditions permit interprotein transfer of radicals; and second, whether the oxidation chains on the individual proteins are comparable in length.

There is limited information available on these factors, particularly the latter. Intrapeptide and protein transfer of radicals has been directly demonstrated and discussed in Chapter 2. Indirect evidence also suggests that such reactions occur in that, as discussed already, aromatic and ring residues are normally damaged more extensively than aliphatic residues, even though all amino acids are usually damaged to a significant degree. Interchain interactions are a prerequisite for cross-linking reactions, some of which, like those involving di-tyrosine formation, require radical-radical reaction. These, unfortunately, give little information as to the extent of radical transfer, other than to indicate that proximity considerations may be permissive.

With Fenton systems and other metal-catalysed oxidations, the location of the active transition metal becomes important, and since residues such as His, Cys, and Met are particularly important in binding metals, they may localize the reactions to their vicinity. The differential capacity of proteins to bind metals often renders them redox inactive (as in the case of some binding sites on specialized proteins such as transferrin, lactoferrin) or conversely may present them in active forms. This will further influence the distribution of damage amongst the population of different proteins present in a solution. Again, few studies have directly addressed the quantitative differences in distribution of damage in such heterogeneous systems.

It is well established that lipid radicals may damage proteins as outlined in Chapter 2 (Roubal and Tappel 1966a, b; Chio and Tappel 1969a, b), reviewed: Tappel 1973). The specificities of such reactions are distinct from those observed in radiolytic systems, even though these processes were initially called radiomimetic (Tappel 1975). This has been revealed, for example, by protein fragmentation patterns in model aqueous-multiphasic systems (Hunt et al. 1988b), even though in the dry state, the cleavages include some due to the α-amidation route (Zirlin and Karel 1969) which seem to be decreased in the presence of water. In reactions with lipid hydroperoxides and soluble proteins present, in which metal-catalysed actions are again central, the selectivity of amino acid consumption in the protein varies somewhat from case to case, as might be expected if site specificity plays a role (Gamage and Matsushita 1973; Gardner 1979). As with radiolytic attack, some interconversions of amino acids are observed after amino acid hydrolysis (e.g. histidine to aspartate (Karel et al. 1975)), and in the dry state, protein radicals ($g = 2.0052$–2.0061 depending on the protein (Schaich and Karel 1975)). Furthermore, protein inactivation by peroxidizing lipid is often associated with the incorporation of lipid components into the protein (e.g. with RNAase and linoleic acid (Gamage and Matsushita 1973)). Thus in a membrane protein one might expect both competition and interaction between protein and lipid oxidation. Early studies have shown that the inactivation of purified and membrane-bound acetylcholinesterase, by redox cycling agents such as ascorbate, or the favism-inducers isouramil and divicine, with copper are rather similar

(Shinar *et al.* 1983; Navok and Chevion 1984). This could be explained if a site-specific metal-ion-catalysed reaction were involved, such that whether free or membrane-bound, the protein localized the functional metal ions on its surface.

In Chapter 2 we also discussed the chemistry of derivatization of proteins by aldehydic end-products of lipid peroxidation, notably MDA and 4-HNE.

Tappel has reviewed the early studies on relationships between lipid and protein oxidative damage in biological membranes (Tappel 1975). He has particularly emphasized the fluorescent cross-links which can form between the lipid oxidation products and proteins, and their possble contribution to ceroid, lipofuschin, and other 'age pigments' found in cells. However, the demonstration of generation of such fluorophores *in vitro* has not generally been followed by the precise chemical definition of the components, such that it can be confirmed that the *in vivo* material is identical to any of them. As we will discuss further in Chapter 5, the detailed constitution of lipofuschin *in vivo* is still unclear. More detailed chemistry of these systems was discussed by Gardner in his careful review (Gardner 1979).

We have more recently undertaken a systematic comparison of radical damage to proteins in the presence or absence of membrane structures, using the soluble protein, albumin, and the membrane-bound protein, monoamine oxidase (MAO). MAO was studied in otherwise intact rat liver mitochondrial outer membranes, by labelling with the radioactive, covalent-binding, site-directed inhibitor pargyline. This, of course, necessitates studying already inactivated molecules of the enzyme. The labelled enzyme can be delipidated, permitting comparison of the reactions in the presence and absence of lipid. In a series of studies (Dean *et al.* 1986*a*, *b*; Dean and Cheeseman 1987; Thomas *et al.* 1989*a*) using both radiolytic and metal-ion-catalysed oxidation, we showed that the presence of lipid diverts some radical reactions from the protein, giving rise to concomitant lipid oxidation. This results in a lower yield of protein fragmentation than observed with either MAO in the absence of lipid, or BSA under similar conditions (in terms of the number of radical hits per mole protein). Furthermore, lipid oxidation products, presumed to be hydroperoxides, can give rise to a further burst of metal-catalysed radical production, which further damages the protein. For example, an irradiated, metal-ion-free, membrane-bound MAO sample, subsequently exposed to added metal ions, gave further fragmentation, which was not nearly as extensive when delipidated MAO was used. Further modification of such proteins by carbonyl-containing products of lipid peroxidation has already been mentioned.

Model systems have been studied in order to further understand these interactions. Thus the influence of the localization of the radical flux in relation to the target, soluble or membrane-bound proteins, has been investigated (Dean *et al.* 1991). This was done using the two commonly used thermolabile peroxyl radical generators, AAPH and AMVN, which are, respectively, hydrophilic and hydrophobic; the latter can therefore be localized within membranes or liposomes. This study assessed amino acid oxidation and fragmentation of BSA and MAO of mitochondrial membranes, and compared these two radical-generating systems. In both cases the peroxyl radicals formed from these initiators in the presence of oxygen were found to fragment the proteins, in agreement with earlier studies on amino acid peroxyl radicals (Wolff and Dean 1986). The AAPH was always found to be effective, whereas the membrane-contained AMVN induced little damage on the BSA present in aqueous solution, or on the MAO present in separate membranes. Trolox C and α-tocopherol could protect the membrane protein, though only the former could protect the soluble protein. Thus, topology is a key influence on radical-protein inter-actions, and it was also shown that lipid radicals contributed to the protein damage in these model systems. A separate study showed that sequestration of copper ions (used as a pseudo Fenton reaction component), or the target protein albumin, within liposomes, restricted their capacity to react with components outside the liposomes, and again indicated roles for lipid peroxidation in protein damage (Hunt and Dean 1989).

Thus the presence of proteins in (or inside) membrane bilayers has dramatic effects on their oxidation reactions, and may also be expected to somewhat stabilize their conformation against changes induced by oxida-tion, making repair of limited damage the more feasible. Many of the same considerations apply to lipoproteins, which are water-soluble, particulate emulsions which contain a high ratio of lipid to protein, often because of extremely hydrophobic cores. The study of peroxidation of low density lipoprotein (LDL), particularly, has received a huge impetus because of its possible importance in atherogenesis, the vessel wall pathology leading to most heart disease. This pathology is discussed in Chapter 5, but here we focus on the purely biochemical and chemical aspects of the reactions of its single protein molecule, apoB.

It is important to appreciate that particulate emulsions have significantly different physical properties from membrane bilayers, and that their interiors have very limited water accessibility, in contrast to membranes through which water can pass. This has significant implications for the transfer of radicals from the external aqueous layer into the particle and *vice versa*. Thus, some regions of an apolipoprotein in a particle are accessible to aqueous oxidants, whereas others are buried inaccessibly in the hydrophobic interior. LDL has been most intensively studied, even though it contains one of the biggest proteins known, apoB, containing 4563 amino acids in a single polypeptide chain. ApoB is extremely difficult to solubilize, so studies like those described earlier comparing lipid-bound and delipidated apoB are essentially impractical, though of course apoB can be delipidated for analytical procedures such as acid hydrolysis, or for resolubilizing (with difficulty) in denaturatants such as guanidine hydrochloride or SDS.

The earliest studies of LDL oxidation were concerned with altered ultra-centrifugal sedimentaion properties caused by oxidation (Ray et al. 1954), and it was shown that both processes could be inhibited by chelators, such as EDTA, and by ascorbate. Data on the UV spectra of the resultant forms were quoted to argue that lipid oxidation must be involved. Hydrogen peroxide was found to be effective only when metal was available, though iron was relatively ineffective. Subsequently, it was found that protein fragmentation also accompanied lipid oxidation in this system; the inhibitory action of EDTA was confirmed, and it was shown that antioxidants, such as BHT, could restrict both processes (Schuh et al. 1978). These workers also indicated that products of the lipid autoxidation were probably responsible for reactions with the protein, including the generation of fluorescent compounds.

Most of the huge number of later studies of LDL oxidation have focused primarily on lipid oxidation, and upon antioxidant consumption, yet a key consequence, and area of interest, of such oxidation is the generation of particles whose apoB has been modified. This is known to affect the lysine residues of the protein, and results in an increased overall negative charge; this is believed to arise from the derivatization of the lysine ε-amino groups, and has important consequences for the interaction of the protein with cellular receptors (Fong et al. 1987; reviewed: Noguchi and Niki 1994). The derivatized apoB binds less well to the native LDL receptor of liver and other cells, which is concerned with its normal function of delivering sterols to cells. On the other hand, it binds better to a range of receptors on cells of peripheral tissues, and on macrophages, including the 'scavenger receptor' which also binds acetylated-LDL (whose lysines have been acetylated chemically). As discussed in Chapter 5, the importance of this is that it offers a means of unregulated sterol uptake, which can lead to the formation of large scale lipid deposits in the cells, generating the 'foam cells' characteristic of the earliest stages of atherosclerosis. This derivatization seems mainly to result from lipid oxidation products, such as MDA and 4-HNE.

However, we are concerned here more with the direct protein oxidation by incident radicals, be they hydroxyl radicals, metal-catalysed radical fluxes, or lipid radicals. It was appreciated early in the study of LDL oxidation that apoB is damaged by modification of amino acids, notably as implied by changed fluorescence properties, largely attributable to the aromatic amino acids (Esterbauer et al. 1992). However, such data are very indirect, since the fluorescence can be influenced not only by the chemical changes in the amino acid, but also by its environment, just as is true of the residues of soluble proteins. Similarly, changed electrophoretic mobility is routinely used to assess the extent of LDL oxidation, and particularly protein modification, but it should be stressed that this is largely an influence of lysine amino-group derivatization by end products. Thus neither kind of data is very informative about the overall extent or nature of the protein oxidation in LDL.

Direct evidence of protein oxidation seems first to have been provided by Steinberg and colleagues, who undertook amino acid analyses of native and oxidized LDL, and demonstrated the loss of some amino acids (for example, proline and histidine, valine and aromatic residues) and, consistent with the discussions in Chapter 2, the increased level in the acid hydrolysates of aspartate and glutamate (Fong *et al.* 1987). Radiolytic studies have examined apoB fragmentation in LDL particles, as a consequence of exposure to known fluxes of well-defined radicals (Bedwell *et al.* 1989). One contrast between soluble proteins and lipid-associated proteins was noted during these studies: the superoxide and hydroperoxyl radicals were quite effective in inducing lipid and protein oxidation in the LDL particles, whereas they were rather ineffective with soluble proteins. This is probably an indirect effect mediated by lipid oxidation. Subseqently, it has been demonstrated that a range of amino acid oxidation products are generated during all stages of LDL oxidation. Furthermore, during hypochlorite oxidation (or reaction of myeloperoxidase with hydrogen peroxide in the presence of chloride ions) the apoB protein has been shown to be commonly the primary target, with extensive alterations to Lys, Trp, Cys, and Met, and lesser changes to other amino acids such as Tyr and His. At lower pHs, such as at inflammatory or intra vacuolar sites, other species e.g. cholesterol, may become a major target (Hazen *et al.* 1996). These reactions give rise to chloramines and their products, as well as di-tyrosines (Hazell *et al.* 1994). Heinecke *et al.* (1993*b*) have shown that if exogenous tyrosine is provided, it can form cross-links with endogenous apoB tyrosines, but whether this re-action occurs with physiological levels of free tyrosine is unclear. Aldehyde oxidation products from tyrosine arising from the action of hypochlorite, have also been described (Hazen *et al.* 1996), confirming earlier studies (Friedman and Morgulis 1936; Nosworthy and Allsop 1956). These re-actions have much in common with the aldehyde-forming autoxidations of tyrosine discussed by Dakin (Dakin 1922*a*), and are analogous to the formation of phenylacetaldehyde from phenyalanine observed by Berlett (Stadtman and Berlett 1991). The detection of these materials may help to distinguish this pathway from other tyrosine oxidation processes *in vivo*.

Limited studies on the oxidation of protein components of other lipoproteins, some of which are much easier to study, being smaller and more hydrophilic, have also been undertaken. Notable are those demon-strating that apoA1 can be selectively oxidized in certain circumstances, with limited methionine modification. As discussed in Chapter 2, some of these methionine oxidation products may arise via molecular, rather than radical, reactions. As with apoB, the function of apoA1 may be transformed upon its oxidation, and it has been suggested that tyrosylated-HDL is a more efficient inducer of cholesterol efflux from fibroblasts and macrophage foam cells than native HDL (Francis *et al.* 1993). Nitration of the endogenous tyrosines is, however, inhibitory.

3.4.2 Protein oxidation as a component of multi-enzyme-system or organelle inactivation

We consider here the role of protein oxidation in the inactivation of small functional units of cells, such as multi-enzyme complexes and membrane electron transport sytems. For historical reasons, we commence with the early studies on phage inactivation by radiation-induced radical fluxes, since these contributed many of the fundamental ideas. We defer consideration of radical-mediated toxicity to other single-celled or multicellular organisms, until Chapter 5 on pathological events.

Radiation-induced, radical-mediated damage to T4 bacteriophage was initially defined by Samuni and colleagues (Samuni *et al.* 1978). They showed that irradiation could cause inactivation, and that the presence of oxygen amplified this effect (the so-called 'oxygen sensitization' effect, which occasioned Schuessler's studies of the oxygen effect in protein radiolysis). They suggested a role for superoxide radicals, as well as hydroxyl radicals, in this process and this was supported by inhibitor/scavenger studies. Subsequently the same group showed that metal-ion-catalysed oxidation was also damaging. The targets studied were phage λ and several of both the T-even and T-odd series, the former apparently showing significantly more rigid surfaces and poorer permeability to reactants such as the transition metal ions. As a result, the T-even series were resistant to such attack, while the other phages were sensitive (Samuni *et al.* 1983, 1984). When the T-odd phages were exposed to copper ions, ascorbate, and hydrogen peroxide it was found that most of the copper ions became bound to the phage, and that oxygen again sensitized the damage. As with the enzyme inactivation studies of this group, this work lead to the concept of 'site-specific' damage, whose location was dependent on the location of the metal ions. In keeping with this, scavengers which compete for potential intermediate radicals, such as the hydroxyl radical, are virtually ineffective, as they fail to reach the appropriate locales in sufficient quantity (somewhat akin to the glutamine synthetase metal-ion catalysed oxidation reactions discussed above). With copper ions plus peroxide, oxygen was not required, again as noted in some of the enzyme inactivation studies discussed above, presumably because oxygen is released during decomposition of the peroxide. The inhibition of infectivity of these species was shown to be due to both decreased phage adsorption and decreased DNA injection.

DNA double strand breaks may also have contributed; the role of phage protein damage was not addressed. Copper could also sensitize the T-odd phages such as T-7 to radiation damage, in a manner consistent with the site-specific proposition (Samuni *et al.* 1984). The importance of protein modification in such events was pointed out by another group (Hartman *et al.* 1979) who showed, also with T-7, that near-UV irradiation damage could be enhanced by non-toxic amounts of hydrogen peroxide, with little DNA double strand breakage, but significant DNA-protein cross-linking. Much more recently, similar observations have been made with RNA phage Q-β exposed to ribose autoxidizing in the presence of copper, in which secondary radical fluxes apparently kill the phages (Carubelli *et al.* 1995). Since the RNA isolated from the damaged phages was still infective, the authors again concluded that protein damage was limiting infectivity.

While phages are unusual systems, functional enzyme complexes and membrane systems in prokaryotic and eukaryotic cells can also be in-activated by oxidative fluxes. We will mention a few examples in which protein oxidation seems involved. Mitochondria seem to have evolved from endosymbiotic bacteria, and hence their inactivation by oxidants is par-alleled by some bacterial responses. Thus hypochlorous acid can damage a plethora of components of *E. coli* (see later), including many cytochromes of electron transport chains, such that aerobic respiration is blocked (Albrich *et al.* 1981). Similarly, rat liver and muscle mitochondria can be damaged by irradation with visible light, or during their own respiratory function, and this has been shown to be enhanced by vitamin E deficiency, involving multiple types of damage including protein alterations (Quintanilha *et al.* 1982). Rat cerebral and cerebellar mitochondria can also be damaged by elevated calcium and sodium exposure, such that complex 1 becomes dys-functional, and mitochondrial generation of reactive radicals is enhanced. NADH-CoQ dehydrogenase is amongst the enzymes damaged, and it has been noted that similar dysfunctional mitochondria can be obtained from humans suffering from Parkinson's, Huntington's and Alzheimer's diseases (Dykens 1994), in which there are also other indications that oxidative damage may be important.

Unlike that of mitochondria, the electron transport system of chloroplasts is continually at risk of photoxidative damage, and several papers have reported on the inactivation of key components of the system during light-induced electron transport. Photosystem II is inactivated by a mechanism which involves degradation of the 32-kDa herbicide binding protein (Ohad *et al.* 1984; Greenberg *et al.* 1987, 1989). Inactivation of this protein seems to be a normal consequence of its activity, but when degradation exceeds synthesis, photoinactivation results. It seems that photo-inactivation then exposes a cleavage site of the respiratory centre (RC) II-D1 protein to degradation, in part by overcoming a regulatory role of plastoquinone in the cleavage process (Gong and Ohad 1991; Zer *et al.* 1994). Ubiquitin is regulated concomitant with this, though its role is not absolutely clear (Wettern *et al.* 1990). Degradation of the RCII-D2 and CP43 proteins may be a secondary process following alterations to the D1 protein (Keren *et al.* 1995; Zer and Ohad 1995).

A special case, revealed recently (Mehta *et al.* 1992), is the abundant soluble chloroplast protein ribulose-1,5-bisphosphate-carboxylase/oxygenase. In plants and algae subjected to a senescence-inducing oxidative stress, the enzyme becomes cross-linked by S–S groups, translocated to the chloroplast membrane, and there rapidly degraded. Translocation to the membrane seems to be an important step in inducing degradation, perhaps as envisaged for translocation of proteins to the lysosomal membrane (Wing *et al.* 1991; Cuervo *et al.* 1995; Dean 1975*b*), but the precise molecular signals for either step, and particularly the role of the disulfide bond formation, remain to be established.

Conversely, the synthesis of some proteins of chloroplasts is light induced, and they may be stabilised until a subsequent dark ('recovery') period, as in the case of the nuclear-encoded thylakoid protein called ELIP (early light-induced protein) (Adamska *et al.* 1992). Indeed, the induction correlates with the inactivation of PSII, and the degradation of D1 protein, and the half-life of ELIP during the recovery period depends on the length of the previous light period. The degradation of ELIP also requires at least low light intensity (Adamska *et al.* 1993). The complexities of this system are only now being determined, and it seems unlikely that photoxidative reactions on the enzyme protein surface are the only important factors.

Like chloroplasts, mitochondria can also, in certain circumstances, undergo self inactivation, in a manner somewhat similar to that described for certain redox enzymes. Electrons which are being transported by the mitochondrial electron transport chains are released unintentionally, resulting in radical formation; these subsequently cause damage. As a consequence there can be disruption of further controlled mitochondrial electron transport, analogous to the chloroplast transport just discussed. However, the initiation of such inactivation has mainly been studied by the addition of external oxidants to isolated mitochondrial preparations, in which situation there is likely to be an interaction between the exogenous oxidants and the endogenous misdirected electron fluxes. We discuss below the literature in which protein damage has been considered, and the reader should bear in mind that there is a much larger literature on lipid peroxidation damage to isolated mitchondria. Indeed, mitochondria are considered the main intracellular radical generation site in physiological conditions, and mitochondrial DNA oxidation has been claimed to occur at a substantially greater rate than in nuclei (Richter *et al.* 1988; Halliwell and Gutteridge 1989; Richter 1992, 1995; Ames *et al.* 1993; Chen, Q. *et al.* 1995).

Thus, isolated rat liver mitochondria exposed to Fe(II)/citrate complexes undergo oxidation, which can be inhibited by EGTA, ruthenium red, and dibucaine (Castilho *et al.* 1994). The authors have interpreted this inhibition in terms of reduction of calcium transport, and it is known that elevations of calcium in the medium bathing mitochondria lead to endogenous radical generation, molecular damage and functional inactivation (Dykens 1994). Similarly, uncouplers seem to lead to mitochondrial permeability dys-regulation by a mechanism depending on calcium elevation, which is followed by radical flux. Castilho *et al.* (1994) have directly demonstrated lipid peroxidation, TBARS formation, and claim to have detected Schiff base adduct formation, and the loss of several mitochondrial membrane proteins (as judged by SDS gel electrophoresis). Together, these changes lead to mitochondrial swelling, inactivation, and lysis. The 'missing' membrane proteins were, surprisingly, found partly in the supernatant of the samples. The loss of such proteins in this complex system cannot simply be equated with oxidation, though this could be a major contributory factor. An interaction with intramitochondrial enzymatic proteolysis, in which a damaged protein is degraded, may also contribute (Desautels and Goldberg 1982; Dean and Pollak 1985; Marcillat *et al.* 1988; Grant *et al.* 1993*a*; Medvedev *et al.* 1993). However, were this the case one would normally expect complete enzymatic catabolism to amino acids and very small peptides, since this is what happens virtually without exception in intact cells.

Reinheckel *et al.* (1995) have studied iron/ascorbate-induced damage to isolated mitochondria, mainly focusing on SDS gel electrophoresis of the proteins, and showed aggregataion, and loss of several of the protein bands, in parallel with inactivation. They also demonstrated formation of TCA-soluble amino groups (expected more extensively from enzymatic hydrolysis than oxidative fragmentation, as discussed earlier in this chapter). Their data suggest, again, an interaction between oxidative damage and proteinase action, though the precise mechanism(s) of protein damage require further study. Others (Parinandi *et al.* 1990, 1991; Zwizinski and Schmid 1992) have focused on the cardiac mitochondrial adenine nucleotide translocase, a 28 kD protein. During copper/*t*-butylhydroper-oxide exposure of mitochondria, this protein initially shows a slight increase in molecular size, as judged by SDS gel electrophoresis, and then is lost from the gel profiles. Subsequent immunological analysis revealed a multistep process, with a gradual increase in molecular size of up to 1.2 kDa, and subsequent fragmentation reactions (Giron-Calle *et al.* 1994). Binding of a selective inhibitor to the translocase before exposure to oxidants could protect it efficiently. The molecular characteristics of the unoxidized and oxidized enzyme have been studied by purification of large quantities, and the incorporation of phosphorus, apparently from oxidized phospholipid, into the oxidized protein has been demonstrated (Zwizinski and Schmid 1992).

Other mechanistic studies on protein damage in isolated mitochondria or mitochondrial membranes have been presented. MAO fragmentation (Dean and Cheeseman 1987) and differential protein modification, as judged by SDS gels and carbonyl assays have been reported (Forsmark et al. 1995). These papers demonstrated a close parallel between lipid peroxidation and protein damage, and their mutual inhibition by, respectively, tocopherol and ubiquinol, and are discussed further in the adjacent section on defences against protein oxidation. Tocotrienols were also effective in restricting oxidation of lipids and proteins of isolated mitochondria by iron/ascorbate, photosensitization, or peroxyl radicals from AAPH (Kamat and Devasagayam 1995), though it is difficult to interpret the relative effectiveness of the tocotrienols vs. tocopherols without more information as to their incorporation into the membranes, and their disposition there, as we demonstrated in earlier systematic studies on roles of tocotrienols in LDL oxidation (Suarna et al. 1993). Mitochondrial vitamin E is not homogeneously distributed in vivo (Quintanilha et al. 1982; Thomas et al. 1989a), and it might be expected that the same will be true for tocotrienol.

In contrast to the studies discussed above in which lipid and protein oxidation seemed to be interdependent, it has been suggested from radiolytic studies that electron transport and ATPase protein inactivation in isolated mitochondria can proceed, even when lipid peroxidation is suppressed by added lipophilic antioxidants (Zhang et al. 1990). However, the measurements of lipid oxidation used were only moderately sensitive, so it is not clear how complete the separation of the two processes is. Protein inactivation was achieved with selectivities characteristic of the individual radical during radiolytic fluxes of either hydroxyl or superoxide radicals (in the presence of oxygen). The significant role of superoxide and hydroperoxyl radicals in protein damage in a lipid environment, as suggested in studies of radiolysis of LDL discussed earlier, was thus confirmed (Zhang et al. 1990). In view of the lack of action of these ambivalent (oxidizing and reducing) radicals on soluble protein functional groups other than SH/S–S systems, one may still wonder whether the action on some of the mitochondrial membrane proteins was secondary to lipid peroxidation, as these two could not be dissociated in the case of LDL.

It is very interesting that Nohl (1979) has argued that age-related losses of function of several mitochondrial proteins are primarily dependent on a changed constitution of their lipid environment, with attendant thermotropic alterations which he has defined. However, direct molecular analysis of the proteins themselves is needed to make such a conclusion firm, and we discuss this issue further in Chapter 5.

Besides physiological ageing, mitochondrial protein damage has also been considered in relation to specific toxins, and two systems in which protein inactivation occurs are relevant here. Oxidation by cerebral mitochondria of paraquat and 1-methylnicotinamide involves complex 1, and as in the case of chloroplasts, leads to both lipid peroxidation and selective damage to a 30 kDa subunit protein of this complex (Fukushima et al. 1995). It is suggested that this may be pertinent to mitochondrial damage in Parkinson's disease, and indeed elevated, mitochondrial, radical fluxes have been claimed to be part of this aetiology. In a somewhat analogous manner, the cardiotoxic side-effects of certain anthracyclines, which are used clinically in the treatment of cancer, are thought to depend on mitochondrial damage induced by redox-cycling of the drug (Davies and Doroshow 1986; Doroshow and Davies 1986), and this has attracted considerable attention. Radical fluxes are known to cause damage to components of the electron transport system, though the relative roles of lipid and protein damage are not clear, and it is apparent that at high anthracyline concentrations, non-oxidative mechanisms may also participate (Marcillat et al. 1989).

Microsomes, representing the endoplasmic reticulum of cells, are the main site of drug and xenobiotic metabolism, and these actions largely involve oxidations carried out by the cytochrome P450 family. Thus, they too perform electron transport functions, and can be the sites of release of radicals. An interaction between endogenous and exogenous radical fluxes, again, can influence protein function in a microsomal system. Thus, Tappel and colleagues (Hu and Tappel 1992a, b) showed that both lipid radical reactions and aldehydic products could inactivate a range of microsomal enzymes including some P450s, with the former mechanism appearing to be quantitatively more important. This inactivation was restricted by both glutathione and tocopherol. Some organic peroxides can be both substrates for P450s and selective in-activators of the system as a result of radical formation (Ando and Tappel 1985b). This inactivation is restricted if the rat microsomes are vitamin E replete (in comparison with microsomes from vitamin-E-deficient animals) (Ando and Tappel 1985a), but the precise relation-ship between lipid and protein damage was not studied in this work. Rat liver microsomes, when exposed to linoleic acid hydroperoxide, lose both cytochrome-P450-family enzymes and glucose-6-phosphatase activity. While MDA formation and enhanced turbidity are concom-itant with this, certain antioxidants, such as tocopherol and N, N'-diphenyl-p-phenylenediamine, can virtually abolish the lipid peroxidation yet hardly affect protein inactivation, suggesting some direct interactions, or some site specificity to the protein damage (Masuda and Murano 1979). This inactivation may be a form of suicidal activation of the hydroperoxide, with the radicals formed from the hydroperoxide damaging the haem moiety of the P450.

The same indication arises from studies of diquat-initiated microsomal oxidation, where a relatively antioxidant-insensitive, protein oxidation path may involve metal catalysis with some site specificity, while another route involves lipid oxidation, and is more amenable to alteration by a lipophilic antioxidant mechanism (Blakeman et al. 1995). Similar implications can be gleaned from studies on the protective action of indolinic and quinolinic aminoxyls against AAPH radical-induced microsomal oxidation (Antosie-wicz et al. 1995): the protection is differential for lipid (as judged by MDA) and protein (as judged by carbonyl formation) oxidation, and in some circumstances lipid oxidation can be virtually obliterated, within the limits of sensitivity of the assays, while protein oxidation remains detectable. Studies with added natural and synthetic ubiquinones, analogous to those described above for mitochondria, have also shown protection against lipid oxidation and enzyme inactivation during oxidant exposure (Wieland et al. 1995). The aqueous antioxidant, ascorbate, can also protect microsomes against P450-dependent protein damage (Mukhopadhyay et al. 1993, 1995). The damage seems to depend on internal metal ions from the cytochrome in a conventional metal-ion-catalysed mechanism (like that earlier defined for microsomal oxidation of soluble glutamine synthetase (Nakamura et al. 1985)); i.e. exogenous metal ions are not required (Mukhopadhyay and Chatterjee 1994a). Mukhopadhyay and colleagues used guinea pig micro-somes, isolated without chelex treatment of reagents and buffers, and the main indication of lack of requirement of exogenous metal was the lack of effect of desferal. They observed time-dependent release of amino-group-containing molecules from the membranes during oxidation, which was inhibited by 60-90 per cent by proteinase inhibitors, suggesting that the majority of the release was enzymatic, though perhaps initiated by oxidative events. Protein carbonyl levels rose from 0.44 nmol/mg protein by about 1 nmol mg^{-1}; α-tocopherol failed to inhibit the events, though this may have simply been due to lack of incorporation, which was not assessed (Mukhopadhyay and Chatterjee 1994). Indeed, it has been reported that metal-catalysed oxidation of guinea pig microsomal membranes, involving both protein carbonyl and lipid peroxide formation, can be inhibited by both GSH and α-tocopherol (Palamanda and Kehrer 1992).

Besides direct induction of protein oxidation chains by lipid radicals (i.e. transfer of damage from a lipid to a protein), as discussed earlier, it is also possible to generate adducts of an attacking radical to the target protein (e.g. hydroxyethyl-protein adducts in alcohol exposure (Clot et al. 1995)), as well as the much discussed aldehyde-protein adducts (Fulceri et al. 1990; French et al. 1993; Moncada et al. 1994). The mobility and function of microsomal membrane proteins can also, like those of mitochondria, be influenced by the state of the lipids: the observed decreased motion of cytochrome P450 concomitant on microsomal oxidation seems to involve first such indirect effects, and then at later stages, protein aggregation, probably depending on more direct protein modification (Gut *et al.* 1985; Richter 1987). As with mitochondria, there have been studies of anthracycline actions on microsomal oxidations, demonstrating lipid oxidation (eg formation of fluorophores) and protein aggregation, whose mechanism of formation was not defined (Fukuda *et al.* 1992).

To summarize, the data on microsomal oxidation parallel that of other organelles, in that endogenous lipid and protein oxidation pathways may be both dependent and independent. Microsomal lipid peroxidation might conceivably inflict damage on nearby non-membrane proteins, as suggested in the studies of glutamine synthetase, and as has been claimed in the case of microtubular tubulin (Miglietta *et al.* 1984), but issues of topology and competition for the reactants will be important *in vivo*, and have not been addressed as yet.

As well as the battery of inactivation mechanisms discussed above, there are also some examples of oxidative *activation* of proteins in microsomes. For example, glutathione-S-transferase is activated by hydrogen peroxide via a mechanism involving SH groups (Aniya and Anders 1992).

Besides electron transport and drug metabolism, another integrated function of microsomes is to participate in protein synthesis. So from the above it is not surprising that there is evidence that radical affronts can inhibit the protein synthetic capacity of microsomes. For example, near-UV or hydrogen peroxide exposure has been shown to inhibit protein synthesis in retinal microsomes and cytosol, in a radical-mediated process, with at least some of this damage arising from protein damage. Both charging of aminoacyl-tRNA (for leucine) and overall protein synthesis were inhibited (Matuk *et al.* 1977). Similar, apparently non-toxic, effects of halogens and *t*-butylhydroperoxide on protein synthesis in liver slices have been reported (Fraga *et al.* 1989). As we will discuss later, evidence for such oxidative inactivation of protein synthesis *in vivo*, in conditions other than those of necrosis, is lacking.

Extracellular matrices can be damaged by radical attack, and consistent with the relative second-order rate constants for reaction of hydroxyl and other radicals with protein in comparison with glycosaminoglycan, we were able to show, as discussed briefly in Chapter 2, that the proteins of intact cartilage discs are preferentially degraded on exposure to radicals in the presence of oxygen (Dean *et al.* 1984a, 1985). This study complemented previous and continuing work on depolymerisation of hyaluronic acid and other cartilage polysaccharides (Hawkins and Davies 1995). For example, in homogenized cartilage slices, copper and hydrogen peroxide could release and then degrade hexosamine-containing materials from proteoglycans, and hydroxyproline-containing peptides from collagen (Chung *et al.* 1984), though the nature of the cleaved bonds was not investigated closely (Hawkins and Davies 1995). Furthermore, other studies, using isolated cartilage proteoglycans in various stages of aggregation, have shown that both protein and polysaccharide can be attacked by radicals, and are consistent with the selectivity of attack we have defined on intact discs (Roberts *et al.* 1987, 1989). In the latter study it was shown that human proteoglycan aggregates, exposed to hydrogen peroxide, undergo selective protein cleavages, notably influenced by the presence of histidine residues (as judged by comparison with rat counterparts in which certain histidines are missing). A cleavage at His 13 of one protein chain is associated with conversion of that histidine to alanine; an additional cleavage nearby occurs between Arg 10 and Ala 11. We return below to the question of whether such oxidative damage affects subsequent inflammatory proteolytic attack (Roberts and Dean 1986).

In this section we have merely described a few examples of the inactivation of complex cellular systems due to radical damage on one or more of their polypeptide components. It must be borne in mind that many, if not all, of the radical damaging systems discussed earlier in this chapter probably cause functional inactivation of membrane systems, whether or not this has been investigated. Furthermore, individual enzymes and proteins do not function in isolation even if they exist as soluble and uncomplexed materials: rather they participate in interactive homeostatic systems. These systems are equally likely to be perturbed as a result of damage to one of their components.

In view of the limited capacities cells have for repairing damaged proteins (Visick and Clarke 1995), it is not surprising that a highly developed proteolytic response exists, making it likely that modest damage can be overcome by removal, and sometimes that excessive fluxes of damaged proteins are sequestered as they are gradually degraded. Only in a few circumstances does the capacity of the degradative system seem to be overcome.

3.4.3 Mechanisms to restrict protein oxidation

Here we discuss the means by which cells limit the extent of protein oxidation, which can be termed primary antioxidant defences, to distinguish them from mechanisms to prevent oxidation products inflicting further damage, which can be termed secondary defences, and which are discussed in later sections.

The first line of defence is the battery of mechanisms which restrict radical generation altogether, and which consume those limited fluxes of radicals which, nevertheless, occur. One can distinguish agents which limit the availability of the transition metals critical for radical generation and transformation, such as the specialized proteins transferrin, ferritin, caeruloplasmin, and the small molecule chelators, such as histidine and citrate (see, for example, discussions in (Halliwell and Gutteridge 1989; Hennet et al. 1992; J. A. Thomas et al. 1995b)).

The roles of these agents are apparently little different in relation to protein oxidation from those in relation to other categories of radical damage. In the case of metal binding, these roles may be ambivalent, in that enhanced solubilization, and sometimes even enhanced rather than reduced redox activity and/or availability, may result from low-molecular-weight chelator association (as discussed for protein oxidation by Stadtman (1993). Metal binding to proteins is an exceptional case (Simpson and Dean 1990). Even the binding of metals to specialized proteins (for example, iron to ferritin) does not necessarily completely preclude their participation in oxidation, as indicated, for example, by the occurrence of oxidized amino acids (containing quinone functions, and so probably DOPA derived from tyrosine) near to the metal-binding sites in purified samples of ferritin (Al-Massad et al. 1992). Metals bound to albumin are also redox active to different degrees, according to their localization and quantity per protein molecule (Marx and Chevion 1986; Simpson and Dean 1990). Non-specialized proteins thus may locate damage to themselves, and affect, positively or negatively, the damage inflicted by a given amount of transition metal upon other nearby targets.

Another unusual preventive mechanism has been proposed by Stadtman and colleagues (Kim et al. 1988) who have identified and purified a thiol-specific antioxidant protein. This soluble protein from S. cerevisiae inhibits metal-catalysed protein oxidation, providing it uses a thiol (e.g. Fe/oxygen/thiol), but not if the thiol is replaced by ascorbate. The protein does not seem to act by sequestering the metal, though it has not been assessed whether it prevents metal ion reduction, nor whether it has an effect on thiol consumption during the reations. Thus, it is not entirely clear whether this protein is preventive, in the sense of removing reactive thiols which might otherwise be sources of radical flux by autoxidation, or whether it is defensive, in the sense of repairing thiyl radicals which would otherwise participate in a chain reaction. Thus, this protein may act like a sulfur counterpart to superoxide dismutase, in that it may dismute $RSSR\cdot^-$ radicals.

In either case, this protein would function in cohort with the system of reversible thiolation which is expressed in many cells during oxidative stress, and which transiently masks protein-thiols which, again, might participate in radical generation. Thiolation of proteins, mainly by glutathione, increases during radical stress (reviewed: (J. A. Thomas et al. 1995a)), and in the case of leukocytes which possess a respiratory burst oxidase, producing a vectorial radical flux toward the interior of phagosomes and towards the extracellular space; triggering this oxidase is also associated with transiently enhanced thiolation (Rokutan *et al.* 1991; Seres *et al.* 1996). This may serve to protect endogenous cellular proteins of the leukocyte from oxidative damage; and the thiolation can subsequently be reversed, thereby regenerating the native form of the protein.

The remaining primary defences are the enzymatic and the sacrificial antioxidants. The enzymatic systems, such as superoxide dismutase, catalase, and the glutathione and phospholipid peroxidases (Halliwell and Gutteridge 1989) act together to remove radicals such as superoxide, and oxidants such as peroxides (hydrogen peroxide or organic, amino acid, and lipid peroxides) which might otherwise undergo decomposition to generate further damaging radicals. Most of these systems are presumed to be in common with defences against damage to lipids and other biological macromolecules, and so are not discussed in great detail here. However, it is worth emphasizing once again that little study has been directed towards the rigourous assessment of protein antioxidation, and hence novelties may well await us. Several specialized systems for proteins may exist, and these possibilities are discussed further in section 3.4.4 on detoxification of oxidized proteins.

The sacrificial antioxidants are those aqueous molecules such as ascorbate and urate, and those lipophilic ones such as vitamin E (tocopherols) and quinols. These can limit peroxidation chains mainly by reducing intermediate radicals to form stable products and a stabilized, less-reactive radical species, such as the tocopheroxyl or ascorbyl radicals, which can be completely detoxified by further conversion ino non-radical species. Here the situation for protein oxidation is very poorly understood, and it is quite possible that antioxidation mechanisms for proteins, especially soluble proteins, are very different from those for lipids. For example, some proteins, such as albumin, contain bound molecules of agents which may acts as antioxidants: in this case bilirubin (BR). As Stocker and colleagues have shown, BR is an important antioxidant in plasma, and when bound to albumin it can restrict damage to the protein. This may be due either to the repair of protein radicals, or scavenging of a proportion of the externally supplied radicals generated by decomposition of AAPH or radiolysis (Neuzil *et al.* 1993). In the case of lipid-bound proteins, in membranes and in lipoproteins, while the lipid antioxidants such as tocopherol may be protective because they limit lipid oxidation chains which might damage proteins, it is less clear whether they interact directly with protein oxidation chains. Evidence from model studies of albumin and MAO, described above, suggests that they may have both actions (Dean *et al.* 1991), since some of their protective actions are maintained even when the only lipids present are saturated, and hence very poorly oxidizable.

Dietary administration of α-tocopherol to rats leads to an increased level in the mitochondrial membranes: this is accompanied by a parallel retardation of both lipid oxidation and monoamine oxidase fragmentation (Dean and Cheeseman 1987). It has also been claimed that ubiquinol can selectively reduce the oxidative Fe (IV) state of haem proteins, thereby protecting other proteins against damage inflicted by this species (Mordente et al. 1994a). A similar defence may operate against the reactions of tyrosyl radicals in these activated haem proteins, particularly preventing intramolecular cross-linking, and the initiation of lipid peroxidation by the radicals (Mordente et al. 1994b). Ascorbate is effective against induction of both lipid and protein oxidation in membranes in some circumstances, for example the apparently metal-ion-independent cases studied by Mukhopadhyay et al. (1995).

The same issue arises more generally: during a protein peroxidation chain reaction, are there antioxidant mechanisms which selectively restrict chain propagation? From the discussion in Chapter 2, it is clear that such antioxidants may not be synonymous with those which interfere with lipid peroxidation chains, since the propagating radicals probably differ between the two systems. In lipid peroxidation, peroxyl radicals are dominant in the propagation phase, and tocopherol, and other lipophilic antioxidants such as $CoQH_2$, are reactive with these radicals. On the other hand, in protein peroxidation, carbon-centred, alkoxyl and peroxyl radicals may all be important, and the possibility exists that there are specialized antioxidants which consume these intermediate radicals, though this has yet to be carefully studied. It is clear, as discussed in Chapter 2, that the water-soluble analogue of vitamin E, Trolox C, and a number of other phenols and related materials, can inhibit protein oxidation induced by a number of attacking radicals (Bisby et al.1982, 1984; Dean et al. 1991; Neuzil et al. 1993). This defence has been shown, in some cases, to be due to the scavenging of exisiting protein radicals, whereas in other cases this action may be due to the removal of radicals which would otherwise initiate protein oxidation. A fertile ground for further study exists in this area.

3.4.4 Detoxification of oxidized proteins

We raised above the possibility of selective interaction with chain inter-mediates in protein oxidation. While the reactions with intermediate radicals are poorly undersood, some information has been gained about detoxifica-tion of somewhat more stable non-radical intermediates, such as the protein hydroperoxides, and the protein-bound reducing species, notably DOPA. Protein and amino acid hydroperoxides are effectively detoxified, ultimately by reduction to stable hydroxides, by a variety of transition metal, enzy-matic and cellular systems (Fu et al. 1995a). Thus, we have shown that incubation of isolated amino acid or protein hydroperoxides with transition metals, with glutathione peroxidase and reductant, or with reductant alone (Simpson *et al.* 1992) leads, at various different rates, to hydroxide formation. In the case of reaction with metals, radical intermediates are detectable (Davies, M. J. *et al.* 1995; Gebicki *et al.* 1995), so that such reactions may not be protective. Indeed, in some cases the extent of fragmentation of a protein containing hydroperoxide groups appears to be enhanced by such processes, suggesting that these materials can initiate further radical reactions. In the other cases, this has not been carefully followed, as yet, but since the conversion to the hydroxide is almost quantitative, it is likely that the reaction is protective.

When cells are exposed to amino acid or protein hydroperoxides in the culture medium, these too are efficiently converted into hydroxides (Fu *et al.* 1995a), and as yet it is not clear whether radical fluxes accompany this. However, it is notable that with some proteins at least, the rate of reduction is much greater than the rate of endocytosis, suggesting that a cell surface system is involved in the hydroperoxide reduction. Several cell surface electron transporting systems which can provide electrons to the exterior are known (Kritharides *et al.* 1995a), and their respective roles in this detoxification remain to be studied. There are clear analogies here with the cell surface and intralipoprotein reduction of lipid hydroperoxides (Christison *et al.* 1994, 1996), though the enzymatic machinery may be distinct.

DOPA is itself a reduced species, being a catechol, but formation of the corresponding quinone does not in itself prevent the molecule from supplying electrons which might initiate further formation of reduced metals, or oxygen radicals, in the manner discussed in Chapter 2. However, a possible detoxification route would be the formation of Michael adducts from DOPA, some of which would be expected to be redox inert. Under physiological conditions, many potential adducts are feasible, notably those formed with glutathione, cysteine, or other amino acids. Cysteinyl-DOPAs have been found in insect proteins, and have been shown to be formed from proteins containing DOPA *in vitro*, but as yet their roles in eukaryotic defence systems have not been studied.

3.5 Cellular metabolism of oxidized proteins: proteolytic removal

The physico-chemical features of oxidized proteins have been discussed earlier in this chapter, where it was pointed out that classically unfolded or denatured proteins have been found to be more rapidly degraded in soluble cell-free systems by many enzymes, such that this phenomenon was often used as a criterion of unfolding. We commence this section by discussing such proteolytic susceptibility in cell free systems, and then continue with more detailed discussions of proteolysis in prokaryotic and eukaryotic intact cells. The general features of proteolysis are reviewed by Goldberg and Dice (1974) and Goldberg and St John (1976).

3.5.1 Proteolytic susceptibility of oxidized proteins to isolated proteinases or lysate cell-free systems

It has been established in many studies that the progressive oxidation of many proteins increases their susceptibility to proteolysis consistent with their partial denaturation (Levine *et al.* 1981; Wolff and Dean 1986; K. J. A. Davies *et al.* 1987*b*), and hence that partially denatured proteins are rapidly degraded. However certain kinds and extents of oxidative modification are associated with decreased susceptibility (Dean *et al.* 1986*b*). More detailed studies have revealed limits to the general trend of progressive increase in susceptibility with increased insult in, for example, hydroxyl radical attack in the absence of oxygen. Thus there appears to be a limit beyond which further oxidation is asssociated with decreased proteolytic susceptibility (K. J. A. Davies *et al.* 1987*b*). In this study it was shown that beyond a molar ratio of hydroxyl radicals to bovine serum albumin of 15, proteolytic susceptibility (to the mixed proteinases of erythrocyte lysates) was decreased, though even at levels of up to 100 radicals per protein molecule it did not decrease below the levels observed for control protein. With hydroxyl radicals in the presence of oxygen, susceptibility in this system increased continuously, in accordance with our earlier findings with trypsin as the proteinase (Wolff and Dean 1986). However, we demonstrated that certain regions in oxidized proteins became relatively resistant to such *in vitro* proteolysis, even at modest levels of oxidation which created an overall enhanced sensitivity (Grant *et al.* 1993*b*). Thus, certain modifications may cause local resistance to enzymatic hydrolysis, and this can often occur during glycoxidation reactions, in which a range of side chain modifications and cross-links can be created (Dean *et al.* 1986*b*; Wolff and Dean 1987*a, b*; Fu *et al.* 1994).

It is relevant here to consider whether modification in proteolytic susceptibility may be imparted by reactions with the aldehyde end products of lipid peroxidation, and/or with other oxidizing systems. In the case of the aqueous soluble MDA, several authors have modified soluble proteins and studied proteolytic susceptibility. For example, Mahmoodi *et al.* (1995) showed that BSA became more susceptible to *in vitro* proteolysis by soluble enzyme preparations from erythrocytes or from mitochondria. However, though we observed an analogous action of MDA on the sensitivity of apoB in LDL to lysosomal lysates, a decreased susceptibility was detected with HNE-modified apoB under identical conditions (Jessup *et al.* 1992*b*).

The range of enzymes and conditions for which these changes in susceptibility apply is quite diverse, but, of course, when one considers lysosomal proteinases, which act at acid pH, one is dealing with a substrate which, if non-lysosomal, usually undergoes a significant pH-induced denaturation in any case. Clearly, the issue of which enzymes really degrade oxidized proteins in intact cells cannot be settled by studies on lysate systems, since the membrane and other more subtle compartmentation barriers of intact cells are missing. For example, a major site of proteolysis in nucleated cells is the membrane-surrounded lysosome, but this is broken in lysates (and absent from procaryotes and erythrocytes).

However, lysate studies have, nevertheless, been used repeatedly to attempt to define the critical enzymatic systems responsible for proteolysis of oxidized proteins. Most notable amongst the studies are those of Stadtman and colleagues, which emphasize the role of an alkaline proteinase, and those of K. J. A. Davies *et al.*, which emphasizes the role of the multicatalytic proteinase complex, or proteasome. It appears that these systems have some enzymes in common. Only the latter studies have yet been followed up with mechanistic degradation studies in intact cells, which will be discussed in a later section.

In the earliest of the studies from Stadtman and colleagues (Levine *et al.* 1981), concerning oxidized glutamine synthetase, an alkaline proteinase was partially purified from *E. coli*, and shown to degrade the oxidized enzyme preferentially in a cell-free system. It was proposed, by analogy with earlier studies on oxidative inactivation and turnover of *B. subtilis* glutamine phosphoribosyl-pyriphosphate amidotransferase (Turnbough and Switzer 1975*a*, *b*) that such a mechanism, whereby oxidation preceded and induced proteolysis, was a feature of normal turnover of the enzyme in intact cells. Subsequently, it has been shown that of the proteinases active in *E. coli* lysates, and mammalian cell lysates, an alkaline proteinase is particularly potent against the oxidized enzyme. Furthermore, inverse correlations between the quantity of active enzyme (lowered) and the quantity of oxidized substrate (increased) in aged tissues have been described (Starke and Oliver 1989). However, these observations might, of course, readily result from a generalized increase in oxidized proteins, amongst which would be inactive proteinase; whether they represent a causal link between the proteinase activity and the increased, oxidized glutamine synthetase is unclear. Furthermore, these same workers observed that short-term *in vivo* oxidative stress (100 per cent oxygen exposure) could initially enhance the amount of inactive glutamine synthetase, and subsequently enhance the alkaline proteinase activities, with concomitant loss of the inactive enzyme molecules, in hepatocytes from rats (Starke and Oliver 1989). Whatever the relative importance of the alkaline proteinases in this loss, the system seems to be an example of a regulatory response to stress, with effective removal of damaged proteins. Treatment of animals with phenytoin, a radical-producing drug, has also been claimed to elevate lipid and protein oxidation products in several sites, though the evidence that the latter also influence *in vivo* protein hydrolysis was limited (Liu and Wells 1994).

Unfortunately, Cutler and his colleagues have reported considerable difficulties in reproducing even the relevant basic observations of Stadtman and colleagues, of increased protein carbonyls and decreased alkaline proteinase activities, in specified aged tissues, reported in these studies (Cao and Cutler 1995*a*, *b*). Whatever the final clarification of these studies, they concern proteolytic activities in cell and tissue lysates, which are not necessarily translateable to intact cell physiological (or pathological) function, as we will discuss further below.

K. J. A. Davies and colleagues have emphasized the role of the proteasome in their extensive lysate studies on degradation of oxidized proteins (Davies 1988; Davies and Lin 1988*a*, *b*; Pacifici *et al.* 1989, 1993; Murakami *et al.* 1990; Salo *et al.* 1990; Grune *et al.* 1995). However experiments from Goldberg and colleagues have been published (Matthews *et al.* 1989), in which complete removal of the proteasomes from cell lysates did not reduce the degradation of haemoglobin, and only inhibited that of radical damaged proteins by 30–40 per cent.

One might wonder whether the information on degradation of proteins in cell-free systems can be directly translated into the situation of the extracellular matrix, parts of which are distant from cells. A significant body of literature on oxidative damage to extracellular proteins exists, compatible with the general features of damage described earlier in this chapter. Furthermore, there have been several studies indicating a synergy between oxidative and proteolytic damage to such matrices, particularly the protein components. Thus, Weiss and colleagues have shown that during neutrophil exposure, radical metabolites damaged connective tissue model-matrices such that subsequent proteolytic damage was enhanced, and this might also positively influence the proteinase/proteinase inhibitor balance (Weiss *et al.* 1986).

Clearly, we must turn to intact cells to understand further the mechanisms of proteolysis of oxidized proteins, particularly for intracellular and endocytosed proteins.

3.5.2 Proteolysis of oxidized proteins in living cells

The intracellular compartmentalization of prokaryotic and eukaryotic, nucleated and non-nucleated cells varies fundamentally, and this is reflected in different kinds of specialization of the degradative apparatus. Most notably, nucleated cells possess lysosomes, intracellular, membrane-bound organelles which contain a high concentration (often up to 1 mM (Dean and Barrett 1976)) of hydrolytic enzymes, active at the acid pH which is actively maintained inside the organelle (see (Lloyd and Mason 1996) for a recent survey of the lysosomal system). These organelles are lacking in bacteria and erythrocytes; yet even in these cells the question of transport of substrates to the degradative machinery exists. Thus, it is known that many of the proteinases present in these cells are membrane bound, and thus not immediately in contact with soluble proteins. Conversely, while there are also cytosolic proteinases, membrane proteins do not necessarily have free access to them. Access may also be influenced by substrate aggregation, as, for example, in the case of Heinz bodies in erythrocytes, which contain especially high concentrations of denatured haemoglobin. As foreshadowed above, these issues mean that observations on cell-free lystate systems, or purified enzymes cannot be immediately assumed to be relevant to intact cells.

Perhaps it is useful to indicate the criteria which would ideally be applied in the process of discriminating the rates and mechanisms of proteolysis of oxidized and normal proteins. One should be able to define both absolute quantities of the proteins which have been catabolized in a given time, and their kinetics. It is also however desirable to know, at the same time, how the pool size of the oxidized proteins and of the normal proteins compare, and what respective half-lives for catabolism are shown by these pools. The half-life is defined in this case as the time for 50 per cent degradation of a pool. Normally, protein pools are degraded with exponential kinetics, which has often been interpreted as indicating that their degradation is random. Random degradation of a homogenenous pool of identical molecules would mean that each molecule has the same likelihood of being degraded at any instant, and also, therefore, in any given period of time. When one deals with a complex mixture of proteins, it is clear that individual proteins possess different half-lives, and yet each shows exponential kinetics, as does the total pool. Thus, each molecule of a given protein normally suffers the same likelihood of degradation. Most proteins in eukaryotic cells have half-lives of the order of 24 hours or longer (Goldberg and Dice 1974), but one can observe, by studies over very short periods, that a much smaller quantity of protein is degraded much more rapidly. Some of these so-called short-half life proteins are well characterized, such as ornithine decarboxylase, which has a half life of a few minutes. Oxidized proteins may have half lives different from their normal counterpart, and knowledge of such information is another way of rephrasing our criteria of knowing both absolute degradation rate and pool size.

It is important, also, to determine whether the conditions which induce the damaged proteins are also damaging to other aspects of cellular metabolism, so as to judge the direct importance of the oxidized protein substrate molecules. Particularly, we need to consider whether the proteolytic systems themselves are damaged, such that a normal enhanced proteolysis of oxidized proteins is submerged through loss of the relevant enzyme activities. Experimentally, it is desirable to study conditions in which the enzymatic proteolysis of endogenous, non-oxidized proteins is not perturbed, and in which the other component of protein turnover, protein synthesis, is not perturbed. Such a balance is difficult to achieve; indeed, as we will see, in many systems it is even difficult to obtain enhanced proteolytic rates of oxidized proteins, and yet maintain the cells in a normally viable state.

Assuming little toxic perturbation of the cells, once we are able to understand the kinetic parameters of particular protein pools, we should be able to assess the mechanistic components of their degradation by perturbation studies, such as the use of selective proteinase inhibitors. In this way, for example, we can ask whether proteinase So of *E. coli* is important, or whether a lysosomal cathpepsin is important. In the case of bacteria, and of yeast, we can also use the tools of molecular genetics to compare protein degradation with and without various enzymatic systems expressed. Such studies often reveal, more clearly than inhibitor studies the redundancy of protein degradation systems. Thus, multiple enzymatic systems are often available for degradation, and deficiency of one of them may not result in an overall deficiency of degradation. Another way of looking at this is that physiological control of protein degradation, which may involve changes in rates of degradation of up to 50 fold, can usually occur without the necessity for changed expression of proteolytic enzyme molecules (Dean 1980*b*). In other words, the proteolytic system is usually present in a considerable excess over the proteolytic capacity required to achieve the physiological degradation rates.

An extension of this is the possibility that oxidative events may sometimes be a trigger for a generalized proteolytic response which is not selective for oxidized proteins. Thus, there may be general regulation of proteolysis during apoptosis, whether induced by oxidants or otherwise; and there most probably is both exaggerated proteolysis by intracellular and intercellular (cell cooperation or phagocytic) mechanisms. This also has to be considered in relation to studies where oxidation is subtoxic, but where the protein substrates, whose catabolism is measured are not definitively oxidized proteins, as in several studies which we will discuss shortly.

There may also be triggering of limited proteolysis as a mediator step in oxidative triggering, which may again not necessarily involve oxidized proteins directly. An example of this has been described in the case of the apparent proteolytic cleavage of the poly-ADP-ribose polymerase (PARP) in RAW 264.7 macrophages, when apoptosis is induced by NO, generated either endogenously or from exogenous NO donors (Messmer *et al.* 1996). In this system p53 expression, and limited PARP cleavage preceded chromatin changes, and in cells transfected with Bcl-2 the PARP cleavage, was largely blocked. Apoptotic systems are discussd further in Chapter 5.

Our understanding of proteolysis of oxidized proteins is obviously still far from complete. In the sections below, in describing a few of the studies in detail, we discuss more of the specific technical problems in fulfilling some of the criteria defined above.

Bacteria

Bacteria exposed to various oxidative affronts have been reported to undergo accelerated catabolism (Davies and Lin 1988*a*,*b*). As a result of the potency of bacterial molecular genetics, this kind of experiment has been undertaken with bacteria with deficiencies of many of the wide rage of characterized proteolytic systems they commonly possess. These studies indicate that the proteinase So and Re systems are particularly important for the proteolysis of oxidized proteins, and that together they provide a heavily redundant system, with an excess of capacity (for example, see Goldberg and Dice 1974; Goldberg and St John 1976). However, the response to cellular oxidized proteins can be reduced in certain mutants, without immediate loss of growth, indicating that the mutant systems are probably, nevertheless, important physiologically. These studies with mutants probably overcome the possible problem that the cells containing oxidized proteins might be simply undergoing necrosis, in which the degradation of their endogenous oxidized proteins, although accelerated, is undertaken by other cells. The efforts to assess this possibility have been limited, but in view of the mutant studies, it is probably reasonable to conclude that this problem is not dominant, otherwise the retention of oxidized protein as cells divide would not occur. However, it needs to be kept in mind as a possible interpretation of such studies.

Erythrocytes

Because of the lack of protein synthesis in erythrocytes, and their lack of lysosomes, they constitute a simplified eukaryotic system, and hence have attracted attention. In some of the earliest studies, Goldberg and colleagues (Goldberg and Boches 1982) used nitrite or phenylhydrazine to induce a putative oxidized protein pool, and then measured a 7–33 fold, enhanced degradation rate, which was dependent on ATP. The measurement of proteolysis did not distinguish normal from oxidized proteins, so that the relative changes in each cannot be established. Other, later studies showed that haemoglobin can be fragmented by exposure to phenylhydrazine, in a haem-mediated process, and it is not clear to what extent this might contribute to subsequent recognition by proteinases (Di Cola *et al.* 1989).

Davies and colleagues (Davies and Goldberg 1987a, b) exposed rabbit erythrocytes to radical fluxes from xanthine plus xanthine oxidase, or from metal-ion-catalysed oxidation, and observed elevated release of the protein degradation product, alanine, within 5 minutes. Haemolysis was observed only after a lag of greater than 2 hours, during which time lipid peroxidation became detectable. Lipophilic antioxidants could inhibit the latter process, but not the enhanced proteolysis. It is difficult to interpret these studies in terms of catabolism of oxidized proteins, since the marker of proteolysis used did not distinguish oxidized from native proteins. Indeed, it might be surprising if a significant oxidized protein pool, such as to contribute the amount of alanine released, could be generated within 5 minutes of attack upon intact cells. There is a possibility that the sensitivity of detection of alanine release is so much greater than that of haemolysis, that the enhanced release might reflect degradation of a very small portion of cells which lysed very rapidly. However, this is not clear, and the interpretation of these data remains to be finalized. In a highly logical and desirable later approach (Giulivi and Davies 1993), it is claimed that di-tyrosine is formed in haemoglobin in erythrocytes exposed to hydrogen peroxide fluxes, and that its subsequent release is a marker of proteolysis of oxidized proteins. The exposed cells clearly undergo accelerated overall proteolysis, as judged by release of alanine, together with at least some toxicity. Unfortunately, the identification and quantitation of di-tyrosine, particularly in the intact cell system, is not always solidly based, for many of the reasons discussed earlier; furthermore, the kinetics and dose-responses of the data presented do not fit the conclusion presented in the abstract to this paper: 'that the elevated rates of proteolysis observed in response to oxidative stress ..reflect selective degradation of oxidatively modified (damaged) proteins'. We have analysed these data in detail in a previous review specific to proteolysis of oxidized proteins, and the reader is referred there for further consideration (Dean et al. 1994).

Other studies showed a similar accelerated proteolysis after exposure to hydrogen peroxide (Salo et al. 1990), though in this case the effect of xanthine and xanthine oxidase was to give rise to up to 50-fold increases in the rate of proteolysis. This response seemed to be ATP independent as judged by studies where cells were depleted of ATP before being exposed to the oxidative stress (Pacifici et al. 1989), and together with the range of lysate studies discussed above, was evidence in favour of the role of a proteasome system in the catabolism of oxidized proteins in these cells. However, other studies of oxidized protein catabolism in erythroctyes and their lysates, while confirming the ATP-independence in intact cells, have argued both for and against a role for the proteasome in lysates (Fagan and Waxman 1992; Matthews et al. 1989; Strack et al. 1996a, b).

Nucleated mammalian cells: proteolysis of oxidized proteins after endocytosis

Endocytosis is the process of internalization of extracellular materials by membrane invagination and intracellular membrane fusion, to form internal, membrane-bound vesicles. These vesicles undergo a wide range of transformations, including fusing with the lysosomal system of degradative enzymes, where their contents may be rapidly degraded under the attack of a high concentration of proteinases and other hydrolases at acid pH.

Endocytosis is also the most important component of 'clearance' of proteins from circulation, which literally means removal to undefined extravascular locations. While there is significant entry into intercellular fluids outside the vascular space, functionally important removal is largely by uptake into liver cells or into tissue leukocytes. It is known that oxidized proteins can often be cleared, and taken into cells, more rapidly than native proteins, consistent with their increased hydrophobicity (Goldberg and Dice 1974; Dean 1978; Dice 1987). For example, IGF1 is cleared more rapidly after oxidation (Francis *et al.* 1988). This may well be due to enhanced adsorptive endocytosis, though in some cases oxidation may generate ligands for specific endocytic receptors

The mechanism of proteolysis of oxidized proteins after endocytosis is, therefore, much easier to approach technically than those concerning intracellular proteins, because one can control the quality and quantity of oxidized proteins supplied to cells for internalization by endocytosis, and hence also control the quality and quantity of the resultant intracellular pools. As we have discussed already, cells detoxify certain of the products of radical-mediated protein oxidation, such as protein hydroperoxides, rather efficiently. But the stable end products such as aliphatic amino acid hydroxides, and species generated from Phe and Tyr (such as DOPA, di-tyrosines, *o*-, and *m*-Tyr isomers, and chloro- and nitro-tyrosines), can be supplied in proteins to cells, and accumulate therein to form significant, intracellular pools.

We have studied the catabolism, by mouse peritoneal macrophages, of the oxidized soluble protein, BSA (Grant *et al.* 1992, 1993*b*), and the oxidized lipoprotein, apoB, in LDL (Jessup *et al.* 1992*b*; Mander *et al.* 1994), in this way. The results with both types of substrate are mutually consistent, but it should be pointed out that in the case of oxidized LDL (oxLDL), cells are exposed to a range of fatty acid and sterol oxidation products, as well as to oxidized protein. For this reason, it is necessary to compare the metabolism of oxLDL with that of an unoxidized, modified form of LDL which is taken up into cells comparably, and which also loads cells with significant quantities of sterols and fatty acids, though is unoxidized; acetylated LDL (AcLDL) is the most commonly used form. This comparison shows that the sterols and fatty acids of both LDL derivatives enter the lysosomal system, and are hydrolysed, such that free sterols and fatty acids (oxidized or unoxidized) are released into the cytoplasm where they become esterified through the action of ACAT. The kinetics of this process are rather similar for the different substrates (oxidized or unoxidized), and both kinds of sterols become similarly distributed amongst cell membranes, as judged by subcellular fractionation studies. Thus, it is clear that the catabolism of the lipid components of the particle is largely independent of that of the protein, and it does not seem that the catabolism of the protein, conversely, is likely to depend primarily on the catabolism of the lipids.

The results obtained with both oxidized BSA and apoB are rather similar: the oxidized proteins are degraded more rapidly than their native counterparts, but they accumulate inside cells to a much higher concentration than their native counterparts. There is a direct relation between the concentration supplied and the rate of proteolysis, which may eventually reach a plateau and even decline if enough substrate is supplied. However, there is also an increase in the intracellular pool in response to increasing supply. Kinetically, the intracellular pool at any given external concentration equilibrates fairly rapidly (within 2–4 hours), as is common in endocytic systems. The salient point is that as the intracellular pool expands past a certain level, overall catabolism no longer increases, so that the efficiency with which the intracellular pool is catabolized falls. In other words, the half-life of the intracellular pool lengthens as loading is increased. This is indicative of inefficient catabolism. Such inefficiency is confirmed during pulse-chase experiments, in which oxidized substrate is supplied during the pulse, but not during the chase. In such an experiment one can directly measure the rate of disappearance of an intracellular pool, gaining another impression of the efficiency with which it is being catabolized. In the case of LDL, the high-uptake, unoxidized, AcLDL is handled efficiently intracellularly, with no substantial accumulation, and rapid removal of the small pool during a chase. Thus, for both BSA and oxLDL it is clear that cellular proteolytic systems are inefficient at catabolism, compared with their native conterparts, and hence there is an intracellular accumulation of substrate, at least when it is supplied in profusion. However, once supply is removed or decreased, the pool size slowly declines. Other data (Lougheed et al. 1991; Roma et al. 1992) is consistent with this conclusion. As with all protein systems, the steady state level is the net of supply (from endocytosis of oxidized proteins) and removal (by catabolism).

Does the inefficiency result from perturbed intracellular transport of the oxidized substrates? Clearly, if these substrates did not reach the lysosomal system, where the degradative machinery is concentrated, then one might expect a failure of normal proteolysis. In the case of LDL we have under-taken detailed subcellular fractionation studies to show that the apoB does indeed reach lysosomes with fairly normal kinetics, and that it is from the lysosomal pool that the slow catabolism is taking place (Mander *et al*. 1994). Thus, the problem seems to be an inability of the proteinases, which remain perfectly active against unoxidized substrates supplied simultaneously to the same cell cultures, to deal with the oxidized substrates. This observation, of course, has parallels in the poor handling of more extensively oxidized proteins in cell free studies with purified enzymes or lysate systems.

Furthermore, it is clear that both direct protein oxidation and certain kinds of protein derivatization can suffice to confer poor susceptibility to the lysosomal proteolytic system. Thus, the catabolism of oxidized BSA only involves oxidized protein; whereas the catabolism of oxLDL might be influenced by the derivatization of the apoB by products of lipid oxidation. This possibility has been directly tested in endocytosis studies, and it has been found that derivatization of LDL with 4-HNE, without overt protein oxidation, also creates a substrate which is poorly handled by cells. This substrate is also poorly handled in cell-free lysate systems, and hence altered proteolytic susceptibility seems to be the main mechanism (Jessup *et al*. 1992*b*). In contrast MDA-LDL is handled relatively well, and these obser-vations on derivatized proteins have parallels in the cell-free studies.

One can summarize by saying that proteins and lipoproteins which are oxidized (and sometimes modified in other ways), traffic through cells after endocytosis normally, but are relatively poorly degraded in the lysosomal system, and hence accumulate. Since the lysosomal system is an important component of the catabolism of the bulk of cellular proteins, particularly those of long half life, one might expect that this finding would be pertinent to the catabolism of intracellular proteins which enter the lysosomal system by autophagy, the intracellular membrane invagination and sequestration mechanism which is in many ways analogous to endocytosis, but deals with intracellular rather than extracellular substrates.

Proteolysis of intracellular oxidized proteins in intact nucleated cells, or their isolated functional mitochondria and chloroplasts
We have previously presented a very detailed review focussed specifically on mammalian cells, to which the reader is referred for further details and examples of the arguments now discussed briefly (Dean *et al*. 1994).

As with bacteria, the first difficulty in studying proteolysis of oxidized intracellular proteins in nucleated cells is how to obtain a measurable pool of such proteins without killing the target cells. There are three main ap-proaches to this: first, to microinject oxidized proteins; second, to damage the cells by oxidative insult, but under limits which allow the cells to survive; and third, to supply oxidized amino acids to cells so that they synthesize proteins containing the oxidized amino acids. These approaches have been attempted successively, and will be discussed in a similar sequence, with the third approach being found in the next subsection of this chapter.

Probably the first approach to be seriously undertaken was that of microinjection, with much effort being expended in the late 1970s and early 1980s in studying the factors which determine the half-lives of normal cellular proteins. The immediate question, which arises from such studies, is whether microinjected proteins are located and handled like their endogenous counterparts. A related issue is whether the function of the recipient cells is disastrously perturbed by the microinjection technique. This, of necessity, involves severe alterations, even if transient, in the plasma membrane function, as a large molecule to which the membrane is not normally permeable must be transported intact across it. Osmotic shock, temporary permeabilization, membrane fusion, and intracellular lysis of endosomes are amongst the most commonly used techniques, and all have such caveats, so that the above question cannot be completely answered satisfactorily. However, all have given useful information, and shown that molecular parameters of protein structure do determine their half-lives. Thus, the application to oxidized proteins seems promising, and a few studies have tried to take advantage of it.

Amongst the most useful and careful are those of Hendil, Hare and Rivett, and of Kulka. Since these studies are very labour intensive, only a limited number of oxidized proteins have been compared with their native counterparts, and these have been generally found to show shorter intra-cellular half-lives than their native counterparts, when injected into the same cell types. A complementary approach is included within Hendil's work (Hendil 1980): here, fibroblasts which had already been microinjected with haemoglobin, radioactively labelled by carbamylation, were exposed to phenylhydrazine, which oxidized haemoglobin to methaemoglobin, and also bound and denatured the globin. This caused roughly a 13-fold increase in its rate of catabolism, with very slight inhibitory effects on the degradation of endogenous proteins, or on cell growth. These data provide one of the clearer examples of oxidation of a limited class of proteins leading to the accelerated catabolism, and they were followed up by analogous experiments with endogenous haemoglobin of rabbit erythrocytes (Gold-berg and Boches 1982), with phenylhydrazine or nitrite as oxidants; indeed, methylene blue, a reductant for the oxidized haemoglobin, could largely reverse this effect.

An obvious limitation of most of the currently available studies is that the pool sizes achieved may not be pertinent to those achieved by endogenously generated, oxidized proteins. Furthermore, the subcellular transport and degradative mechanisms of these proteins have not been fully elucidated. However, the studied proteins were, apparently, moderately oxidized, and as such, the observation that they show accelerated degradation compared with their native counterpart is compatible with the interpretations put forward already, granted that this is achieved by a moderate elevation of their pool size compared with that normally reached by their oxidized counterparts.

The second approach, as with bacteria and erythrocytes, is to expose cells to an oxidative affront, of moderate extent so that the cells survive, and then study the proteolysis of the resultant substrates, which include oxidized proteins. In assessing proteolysis with nucleated cells, this approach was first undertaken with isolated mitochondria from rat liver (Dean and Pollak 1985), whose radical flux can be manipulated by un-couplers and agents which isolate segments of the electron transport chain (by blocking transfer to other segments), so that enhanced radical flux from the CoQ or other sites results. These manipulations resulted in roughly a 20 per cent increase in the rate of proteolysis of prelabelled mitochondrial proteins, which were labelled through their own synthetic efforts, using radioactive precursor amino acids. Again, while the pool size of labelled protein was known, that of the oxidized proteins was not, indeed oxidation of endogenous proteins was not directly demonstrated, as in many of the studies mentioned above. On the other hand, it was shown that inactivation of phospho-enol pyruvate kinase (GTP) of rat liver (Ballard and Hopgood 1976) could be effected by a liver extract, by means of S–S formation on the enzyme. The degradation rates of the enzyme in intact cells paralleled the inactivation rates, suggesting, as also argued by Levine and colleagues (Levine et al. 1981), that oxidative inactivation might be a controlling step in overall catabolism.

To assess the impact of oxidative stresses more directly, studies were undertaken with intact cells using a very wide range of radical affronts, and taking care not to exceed the dose and duration of exposure which the cells could survive (Dean et al. 1986b; Vince and Dean 1987). Again, these studies indicated only modest increments in the rate of degradation of pre-labelled proteins, be they of long or short half life. Biphasic responses were found, so that after a limited attack increased oxidative exposure resulted in a decrease in degradation rate, though this could often not be absolutely distinguished from the concomitant toxic effects. Thus it is possible, but not established, that the biphasic enhancement and then regression of susceptibility to turnover described above for endocytosed proteins, and for lysate studies, applies to endogenous, oxidized proteins.

The key limitation in all the studies just described is that proteins which contain oxidized moieties could not be absolutely distinguished from those which do not. The studies (discussed earlier) on di-tyrosine formation in erythrocytes, and the catabolism of the proteins containing di-tyrosine, though technically difficult to interpret, seek a direct distinction of this kind. The next section describes an incipient alternative approach, which is physiologically relevant and simpler to interpret.

A variety of degradative systems seems to participate in degradation of abnormal proteins, including those containing amino acid analogues, or those carrying products of errors in protein synthesis. These include the ubiquitin-dependent system, the lysosomal system, and the multimolecular cytoplasmic complex, the proteasome. Mainly by virtue of lysate studies, Davies and colleagues have argued that the proteasome is critical for degradation of oxidized proteins, but converse evidence, that the removal of the proteasome makes no difference to the preferential susceptibility of oxidized proteins in such lysates, has been presented by Goldberg and colleagues (Matthews *et al.* 1989). Their recent review of this topic (Coux *et al.* 1996) concludes that the role of the proteasome, if significant, is complemented by a plethora of other mechanisms. There may therefore be sufficient redundancy in the system for the contribution of the proteasome to be replaced, when necessary.

Most recently, Davies and colleages have used a very logical approach to resolving this issue, using antisense RNAs to inhibit proteasome expression in clone 9 liver (Grune *et al.* 1995) and K562 (Grune *et al.* 1996) cells. Degradation of short and long half-life proteins in clone 9 cells (biosynthetically labelled) was measured as release of low-molecular-weight (TCA-soluble) isotope, and reported as accelerated by a variety of oxidative treatments of the cells. This claim supports earlier data for nucleated eukaryotic cells, such as our own for long half-life proteins (Dean *et al.* 1986*b*; Vince and Dean 1987). The accelerations reported in the more recent data are very varied, but in some cases up to 2.5 fold the basal level, rather greater than found previously. Unfortunately, the data (Grune *et al.* 1995) cannot be interpreted in terms of proteolysis, since isotope reutilization is the largest factor at work. This can be seen from the fact that 2 hour labelling with ^{35}S-cysteine/methionine, followed by a wash period, gives rise to no more than 20 per cent degradation of the labelled pool in 24 hours, and there is a clear plateau effect in some data, such that the ongoing percentage rate of degradation is virtually zero. These data are not compatible with measuring the degradation of the 'short half-life proteins' which are inevitably selectively labelled by such a short pulse of isotope (the measured half-life should be approx. 2 hours); they could only arise if isotope reutilization (re-incorporation into protein by protein synthesis) is substantial, thereby vastly decreasing the apparent rate of proteolysis. Greater overall degradation of 'long half-life proteins' (labelled over a 16 hour period, then chased for 2 hours) is achieved than of 'short', again consistent with reutilization.

Even if the data represent degradation to some degree, there are many complicating features. For example, after a bolus of hydrogen peroxide, 'short half-life protein degradation' was delayed in relation to the degradation in controls, and its maximum rate in a 1 hour period (between 1–2 hours after exposure) was never as great as the rate of degradation in the controls in the first hour. Secondly, with 'long half-life proteins' there are no differences in rate for the first 6 hours at least between cultures exposed or not exposed to a peroxide bolus (Grune et al. 1995, Fig. 4); but there is inter-experimental variation (Grune et al. 1995 Fig. 9 shows a 2.5-fold enhanced 'long half-life' proteolysis at 6 hours after exposure to a peroxide bolus). It is also notable that it is claimed that several non-oxidative stresses (exposure to 4-hydroxy-nonenal and other aldehydes) also accelerate degradation of short half-life proteins, making it quite clear that effects on degradation other than oxidation of the newly synthesized protein substrates can be important: these agents, like the oxidative stresses, probably alter protein synthesis rates, and hence reutilization, and hence the observed release of soluble isotope.

The 'degradation' of oxidized proteins in the living cells, of both 'short' and 'long half-life', is depressed by the antisense RNA treatment, which duly suppresses proteasome expression substantially. Clearly, these data cannot be interpreted; though there was evidence presented from lysate experiments that the proteasome can play a role in degradation. Proteinase inhibitor experiments presented using the lysate indicate roles for -cysteinyl and -metallo proteinases, but no experiments were undertaken at acid pH, so the capacities of lysosomal enzymes were not studied. However, note that in the experiments with clone-9-labelled proteins as substrates, no evidence that these substrates became oxidized was presented.

Thus, the common problem of incomplete definition of pool sizes of the native and oxidized proteins remains. Thus, the role of the proteasome in catabolism of oxidized proteins is still subject to question, and the conservative interpretation of Goldberg and colleagues seems appropriate. That is, that proteloytic redundancy is substantial, and while the proteasome may play a role in catabolism of short half-life proteins in general, and oxidized proteins in particular, this role can be taken over by other cellular components when needed (Matthews et al. 1989; Coux et al. 1996).

Reutilization of oxidized amino acids

It is interesting to consider what might happen to the products of proteolysis of oxidized proteins. If protein synthesis can use a particular oxidized amino acid, then once released as a result of degradation it may enter the pool for reutilization, just as does its parent amino acid, or the amino acid whose structure it most resembles. Thus, hydroxyvaline might be expected to be handled like valine, whereas o- and m-tyrosine (from phenylalanine) might be handled like tyrosine, rather than phenylalanine. Many studies have been published on the incorporation of amino acid analogues by protein synthesis, and it is clear that there can be discrimination against abnormal amino acids at the level of tRNA charging, by hydrolysis at the time of formation of the acyl bond, or there can be successful incorporation and removal by proteolysis. While it seems that DOPA can be incorporated by protein synthesis (Agrup *et al.* 1978), the metabolism of the resultant proteins has not been studied. Similarly, several hydroxyleucines and hydroxyvalines, including some, but not all, of those arising from oxidation, and in the case of leucine including some which are not products of oxidation, have been studied. They often cause abnormal folding, abnormal secretion, and in some cases abnormal catabolism of the resultant proteins. Modified leucines may have particular relevance to the processing of signal peptides, in view of their frequent occurrence in signal sequences, and previous data on altered viral polyprotein and secretory protein expression (Green 1982; Schwartz 1988; McAndrew *et al.* 1991).

We have demonstrated the incorporation of 3-hydroxyvaline, 4-hydroxyleucine, DOPA, *m*- and *o*-tyrosine into mouse macrophages in culture, even in the presence of the parent amino acid (Fu, unpublished data). The levels achieved can be controlled, and we envisage that this will permit the detailed study of catabolism of oxidized proteins. It might be argued that protein oxidation is unlikely to generate a narrow range of products on the oxidized species, but, in fact, at low extents of oxidation, the number of modified amino acids per individual protein molecule is probably around 1 (and this number is consistent even with the exaggerated determinations of carbonyl levels in proteins discussed by Halliwell *et al.* (1992)). Thus, in studying proteins containing only one modified amino acid, one may be modelling the behaviour of individual molecules rather well. Furthermore, physiological reutilization of the small quantities of oxidized amino acids released from degradation is likely to occur in at least some cases, since this is exactly what happens when tracer radioactive amino acids are given experimentally to cells in the presence of physiological concentrations of the parent (non-radioactive) amino acid. This approach seems to be a highly promising way to resolve the open questions concerning the kinetics and mechanisms of degradation of oxidized proteins.

3.6 Oxidized proteins as control and trigger mechanisms in cell growth and programmed cell death

Although, so far in this chapter, we have emphasized damaging aspects of radical-mediated protein oxidation, there are examples of protein activation by radicals, as well, of course, as radical-mediated catalysis. In addition, we will discuss here the oxidation of specific proteins which may be part of control processes, or the triggering of programmed cell death.

The simplest relevant molecular examples of protein activation would be if certain enzymes are converted into active forms by oxidant exposure. A few such clear-cut molecular examples have been defined in cell-free experiments. Microsomally-bound glutathione-S-transferase can be activated by dimer formation upon exposure *in vitro* to hydrogen peroxide (Aniya and Anders 1992). The single-chain, urokinase zymogen of plasma can be activated *in vitro* by chloramines generated from hypochlorite, apparently through the intermediacy of singlet oxygen (Stief *et al.* 1991). The relevance of this to activation during fibrinolysis, or during exposure to activated neutrophils, is not yet clear. However, in other experiments with triggered neutrophils, it was shown that components of the hypochlorite-generating systems, which use MPO to convert superoxide primary products of the respiratory burst into hypochlorite, lead to the conversion of several metalloproteinase (MP) zymogens into their active forms in the cell supernatants (Ottonello *et al.* 1994). The evidence for this was that genetic removal, or chemical inhibition, of some of the components, notably the myeloperoxidase (MPO), leads to the MPs remaining as zymogens in the supernatants. Although inactivation of α-1-PI was also detected in these experiments, this was not well inversely correlated with the activation of the zymogens, suggesting that the actions of the zymogens were more direct. However, the precise molecular basis of this was not clarified. In a related study, it has been suggested that the cysteinyl proteinase, calpain, in cultured rat lenses, is activated by exposure of the cells to hydrogen peroxide, since enhanced cleavage of one of its most rapidly removed substrates, and enhanced autolysis of the enzyme, which normally accompanies activation, was observed (Kadoya *et al.* 1993). The precise chemistry of the enzyme activation was not studied, and it may represent an indirect rather than direct action of the radicals generated from hydrogen peroxide.

Several studies have indicated that soluble guanylate cyclase may be reversibly activated by oxidation. For example, *in vitro*, reagents which oxidize thiols show a biphasic effect on the activity of the form of this enzyme from human platelets, and at the intermediate levels of activation, the response of the enzyme to further stimulation by NO is also enhanced (Wu *et al.* 1992). Activation was associated with protein-glutathione adduct formation via a disulfide link. Similarly, ascorbate can activate the purified bovine lung enzyme, provided that a range of other reactants are present, notably catalase, and the available evidence would be consistent with a role for Compound 1 of catalase in the activation events, and its inhibition by superoxide per se (Cherry and Wolin 1989).

The possible activation of certain enzymes by methionine oxidation has been discussed (Vogt 1995), but evidence that such reactions are important physiologically is limited. Conversion of quite a substantial group of oxidases into their active form appears to involve copper-mediated autoxidation of a specific tyrosine to form TOPA (Choi *et al.* 1995). It does not seem that such specific and limited mechanisms will be widespread, in view of the risks that vicinal or distal protein damage will be concomitant with the oxidative step.

In the special cases of small peptide hormones and effectors, oxidative modification sometimes enhances activity; this may reflect the greater flexibility of secondary and tertiary structure of these peptides in comparison with larger proteins, and the lesser dependence on maintaining a limited range of conformations. In any case, Met-enkephalin can be oxidized at methionine, tyrosine, and phenylalanine moieties, and both hydroxylation and cross-linking can occur at the aromatic residues (Rabgaoui *et al.* 1993). The consequence of hydroxylation due to a neutrophil respiratory burst is activation of the physiological function, though this is not true of cross-linking by di-tyrosine formation.

p53 is a selective DNA-binding, tumour-suppressive gene-product, whose nuclear expression is induced during apoptosis, and which is associated with some cancers. Its site-specific DNA binding depends on zinc coordination and redox regulation, which are separable determinants as judged by protein engineering substitution of several systems by serine (Rainwater *et al.* 1995). Furthermore, a copper redox inhibitory mechanism may be important, in which Cu(I) becomes bound to the DNA, as judged by EPR studies; the selective Cu(I) chelator, bathocuproine-disulfonic acid, can protect against this, though not radical scavengers. It is difficult to interpret this other than in terms of a site-specific binding or damaging mechanism of the copper redox conversion to the Cu(I) form (Hainaut *et al.* 1995b). p53 can also be regulated by phosphorylation, both *in vitro* and in living cells, by a member of the stress-activated subfamily of MAP kinases (Hainaut and Milner 1993), and its conformation is highly temperature dependent (Hainaut *et al.* 1995a). While this and other selective protein oxidation is quite possibly critical in message mediation in programmed cell death, and in necrosis, little more can be said of the specific molecular changes involved, and the discussion of the biological aspects of these issues is deferred until Chapter 5. Discussion of NF-κB is also delayed until then.

4 The physiology of protein oxidation

We now focus on tissues and organisms, and address the issue of how to demonstrate and interpret the presence of oxidized proteins, and in particular, how to assess whether they have a physiological role to play. Because of the additional complexity of assaying protein oxidation in samples which have as much internal heterogeneity as biology provides, we have also centred our discussion of the validity and precision of such assays here, though comments on this issue are of necessity to be found throughout the book.

4.1 Criteria of involvement of protein oxidation in physiological processes

As in some previous chapters, it appears worthwhile to assemble and discuss the key criteria that need to be applied in assessing physiological roles of oxidized proteins. First, of course, it is essential to be able to demonstrate that production of oxidized proteins does occur in a particular biological system, and under non-toxic, physiological conditions. It follows that the sensitivity of assays may be a limiting factor in such investigations, since a pool of oxidized protein at levels lower than can be detected, will be effectively invisible, yet might be of great functional importance. Thus the lack of demonstration of an oxidized protein pool cannot rule out a role, while a positive demonstration is but a first, necessary, but far from sufficient, condition. Further assessment would involve kinetic relationships: is the production and pool size of oxidized protein(s) varying in a precursor-result relationship with the putative function? Or is its production indifferent to the progress of the function? Might the pool be an innocent bystander, or a consequence of incomplete control, rather than an active player? May there be ancillary toxic, but sublethal, events, which involve protein oxidation?

Some similar criteria must be applied carefully to the assay methods themselves: it is crucial that artifactual generation of oxidized proteins during the chemical processing be distinguished from *in vivo* products. A recent example of this has come in studies of mutant haemoglobins, in which an unusual mutant (Haemoglobin Atlanta-Coventry), apparently lacking leucine residue 141 in the beta-chain, was actually shown to be replaced by a new residue with a molecular weight of 129 Da (Brennan *et al.* 1992); this change was also found in two other mutants (Fay *et al.* 1993). This residue was defined in the isolated protein as being a hydroxyleucine, on the basis of mass spectroscopy, and was thought to result from the mutation of Pro to Leu at position 75, and consequent structural changes (Brennan *et al.* 1993). The authors suggested that β-hydroxyleucine (3-hydroxyleucine) was likely, though our characterization of leucine hydroxides, discussed in Chapter 2, would indicate that one or more γ-hydroxyleucines (4-hydroxyleucines) are more likely, on the grounds of stability. Subsequently (Wilson *et al.* 1993), this group noticed that residue 9 (Leu) of the γ-T-15 peptide of the minor M-chain of fetal haemoglobin (F) can also be replaced by a residue of molecular weight 129. They found that the original leucine is maintained in some samples, but that it is rare when isolated from erythrocytes which have been exposed to carbon tetrachloride. Further experiments indicated that the hydroxyleucine can be generated during processsing, and this can be blocked by conversion of the haemoglobin to carbon monoxyhaemoglobin prior to exposure to carbon tetrachloride. The authors concluded that an artifactual oxidation reaction is probably the main source of this moiety in haemoglobins. This can probably be explained on the basis of the proximity of the particular leucines to the iron atom of the haem group, which might confer serious risk of artifactual oxidation in an iron-mediated reaction. Such studies, to check for artifactual generation, must be undertaken routinely and extensively. In addition, it is important to assess the extent to which a particular oxidation product is preserved during the analytical processes, by adding known amounts of preferably protein-bound material, and determining the extent of recovery.

With these issues in mind we can summarize and assess the available methods. We can first consider assays of the transient intermediates in protein oxidation, the protein radicals. In biological samples, the concentrations of these radicals are normally far too low for direct detection, though some exceptions have been noted. These tend to be the least reactive and hence most stable (and non-damaging?) radicals (Chapter 2). Reports where radicals have been directly observed must be interpreted with care, as in many cases the samples have been subjected to quite considerable processing before analysis. Thus, though signals have been detected in both rapidly frozen, powdered (or chopped) samples and lyophilized materials, both of these techniques are known to give artifactual signals very readily. In some cases there is good evidence that the observed signals are not artifacts, but there can be doubt as to the nature of the species giving rise to the observed signal. The best characterized and most reliable data from direct EPR experiments arise from studies on antioxidant- and drug-derived-radicals, and the changes in the concentrations of these during acute oxidative insults. More commonly, the only feasible approach is that of spin trapping, discussed earlier in this book (Chapter 2), which allows a gradual cumulation of radical species in the form of relatively stable spin adducts. The EPR spectra of these adducts give information which, with care, can often reveal the initial radical species.

The relatively unstable intermediates which we have discussed above as the reactive species produced by protein oxidation, such as the protein hydroperoxides, present almost as much difficulty. No direct determination of these materials, endogenous to a biological sample, has yet been achieved. However, because the hydroperoxides can be reduced to hydroxides (as discussed very shortly), it should, in theory, be possible to undertake determinations with and without a hydroperoxide reduction step, so as to establish how much hydroperoxide might be present as such, and how much is present in the already reduced hydroxide form. For example, a biological sample can be split into two portions, one of which is immediately reduced (giving the total of hydroperoxides and hydroxides), while the other is treated to a step which removes hydroperoxides as forms other than hydroxides and no longer reducible into hydroxides (if possible), prior to the reduction step. Preliminary data indicate that acid hydrolysis may meet these requirements.

Similarly, the reductant reactive-intermediates, DOPA and its congeners the indoles, may be present partly as Michael adducts, for example cysteinyl-DOPA, and partly as unreacted materials. One approach to analysing the sum of the DOPA and the indoles which are still catechol-o-quinone redox couples, has been studied in our labs. This is the derivatization of such o-quinones with ethylene diamine (Armstrong and Dean 1995). Such assays are hard to make absolute, in the same way that the Lowry protein assay is, since they assay a wide range of different compounds by virtue of a group of shared reactive features. This means that determination of the quantity of material is imprecise by a factor of about four, as judged by comparing a range of different individual protein-DOPA/indole systems (Armstrong and Dean 1995), which is not quite as variable as the Lowry assay (whose range of precision is about five fold). This approach can be applied successfully to systems of the complexity of LDL, but we have yet to pursue it carefully with complex tissue samples.

Thus, we are currently faced mainly with information on the determination of stable end-products. So we next comment on the various assays used. The most widely used are those for carbonyl functions on proteins (Jayko and Garrison 1958), deriving mainly from amino acids such as histidine, lysine, proline, and arginine (Amici *et al.* 1989), but also from the aliphatic side chains, in which the carbonyl functions may be derivatized by 2,4-dinitrophenylhydrazine, generating a readily measurable, optically absorbing species, a hydrazone with a large extinction coefficient (Levine *et al.* 1990, 1994). These may alternatively be reduced by radioactive borohydride, thus becoming radioactively labelled (Amici *et al.* 1989; Lenz *et al.* 1989). One possible means of reducing the interference from carbonyls other than those on proteins, is to hydrolyse the labelled samples, and rapidly separate the amino acids by Dowex ion exchange; it is not clear whether any interference remains after this procedure. On gels, these DNP-hydrazones may also be detected by means of anti-DNP antibodies (Keller *et al.* 1993) and carbonyls by reaction with fluorophores such as fluoresceine hydrazide or semicarbazide (Ahn *et al.* 1987). In addition, the γ-glutamyl semialdehyde in oxidized glutamine synthetase (derived from arginine) can be detected selectively by reaction with fluoresceinamine, and this approach may be of more general utility (Climent *et al.* 1989; Climent and Levine 1991). Carbonyl functions may be lesser products from aliphatic amino acids, and they may form internal Schiff bases or other products, depending on their location and hence the availability of suitable co-reactants (Fu and Dean 1997). There will normally be a basal protein-carbonyl level contributed at the very least by quino- and other post-translationally modified proteins, but it is not clear precisely what the magnitude of this is.

Halliwell and colleagues (Lyras *et al.* 1996) have discussed and analysed the wide variation of reported basal protein carbonyl values from human brain. In five prior papers (Oliver *et al.* 1990; Smith *et al.* 1991; Bowling *et al.* 1993; Stafford *et al.* 1993; Shaw *et al.* 1995) they find a range of control values from 0.73 to 6.8 nmol/mg protein. Their own determinations suggest that the final protein-dinitrophenylhydrazone samples they obtain contain only about 15 per cent of the starting protein, and on the assumption that they might, nevertheless, contain all the original protein-carbonyls, they also present figures as low as 0.28 nmol mg protein. On the simplifying, but reasonable, approximation that protein molecular sizes are normally distributed around a mean of 50 000 Da, a value of 5 nmol mg^{-1} corresponds to 0.25 mol carbonyl per mol protein, which would also imply that almost 25 per cent of protein molecules contain one carbonyl, and a few per cent might contain more. This seems a remarkably high value, especially in comparison with estimates of the frequencies of amino acid misincorporation by errors which are generally in the order of one in 10 000 amino acids. This latter frequency corresponds, on the assumption that the average amino acid molecular weight is 100 Da, and hence 500 amino acids per average protein molecule, to one in 20 protein molecules, i.e. 5 per cent. The carbonyl figures also are much higher than the specific protein modifications to be discussed later, which centre around less than one in 100 000 amino acids in controls (i.e. 0.5 per cent of protein molecules). While protein carbonyl assays may quantify considerably more protein oxidation events than other individual markers, these carbonyls may be formed on amino acids which are not the most susceptible targets for oxidation, and so it does not seem likely that the realistic values are even five times higher than those of the specific modifications. Indeed, there are some reports of even lower carbonyl values than summarized above. We prefer to restrict the use of this assay to studies with purified proteins.

Halliwell and colleagues point out that some, but not all, of the published inter-investigator variation derives from the *choice* of which protein fraction of the tissue to assay and use as the basis of standardization for protein quantity itself; but other variation is within the carbonyl assay procedures themselves, as also emphasized by Cao and Cutler (1995b). The recovery of protein in the final assayed fraction is clearly an important factor, and if the evidence mentioned above, that in brain this is only 15 per cent can be generalized, then it cannot be representative of the whole protein of the tissue, and may well be very variable. These assays run the risk of being overwritten by carbonyl functions deriving from non-protein molecules, such as nucleic acids, so a streptomycin precipitation step is commonly included to reduce this contamination (Levine *et al.* 1990, 1994). The reliability and precision may depend in some circumstances on the degree to which such molecules are excluded (Cao and Cutler 1995b).

The assays of hydroxide functions are much more complicated, but by the same token much more specific. They also indicate much lower occurrence of the modified moiety in oxidized proteins. Even if one aggregates the likely occurrence of all the known hydroxides, at the rate measured for β-hydroxyvaline (3-hydroxyvaline), this leads to estimates of the order of one function per 1000 protein molecules in normal samples. It is likely that these values for hydroxides are more realistic.

The same conclusion is reached on the basis of determined values from the aliphatic and aromatic amino acids, that the frequency of occurrence of each individual moiety is of the order of one per 10 000 in normal samples, in spite of the fact that the aromatic amino acids are significantly more reactive with most radicals. This, again, reinforces the implication that the measured carbonyl values may be unrealistically high.

A general problem is obvious from these comments: no individual determination can represent even the frequency of overall protein oxidation events. Thus, a Fenton site-specific *in vivo* oxidative event may well have quite different real and observed yields from those of a lipid peroxidation reaction. It is important to keep this limitation of current data in mind in assessing their implications.

4.2 Criteria for defining protein oxidation routes responsible for *in vivo* protein oxidation

The same issue arises in consideration of the relative contribution of different oxidative mechanisms: the relative efficiency with which they are measured may vary from case to case. More important still is that many of the products can be the results of several different pathways (cf. Chapter 2). For example, there are a large number of different pathways which can generate DOPA, such as reaction of tyrosine with hydroxyl radicals, with Fenton systems, and with peroxynitrite, amongst others. To distinguish these various routes it may be possible to use the determination of the relative quantities of 3,4- and 2,4-DOPA (Dizdaroglu *et al.* 1983), though this has not been carefully assessed yet. Similarly, di-tyrosine, resulting from the coupling of phenoxyl radicals, may be generated during hydroxyl radical attack, especially if oxygen and superoxide radicals are absent or limiting. Fluorescence spectra are not a satisfactory way of identifying di-tyrosine in proteins, as other products possess similar spectra. It is relatively stable, and can be conveniently assayed by well characterized HPLC techniques (Hazen *et al.* 1996). Di-tyrosine may also result from reactive nitrogen species, hypochlorite, or myeloperoxidase plus hydrogen peroxide in the presence of chloride ions (though in the latter cases this is disputed (Hazen *et al.* 1996)). The interpretation of its mechanism of formation is another matter, since any oxidant generating a phenoxyl radical may potentially give rise to it. An additional complication in using di-tyrosine as a marker of *in vivo* oxidation is that compound 1 and 2 of haem proteins (e.g. myeloperoxidase) can further oxidize this material (Marquez and Dunford 1995).

Which products currently seem most likely to be diagnostic of individual reaction routes? It might seem that one of the most clear-cut is 3-nitrotyrosine (van der Vliet *et al.* 1995), which obviously requires the action of reactive nitrogen species. But even in this case it must be noted that both NO itself and peroxynitrite (Ischiropoulos and al-Mehdi 1995) have been suggested to give rise to this species. Similarly, 3-chlorotyrosine is believed to be generated solely by hypochlorite, or chlorine/chloride-dependent mechanisms, though, again, this may also not be as straightforward as it seems (Domigan *et al.* 1995; Kettle 1996). Recent studies showed that nitrating and chlorinating species can be formed by the reaction of nitrite with hypochlorous acid (Eiserich *et al.* 1996), the former of which is generally available, while hypochlorite is provided by the action of activated phagocytes, notably neutrophils. It was shown that nitration of tyrosine residues in proteins can be effected by these reagents, and that a modest production of di-tyrosine also results. Thus, the detection of 3-nitrotyrosine can not be used to immediately incriminate peroxynitrite, or the other routes. Furthermore, the possibility exists that the tyrosyl radical, viewed as an intermediate in both the dimerisation and the generation of the nitrated species, may give rise by disproportionation to DOPA (see Chapter 2). This possibility was not assessed in the work of Eiserich *et al.*

Likewise, a wide variety of reactive species (e.g. Fenton chemistry, peroxyl radical chemistry, and others) appears to give rise to the aliphatic side chain products.

There are some other reports of widespread cellular modification of proteins directly consequent on oxidative events, notably in neutrophils upon activation of the respiratory burst. Not only is there stimulation of reversible methionine modification, as discussed in Chapter 3, but also incorporation of tyrosyl residues into proteins (Nath *et al.* 1992), particularly of membranes. This apparently results in formation of protein carbonyls, and does not occur in chronic granulomatous disease cells, which lack the respiratory burst. Phenylalanine is not similarly incorporated, so the reaction may well depend on the phenolic hydroxyl of tyrosine.

A future aim of protein oxidation studies must be to elucidate the pathways responsible for the oxidized protein moieties observed *in vivo* much more fully.

4.3 Oxidized amino acids in physiological conditions

4.3.1 Adhesive proteins, melanins, and lignins

Extracellular proteins of marine organisms often use oxidized amino acids as 'glues and varnishes' (Rzepecki and Waite 1995). Many modified amino acids are involved, including hydroxyarginines (Papov *et al.* 1995), though DOPA is quantitatively one of the most important (Taylor *et al.* 1991; Rzepecki and Waite 1993). TOPA may also be formed (Taylor *et al.* 1995). It seems that these catecholic compounds, forming a range of polyphenolics, are formed non-enzymatically, and may be present as a large proportion of total tyrosines, which themselves are an unusually large proportion of amino acids. For example, in the byssus of mussels, so much DOPA is present that it can be detected histochemically in the foot proteins. Some excellent biochemical work has been done on these proteins, but as yet the degree to which its insights translate to intracellular proteins and higher organisms is not clear.

There is a well defined example of the formation of a protective coat by means of protein oxidation, during the fertilization of sea urchin eggs (reviewed: Shapiro 1991). Within a few minutes of fertilization, there is a respiratory burst, generating extracellular hydrogen peroxide. The contents of intracellular 'cortical granules' are released onto the external egg surface, placing protein tyrosine residues in close apposition, and forming the 'soft fertilization envelope'. Some of these tyrosines are then crosslinked as di-tyrosine, forming the 'hard' envelope, which is resistant to further sperm, and to acids and alkalis. Crosslinking may also generate tri-tyrosine and higher oligomers (Nomura and Suzuki 1995). The crosslinking is effected by another cortical granule secretion, the heme enzyme ovoperoxidase, acting on hydrogen peroxide. The egg itself is protected against oxidation by approximately 5 mM levels of ovothiol, a 1-methyl-4-mercapto-histidine derivative capable of both one- and two-electron antioxidation. Like glutathione, this does not readily reduce transition metals or cytochrome c.

Melanins are formed in the pigment cells of the skin as the result of a multiplicity of polymerization/cross-linking reactions involving catechol/quinones systems derived from DOPA and cysteinyl-DOPAs. The resultant polymers are unusual in their continuous possession of radical signals. The polymers are not proteins, though they contain amino acid-derived components. The specialized chemistry of this system has been studied a great deal (Enochs et al. 1994; Cooksey et al. 1995; Schmitz et al. 1995; Sugumaran et al. 1996), and cannot be pursued further in this book. Similarly, lignin is a polymer formed from phenolic compounds by oxidative mechanisms (Ortiz de Montellano 1992), and protein components can be bound up with it; little specific to protein oxidation within lignin seems to be in the literature, and hence it will not be discussed here.

4.3.2 Some radical-mediated control mechanisms involving enzymes or other proteins

A body of evidence has been amassed to argue that radicals are important in the control of cell growth. For example, low doses of hydrogen peroxide often stimulate the growth of cultured cells (Wiese et al. 1995), and it can be argued that radicals are necessary intermediates in such triggering (Abe et al. 1994). Related mechanisms may also be important in physiological responses to stress, such as the triggering of heat shock protein synthesis, and the generation of other complements of proteins which defend against subsequent oxidative stress (such as the OxyR response (Storz and Tartaglia 1992)), and often minimize its effect (Davies, J. M. et al. 1995). There are also analogous, pathological triggering mechanisms, to which we return in the next chapter. These topics are very large, and will not be reviewed in detail here, since what concerns us is the more specific question of whether protein oxidation is amongst the participating mediator or effector mechanisms. Again, it is important to bear in mind that biological systems often have considerable redundancy, which is sometimes an insurance against the failure or absence of one constituent mechanism. In such circumstances, the role of an important contributory mechanism can be circumvented even if it is inhibited. Thus, the interpretation of the roles of component mediators and effectors is always difficult, unless positive results ensue, where the absence of a path is always associated with a lack of response. The experience with gene knock-out animals to date confirms our need for wariness in these issues of interpretation.

In the case of cell division, signs of triggering include expression of early response genes, such as c-jun, and of late response genes, such as the very short half-life ornithine decarboxylase. At these stages of the response, normal triggering and transformation (to which we will return in the next chapter) have much in common (reviewed: Kensler *et al.* 1995). On the other hand, the *in vitro* life span of limited population-doubling cells, such as human IMR-90 fibroblasts, can be extended by lowering the oxygen tension of cultures, or by supply of the spin trap PBN, suggesting an important role for oxygen radical events (Chen, Q. *et al.* 1995).

A role for a protein oxidation product as mediator in the control messages of cell growth would be indicated by evidence of changes in concentration of the product being required to precede the response, and by re-equilibration of the oxidized species at some point after the response had commenced. As indicated in the Preface, we will not discuss in detail the role of those enzymes whose action involves protein radicals, of which ribonucleotide reductase (Sahlin *et al.* 1994; Lassmann and Potsch 1995) and others are important in effecting components of the growth response. Unfortunately, relatively little information is available which is specific to this question. There is much evidence that the transcription factor AP-1, whose activity is important in regulation of cell growth, is redox activated (Barchowsky *et al.* 1995). Some perturbation experiments have tested aspects of the possible precursor-consequence role of this factor: thus, selenite and seleno-diglutathione restrict mammalian cell growth, oxidize thioredoxin, and have been found to inhibit the binding of AP-1 to DNA from 3B6 lympho-cyte nuclear extracts (Spyrou *et al.* 1995). Furthermore, binding of the trans-activators AP-1 and NF-κB to nuclear DNA extracted from endothelial cells at various stages after exposure to hydrogen peroxide, shows a vari-ation consistent with a role in the resultant growth triggering (Barchow-sky *et al.* 1995), with enhanced binding resolving by 24 hours. This may indicate a mediator role for the transcription factors in the control of cell growth. The relevance of the reduced and oxidized forms, and hence their sensitivity to reductant thiols, and oxidants such as peroxides, varies between AP-1 and NF-κB (Frame *et al.* 1991; Das *et al.* 1995*a, b*). This may also vary between regulatory sites or systems, since in lymphocytes the antioxidant reductant, cysteamine, decreased AP-1 and NF-κB binding to sites involved in regulation of IL-2 expression, but was indifferent to the binding of two other transcription factors (Goldstone *et al.* 1995). These issues are discussed by Meyer *et al.* (1994) and Sen and Packer (1996).

The relevance of protein oxidation products beyond the thiol/disulfide system does not yet seem to have been considered. Organic hydroperoxides are common agents of tumour promotion, and protein hydroperoxides probably share this property. Further, it is apparent that the protein quinone systems, such as DOPA, and the precursor phenols may have mechanisms in common with butylated-hydroxytoluene (BHT). BHT hydroperoxides are formed *in vivo*, and have been shown to give rise to quinone methides which appear to be important in cell transformation and mitogenesis by way of alteration of signalling processes involving protein SH groups, such as on AP-1 (Kensler *et al.* 1995).

Protein oxidation products might also function as effectors of cell growth changes, in which case their expression would be concomitant with the response, rather than a precursor to it; but again they might be necessary components of the response, whose absence (inhibition of formation/ prevention of maintenance) would be accompanied by no response. The levels of protein carbonyls in IMR-90s at various population doublings are not significantly different (Chen, Q. *et al.* 1995), and those in fibroblasts taken from humans of various ages are only elevated after age 60 (Oliver *et al.* 1987), though they are higher in Werner's and Progeria fibroblasts than in normal controls. In sum, these data suggest that protein oxidation may not be a necessary effector, as contrasted with mediator, mechanism.

However, the level of protein carbonyls (measured in nmol mg^{-1} cell protein) of course depends on the relative rates of input and output. Thus, there might be a continuously enhanced input, with which the removal mechanisms, notably protein degradation, keep pace. Similarly, cell growth requires a nett positive balance between protein synthesis and degradation. Thus, the question arises as to whether oxidant-mediated changes in protein synthesis or degradation are part of their triggering actions on the control of cellular concentrations of individual proteins, or even, more grossly, on organismal growth. On the other hand, they may merely express toxic and inhibitory actions on both components of protein turnover. We have discussed the complexities of the cellular biochemistry of protein degradation during oxidative damage in Chapter 3. Here, we focus specifically on its possible relation with control of organismal protein turnover (and we will discuss its involvement with ageing in the next chapter).

The only well studied cases of a possible physiological control of protein degradation by oxidative modification of a protein are those stemming from the studies of Switzer (Turnbough and Switzer 1975*a*, *b*; Ruppen and Switzer 1983;) and Levine and Stadtman (Levine *et al.* 1981). These led to the idea that metal-catalysed inactivation of bacterial glutamine synthetase and other enzymes might be such a control, especially as it could be shown to be influenced by the adenylation state of the enzyme, which was already known to be such a physiological control. We have discussed the mechanistic and structural complexities of the relation between inactivation and cell-free proteolytic sensitivity of this enzyme in Chapter 3. The studies of Switzer were an important antecedent to these, and in the 1983 paper (Ruppen and Switzer 1983) it is shown that in intact *B. subtilis* stationary phase cultures, there is a rapid oxygen-dependent inactivation of the amido-transferase, and that inactive enzyme accumulates if chloramphenicol is provided, blocking protein synthesis and also degradation. No direct evidence was provided to show that the inactive enzyme was indeed oxidized, though the in vitro model studies and oxygen dependence would suggest this (Turnbough and Switzer 1975*a, b*). In the absence of chloramphenicol the inactive enzyme is rapidly degraded, and loss of activity parallels very closely the loss of immunologically detectable enzyme protein ('cross-reactive material': CRM). There are no degradation intermediates detectable in SDS gels of immunoprecipitates, as is normally the case with proteolytic degradation *in vivo*. In this case there is no sign of inactivation preceding degradation, and direct evidence to distinguish inactivation from degradation *in vivo* is not available.

Here, we focus mainly on two studies (Fulks and Stadtman 1985; Chevalier *et al.* 1990) which have made the very difficult attempt to carry these ideas further into functioning organisms (these are also the only two relevant studies which study protein turnover in intact cells in relation to *metal-ion*-catalysed oxidative inactivation). These interesting papers concern *Klebsiella pneumoniae* and *K. aerogenes*, respectively, and they deserve quite detailed presentation.

Fulks and Stadtman studied the loss of aspartokinases III (lysine-sensitive) and I which occurs when *K. aerogenes* suspensions are incubated in a nitrogen-lacking medium, describing it clearly as 'regulation'. While this occurs, glutamine synthetase levels rise, and then remain constant. Synthesis of glutamine synthetase continues, as judged by several criteria, and can be inhibited by chloramphenicol. Chloramphenicol causes a loss of total glutamine synthetase activity and immunologically detectable protein; and accelerates the loss of the aspartokinase activities (though their synthesis and protein levels were not studied). Glucose stimulates the chloramphenicol-triggered loss of all three enzymes in the nitrogen-restricted conditions. The authors quote preliminary data (given in (Levine *et al.* 1981)) as indicating that in the presence of chloramphenicol the glutamine synthetase inactivation precedes loss of the enzyme protein (i.e. immunologically cross-reactive material), though such data are not presented again or extended.

Unfortunately, the data concerned (Levine *et al.* 1981) are very limited and seem to be misinterpreted. The comparison is made of loss of enzyme activity and Ouchterlony double-immunodiffusion detection of CRM, in each case showing data for 0, 1.5, 3, and 4.5 hours of incubation of the cells.

By 3 hours, and after activity is almost zero, the precipitin line is virtually invisible. The apparent lack of parallel between the two data sets is at 1.5 hours where the precipitin is quite visible, yet 75 per cent of the enzyme activity has been lost. However, the basis of formation of precipitins in gel diffusion is the establishment of antigen:antibody equivalence, at which insoluble aggregates of the complexes precipitate as antigen and antibody diffuse towards each other; it is not the complete precipitation of all antigen in a line whose density indicates the quantity of antigen present. The position of the precipitin in relation to the origin of the antibodies and the antigen is more indicative of the relative concentration of different antigen samples. In this case, the antibody is provided from a single trough, and the separate antigen samples start in wells facing it. The distance between the edge of the antigen well and the precipitin line is directly related to the quantity of immunologically recognizable antigen diffusing; measurement from the published photograph indicates that the precipitin is closer to the well of the 1.5 hour antigen than of the 0 hour, indicating significant loss of CRM has indeed occurred. This method is not quantitative, but the data do not support the contention of a clear antecedence of inactivation over degradation; on the contrary, the system seems like that of Switzer's *B. subtilis* experiments, in which the kinetics of degradation and inactivation are indistinguishable.

The authors then proceed to detailed studies (Fulks and Stadtman 1985) of the mechanism of inactivation of purified *K. aerogenes* glutamine synthetase, when added to cell-free extracts of the organism (mostly at pH 8.0), arguing for a major role of the metal-catalysed oxidation system. There are indications that an oxidative system is involved, most notably the fact that inactivation is inhibited by 50 per cent in an anoxic, argon environment; indeed the earlier paper (Levine *et al.* 1981) had indicated a figure of 100 per cent . However, selective serine proteinase inhibitors reduced the inactivation by up to 50 per cent; and sulfydryl agents, which would act both on cysteine and serine proteinases, could do so by 85–90 per cent. At pH 8, the only other of the four major catalytic groups of proteinases which would be expected to be active are the metalloproteinases. Accordingly, a range of metal chelators are effective inhibitors (up to 90 per cent), though in the case of *o*-phenanthroline further iron ions overcame the inhibition, while further additions of the main metalloproteinase cofactor, zinc, did not. Nevertheless, the addition of key components of metal-catalysed oxidation at supraphysiological levels will inevitably accentuate oxidative damage. Thus the most economical interpretation of the data discussed so far is that proteinases are key agents of inactivation, while metal-catalysed oxidation may play an additional role.

Consistent with this is the fact that boiling the extracts prior to addition to the glutamine synthetase virtually blocks inactivation: a property expected of an enzymatic inactivation system, but not of a metal-catalysed inactivation. The authors show that the cell-free inactivation does not involve loss of cross-reactive material, by immunotitration of the enzyme activity, and imply that this also indicates that proteolysis is not important. However, these data are neutral to the issue, since they simply show that whatever range of fragments of glutamine synthetase are present, they cross-react like the intact enzyme with the polyclonal antibodies to the enzyme: in a cell-free system, it is not to be expected that complete degradation to amino acids would necessarily occur, since this usually requires the coordinated action of many enzymes, and often specialized, intracellular transport into degradative sites.

Fulks and Stadtman conclude with the suggestion that the cell-free inactivation is a component of the triggering of degradation in the intact cells, and propose, again, that the oxidative inactivation is critical, and precedes proteolytic degradation (Fulks and Stadtman 1985). However, as we have just illustrated, the data do not point strongly in favour of that interpretation, and there is no evidence that inactivation in the living cells is oxidative, and not much that it precedes enzymatic proteolysis. These particular issues were taken up carefully in the other paper under discussion, albeit with a different organism (Chevalier *et al.* 1990).

K. pneumoniae uses different pathways for glycerol metabolism in aerobic and anaerobic conditions. So when anaerobic organisms are moved to oxic conditions, synthesis of glycerol dehydrogenase is repressed, the enzyme is inactivated, and the protein is degraded. Two other enzymes behave similarly. The same three enzymes are inactivated when anaerobic cells are exposed to low concentrations of hydrogen peroxide. Chevalier and colleagues addressed the question of the state of the glycerol dehydrogenase in the cells, before and after *in vivo* exposure of the cells to peroxide, by purifying samples from the two conditions. They state that 'loss of cross-reacting material generally paralleled loss of activity, although inactivation appeared to occur slightly faster than loss of cross-reacting material'; but the data presented do not show this convincingly, and if there is a difference, it is very slight. Although the enzyme from the peroxide-exposed cells had only 10 per cent of the specific activity of the native form, it was similar in terms of molecular weight and amino acid composition, though slightly different in hydrophobicity as discussed in Chapter 3. However, it was very susceptible to degradation by subtilisin, while the native enzyme was resistant. This is a key observation, in favour of the idea that inactivation precedes proteolysis in this case; but, as concluded in Chapter 3, the case that the inactivation was due to oxidative modification of the enzyme was not made.

There are some other very interesting observations in this study. Notably, chloramphenicol, an inhibitor of protein synthesis, prevented the inactivation and degradation of glycerol dehydrogenase caused by oxygen exposure, but not that due to peroxide. This suggests that some newly synthesized protein is necessary for the inactivation step triggered by oxygen exposure. This is not a feature which would obviously be predicted for a metal-ion-catalysed inactivation system, which would rather be expected to be independent of protein synthesis, but it makes the experimental system absolutely fascinating. The case remains open whether oxidative modification is important in control of degradation of this enzyme; and therefore, also open as to whether this has more general regulatory implications.

We turn, finally, to gross protein turnover in organisms. In the late 1970s and early 1980s, the idea that oxidation of protein SH groups, by sensing overall cellular redox status, might be a large-scale regulator of protein degradation was considered quite extensively (reviewed: Goldberg and Dice 1974; Goldberg and St John 1976), as mentioned briefly in Chapter 3. While there are individual examples of the influence of protein SH groups, the most detailed evidence on the importance of redox status has come from studies on isolated muscles (Fagan and Goldberg 1985), and it argues against such a general role. Bulk proteolysis can be regulated independently of redox status, and redox status altered without altering proteolysis.

However, there are some interesting data concerning turnover of (bulk) proteins modified as a result of lipid oxidation in rats which were made vitamin E deficient, or fed iron nitrilotriacetate, or treated with carbon tetrachloride, compared to normal controls (Mahmoodi et al. 1995). The animals were fed an MDA-free diet, and the levels of MDA (malondialdehyde), lysine-MDA adduct, and its N-acetyl derivative were increased in urine. Urinary *fluxes* of these products were increased, so that unless significant amounts of free lysine-MDA were formed initially, the absolute turnover of proteins containing MDA must also be greater in the dosed than the control animals. Since there were no determinations of tissue pools of MDA-protein adducts, the data obtained do not permit an estimation of the average tissue MDA-protein half-life, but simply suggest that the absolute rate of catabolism (as judged by excretion) rose. However, in diabetes, some tissues show elevated MDA-protein levels, others reduced (Shah et al. 1994), so the situation is likely to be complex even in the studies of Mahmoodi et al.

These authors also showed that in cell-free experiments, BSA-MDA adducts were degraded more rapidly by erythrocyte and mitochondrial extracts, as described earlier. As discussed in Chapter 3, this may not be a general effect of lipid aldehyde derivatization, since the converse is observed with apoB derivatized with 4-hydroxynonenal, and it is also found with glucose-6-phosphate dehydrogenase from *Leuconostoc mesenteroides*, which becomes cross-linked (Friguet et al. 1994a, b). The effect of modification may depend both on the nature of the substrate and on the degradation mechanism(s) most involved. In view of the deposition of protein-adducts in tissues, detected in the work of Draper and colleagues (Mahmoodi *et al.* 1995), and also the claim that MDA-apoB is in circulation in normal humans (Lecomte *et al.* 1993), it is unlikely that erythrocyte or mitochondrial degradation mechanisms are important, and likely that lysosomal ones play a role, after autophagy or endocytosis, respectively. This approach is very promising, and the authors point out that there are obvious parallels between the MDA-proteins and hydroxyl-radical-modified proteins; a similar approach to studying the *in vivo* turnover of the latter would be very interesting.

One additional possible fate of oxidized proteins in lysosomes, especially in the liver, is excretion into the bile. An interesting study concerning Fischer 344 rats, oxidatively stressed by diquat, has indeed demonstrated enhanced release of oxidized proteins into bile, both in terms of absolute amount, and relative to total protein present in bile (Gupta *et al.* 1994). Total protein and lysosomal enzymes in bile (which mainly derive from hepatocytes) were also elevated. While this might simply reflect toxicity, it is also possible that triggered lysosomal exocytosis into bile, a known phenomenon, plays a role. In this way, protein oxidation might be coupled to excretion of excess oxidized protein.

At an extreme of regulation of tissue growth and protein accretion, is the specialized process of programmed cell death, apoptosis, which has become a major thrust in recent research. The characteristic changes which occur during this phenomenon, such as cellular and organelle shrinkage, DNA laddering, and the exposure of phosphatidyl serine on cell surfaces, seem to be part of a mechanism by which apoptotic cells are removed for catabolism by other, viable cells (Aupeix *et al.* 1996). We will consider here whether protein oxidation is an initiator, mediator, or effector of apoptosis, extending the brief reference to protein oxidation molecular events during apoptosis given in Chapter 3.

The initiation of apoptosis is clearly often a programmed developmental event, but sometimes a physiological response to hormonal conditions, as in the case of lymphocytes (Castedo *et al.* 1995). Some instances of apoptosis may be induced by toxins, even though necrosis (usually involving cell swelling and ultimate rupture through osmotic imbalance) is more common as a toxic mechanism. It is most convenient to consider all cases of apoptosis here, since as far as we know they share common mechanisms; necrosis is considered in the next chapter.

Certain oxidized moieties, notably heavily oxidized LDL (Bjorkerud and Bjorkerud 1996), can trigger apoptosis in a range of cells. The active ingredients in the LDL are not clear (Yang *et al.* 1996), though oxysterols may be important in this regard (Aupeix *et al.* 1996; Lizard *et al.* 1996;

Palladini *et al.* 1996). The delivery mode of oxysterols is important for their toxic actions, and has not been fully elucidated. For example, oxysterols delivered in organic solution to cells are much more toxic than equivalent quantities delivered by way of lipoproteins (Jessup *et al.*, unpublished data). In several situations NO or resultant reactive nitrogen or oxygen inter-mediates, can induce apoptosis (Fehsel *et al.* 1995; Fukuo *et al.* 1996; Geng *et al.* 1996; Yamada *et al.* 1996). As discussed in Chapter 3, p53 may par-ticipate in this (Messmer *et al.* 1994*a, b*; Ho *et al.* 1996), and cleavage of poly-ADP-ribose polymerase, by an undefined mechanism, occurs during apoptosis (Messmer *et al.* 1996). Natural killer (NK) cells are even more sensitive than lymphocytes to oxidatively induced apoptosis (Hansson *et al.* 1996). Radiation exposure can also initiate apoptosis by mechanisms in-volving p53 (Rosselli *et al.* 1995); glutathione affords significant protection against this process, suggesting that protein thiols may be involved (Bump and Brown 1990). Indeed, low-molecular-weight thiols, which have been shown to be radio-protective, can initiate toxicity (necrosis) or apoptosis, depending on their concentration (Held *et al.* 1996). Down's syndrome neurons differentiate in culture, but then, unlike normal neurons, undergo apoptosis which can be inhibited by catalase and certain antioxidants. This suggests that these cells may have a deficiency in antioxidant defences which can be overwhelmed, and hence permits an oxidative mechanism for the induction of apoptosis, but the role of protein oxidation in this is again unknown (Busciglio and Yankner 1995). Richter has suggested that alterations in mitochondrial function are imporant in apoptosis induced by both RNIs and oxygen radicals via control of cellular ATP (Richter *et al.* 1995).

Antioxidants can protect against a wide range of inducers of apoptosis (Quillet *et al.* 1996). For example, the glutathione peroxidase mimic, ebselen, can protect against radiation induced apoptosis, and in the process it decreases intracellular oxidant generation or availability, as judged both by the dichlorofluorescein reaction and by the occurrence of membrane lipid peroxidation, which are induced by radiation and suppressed by ebselen (Ramakrishnan *et al.* 1996). Indeed, endogenous Bcl2 expression is thought to be a key cellular defence against apoptosis (Messmer *et al.* 1996) and to operate also by restricting oxidative events (Ivanov *et al.* 1995), but the evidence for this is quite indirect, and there is no specific information on protein oxidation in this process. While radicals and oxidative events are indeed normally considered pro-apoptotic (Slater *et al.* 1995), and down-regulation of superoxide dismutase by an antisense nucleotide predisposes certain cells to apoptosis (Troy *et al.* 1996*a, b*), nevertheless apoptosis mediated by the surface receptor Fas (Um *et al.* 1996) can be inhibited in conditions in which intracellular superoxide seems elevated, and this has been proposed as a physiological control (Clement and Stamenkovic 1996).

The possible mediation of apoptosis by oxidation has received limited attention. During non-oxidative triggering of apoptosis, intracellular oxidative events, including DNA damage and GSH depletion, can often be observed (Slater *et al.* 1995; Kohno *et al.* 1996). For example, in fetal hepatocytes the induction of apoptosis by TGFβ involves oxidative events, including the induction of the redox sensitive cFos (Sanchez *et al.* 1996). In all these cases, it is not clear whether oxidation is functional or incidental, and the evidence of protein oxidation, beyond the changes in p53 discussed in Chapter 3, is very limited. Indeed, it has been pointed out that several apoptosis initiators can act even in hypoxic conditions (Slater *et al.* 1995), though this is a weak argument against the role of oxidative events. The importance of oxidation as mediator remains unresolved, and the possible participation as effector mechanism does not seem to have been investigated directly; for example, it is not yet known whether the reactive products of protein oxidation can be found during apoptosis.

Cellular differentiation processes in some cases may involve protein oxidation as mediator. A very interesting series of studies by Hansberg and colleagues on conidiation in *N. crassa* illustrates this (reviewed: Hansberg and Aguirre 1990; Hansberg 1996). Conidiation involves, successively, the germination of the asexual spore (conidium) to form filaments (hyphae), by apical growth. Masses of hyphae form the so called mycelium, and when growth is restricted, hyphae may mutually adhere. Subsequent to this, aerial hyphae grow, and when the adherent mycelium becomes limiting for such growth, conidia form at the tips of the aerial hyphae. Thus, there are three transitions, between intermediate, 'unstable' states: from growing hyphae to adhered; from adhered to aerial; and from aerial to conidia (Hansberg and Aguirre 1990; Hansberg 1996). Each of the three steps seems to involve a hyperoxidant state, judged by chemiluminescence detection of reactive oxygen species in the cultures (Hansberg *et al.* 1993), alteration of the redox couples (GSH/GSSG and NAD(P)H/NAD(P)) of the cells (Toledo *et al.* 1995), and excretion of GSSG (Toledo *et al.* 1991). Protein oxidation is specifically related with these steps, both in time and in space.

To establish this relationship, Hansberg and colleagues undertook an elegant series of studies, specifically influenced by the ideas of metal-ion-catalysed oxidation and its possible relation to proteolysis, as generated by Levine and Stadtman, and discussed above. Using the 2,4-dinitrophenyl-hydrazine method to measure protein carbonyls, with special care taken to avoid interference by the substantial and localized carotenoid concentrations, they observed substantial peaks of protein carbonyls coincident with the commencement of adhesion, and slightly preceding formation of aerial hyphae and conidia (Toledo and Hansberg 1990). The basal values of carbonyls were reported as around 10 nmol mg^{-1} protein, which on the basis of the arguments discussed above would correspond to 0.5 mol carbonyl per mol protein, a huge value. In periods of 30–60 minutes, depending on the particular transition, the carbonyl levels increased by a factor of 1.8–2.5. Similarly, the return to basal values which follows each peak operated on the same time-scale. Unless these organisms possess some special protein carbonyl blocking, repair, or redistribution mechanism, which has not been observed, then at a minimum these recoveries require very fast proteolysis of the oxidized proteins, even if there is no further generation of protein carbonyls at that point. A half-life for the protein pool containing carbonyls of the order of 30 minutes would be required.

In vivo protein inactivation and turnover was investigated in more detail in a subsequent paper by Toledo *et al.* (1994). This took advantage of the information from their own previous in vitro studies of oxidative inactivation of glutamine synthetase (Aguirre and Hansberg 1986) and glutamate dehydrogenase (Aguirre *et al.* 1989) in this organism. These studies had shown that metal-ion-catalysed oxidation could inactivate both enzymes, with limited structural changes. The products from glutamate dehydrogenase were quite heterogeneous, but from glutamine synthetase a significant portion of more acidic polypeptides of the same molecular size as the parent polypeptides could be detected in two-dimensional gels of inactivated enzyme. Most importantly, and unlike the cases of glutamine synthetase inactivation discussed earlier, these charge-modified polypeptides could be detected *in vivo* in hyper-aerated cultures (Aguirre and Hansberg 1986). It is clearly the most economical interpretation to envisage that these *in vivo* polypeptides *are* oxidatively generated, though again no *specific* marker of oxidation has been detected. Furthermore, the *in vitro* oxidized glutamate synthetase was also rendered more susceptible to some endogenous proteinases of the organism.

In the more recent study, the relationship between carbonyls, enzyme inactivation and protein turnover was addressed (Toledo *et al.* 1994). Loss of glutamine synthetase activity occurred prior to each differentiation step, and coincided with each increase in protein carbonyls. Again, charge-modified, presumably oxidized glutamine synthetase polypeptides could be detected *in vivo*, and this was shown during hyphal adhesion. The GDH(NADP) (NADP-dependent glutamate dehydrogenase) activity was also lost, in this case during adhesion and before aerial hyphal formation, and the catabolic GDH(NAD) behaved in an opposite manner, which would be physiologically beneficial. Total protein turnover was measured by incorporating radioactive leucine into cultures for 3.5 hours (thus focusing on proteins of fairly short half life), and following the loss of specific activity of the proteins in subsequent chases in the absence of radioactive leucine. It is not clear to what degree isotope reutilization would occur, but during hyphal adhesion significant degradation could be detected within 10 minutes, and reached about 50 per cent in 60 minutes. In the non-adhered portion of these cultures, the protein degradation was much slower (less than 10 per cent at 60 minutes) but there was a dramatic loss of protein carbonyls, from 10 to virtually 0 nmol mg^{-1} protein, over a period of 20 minutes. If degradation is responsible for this loss, then it is highly selective.

It seems very plausible that in this fascinating system protein oxidation is an important mediator of the degradative/synthetic remodelling of enzyme systems which occurs during the differentiation steps. The data offer by far the best studied example of such a role. Hansberg and colleagues have offered a theoretical perspective in which they suggest that a common thread is 'dioxygen avoidance' (Hansberg and Aguirre 1990), based on the idea that cells maintain intracellular oxygen concentrations only of around 10 μM, much lower than the solubility of oxygen in water (*c*. 250μM). In this theory hyperoxidant states are viewed as central to differentiation steps, and in order to stabilize the resultant, differentiated state, necessary features are: the limitation of oxygen entry, through structural changes; the consumption of oxygen, through the action of reductants; and the restriction of oxygen radical activity, through defence mechanisms (e.g. by means of antioxidant enzymes (Lamboy *et al.* 1995)) so that another hyperoxidant state is not immediately generated. It is argued that hyperoxidant states may quite commonly characterize microbial cell differentiation. A few examples implying protein oxidation in these events in other organisms are given, and the field is one of great potential.

Situations in which radical production is more substantially triggered are also ones in which the issue of possible protein oxidation mediators need to be addressed more carefully. Thus, the leukocyte respiratory burst is a radical flux which may interact with control mechanisms, and to some degree this has been assessed. We will discuss protein oxidation during cytolytic actions of triggered radical fluxes in the subsequent section. The conditions in which radical fluxes are triggered are often those in which an extracellular particle or the extracellular matrix needs to be degraded, so that tissue regeneration can take place. Thus, an interaction at the cell surface of mononuclear phagocytes, between the radical-mediated degradative mechanisms and the proteolytic enzyme systems, has been considered (Roberts and Dean 1986; Vissers and Winterbourn 1986). Pre-exposure of albumin or glomerular basement membrane to neutrophil MPO in the presence of hydrogen peroxide and chloride enhanced their susceptibility to neutrophil proteinases. In a model system in which neutrophils adhered to basement membrane via immune complexes, degradation was largely due to proteinases, and oxidants did not affect overall degradation, as judged by a lack of action of scavengers and inhibitors. However, this was deceptive, as simultaneously the oxidants inactivated the released elastase, lysozyme, and β-glucuronidase by up to 50 per cent, judged by the same criteria.

Thus, a smaller amount of active proteinase effected the same degree of degradation of collagen (measured as hydroxyproline release) after oxidation than before, so that the substrate was apparently sensitized to proteolysis (Vissers and Winterbourn 1986). In a macrophage-cartilage disc system, a cell surface machinery was implicated (Roberts and Dean 1986), and again both oxidative and proteolytic events may contribute to degradation.

A subsequent paper (Mukhopadhyay and Chatterjee 1994*b*) has made a major contribution to this issue. Using buffers and reagents, in which free transition metal availability was restricted by chelators, these authors showed that PMA-triggered guinea pig macrophages (but not their lysates, nor their untriggered counterparts), could degrade calf skin collagen suspensions, by a mechanism involving a brief respiratory burst and concomitant substrate oxidation, followed by proteolytic digestion. The proteolytic digestion could be inhibited by selective proteinase inhibitors, while the first phase was unaffected. The oxidative phase could be dramatically inhibited by 20–50 µM ascorbate, in contrast to its pro-oxidant action at these concentrations in free-metal catalysed systems. SOD was also a potent inhibitor. A very similar inhibitor sensitivity and action was observed for xanthine oxidase plus its substrate, when exposed to collagen. It seemed, in this case, that enzyme-bound functional metal participated in the generation of effective oxidants, probably hydroxyl radicals, from the primary superoxide product of the enzyme, and that this step was blocked by ascorbate; in the cell system, superoxide is also the primary product of the respiratory burst, and the authors argued that macrophages release metalloproteins such as cytochromes containing similarly functional metal.

Besides action on the degradative enzymes and their substrates, there may be an inhibition by neutrophils of proteoglycan synthesis via hydrogen peroxide, while hypochlorite and the neutrophil elastase are active in degradative events (Kowanko *et al.* 1989). Interactions via the oxidation-sensitive proteinase inhibitors have been described already, and examples of enzyme activation by radicals also. These systems may be integrated to permit effective matrix degradation. For example, the single chain protein urokinase, released by triggered neutrophils, can be activated by chlor-amines and hypochlorite produced by the same cells, apparently in an indirect mechanism involving oxidative inactivation of proteinase inhibitors (Stief *et al.* 1991). This may be a prototype of a more general mechanism. Furthermore, such matrix degradation may influence cell growth, just as much as may intracellular oxidative events, through cell surface signals from the interaction of glycosaminoglycans or proteoglycans and membrane receptors. This kind of sensing of the extracellular milieu may well involve oxidative degradation events.

4.4 Protein oxidation, cell damage, and defensive cytolysis

It is well established that the respiratory burst of leukocytes, such as mononuclear phagocytes and polymorphonuclear neutrophils, is an important mechanism of killing invading organisms in the extracellular space. Similarly, intracellular killing of parasites, such as a range of protozoa, may involve oxidative mechanisms. It is clear that oxygen-independent mechanisms also exist, so there is commonly an interaction between oxidative and enzymatic hydrolytic mechanisms. Our specific topic here is what role protein oxidation has in these events.

There are two aspects of this question: whether protein oxidation is important in the lytic events themselves, and what role it has to play in the consequent catabolic removal of dead organisms. As also discussed in Chapter 5 in relation to radical toxicity to host cells, permeability changes in the target organism (Sips and Hamers 1981), in the case of *E. coli* exposed to myeloperoxidase or to reagent hypochlorite, are often central to osmotic derangement and subsequent lysis. Key protein targets include the ionic pump proteins necessary to maintain ionic and osmotic equilibrium of cells. In some circumstances the direct inactivation of a plasma (or other) membrane transporter may be a key step in the derangements which lead to lysis. For example, amino acid hydroperoxides and other organic hydroperoxides can inactivate the glutathione-S-conjugate pump, which removes oxidized glutathione from cells as part of cellular detoxification (Soszynski *et al.* 1995), and radiation-induced radicals can also inactivate transporters (Grzelinska *et al.* 1982). Photodynamic inactivation of yeast also involves inactivation of membrane carriers for sugars, amino acids, and phosphate, and reconstitution studies have shown that this involves an effect on the carrier proteins, and not solely on membrane lipids (Paardekooper *et al.* 1993). During photodamage to mammalian cells, the $Na^+/K^+/ATPase$ ion pump seems to be an important target (Ben *et al.* 1992*a*). This seems also to be true during radical attack induced by Fenton systems (Richards *et al.* 1988), and it can be expected that transporter inactivation is generally important in cytolytic attack on invading organisms.

In the microbicidal mechanisms of leukocytes, hypochlorite seems to be very important (Albrich *et al.* 1981). Similarly, in the hydrolysis of macromolecules of the pathogen which follows cell death, oxidative damage may play a role. For example, hypochlorite, produced by neutrophils from the myeloperoxidase-catalysed action of hydrogen peroxide (formed from the dismutation of superoxide radicals generated by the respiratory burst) upon chloride ions, can fragment proteins effectively (Selvaraj *et al.* 1974). This is judged by release of radioactive carbon dioxide from bacterial macromolecules into which $(1,7-^{14}C)$-diaminopimelic acid had been incorporated biosynthetically. HOCl also decarboxylates and deaminates most free amino acids and in proteins, particularly, attacks tyrosine, tryptophan, and lysine (Adeniyi et al. 1981). The decarboxylation pathway is associated with the formation of aldehydes, rather as shown in other systems by Dakin (see Chapter 1), and these have potential cytotoxic activities also (Strauss et al. 1970). The fragmentation, in particular, may facilitate the structural opening up of the organisms, and hence access of larger proteolytic enzymes to the protein substrates. Thomas and colleagues undertook very detailed early work on such actions of hypochlorite, and also other hypo-acids (Aune and Thomas 1978). They showed that free and protein sulfydryls in bacteria were particularly sensitive (Thomas and Aune 1978a, b). N-Cl compounds, as also foreshadowed by Dakin (see Chapter 1), were important effectors when amino acids were supplied, as well as products of hypochlorite attack on the bacteria (Thomas 1979a, b). The action of these compounds was long lasting, continuing well after the supply of hydrogen peroxide to the enzyme system ceased. In addition, this process (like that due to hypochlorite itself) was accompanied by drastic release of protein fragments from the organisms (Thomas 1979a). 30–50 per cent of the HOCl supplied could be detected as N-Cl derivatives of such released peptides. Their size distributions, in comparison with those extracted from the host organism, suggested that they resulted from direct protein fragmentation, and in experiments with polylysine the authors directly demonstrated such extensive fragmentation by HOCl (Thomas 1979a). In model systems, treatment of target proteins with $RNCl_2$ resulted in the incorporation of amines into target proteins, though it was argued that this would not necessarily be relevant to the bactericidal activity (Thomas et al. 1982).

Removal of lysed micro-organisms normally involves phagocytosis by leukocytes. Lysed, aggregated, particulate materials are very good substrates for phagocytosis, but there also may be some specialized, oxidative mechanisms for enhancing uptake. These comprise both chemical cross-linking (enhancing aggregate formation) and fixation of immuno-globulin molecules onto the micro-organism, such that the phagocytes can recognize the immunoglobulin as a selective ligand for their surface endocytic receptors. One interesting study demonstrated a monocyte-mediated crosslinking mechanism for immunoglobulin which could utilize exogenously added catechol (Jasin 1987). This apparently involved the action of myeloperoxidase and peroxide, and could be inhibited by azide and catalase. It seemed that the quinone derived from catechol was important, which points to the relevance of protein-bound DOPA generated by oxidation in such reactions.

4.5 Intracellular and extracellular accumulation or storage of oxidized proteins: comparison between stable and reactive products of protein oxidation

There are now many examples of the detection of significant quantities of oxidized proteins in normal living tissues. Protein carbonyls, of undefined nature are most commonly detected (see Table 4.1) and, as mentioned above, there are serious difficulties in interpreting these data reliably because of variability between methods, and also because of problems with the presence of other, non-protein, carbonyl-containing materials. However, the data give some weight to the idea that even in physiological conditions, significant pools of oxidized proteins exist.

There is currently considerable interest in whether, and to what degree, other specific oxidation products of proteins occur *in vivo*. In particular, to what extent are the other the reactive products we have already discussed, such as hydroperoxides and catechol/quinone systems present? Table 4.1. cumulates some of these new data, and supports the general idea, from studies of carbonyls, that significant, oxidized pools exist normally. The arguments discussed above indicate that there might be as many as one carbonyl per 250 candidate amino acid sites. The value for individual oxidation products expressed per parent amino acid, is not suprisingly much lower. For example, values of roughly one oxidation product per 10 000 parent amino acids are now common, with the frequency being notably higher for the products from the more reactive aromatic residues than from the aliphatic amino acids, as one might predict.

How can these two incomplete sets of data be reconciled? One approach would be to integrate the estimated frequency of each individual specific product with that of the parent amino acid, and thereby deduce the overall frequency; data limitations make this, as yet, inappropriate. An alternative approach is to assume that the average frequency with which *any* amino acids is found oxidized, is intermediate between the two ranges for aromatic and aliphatic residues, i.e. one might take a figure of one in 5000. A 50 kDa protein normally contains about 500 amino acids, and hence this argument would suggest that around one in 10 protein molecules would contain one or more oxidized amino acids. In summary, these data indicate that under steady state physiological conditions, 10 per cent of protein molecules probably contain one or more oxidized amino acids.

Most of the data relate to intracellular proteins or to total tissue proteins in which intracellular and extracellular components are not distinguished. With extracellular proteins, some of which are notably long lived, such as connective tissue collagens and lens crystallins, the values may be much higher. An important feature of these proteins is that unless a pathological

Table 4.1 Selected data on concentrations of oxidized amino acids in normal tissue proteins

Product	Physiological levels	Source of data
DOPA	85 pmol mg LDL protein (6 per 10 000 tyrosines)	Unpublished
o-, m-tyrosine	62 and 35 pmol mg^{-1} LDL protein, (5 and 3 per 10 000 phenylalanines respectively	Unpublished
	3 and 1 per 10 000 human plasma protein phenylalanines	(Heinecke et al., in press)
	5 per 10 000 phenylalanines in human lenses of any age	(Wells-Knecht et al. 1993)
N-formylkynurenine; kynurenine	ND	
di-tyrosine	0.2 pmol mg^{-1} LDL protein (0.02 per 10 000 tyrosines)	Unpublished
	0.02 per 10 000 plasma protein tyrosines	(Heinecke et al., in press)
	0.01 per 10 000 tyrosines in human lens proteins from young people	(Wells-Knecht et al. 1993)
dimers of hydroxylated aromatic amino acids	ND	
2-oxo-histidine	ND	
hydro(pero)xyleucines	leucine hydroxide: 5 pmol mg^{-1} LDL protein (0.1 per 10 000 leucines)	Unpublished
hydro(pero)xyvalines	valine hydroxide: 5 pmol mg^{-1} LDL protein (0.1 per 10 000 valines)	Unpublished
3-chlorotyrosine	Normal aorta: 0.8 per 10 000 protein tyrosines Normal plasma: 0.1 per 10 000 protein tyrosines	(Heinecke et al., in press)
3-nitrotyrosine	< 10 pmol mg^{-1} LDL protein (< 1 per 10 000 tyrosines)	Unpublished
	0.09 per 10 000 plasma protein tyrosines	(Heinecke et al., in press)
p-hydroxyphenyl-acetaldehyde	ND	
Aminomalonic acid	0.04–0.3 per 1000 total amino acids in two E. coli strains	(Van Buskirk et al. 1984)
5-hydroxy-2-amino-valeric acid	0.15 nmol mg^{-1} protein in 100 000 g supernatants from young mouse liver	(Ayala and Cutler 1996a)
Protein carbonyls	approx 1 nmol mg^{-1} protein in many physiological tissue samples	(Levine et al. 1994; Lyras et al. 1996)

Unpublished refers to work of the present authors in collaboration with Dr Shanlin Fu: means of three advanced human atherosclerotic plaque and three human LDL samples obtained freshly. In these studies, levels of the measured species in fresh human plasma expressed per parent amino acid were, in most cases, very slightly lower. The aorta samples used in the studies of Heinecke et al., were obtained post mortem. ND: detailed data not found.

circumstance supervenes, such as the inflammatory invasion of leukocytes, they remain relatively distal to normal enzymatic turnover mechanisms. Once access is gained, they are probably commonly efficiently removed.

Current evidence suggests that the levels of the reactive products, such as the catechols, and of the other products are comparable in magnitude. Thus, the figures for DOPA presented in Table 4.1. are of the same order as those for *o*- and *m*-tyrosine and the highest of those for di-tyrosine. Similarly, those for the protein hydroxides are comparable with some of the values for protein carbonyls. An unresolved issue, as discussed earlier, is the distribution of side chain oxidation products between hydroperoxides and hydroxides. The pool size of these species depends on the net of input (oxidation plus reincorporation by protein synthesis) and removal (detoxification/chemical decay plus enzymatic hydrolysis followed by excretion). Unless detoxification/decay were processes which operate *much* faster than the other processes, it would be expected that the reactive intermediates would be found at a concentration of the same order as that of the carbonyls, di-tyrosine, etc., as is observed. The studies on *N. crassa* discussed above indicate that hydrolysis of the protein carbonyl pools can sometimes indeed be fast, and probably at least as fast as any detoxification path, in agreement with this argument.

Taken together, the available data indicate that both the stable and the reactive products of protein oxidation accumulate physiologically, to comparable levels, and such that roughly 10 per cent of protein molecules may contain at least one oxidized amino acid. Clearly, they have the potential for significant actions in the physiology of the organism, and equally, their actions might be significantly deranged in pathological circumstances, if their concentrations are drastically changed. The pathological effects of such species are considered in the next chapter.

5 The pathology of protein oxidation

We will devote most of this chapter to focusing on a limited number of pathologies in which it has been possible to make some analysis of the *importance* of protein oxidation. However, we first wish to summarize the occurrence of products of protein oxidation in a range of pathological situations (Table 5.1), to complement the discussion of Chaper 4. Many, but not all, pathologies are accompanied by the presence of oxidized proteins at levels beyond the physiological. The difficulty, as always, is in distinguishing 'bystander' oxidation, which is a quite secondary *consequence* of the pathology, from that which might be important in its progression.

However, it is encouraging that, when the data are assessed critically, it is apparent that some pathological locales do not display elevated protein oxidation products. If this is, for the purposes of argument, assumed to indicate that they also show no elevated rate of production of such moieties, then one can argue that protein oxidation is not a necessary side-effect of all pathology. Of course it could be, conversely, that those situations in which no accumulation occurs are simply those in which oxidation products are most successfully removed, having nevertheless been generated in an exaggerated manner as a result of the pathology.

Only in a few cases can one currently begin to make the distinctions required for further assessment of these issues, and it is these cases that we have chosen to analyse in a little more detail.

5.1 Toxic and lytic damage to host cells: roles of oxidized proteins

We discussed in Chapter 4 the role of protein oxidation in radical-mediated killing of invading pathogens. As pointed out there, radical damage to proteins is usually concomitant with damage to membrane lipids, and sometimes to nuclear DNA. Thus, an important issue is to distinguish the relative importance of these several actions for toxicity. The same issues arise in considering toxic events which act on the host rather than the invader.

Clearly, events which damage lipids, DNA, or protein may all be seriously deleterious. For example, a gross disruption of membrane structure through

Table 5.1　Selected data on concentrations of oxidized amino acids in tissue proteins from pathological circumstances

Product	Approximate physiological levels (see Table 4.1)	Pathological levels	Source of pathological data
DOPA	85 pmol mg^{-1} protein (6 per 10 000 tyrosines)	410 pmol mg^{-1} protein (14 per 10 000 tyrosines) in advanced human atherosclerotic plaques.	Unpublished
		Elevated 15–25 fold over physiological (or normal lens) levels in type IV cataractous human lens proteins.	(Fu *et al.*, unpublished data)
o-, *m*-tyrosine	62 and 35 pmol mg^{-1} protein, (5 and 3 per 10 000 phenylalanines) respectively	105 and 175 pmol mg^{-1} protein, (3.5 and 6 per 10 000 phenylalanines) respectively, in plaques.	Unpublished
		No increase in atherosclerotic aorta samples compared with normal.	(Heinecke *et al.*, in press)
		Elevated > 70 fold in type IV cataractous human lens proteins compared with physiological (or normal lens) levels	(Fu *et al.*, unpublished data)
N-formylkynurenine; kynuernine	ND	ND	
di-tyrosine	0.2 pmol mg^{-1} protein (0.02 per 10 000 tyrosines)	150 pmol mg^{-1} protein (5 per 10 000 tyrosines) in plaques.	Unpublished
		Elevated 10 fold in aortic lesions in comparison with normal aortic samples.	(Heinecke *et al.*, in press)
		0.5 per 10 000 tyrosines in type IV cataractous human lens	(Fu *et al.*, unpublished data)
dimers of hydroxylated aromatic amino acids	ND	ND	

2-oxo-histidine	ND	ND	
hydro(pero)xyleucines	leucine hydroxide: 5 pmol mg^{-1} protein (0.1 per 10 000 leucines)	Leucine hydroxide: 20 pmol mg^{-1} protein (0.2 per 10 000 leucines) in plaques. Elevated > 10 fold in type IV human cataractous lens proteins compared with physiological or with normal lens.	Unpublished (Fu et al., unpublished data)
hydro(pero)xyvalines	valine hydroxide: 5 pmol mg^{-1} protein (0.1 per 10 000 valines)	Valine hydroxide: 10 pmol mg^{-1} protein (0.1 per 10 000 valines) in plaques. Elevated > 10 fold in type IV human cataractous lens proteins compared with physiological or with normal lens.	Unpublished (Fu et al., unpublished data)
3-chlorotyrosine	0.1–0.8 per 10 000 tyrosines	Atherosclerotic aorta 3 per 10 000 tyrosines	(Heinecke et al., in press)
3-nitrotyrosine	< 10 pmol mg^{-1} protein < 1 per 10 000 tyrosines)	< 10 pmol mg^{-1} protein (< 0.3 per 10 000 tyrosines) in plaques. Elevated 100 fold in aortic lesions LDL in comparison with normal plasma LDL.	Unpublished (Heinecke et al., in press)
p-hydroxyphenyl-acetaldehyde	ND	ND	
Aminomalonic acid	0.04–0.3 per 1000 total amino acids	0.2 per 1000 glycines in post-mortem human plaque.	(Van Buskirk et al. 1984)
5-hydroxy-2-amino-valeric acid	0.15 nomol mg^{-1} protein	Unchanged in old mouse livers. Elevated by hyperoxic exposure.	(Ayala and Cutler 1996a)
Protein carbonyls	approx 1 nmol mg^{-1} protein	up to 8 nmol mg^{-1} protein in diseased brain samples	(Levin et al. 1994; Lyras et al. 1996)

Unpublished refers to work of the present authors in collaboration with Dr Shanlin Fu: means of three advanced human atherosclerotic plaque and three human LDL samples obtained freshly. In these studies, levels of the measured species in fresh human plasma expressed per parent amino acid were, in most cases, very slightly lower. The aorta samples used in the studies of Heinecke et al. were obtained post mortem. ND: detailed data not found.

lipid alterations may prevent its proper function as a permeability and transport control site. Similarly, extreme DNA damage, as observed in apoptosis, must preclude further division by the cell, and ultimately lead to death. However, proteins are possibly the most immediate vehicle for inflicting toxic damage on cells, since they are often catalysts, rather than stoichiometric mediators, and hence the effect of damage to one molecule is greater than stoichiometric. For example, inactivating 10 per cent of an individual ion transporter protein in a membrane may well be much more drastic in its effects on homeostasis (as opposed to physiological triggering) than modifying 10 per cent of the membrane cholesterol molecules. The effects in non dividing cells of protein damage may also be much more immediate than those of DNA or possibly lipid damage.

Thus, several studies have attempted to distinguish the relative importance of protein and lipid damage in toxic events which lead to osmotic lysis, the major form of toxic necrosis of cells. Osmotic lysis ultimately involves influx of water, through deranged ion transport, which leads to swelling and cell rupture. Can protein damage be separated from lipid damage in these circumstances? A range of studies summarized argues that lipophilic antioxidants may be able to prevent or largely restrict lipid oxidation during an oxidative affront, and yet cell toxicity remains: in some cases direct evidence of protein damage is available, and damage to transporters and pumps has been observed. In other studies, functional changes in membrane potential have been observed, even while lipid oxidation is blocked, and these are followed, after a lag of the order of 1–2 hours, by cell death. Such studies indicate that membrane protein damage may be a primary aspect of toxicity in these circumstances.

There may be no generality to this conclusion, however, since several oxidative affronts act selectively at intracellular sites, and may involve different mechanisms. For example, photosensitizers often induce membrane lipid damage when irradiated, but membrane protein damage seems normally more important in what is usually an eventual osmotic lysis (Cardenas et al. 1992). But some photosensitizers accumulate in the low pH interior of lysosomes of cells, often because of weakly basic functions (Dean et al. 1984a). Light exposure may cause toxic actions as a consequence of this location. This process may involve lysosomal rupture and subsequent toxic events, though the initial view of the lysosome as a 'suicide' bag, propounded by de Duve and his colleagues in the 1950s and early 1960s, is no longer tenable, since it is appreciated that the cytoplasm of cells is richly endowed with hydrolase inhibitors, such as proteinase inhibitors, so that the release of lysosomal enzymes into the cytoplasm can normally be neutralized through enzyme inactivation (reviewed: Dean and Barrett 1976; Lloyd and Mason 1996). In such cases membrane lipid oxidation might be very central, though more subtle changes involving ionic homeostasis may be important, and involve oxidation of critical proteins, though they have not been resolved in most cases.

Thus, protein oxidation is intrinsic to much cytotoxicity, and may be of primary importance in many cases. A secondary reason why protein damage should ideally be restricted in defending against such toxic attack is that proteins are the effectors of the removal/repair mechanisms which are potent in the case of lipid and DNA oxidation, though less so for proteins themselves. Although protein oxidation may be followed by repair in the rare case that methionine only is oxidized (as discussed earlier), it is normally succeeded by degradation, yet the accumulation of oxidized proteins shows that this process is incompletely efficient. Furthermore, oxidized amino acids may be reutilised, thus regenerating the oxidized proteins to some extent. Therefore, the prevention of protein oxidation may be the best method of minimizing oxidative toxicity, through both these primary and secondary factors.

5.2 Inflammatory generation of oxidized proteins in the host

Host protein oxidation may occur during host defence reactions, as well as during the action of exogenous oxidative affronts. Thus, it is clear that triggered neutrophils, while vectorially releasing their superoxide flux into the location of a foreign organism or other trigger of the respiratory burst (Rossi *et al.* 1983), may also damage some host molecules (Kowanko *et al.* 1989; Kurtel *et al.* 1992). Thus, proteins found in broncheoalveolar lavage fluid have been shown to have elevated methionine sulfoxide:methionine ratios (Costabel *et al.* 1992).

Evidence for host DNA and protein damage in these circumstances is available (Oliver 1987; Krsek and Webster 1993; Fliss and Menard 1994). Protein carbonyls are formed in triggered neutrophils (Oliver 1987), and internal and external chlorination and nitration of tyrosines can occur through the action of the myeloperoxidase/hyphochlorite and NO/peroxynitrite pathways respectively (Domigan *et al.* 1995; Salman *et al.* 1995; Kettle 1996). Some of the proteins which are damaged are probably co-located with the target organisms, either in the immediate extracellular space, or in the phagosomes (Krsek and Webster 1993). However, more distal damage can occur (Lundqvist *et al.* 1996), as indicated by failures of the intracellular actin contractile systems (DalleDonne *et al.* 1995), inhibition of chemotactic responses (Till *et al.* 1987), and by the nuclear DNA damage observed in some studies (Shacter *et al.* 1990). System damage, such as glomerular injury (Couser 1990), is probably consequent on this, and may be very important in the leukocyte-dependent ischemia-reperfusion damage in many organs (Werns and Lucchesi 1990). Since plants (Dwyer *et al.* 1996) and probably other organisms possess protein systems related to the human respiratory burst oxidase complex, it might be expected that damage to host proteins through such triggering will be widespread. Several systems (Nakamura *et al.* 1994), notably the reversible thiolation system discussed earlier, exist to buffer intracellular proteins against such changes (Chai *et al.* 1994*a, b*; Seres *et al.* 1996).

Several studies point to such inflammatory damage to host proteins. It has been argued that chronic inflammation is a major source of oxidative mutation, and hence a contributor to cancer. This is an important issue, since the vast majority of the world's population has chronic periodontal disease, and many suffer other chronic inflammatory conditions and their oxidative consequences (Dillard *et al.* 1982*b*), which in themselves are containable. The possibility exists that such mechanisms are also important in the accumulation of oxidized proteins in ageing tissues, as will be discussed later. They may be particularly relevant to accumulation of extracellular, oxidized proteins, in view of the primary action of the leukocyte respiratory burst on molecules exposed outside the cell surface.

Chronic inflammation is accompanied by accelerated catabolism of extracellular connective tissue macromolecules, including proteoglycans and collagens, as well as hyaluronic acid. These pathways have been the subject of many studies, and it is clear that both oxidative fragmentation and modification of the extracellular proteins and proteoglycans, and enzymatic hydrolysis occur (as discussed in Chapter 4). Some studies have indicated a synergy between the two processes, where oxidation of connective tissue components may accelerate subsequent enzymatic proteolysis, both by increasing accessibility and by enhancing proteolytic susceptibility of some components (Dean *et al.* 1984*b*; Roberts *et al.* 1987). For example, hypochlorite and collagenase may so interact in facilitating connective tissue degradation (Davies, J. M. *et al.* 1993). Such interactions are, however, confusing, since radicals can inactivate both the proteinases and the proteinase inhibitors relevant to inflammatory catabolism, for instance, those of neutrophils (Dean *et al.* 1989*b*). Similarly, *N*-chlorotaurine, though not several other *N*-chloro-amino acids, can inhibit collagenase (Davies *et al.* 1994). As yet, no studies have applied the recent understanding of specific products of protein oxidation to estimate its quantitative involvement. For example, the extent of oxidative, as opposed to hydrolytic, fragmentation could now be measured, since the products are largely distinct ((Roberts *et al.* 1989) and see Chapter 2). The oxidative component could then be correlated with the extent of oxidative modification of amino acids to substantiate the estimates of oxidative fragmentation.

Such studies will be valuable, since the situation of chronic inflammation is a complex one (Fig. 5.1), in which disentangling different roles is difficult.

In the case of protein degradation, the oxidative mechanisms may contribute directly to protein damage; but in so doing they may also change the proteinase-proteinase inhibitor balance by inactivating either or both components. This, in turn, would result in the oxidative process altering the activity of the proteolytic machinery itself, as well as providing modified connective tissue protein substrates which might be more accessible and readily hydrolysed. Clearly these actions can be synergistic or conflicting.

The issue of interaction between radicals and proteinases has often been treated rather simplistically in the literature, with a largely single-minded focus on the idea that proteinase inhibitors can be selectively inactivated, and that radical fluxes will thus enhance the available proteinase activity by reducing its inhibition. However, this idea is based on the stereotypic idea that proteinase inhibitors are all like α-1-proteinase inhibitor (α-1-PI) in having a selectively sensitive methionine residue essential for inhibitor function. It also depends on the assumption that the radical fluxes which occur comprise radicals selective for methionine, and many oxidants show

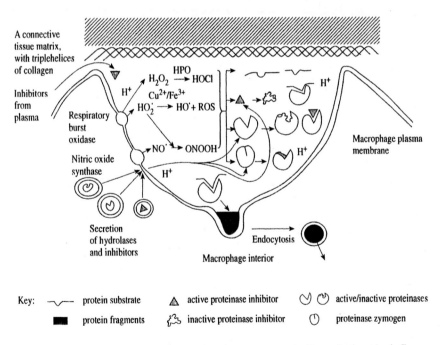

Figure 5.1   Radical-damage to proteins in sequestered sites of chronic inflammation. Protein breakdown in chronic inflammatory sites is influenced by a complex of opposing actions. These include matrix degradation by radicals which release diffusible fragments, and inactivation or activation of proteinases and their inhibitors, altering the balance between them. Extracellular degradation is completed intracellularly after endocytosis.

only modest (if any) selectivity for this amino acid. Thus, we showed that on exposure to Fenton systems, several proteinase inhibitors with or without methionine active sites, and their target proteinase, human neutrophil elastase, are comparably sensitive to inactivation (Dean *et al.* 1989*b*. Furthermore, it is well established (Chapter 3) that most enzymes are highly sensitive to oxidative inactivation (and a few proteinases contain functionally important and sensitive methionines, while there is a whole catalytic group of cysteine-proteinases). Thus it is impossible to predict what effect an oxidative flux in an inflammatory site will have on the proteinase/proteinase inhibitor balance, and no studies seem to have been undertaken to assess this carefully with respect to overall proteolysis, rather than with respect to the action of individual proteinases.

In sum, oxidative damage to proteins frequently occurs at inflammatory sites. This may make the protein substrates more available to the local proteolytic assemblage. At the same time that assemblage may be altered in an unpredictable direction, depending on the constitution of the proteinase/ proteinase inhibitor system, and equally on the nature of the radical fluxes. This very unpredictability may be an important feature which contributes to an unstable, yet chronic, evolution of the lesion.

For this reason, it would clearly be desirable to prevent the ongoing oxidation in these sites, and many pharmaceutical studies have been undertaken along these lines, though protein oxidation was assessed in few. As we will discuss further in the final chapter, no antioxidants have yet been successfully targeted specifically at protein oxidation, and it is only now that we can approach this possibility logically. Thus, it is not surprising that the interventions summarized have met limited success. However, the case of connective tissue catabolism in chronic inflammation is perhaps a key case in which protein metabolism is central, and in which a selective inhibitor of the oxidative component might be most useful, since it could permit most other oxidative, physiological processes to continue unperturbed. However, localized blockage of *all* the oxidative events at an early stage, and relevant to all macromolecular targets, might also be desirable. This is more likely to be achieved by control of radical generation than selective control of one of the actions of the radical flux, protein oxidation.

5.3 Transfer of damage from proteins to other targets

In this section we wish to analyse further the general theme that primary protein oxidative damage may affect the action of other proteins and other systems. The toxic actions of a few of the oxidized free amino acids we have considered are well established: for example, TOPA (2,4,5-trihydroxyphenylalanine; Skaper *et al.* 1992, 1993*a*, *b*). However, the relevance of comparable mechanisms, when the oxidized amino acids are present on proteins, is less well understood, and will be assessed in what follows. In so doing, we generalize ideas which have been expressed already, but distinguish damage which results from perturbed action of proteins, from that which results from an oxidized protein chemically modifying another molecule (e.g. forming a DNA-protein cross-link). We have chosen a limited range of examples to summarize these more general ideas.

5.3.1 Protein oxidation causing malfunction of protein systems: cardiac arrhythmias and ischemia/reperfusion

The essential feature of this case is similar to that discussed earlier in this chapter in the context of osmotic cell lysis: that damage to protein ion pumps and channels may have catastrophic, magnified actions on cellular and organism homeostasis. Here, we deal not solely with immediate cellular toxicity, but also with a derangement of the mechanical function of an organ caused by similar, fundamental damage. Leukocyte infiltration normally follows an ischemic period, and is important at least in the first few minutes (Galinanes *et al.* 1993) in subsequent, continuing damage and repair (reviewed: Werns and Lucchesi 1990). The derangements can quite often be fatal, leading to heart failure. In considering the probable importance of the proteins involved in ionic homeostasis, it will not always be appropriate to distinguish between the different mechanistic categories of pumps, channels, transporters, and their fellows: we will then use the term 'ion transporters' more loosely, without implication as to whether transport is active, passive, facilitated, etc.

Studies by Hearse and colleagues have generated elegant systems for the study of well-directed oxidative affronts to the heart and cardiac cells, using photosensitization by rose bengal to generate singlet oxygen and superoxide radicals (Kusama *et al.* 1989; Vandeplassche *et al.* 1990) and sometimes other photosensitizers to localize the action and to permit singlet oxygen generation alone (Kusama *et al.* 1990). These allow the demonstration that alteration of protein effectors of ionic homeostasis can be critical in leading to cardiac pathology. We will discuss the model experiments first, and then consider to what degree they can be applied to the *in vivo* cardiac pathologies.

Perfusion of hearts with rose bengal, followed by illumination leads to immediate alterations in transport, membrane electrophysiology, and to arrythmias (reviewed: Bernier *et al.* 1991; Hearse 1991*b*). Related effects are achieved on isolated ventricular muscle (Shattock *et al.* 1991). The kinetics of damage, which occurs within a few seconds of exposure to light, and their sensitivity to antioxidants (Bernier *et al.* 1989), are consistent with a primary protein damage which at least involves specific, selective ion transporters. The perturbation of the transporters leads to subsequent derangement of ionic events required for synchronous tissue contraction, and effective pumping: for example the Na^+/H^+ exchanger seems important (Yasutake *et al.* 1994). The resultant arrhythmias may ultimately lead to complete asynchrony and failure.

In isolated heavy sarcoplasmic reticulum vesicles, the photosensitized attack leads to direct alterations in ryanodine binding to the calcium release channels, the concomitant degradation of high-molecular-weight membrane proteins, and alterations in the release channel function (Holmberg *et al.* 1991). Comparative studies on different species and ages underscore the possible importance of the calcium control mechanisms (Nakata and Hearse 1990). The specific proteins which are involved in oxidative arrhythmogenicity *in vivo* have not yet been definitively identified, though there is already evidence of membrane protein-SH oxidation and several examples of proteins of ion channels with SH sensitivity (Lacampagne *et al.* 1995). Thus, the activity of the Na^+/Ca^{2+} exchanger can be altered during exposure of either cardiac sarcolemmal vesicles or cardiac myocytes to oxidative conditions (Reeves 1986; Kim *et al.* 1988; Coetzee *et al.* 1994), apparently through effects on the redox activity of its SH group (Reeves 1986; Coetzee *et al.* 1994). Similarly, the regulation of the Na^+/K^+ ATPase activity depends on the cellular glutathione levels being altered when these are directly manipulated *in vivo* (Haddock *et al.* 1995b) or *in vitro* (Kako 1987). This indicates that besides direct sensitivity of transport proteins to regulation by their own SH status (see (Haddock *et al.* 1995a) for the case of Na^+/K^+ ATPase) and the levels of defence against this offered by cellular reductants, indirect mechanisms following reductant depletion might be important. Depression of the activity of the Na^+/K^+-ATPase of pig kidneys has been observed as a result of ischemia, and this has been ascribed to free radical reactions and a decrease in SH content.

Another example of a transport system with oxidation-sensitive protein components which has been extensively studied is the Na^+/Ca^{2+} cardiac exchanger (Hilgemann and Collins 1992). Even in this case, the nature of oxidative impact is, as yet, unclear. However, it is clear that common amongst the early effects of a failure in ionic homeostasis are alterations in intracellular calcium, which is normally regulated at around 500 nM in most cells. This can readily cause alterations in proteolysis (Geeraerts *et al.* 1991) and other aspects of membrane function (Penning *et al.* 1992).

The studies just described were designed partly as models for the oxidative attack which clearly accompanies reperfusion of previously ischemic tissue, for example following a heart attack precipitated by deposition of a clot in one of the essential vessels supplying the heart. The clot causes a failure of flow and hence deoxygenation of a region of tissue; during such reduced oxygen supply a range of oxidative events, nevertheless, takes place, several showing accentuation at low oxygen tensions. Radical formation during such an ischemic phase has been demonstrated by EPR studies (Blasig *et al.* 1986; Arroyo *et al.* 1987*a, b*). Further, during the ischemia there is slow but progressive cell death. Subsequent reperfusion, which is absolutely essential for the survival of any of the affected tissue, may be achieved physiologically, or through therapy with clot-dissolving enzymes such as plasminogen activators. During reperfusion there is not only recommencement of flow, together with a rapid increase in the oxygen concentration (Yamada, M. *et al.* 1990), but also release of redox-active transition metals from the tissue (Chevion *et al.* 1993), and of radicals (Garlick *et al.* 1987) into the perfusate itself. The latter have been detected directly in animal models, such as the Langendorff-perfused or working rat heart or anaesthetized, intact dogs (Arroyo *et al.* 1987*a, b*; Garlick *et al.* 1987; Kramer *et al.* 1987; Zweier *et al.* 1987; Bolli *et al.* 1988; Zweier 1988; Pietri *et al.* 1989), by use of EPR spin trapping. This burst has been shown not to occur on reperfusion with anoxic buffer, suggesting that the observed species are either oxygen derived or produced by an oxygen-dependent process (Garlick *et al.* 1987). In the latter study, and that of Bolli *et al.* (1988), the hyperfine coupling constants of adducts were consistent with the presence of either carbon-centred or alkoxyl radicals, both of which are easy to envisage as generated during (lipid ?) peroxidation processes. In lysates of cardiac myocytes, it could be shown that the ferryl myoglobin species may act as initiators of radical damage and hence contribute to the generation of radical signals from these cells (Turner *et al.* 1991).

The presence of radicals in the myocardial tissue itself, during both the ischemic and reperfusion phases, has also been investigated in a number of studies by direct, low-temperature, EPR (Zweier *et al.* 1987; Baker *et al.* 1988; Nakazawa *et al.* 1988; Zweier 1988; Baker and Kalyanaraman 1989; Shuter *et al.* 1990*a*), though in some of these studies the observed species probably arise as a result of the methods used to process the tissue samples, i.e. they are artifactual. It has been shown that considerable technical care is required to avoid artefactual radical generation in such studies (Shuter *et al.* 1990*a*). In those cases where precautions have been taken, the observed changes are much less significant, with the major species present being assigned to a mitchondrial electron transport chain semi-quinone radical species (Baker 1988; Nakazawa *et al.* 1988; Baker and Kalyanaraman 1989).

Thus reperfusion of previously ischemic tissue, which is essential for the salvage of any of the affected area, can result in significant levels of oxidative damage. During reperfusion in working rat hearts, protein carbonyls in soluble proteins have been shown to rise after 22 minutes of ischemia followed by 5 minutes of reperfusion to 4 times basal values, and to return within the following 15 minutes to only 1.5 times basal (Poston and Parenteau 1992). Whether they were degraded, lost into the perfusate, in dead cells or otherwise, was not established (cf. indications of loss in Wickens *et al.* 1987).

Cardiac arrest and subsequent treatment can also lead to distal reperfusion damage in tissues such as the brain which are highly oxygen demanding. This has been shown clearly in studies with dogs, in which carbonyls of the brain are increased in the soluble proteins of the frontal cortex after 10 minutes of arrest followed by 2 or 24 hours of reperfusion (Liu *et al.* 1993). *N*-acetyl-L-carnitine, which improves neurological recovery when given intravenously, also reduced the level of protein carbonyls after 24 hours (though not after 2 hours). These results are impressive, even though changes in protein population and cellular infiltration may be occurring simultaneously with oxidation during the reperfusion phase. On the other hand, other authors using 20 minutes of cardiac arrest followed by 2 or 8 hours of reperfusion in dogs, found no significant changes in protein carbonyls in soluble and ribosomal fractions, and only modest changes in a synaptosomal fraction at 8 hours (and not at 2 hours) (Krause *et al.* 1992). The proteins under study were shown to be susceptible to *in vitro* Fenton-induced oxidation, but ribosomal RNA was not significantly damaged *in vivo*, leaving the impression that oxidative events were of limited significance. In studies on ischemia/reperfusion of Mongolian Gerbil brains, it was noted that a variety of oxidative parameters were elevated, including the levels of protein carbonyls, and these changes could be remarkably repressed by the spin trap PBN (Carney and Floyd 1991).

As yet, the differences between these results on reperfusion of the brain cannot be readily explained, and so the significance of the described oxidative events is unsettled (see discussion in Levine 1993). However, other authors have also observed oxidative damage to proteins in similar situations, and addressed further the possible antioxidative actions of some agents. Thus L- and D-propionyl carnitines could also suppress protein carbonyl accumulation during reperfusion of previously ischemic hearts (Reznick *et al.* 1992*a*), as well as improving recovery. Enhanced recovery due to the presence of the physiological L-form seems to involve both inhibition of Fenton chemistry, as a result of metal chelation, and metabolic stimulation. Site-specific damage may also be important in such distal effects of cardiac arrest, since again using dogs it has been found that activity of pyruvate dehydrogenase (PDH), an important control enzyme in mitochondrial metabolism, is lost by up to 72 per cent shortly after the onset of reperfusion (though not during the ischemic phase), and it is still reduced by 65 per cent at 24 hours (Bogaert *et al.* 1994). In contrast, there were no significant changes detected in LDH activities during these manipulations; unfortunately, the effects on PDH activity of the carnitine derivatives tested so far were unimpressive. Confirmatory evidence as to the selective inactivation of PDH has been obtained with cultured cardiac myocytes exposed to modest quantities of peroxide, and undergoing limited energy metabolite depletion prior to the decline in PDH (Vlessis *et al.* 1991). In Triton-X-100 treated cardiac muscle fibres (which are still contractile), selective inactivation of creatine kinase, apparently via its essential SH groups, has been observed (Mekhfi *et al.* 1996).

Cardiac adaptation after oxidative stress may well involve altered gene expression, and the oxidant-sensitive transcription factors AP-1 and NF-κB have indeed been found responsive to oxidants in isolated cardiac myocytes (Peng *et al.* 1995). However, therapy is currently largely directed towards ensuring that reperfusion is as rapid and early as possible, so that ischemic death is minimized. More recently, it has also been appreciated that minimizing damage during the reperfusion phase, mainly through regimes which minimize oxidative attack, would be a valuable supplement.

The approaches to this have been of limited success, probably mainly because it is not understood what molecular targets should ideally be protected. There is evidence of reperfusion damage to all the major groups of macromolecules, and protein oxidation is fairly well demonstrated, though the specific mechanisms are not known. Neither reperfusion arrhythmias nor subsequent functional recovery of rat hearts appear to be affected by varying the heart vitamin E levels by a factor of five, from suppressed by dietary deprivation, through normal, to elevated roughly two fold by chronic supplementation (Shuter *et al.* 1989). On the other hand, supply of catalase and allopurinol could effectively suppress the radical burst observed in the reperfusate, though SOD and desferal had more subtle effects (Shuter *et al.* 1990*b*). The mechanism of allopurinol's beneficial action on rat hearts does not seem to involve inhibition of tissue xanthine oxidase (Chambers *et al.* 1992) and remains unresolved. Superoxide dismutase, particularly when supplied as a PEG conjugate to extend availability, suppresses reperfusion damage in blood-perfused rabbit hearts, and this is associated with improved redox status of the tissue (e.g. GSH levels), though MDA values are unchanged, and it is not clear what effects the regime has on protein oxidation per se (Galinanes *et al.* 1992*a, b*; Qiu *et al.* 1992). Slight improvement due to the supply of *N*-acetyl-cysteine may also be related to improvements in intracellular redox status (Qiu *et al.* 1990).

Modest benefits have been achieved with the spin traps DMPO and PBN (Hearse and Tosaki 1987*a, b*), the latter apparently interacting with control of calcium levels (Hearse and Tosaki 1988). It must be noted that there are several circumstances in which regimes expected to limit oxidative events have no benefit for organ recovery: for example, with deferoxamine (Maxwell *et al.* 1989; Galinanes and Hearse 1990) and some reducing agents and scavengers (Chambers *et al.* 1989). The evidence as to the overall-importance of oxygen-radical-mediated events in either arrhythmogenicity or reperfusion damage, in sum, is quite ambiguous because it is so complex.

From the perspective of this book, the important issue is whether there are specific proteins which should be protected, as implied by the studies of Hearse and colleagues, and whether these are of predominant importance over the lipid oxidation. The arguments given earlier of the exaggerated importance of proteins because of their catalytic function and the observed kinetics of oxidant damage, may well be relevant, and hence a future, specific defence against protein oxidation may be valuable (see Chapter 6). Such highly specific studies may also be the only way forward in resolving the more general issue of the global significance of the oxidative damage in pathology of cardiac arrest.

5.3.2 Protein oxidation causing malfunction of gene expression or mutation: cancer, p53

Radicals are often found in association with tumour tissue, and the mediation of macromolecule oxidation in carcinogenesis has often been discussed (Sahu 1990; Ames *et al.* 1993). For example, Drake *et al.* (1996) showed the presence of radicals in gastric tumours and the conversion of signals into ascorbyl radicals on the addition of ascorbate, suggesting the likely protective role of ascorbate in the tumour-associated damaging processes.

Evidence of protein oxidation being associated with cancer is only modest. For example, during experimental hepatocarcinogenesis induced in rats by diethylnitrosamine (Sarkar *et al.* 1995) there is evidence of progressive erythrocyte lipid peroxidation. However, the authors adduce as evidence for protein oxidation the increased release *in vitro* of alanine from the cells. Such release is associated with enzymatic proteolysis, rather than directly with oxidation. As discussed in Chapter 3, it is not absolutely clear that enhanced oxidation of erythrocyte proteins is responsible for enhanced alanine release; conversely, such enhanced release cannot be safely used as a criterion of enhanced protein oxidation, even though it was reduced by elevations of β-carotene, as was lipid peroxidation. In the induction of renal cell carcinomas in rats by iron-nitriloacetate (Nishiyama *et al.* 1995), formation of aldehyde-protein adducts (through incompletely defined mechanisms, amongst those discussed) accompanies 8-OH-deoxyguanosine production in early stages (Toyokuni *et al.* 1994). However, mutations in p53 and several other oncogenes do not occur frequently in this system, nor in mouse liver cancers (Rumsby *et al.* 1994). Nickel carcinogenicity seems to be associated with both intracellular protein oxidation and, because of selective binding of nickel ions to amino acids rather than DNA, protein is the locale for the launching of DNA oxidation by Ni, which involves protein-DNA cross-links, as studied in cellular models (Costa *et al.* 1994). Chromium carcinogenicity also seems to involve oxidative components (Molyneux and Davies 1995), though the role of protein oxidation has not yet been studied to any extent. In some cases (Wogan 1989) the generation of 'hydroxyvalines' during carcinogenesis has been described incorrectly, since what was detected was a non-oxidative adduct of valine.

Suggestions of oxidation of nuclear transcription factors during carcinogenesis, notably p53 and NF-κB, abound, and SH regulation is apparently important (Yao *et al.* 1994; Das *et al.* 1995a, b; Rainwater *et al.* 1995). These actions may transduce into proliferation/cycle control mechanisms which influence carcinogenesis (Iijima *et al.* 1996; Sen and Packer 1996), and may involve nuclear accumulation of the transcription factors triggered by oxidant stress (Sugano *et al.* 1995). For example, it is claimed that the most common HIV-associated cancer, Kaposi's sarcoma, is associated with changed cycle control (Mallery *et al.* 1995), and that there are also other factors tending to lead to a cellular deficit of reducing components, and enhanced protein disulfides.

Though the evidence is weaker than one might have imagined, it seems reasonable to anticipate that enhanced protein oxidation is commonly associated with carcinogenesis. Some of the data mentioned so far only indicate an association which might be secondary. In what ways might protein oxidation be more fundamental to carcinogenesis? There are probably two main possibilities: one under intensive study, one so far rather neglected. The first, mentioned above for NF-κB, is that proteins which are key transducers of the information controlling cell proliferation may become oxidized, and the chemistry of such modification of p53 has been discussed already. The second is that protein oxidation reactions might inflict damage on DNA which leads to mutation, and hence ultimately to transformation. We will discuss these two aspects in sequence.

First, the question of oxidation of transducer proteins. Amongst the transcription factors, the zinc finger proteins, such as Sp1, are probably quite well protected against oxidative damage in several ways. First, the Zn site preferentially binds the redox-inactive transition metal ion, Zn^{2+}, and much less well than other more redox-active metals, such as Cu^{2+} or Ni^{2+}; secondly, the bound metal ions are rendered relatively redox inactive; thirdly, metallothionein and other metal-ion-binding proteins probably act to reduce the likelihood of substitution of other metal ions for zinc, by sequestering the Cu^{2+} or Ni^{2+} in preference to Zn^{2+} (Posewitz and Wilcox 1995).

Second, the possibility of DNA damage being caused by protein oxidation. We have indicated in earlier sections that protein-derived radicals, such as phenoxyl, alkoxyl, and peroxyl radicals, may inflict damage on other macromolecules. Evidence for such transfer to DNA is mainly that of formation of protein-DNA cross-links (such as summarized in Dizdaroglu

1991, 1992; Nackerdien *et al.* 1991; Olinski *et al.* 1992). For example, during the ferric-nitrilotriacetate renal carcinogenesis mentioned above tyrosine-thymine cross-links are observed (Toyokuni *et al.* 1995). In addition the possibility of protein radical abstraction mechanisms acting on DNA and so creating DNA damage without cross-links exists, and has hardly been studied. From the chemical similarities between the protein-bound radicals and those more commonly used experimentally (e.g. peroxyl and alkoxyl radicals from hydroperoxides and thermolabile azo compounds) which are known to damage DNA in this manner (Hazlewood and Davies 1995*a*, *b*), it is probable that only spatial considerations may limit such attack. A detailed study of these possibilities is needed. Some data on free DOPA interacting with DNA (Spencer *et al.* 1994; Husain and Hadi 1995), and preliminary evidence on protein-bound DOPA and protein hydroperoxides (Davies *et al.*, unpublished data), are in accord with this idea.

Thus, evidence that reactive intermediates in protein oxidation can damage DNA exists, and there is also the possibility that the stable end-products, for example the oxidized amino acids, might influence DNA metabolism. This might, in turn, have effects on DNA repair and, ultimately, mutation. Such possible actions remain to be investigated for the novel products of oxidation of protein-bound amino acids discussed earlier in the book. These demonstrated or probable modes of attack upon DNA by oxidizing, or oxidized, proteins may be associated with base modification, and hence at least with the risk of mutation, which is behind many cancers. While model studies have demonstrated that the formation of 8-OH-guanine may lead to mutation, as a result of error correction being incomplete, such studies have not been carefully made with protein radicals as the oxidizing species. This area is currently moving very rapidly, so this summary will be outdated by the time of publication.

Radicals and protein oxidation may also play a role during metastasis. For example, the metastatic potential of some sets of related cell lines appears to correlate with their capacity for radical production (Soares *et al.* 1994). Furthermore, Shaughnessy *et al.* (1993) argue that radical-mediated activation of a gelatinase might be important for matrix degradation associated with certain tumour cells' capacities to migrate through vessel walls. The generality of these ideas is not clear.

5.4 Oxidized proteins during ageing

It is well established that inactive forms of many proteins accumulate in ageing cells in culture, and in aged tissues. One of the most careful of such early studies was that of the Gershons, in which careful comparisons of isocitrate lyase activities and quantities of cross-reactive antigen in the nematode *Turbatrix aceti* were compared (Gershon and Gershon 1970).

These authors had the advantage not only of precipitating but also inactivating antisera, and suggested that even 50 per cent of the enzyme molecules might be inactive in aged organisms. However, without precise knowledge of the chemistry of both native and modified antigens, this figure cannot be firmly established, because of the complexities of immuno-compexation and immuno-precipitation.

Age pigments, such as lipofuschin, also seem often to contain protein components, though whether they are usually oxidized *in vivo* is not absolutely clear, since they are normally demonstrated by spectrofluorometric methods (Marzabadi *et al.* 1988; Sohal and Brunk 1989; Brunk *et al.* 1992; Yin 1992). Several studies have claimed to demonstrate the presence of oxidized proteins in similar circumstances, and they have suggested that a significant portion of the inactive proteins may be inactive because of oxidation. Oxidative conditions do seem also to generate lipofuscin-like pigments very rapidly in model systems (Marzabadi *et al.* 1990, 1991; Yin 1992; Yin *et al.* 1995).

Both links of this argument, that inactivation of proteins is exaggerated in ageing and oxidative in nature, require caution, and may be less than general in applicability. We will consider first studies of rodents and man, which have obvious restrictions as far as end points and genetic manipulation. Then, in a separate subsection, we will consider the substantial and interesting body of data (largely from Sohal and colleagues) on the housefly, *Drosophila*, which does not present such restrictions.

Table 5.1 mentions some of the available data concerning protein oxidation product levels in ageing organisms. Little has been measured but for protein carbonyls, and as discussed earlier these measurements are difficult and somewhat dangerous (see Stadtman 1988*a*, *b*) for a discussion of molecular parameters of protein oxidation and modification in ageing). However, in several tissues of gerbils it seems that protein carbonyl levels do rise with ageing (Carney and Floyd 1991; Sohal *et al.* 1995*b*). Rat plasma and splenic lymphocyte proteins also show an increase in protein carbonyls with age (Tian *et al.* 1995). Similarly, in rat and gerbil erythrocytes, certain membrane proteins become deranged during ageing in terms of conformational parameters determined by an EPR probe (Hensley *et al.* 1995*d*), and there are complementary data for SH reagent accessibility of human erythrocyte proteins (Seppi *et al.* 1991) and for liver mitochondrial membrane proteins of certain rat strains (Salganik *et al.* 1994). In accord with this, normal mouse erythrocytes separated on the basis of density, with the denser representing the older, show increasing protein oxidation products with density (He and Yasumoto 1992). Indeed the so called 'senescence' antigen of band III of erythrocytes and other cells, can be generated by oxidation, though how big a role it plays in this is not entirely clear (Kay *et al.* 1995).

Nevertheless, several authors have either found little or no sign of increased protein carbonyls in aged human diploid fibroblast cultures (Chen, Q. *et al.* 1995) except when obtained *ex vivo* from people aged more than 60, or from Werner's and Progeria cases (Oliver *et al.* 1987). Some report little change in rat brains (Cini and Moretti 1995) or note particular technical difficulties in reproducing the positive studies on ageing tissues (Cao and Cutler 1995*a*). No studies of the specific amino acid oxidation products in aged cultures have yet been published.

On the other hand, in the case of glutamine synthetase the evidence of decreased *activity* in aged cells and tissues is strong (Stadtman *et al.* 1992). For example, in a comparison of rat hepatocyte proteins from animals between 3 and 36 months of age, it was found that protein carbonyls accumulate progressively, and that glutamine synthetase and glucose-6-phosphate dehydrogenase activities decline. Furthermore, there was not a proportional decline in immunologically detected enzyme protein in these cases, indicating that the molecules present were, on average, less active (Starke and Oliver 1989). There are relatively few other cases where such sound evidence of an accumulation of inactive enzyme is available, even though there are several cases in which a loss of glutamine synthetase activity is reported with ageing (Carney *et al.* 1991). However, as discussed in Chapter 4, the question remains whether the inactive enzyme molecules were oxidatively inactivated; no evidence on this was adduced in most cases, though it has been claimed that chronic administration of the spin trap PBN to rats prevents both the accumulation of protein carbonyls, the loss of this enzyme and of a neutral proteinase(s) activity, and certain behavioral decrements, all of which might therefore reflect oxidative affront (Carney *et al.* 1991; reviewed: Floyd and Carney 1992). Counter-claims exist (Cao and Cutler 1995*a*), but have been forcefully questioned by others (Dubey *et al.* 1995). The latter study observed levels of protein carbonyls in 15-month-old gerbil brains averaging 1.8 nmol mg^{-1} protein; different regions of the brain varied in level by a factor of up to 1.8. Arguing in support of Carney et al, these authors state that age (between 3 and 15 months) had a significant 'overall effect' (an increase of about 20 per cent) on carbonyl levels, using analysis of variance in relation to six separately studied regions; amongst these regions several showed no change. What they neglect to point out is that these changes are negligible in comparison with the 85 per cent increases presented by Carney and colleagues. In addition, Dubey *et al.* do not discuss the considerable variation in control levels (without PBN) observed in the different experiments for animals of 15 months: it seems that these differences might well be so great as to undermine the idea of a significant 20 per cent rise with age. Dubey *et al.* found no effect of PBN on mouse brain levels, or *Drosophila* life span (except for toxicity at high concentrations), but they did find a 34 per cent decrease of gerbil carbonyls due to PBN (in relation to levels which are already much lower than previously reported), which they compared with the 50 per cent decrease quoted by Carney. It is very difficult to be confident of biological significance in any of these data, and indeed in some cases the statistical complexity of the analysis needed to point to any differences at all is perturbing. Indeed, Dubey *et al.* pointed out that the levels achieved in tissues were unlikely to be high enough to provide substantial competition for radicals, in the light of known kinetic parameters, so that if PBN has an action, it is unlikely to be a directly antioxidative one.

The accumulation of protein carbonyls, and the loss of both glutamine synthetase and creatine kinase in aged and age-matched Alzheimer's human brain regions, have also been described (Smith *et al.* 1991). The loss of cognitive and motor abilities in ageing mice seem to proceed differentially, though in both cases paralleling regio-specific increments in protein carbonyls (Forster *et al.* 1996). Whether antioxidants generally will interfere with protein oxidation in ageing, or retard age-related changes, has long been debated (Tappel 1968) and remains unresolved.

Thus, the relationship between glutamine synthetase loss and oxidation is more assumed than demonstrated; but it is so relied upon that some authors even present evidence of decreased glutamine synthetase activity as evidence of protein oxidation (Mo *et al.* 1995), which is, of course, mistaken. Phosphoglycerate kinase purified from muscles of aged rats is claimed to show properties in common with the 'young' enzyme which has been inactivated by metal-catalysed oxidation (Zhou and Gafni 1991), but no specific lesion is determined to confirm this.

Nevertheless, the balance of evidence is in favour of an accumulation of oxidized protein species in these aged tissues and in cells therefrom, and this is supported by some notable studies of insect ageing, which we will discuss. The evidence is strongest for slow turnover tissues such as the lens, and early reports (Truscott and Augusteyn 1977*a*, *b*, *c*; Garcia-Castineiras *et al.* 1978) of di-tyrosine in lens proteins included mass spectral definition of the presence of the compound (Garcia-Castineiras *et al.* 1978), together with anthranilic acid, though they may be questioned in quantitative terms. Selective oxidation of up to 60 per cent of cysteine and methionine, and accumulation of GSSG, was described in aged and cataractous lens proteins (Garner and Spector 1980). These data were complemented by *in vitro* studies of the action of up to 1 mM hydrogen peroxide on lens proteins during incubations for up to 2 weeks. Rapid oxidation of as much as 100 per cent of cysteine and 45 per cent of methionine was observed, together with enhanced 'non-tryptophan' fluorescence (McNamara and Augusteyn 1984). Protein conformational changes were detected, as well as an increase in average size measured in urea, consistent with opacification. Other amino acids apparently were not lost, though data were not presented. In agreement with these earlier studies, Garland and colleagues found modest elevations in total metal levels in cataract and aged lens, and small increments in lens protein carbonyls, non-tryptophan fluorescence, and aggregation due to exposure of bovine crystallins to ascorbate and metal (Garland et al. 1986; Garland 1990).

These studies are supported by more detailed recent studies of a wide range of specific protein oxidation products in different regions of the human lens and their relation to cataract (see Table 5.1). For example, in proteins of human non-cataractous lenses, while there is no increase with age of o-tyrosine, there is a 33 per cent increase in di-tyrosine (measured by selective ion monitoring mass spectroscopy (Wells-Knecht et al. 1993)). The 'di-tyrosine' fluorescence of the tissue rises by 11 fold, indicating again the unsuitability of such tissue (or protein) fluorescence approaches to determining this moiety. There are no significant changes in protein-SH/mixed disulfides in lenses from old rats (Lou et al. 1995), though in the trabecular mesh of the human eye, the concentration of methionine sulfoxide rises with age (Horstmann et al. 1983).

The issue immediately arises as to how enlarged pools of oxidized protein are sustained. As discussed in Chapter 3, the pools are the net of production (oxidation, plus reutilization of oxidized amino acids) and consumption (chemical decay in the case of the reactive species; otherwise degradation and excretion). Reutilization has not been studied in relation to this issue as yet, but it is likely that it is only changed as a secondary consequence of the oxidized pool size, since it will depend on competition between the parent amino acid and the modified amino acid for binding to tRNA and other stages of protein synthesis. The concentration from competing, native amino acid levels will probably be relatively unchanged.

Thus, the potentially important factors are the rate of protein oxidation and the rate of removal of the products. Several authors have presented data to indicate that mitochondrial, or more generalized, rates of radical production increase in aged tissues (Sohal et al. 1995b). It is a matter of debate as to how meaningful the measures of oxygen radical generation by isolated mitochondria are for the function of intact mitochondria in living cells. If they do correspond, then the rate of protein oxidation might well increase too. Furthermore, an interesting experiment has compared the sensitivity of cell extracts from gerbil tissues of various ages to radiolytic protein oxidation, and revealed signficantly increased sensitivity in the older tissues (Sohal et al. 1995b), though this was not found in extracts of rat tissues using endogenous, or exogenous, metal-catalysed oxidation (Cini and Moretti 1995). Enhanced availability of iron ions for redox reactions, including protein carbonyl formation, has been claimed to characterize hepatocytes from aged versus young rats (Rikans and Cai 1993). Increases in protein oxidation under given conditions might reflect a decreased aggregate of antioxidant defences, or decreased competition from other macromolecules for oxidizing species, such that protein oxidation is proportionally enhanced. That the rate of macromolecule oxidation might be an important determinant of the observed levels could also be implied by experiments on protein- or calorie-restriction of the diets of rats, which confirm an age-related increase in protein carbonyls, as well as DNA-oxidation products, and demonstrate its reduction by the dietary restrictions (Youngman et al. 1992; Tian et al. 1995). The mechanism of this effect is unclear, but such restrictions also decrease another possibly oxidative process, cataract generation in the Emory mouse (Taylor et al. 1989). Calorie restriction can also lengthen mammalian life span (Sohal and Weindruch 1996).

Sohal and colleagues have reviewed the modest variations in levels of antioxidant defensive enzymes (such as SOD, catalase, glutathione peroxidase, etc.) in mammals of various ages, and also the apparent rates of radical production (such as from mitochondrial metabolism (Ku et al. 1993; Ku and Sohal 1993)) and their apparent enhancement in aged tissues. They argue that the latter is likely to be a more important factor (Sohal and Orr 1992). This may be part of a vicious circle in which mitochondrial damage leads to poor respiratory control and enhanced radical release (Ames et al. 1995).

Elevated protein oxidation rates may therefore suffice to explain the accumulation of oxidized proteins in ageing. It may not be necessary to postulate changes in the degradation half-lives of oxidized proteins in order to explain an observed accumulation. But since moderately oxidized proteins, at least, are usually more susceptible to enzymatic degradation than the native proteins, one might expect that there would be great scope for alteration of pool size through changes in catabolism (indeed, proteins whose concentrations are regulated by degradation mainly have short half-lives). However, the proteolytic systems of the cell are usually both redundant and in excess, so such regulation may not occur for oxidized proteins.

In spite of these considerations, Stadtman and colleagues have presented data to indicate that an alkaline proteinase(s) which has some selectivity for oxidized proteins is reduced in certain aged tisses, and suggested that this might explain in part the accumulation of oxidized proteins in those tissues (reviewed: Stadtman 1992). For example, in hepatocytes of aged rats the alkaline activity is decreased to about 20 per cent of its value in young (Starke and Oliver 1989), and furthermore, the activity is not induced during hyperoxic exposure, unlike that of the young animals (though again, technical queries about the assays have been raised (Cao and Cutler 1995b)). Others found a comparable drop in liver, none in brain, and an even greater drop in heart, in Sprague-Dawley rats of increasing age (Agarwal and Sohal 1994a). In contrast, in a careful study of Fischer 344 rats (from both Japan and the USA), Levine and colleagues found no loss of activity of either neutral or alkaline proteinase activities, including those of the multicatalytic proteinase, and carefully documented that these systems maintained the capacity to selectively degrade glutamine synthetase which had undergone limited oxidation and modification *in vitro* (Sahakian *et al.* 1995).

The idea of reduced proteinase activity assisting the accumulation of oxidized protein is, nevertheless, very interesting, but it relies on the particular proteinase(s) assayed being of dominant quantitative importance in the degradation of oxidized proteins, which has not been demonstrated, and might be expected to be unlikely. No measurements of turnover (i.e. *in vivo*) of oxidized proteins have been made in these systems to confirm or refute the hypothesis, but Cutler and colleagues have reported their inability to confirm the loss of the proteinase in rats (Cao and Cutler 1995*b*), and the alkaline activity is also found to be maintained in aged gerbil tissues, as judged both by conventional assay and in terms of the ability of the tissue to degrade oxidized proteins (Sohal *et al.* 1995*b*). One should keep in mind the different catabolic routes for endogenous intracellular proteins, endocytosed proteins, and extracellular matrix proteins, which implies that the same issues may be just as relevant to the accumulation of these proteins in oxidized forms.

If the *generation* of oxidized proteins is likely to be the key determinant of pool sizes of the products, then perturbation of oxidative fluxes should alter these pools. Sohal and colleagues have initiated an elegant and desirable approach to these questions, in their system of ageing *Drosophila* flies.

5.4.1 Protein oxidation and ageing in *Drosophila*

Sohal and colleagues have taken advantage of the flexibility of the fly as an experimental system to perturb oxidant exposure, physical activity levels (on the expectation that oxidant generation would be proportional to activity), and genetically-controlled antioxidant enzymes, in order to assess their importance in ageing and in protein and other macromolecule oxidation. They have made a comparative study of five different fly species, which vary more than two-fold in life span, to support the general relevance of such considerations (Sohal *et al.* 1995*c*). They found that life span correlated inversely with oxidant generation (superoxide and hydrogen peroxide) as measured from isolated mitochondria, though as noted above, how relevant this is to *in vivo* oxidant generation is not clear. Life span was also inversely correlated with protein carbonyl concentrations measured in homogenates of the (young) flies, but positively correlated with cytochrome *c* oxidase activities. The most economical interpretation of these findings is indeed that longer life-span is related to lower oxidant flux, and this can be argued to fit equally with the information available about differential life spans of small and large mammals (Sohal *et al.* 1995*c*). As an experimental organism in ageing studies, *D. melanogaster* has a very long history, and it shows some of the classic features such as accumulation of fluorescent age pigments like lipofuscin, usually within lysosomes (Miquel *et al.* 1974; Sheldahl and Tappel 1974).

There is an age-related increase in oxidant production from mitochondria obtained from the flight muscle of the organism, and protein carbonyl levels and indices of DNA damage also increase with age (Sohal and Dubey 1994). Thus, it is possible that the vicious cycle emphasized by Ames, in which oxidative damage to mitochondria cumulates to exaggerate its own oxidant production, is in action in these organisms. The importance of such mechanisms can only be approached by perturbing the several individual components which seem important, and a number of pertinent attempts have been so made.

One can directly manipulate the oxidant exposure of the flies. Sub-lethal hyperoxic exposure of flies caused a subsequent decrease in oxygen consumption, and an increment in protein carbonyl levels which seemed irreversible (Sohal *et al.* 1993*b*). This latter is surprising in view of the evidence (below) that the proteolytic systems able to selectively act on the oxidized proteins are normally intact throughout the insect's life span.

Physical activity levels also influence oxygen consumption. On the theory that oxidant/radical production is a small leak from the main flux, physical activity would be expected to control oxidant generation too. Activity levels can be controlled in cultivated flies, for example by determining the extent of airborne activity. Thus, it has been found that decreased physical activity is associated with decreased accumulation of oxidized DNA products, and of protein carbonyls, together with enhanced life span (Agarwal and Sohal 1994*b*). However, the time courses of the carbonyl levels, and the variations between different conditions and experiments, make these data quite difficult to interpret in a simple manner. There seem to be some disjunctions between the oxidative events and the change in life span.

The next level of analysis of the influence of oxidation processes concerns the influence of antioxidant defence mechanisms, which might limit the impact of a given flux of oxidants to varying degrees. Aged flies and fly homogenates were more susceptible to protein carbonyl generation and inactivation of glucose-6-phosphate dehydrogenase by exposure to X-rays than their younger counterparts (Agarwal and Sohal 1993), suggesting either a changed ratio of protein concentration to that of other (oxidizable) macromolecules, or a decrement in the antioxidant defence systems. The latter possibility seems not to have been tested directly, but the spin trap PBN, while effective in some mammalian systems in reducing protein oxidation product accumulation with age or acute oxidative stress, had no effect on the life span of the fly (Dubey *et al.* 1995).

Mutant flies with various levels of catalase have been studied, and it seems that even 14 per cent of the normal level of catalase is sufficient for optimal antioxidant protection, in spite of the fact that the flies lack glutathione peroxidase, so that catalase is the main agent for enzymatic detoxification of hydrogen peroxide. Consistent with this, enhanced catalase expression in transgenic flies has no impact on life span (Orr *et al.* 1992; Orr and Sohal 1992). Overexpression of SOD also had little effect (Orr and Sohal 1993). The most striking data, which is as yet still difficult to interpret, were obtained when it was found that simultaneous overexpression of Cu,Zn-SOD and catalase in the flies leads to elongated life span (Orr and Sohal 1994; Sohal *et al.* 1995a). Multiple copy overexpression enhanced life span and aggregate physical activity, and this was associated with lower levels of protein carbonyls at various stages of the life span (Orr and Sohal 1994). Single-copy overexpression was associated with decreased DNA oxidation product levels and slower decline in glucose-6-phosphate dehydrogenase (G6PDH) activities, and a slower rate of the progressive rise in oxidant release by mitochondrial preparations from the flies as they age. All these observations could readily be interpreted as defensive actions of the overexpressed antioxidant enzymes, though evidence that the loss of G6PDH is oxidative is not available. However, there was also enhanced oxygen consumption in the last two-thirds of the life span, so that in an average life the transgenic flies consumed 30 per cent more oxygen overall. That they could resist the associated radical and oxidant production can be understood in terms of their enhanced defences, but the reason for the enhanced consumption in the latter period of life is not so obvious, and suggests more complicated levels of regulation (Sohal *et al.* 1995a).

The variable rates of removal of oxidized moieties is, of course, one complicating factor which makes it quite difficult to interpret the pool sizes of the moieties at different ages (as opposed to measurement of the generation rate of these materials). The possible influence of the removal mechanisms of proteolysis on the accumulation of oxidized proteins in the flies has so far only been addressed by measurement of enzyme activities, not by *in vivo* turnover studies. Albumin which had been oxidized to various degrees by radiolysis was used as substrate, and it was found that alkaline proteinase(s) active in fly homogenates could selectively cleave the oxidized protein, with the rate of cleavage paralleling the extent of carbonyl modification of the substrate. The activity of these alkaline proteinase(s) in fly homogenates was unchanged with respect to age (Agarwal and Sohal 1994a), though the possible influence of the proteinase/proteinase inhibitor balance has not been carefully studied as yet.

The yield of reactive carbonyl materials (thiobarbituric acid-reactive substances) seems to decline in concentration with ageing in the fly, while 'inorganic peroxides' (which were not fully characterized) rise early and then stay roughly constant (Sohal *et al.* 1990a). Thus it is apparent that oxidative events are unlikely to occur homogeneously in time or in space within the organism. This emphasizes that what will be needed for full elucidation of the relationships implied between oxygen consumption, oxidant generation, oxidized product levels, physical activity, and ageing, will be detailed, kinetic studies, which will be both very difficult and very labour intensive. However, the fly system seems to offer one of the best opportunities for undertaking such elaborate work (reviewed: Sohal and Weindruch 1996).

5.4.2 Protein oxidation in ageing: conclusions

In sum, the perturbation studies do not yet convincingly demonstrate that protein oxidation, or even other oxidative events, are critical influences on the progresssion of ageing; but they are highly suggestive and exciting. The restriction of these oxidative events does not definitively restrict ageing, though ageing in flies, at least, can be perturbed by manipulation of anti-oxidant enzyme expression. Mechanistic possibilities within this thesis, for example of the protein radicals generated from the reactive products inter-fering with cellular metabolism in a manner which can progress the ageing process (Dean *et al.* 1992), have yet to be assessed directly. However, in some of the age-related diseases we consider in the next section, more endeavour has been applied, and there is now some such information available.

5.5 Oxidized proteins during age-related diseases: diabetes, atherosclerosis, and neurodegenerative diseases

Rather than catalogue age-related diseases, we focus here on a limited selection: diabetes, atherosclerosis, and Alzheimer's have been chosen because the most relevant studies have been undertaken in these fields.

Diabetes is one of the most common inherited diseases, caused by the impaired production of insulin by pancreatic islet β-cells, and/or by dimin-ished tissue responses to insulin (insulin resistance). The consquence of this is that circulating blood glucose levels are chronically elevated and this appears mainly responsible for the major problems of diabetes, blindness, gangrene, and kidney failure. The identification of genes responsible for diabetes has developed considerably recently (Yamagata *et al.* 1996), but understanding of the consequences of hyperglycaemia has lagged behind.

Glycation reactions between glucose and proteins and other biological molecules, notably the Maillard (browning) reaction, have long been considered a potential major part of these consequences. 'Autoxidative glycosylation', involving both autoxidation of glucose via di-carbonyl intermediates and of protein-bound sugars, was proposed to be important (Wolff and Dean 1987*a*, *b*), following earlier studies of sugar autoxidation and oxyhaemoglobin oxidation by glyceraldehyde (Thornalley *et al.* 1984). This has lead to a continued assessment of the role of oxidative processes in the secondary consequences of diabetes (reviewed: Baynes 1996). Here we only consider the specific relevance of protein oxidation.

Metal-catalysed autoxidation of sugars and products of protein-glycation can generate radicals which initiate and propagate protein damage (Wolff and Dean 1987*a*, *b*, 1988; Hicks *et al.* 1988; Hunt *et al.* 1988*a*, *b*; Wolff *et al.* 1989, 1991). Cross-linking of collagen *in vitro* by exposure to glucose is virtually blocked under nitrogen and in the presence of chelators, confirming the important role of oxidative events (Chace *et al.* 1991). We observed that proteins exposed to autoxidizing glucose contain the protein-bound oxidizing and reducing reactive species subsequently characterized as hydroperoxides and DOPA (Dean *et al.* 1992, 1993, 1996; Simpson *et al.* 1992, 1993; Gieseg *et al.* 1993). In more recent unpublished work (in collaboration with Thorpe and Baynes) we have also quantitated formation of a range of aliphatic amino acid hydroxides, DOPA, di-tyrosine, and hydroxylation products of phenylalanine during exposure of proteins to glucose.

Glyoxal and arabinose are autoxidation products of glucose (M. C. Wells-Knecht *et al.* 1995); the former can form N-ε-(carboxymethyl)lysine (CML) (Dunn *et al.* 1991) and the latter can participate in the generation of the fluorescent pentosidine cross-links in proteins (Sell and Monnier 1989). Ascorbate, and dicarbonyl sugars such as methylglyoxal and 3-dexoyglucosone, which are observed *in vivo* (Wells-Knecht *et al.* 1994), may participate in autoxidative reactions contributing to browning; and there are other sources of glyoxal and related aldehydes such as from amino acids (Dakin 1906, 1908*a*, *b*, *c*, 1909) or lipids (Fu *et al.* 1996). The protein-bound Amadori intermediates are generally more readily autoxidizable than the free sugars (Zu *et al.* 1996), so the relative importance of autoxidation before and after protein binding may vary with the relative concentrations of the reactive components and the catalyst metal ions (K. J. Wells-Knecht *et al.* 1995*b*), and cannot be readily predicted. Some of the protein-bound intermediates may be stabilized as radicals during cross-linking reactions, as in the case of the cross-linked methylglyoxal-dialkylimine radical-cation formed during the reaction of methylglyoxal with amino acids (Yim *et al.* 1995), and presumably also with proteins. Similar reactions are likely with glyoxal, a demonstrated major product of glucose autoxidation (M. C. Wells-Knecht *et al.* 1995), as well as a product of lipid and protein oxidation. Another major product of glucose autoxidation is arabinose, a precursor of the fructosyl-lysine intermediate and hence pentosidine (M. C. Wells-Knecht *et al.* 1995). N-E-carboxymethyllysine and pentosidine accumulate *in vivo* with ageing, and their levels can be elevated in diabetes, and restricted in animal models by certain antioxidant regimes (Baynes 1996*a*, *b*). Whereas the former can be produced by reactions of lipids, through glyoxal, it seems unlikely that the latter can (Zu *et al.* 1996). Rather, the best characterized route for pentosidine formation is through fructosyl-lysine. The evidence to date points towards a significant role of sugar autoxidation, be it of free or protein-bound sugars, in the complications of diabetes.

Diabetes predisposes towards atherosclerosis, and the evidence that macromolecule oxidation accompanies atherogenesis is now very strong. Early events in atherogenesis involve the enhanced adherence of peripheral blood monocytes to the endothelial lining of the blood vessel, and their transmigration between the cells into the intima (reviewed: Schwartz *et al.* 1993). Once in the intima, instead of continuing to journey to the peripheral tissues as occurs in most inflammatory responses, at least some of the cells remain, and become lipid-laden 'foam cells', the first morphological hall-mark of atherosclerosis (Rosenfeld *et al.* 1990). Oxidised fatty acids and sterols of (at least partially) defined nature, and quantity, are present in animal models of the disease (De Meyer *et al.* 1991), and accumulate in human lesions. For example, around 30 per cent of the cholesteryl linoleate found in advanced human lesions is in oxidized forms (Suarna *et al.* 1995).

The main donor of the lipid which accumulates seems to be modified low density lipoprotein, and hence there has been a major thrust to understand how this particle, and its other lipoprotein relatives, becomes oxidized, since oxidation generates forms with modified apoB protein molecules (with their lysine residues derivatized), which are high-uptake lipid donors via either the so-called 'scavenger' or other receptors and routes (Ramprasad *et al.* 1995). Furthermore, the idea of lipoprotein oxidation pointed to the likelihood that the protein component of LDL, apoB, would also become oxidized in atherogenesis. It was also apparent that significant apoB modification might result from the lipid oxidation products themselves, for example through lysine derivatization by aldehyde end-products of lipid oxidation (Yla-Herttuala *et al.* 1995). It is important to keep in mind the distinction between direct radical-induced protein oxidation and secondary protein modification by such addition reactions.

We will consider the *in vivo* evidence that modified proteins accumulate in atherogenesis, and then the mechanisms which may contribute to oxidation. Evidence was first sought by immunological approaches, in which anti-bodies to LDL derivatized with lipid aldehydes were raised, and tested immunohistochemically on atherosclerotic tissue samples (Rosenfeld *et al.* 1991; Yla-Herttuala *et al.* 1991). Several controls were undertaken, such as the generation of antibodies to derivatized albumin or other lipid-free proteins, and their application in the histochemistry; and limited attempts to determine whether the anti-lipoprotein antibodies were specific for the apoprotein derivative. Virtually all of these studies show or leave open the possibility that the specificity of the antisera are quite broad (Uchida *et al.*

1995). The resulting immunohistochemical data are therefore supportive of the idea that derivatization of proteins by aldehydes can occur, but do not clarify what protein(s) are involved. It is easy to appreciate that a 4-hydroxynonenal (HNE) side chain on a peptide may be the dominant component of the resulting epitope, such that an HNE on a different peptide is quite well recognized also, and experimental evidence confirms this (Uchida *et al.* 1994).

Analogous histochemical studies have claimed to demonstrate large amounts of 3-nitrotyrosine bearing oxidized proteins in plaque (Beckman *et al.* 1994), though these are subject to similar criticisms, and chemical determinations of 3-nitrotyrosine do not support the conclusion. A more detailed study of hypochlorite-oxidized proteins has also recently been published using an immunological approach, in which the specificity of the antisera has been more carefully assessed and vindicated (Malle *et al.* 1995). The data (Hazell *et al.* 1996) indicate the widespread presence of hypochlorite-oxidized proteins in and around cells of the lesion; these seem to include oxidized apoB. This is supported by the detection of catalytically active myeloperoxidase in plaque (Daugherty *et al.* 1994). Gel electrophoresis and Western blotting of the plaque-extracted proteins confirmed the presence of epitopes on a significant number of different proteins, including apoB aggregates which are a significant component of advanced human plaques. Another set of data have assessed the presence of fragments of apoB by Western blotting of extracts of plaque. It is clear that such fragments are present, but the mechanism by which they are produced may well be proteolytic as well as, or in place of, oxidative.

One very notable early paper used chemical means to identify aminomalonic acid (which in chemical systems can be a product of radical-mediated carboxylation of glycine (Wheelan *et al.* 1989)) in atherosclerotic plaque (Van Buskirk *et al.* 1984). Using post-mortem human samples, 0.2 Ama (aminomalonic acid) per 1000 glycine residues were detected in alkaline hydrolysates; in addition, carboxylated derivatives of aspartate and glutamate were found. The proteins on which these derivatives were present were not identified, and it is notable that these workers later attempted, in model experiments, to form Ama on LDL, without success (Wheelan *et al.* 1989). However, great care has been taken in subsequent work by these authors (Copley *et al.* 1992) to show that in *E. coli* Ama is a genuine component, and not an artefact of processing. The chemical method which has been used to generate these species involves the reaction between a $CO_2 \cdot^-$ and a glycyl α-carbon radical (Wheelan *et al.* 1989). As both these radicals react very rapidly with oxygen, their concentrations *in vivo* will probably be very low, so it is doubtful that this pathway operates *in vivo*, and this may also explain why the reaction was not successful with LDL. An alternative interpretation of the presence of the carboxylated amino acids could be that they arise from further oxidation of oxidized derivatives of amino acids. For example in the case of aminomalonate, oxidation of the aldehyde (1) produced from serine (Chapter 2) could be the mechanism. Derivatives of valine and leucine may be the source of the other carboxylated species mentioned above. As originally suggested (Van Buskirk *et al.* 1984), the formation of such carboxylated sites in proteins *in vivo* may cause some accumulation of bound calcium, as is observed in many advanced, atherosclerotic plaques.

Only more recently has it been possible to address the question of accumulation of oxidized proteins in plaque by a wide range of specific chemical assays, including those for the reactive species (Table 5.1). In general, these studies confirm the presence of oxidized amino acids within the proteins of plaque, but show that only certain of these are present at significantly higher levels than in normal, undiseased vessels, or normal plasma. The 3-nitro- and 3-chloro- derivatives of tyrosine do not seem to be elevated, whereas di-tyrosine and some other tyrosine derivatives do. The oxidized side chains of the aliphatic amino acids are also present, but not in drastically enhanced quantities compared with normal vessels.

It is difficult currently to interpret these data in terms of likely contributing mechanisms. For example, the pool size (as experimentally determined and just summarized) is the net of production and removal, and there is no information as yet about the latter. Furthermore, it is quite possible that removal is differential with respect to different oxidation products, whether through chemical detoxification or through proteolysis. In the case of a complex tissue such as plaque, there is also the question of removal of macromolecules (even lipoprotein particles) into the media, or back into the blood stream; both processes are known to occur. Thus the relative roles of different oxidative pathways cannot be decided on the basis of the present evidence, though the presence of several different components indicates that at least these pathways are operative at sites which can feed the plaque pool, probably in the intima itself.

What might these mechanisms be? The most likely candidates seem to be initiation by free (delocalized) transition metal ions; or cell-mediated oxidation (of which virtually all examples demonstrated to date have been metal-ion dependent). Many cell types are capable of enhancing LDL oxidation, in the presence of transition metals, though it has recently been pointed out (Kritharides *et al.* 1995*a*) that they can also be inhibitory to the process, probably by metal sequestration. Some mechanisms, such as the generation of hypochlorite by triggered leukocytes, could lead (at least initially) to two-electron, non-radical oxidation, which might be independent of metals. The full range of possibilities are critically discussed by Stocker (1994).

Are metals available in the intima? A series of studies (Hunter *et al.* 1991) have made bold positive claims in this regard. However, the data presented do not confirm the interpretations claimed, because of inappropriate (or in some cases lack of) comparisons with normal vessel samples, the possible release of metal ions during homogenization and processing, and the variability of data obtained. We have found that metal availability in normal tissues, resulting from homogenization, however carefully controlled, is often greater than that in plaque. Electron microprobe analysis studies are indicative of progressive accumulation of copper, and reduction in zinc ions in plaques during atherogenesis; and the absolute quantities of metals also increase per gram of tissue. A new range of techniques, such as EPR on whole pieces of tissue, will be needed to clarify these questions, but currently it remains at least feasible that free transition metals are available.

That being the case, it is reasonable to consider further the two possibilities for radical-mediated oxidation mentioned earlier: direct metal-ion-initiated oxidation and cell-mediated oxidation. A system of metal-induced lipid peroxidation generates a secondary radical flux (e.g. peroxyl radicals) which can oxidize protein, as defined already. In addition it may generate stable, yet reactive, end-products such as aldehydes which can modify protein. Metal ions induce LDL oxidation, and this provides all the ingredients necessary for protein oxidation.

It has been argued on the basis of *in vitro* experiments that extracellular fluid, such as that in the intima, would completely prevent cell-mediated oxidation, metal-ion-induced or otherwise (Dabbagh and Frei 1995). Suction blister fluid contains concentrations of ascorbate and urate equal to or greater than those in plasma, and these, like serum components (Kalant and McCormick 1992), very efficiently inhibit LDL oxidation in model systems, with and without cells (Dabbagh and Frei 1995). It has been pointed out that the absolute concentration of the lipophilic antioxidants in blister fluid is much lower than in plasma (Dabbagh and Frei 1995), but when expressed per oxidizable bis-allylic fatty acid this is no longer the case. Indeed, we have found that neither aqueous nor lipophilic antioxidants are depleted in advanced human plaque samples (Suarna *et al.* 1995), so it is possible that oxidation is occurring in the presence of antioxidants, perhaps by tocopherol-mediated peroxidation (Stocker 1994; Bowry *et al.* 1995; Thomas, S. R. *et al.* 1995), or that it occurs separated in time or space from the antioxidant availability. Furthermore, there is no doubt the intercellar fluid can be oxidized by peroxyl radical fluxes (Kurtel *et al.* 1992).

The study of oxidation of apoB has lagged vastly behind that of the lipid components of LDL, largely because of the greater difficulty of analysing it. Many early studies have measured UV fluorescence spectra of the particle, in order to demonstrate tryptophan consumption (Giessauf *et al.* 1995). The evidence is clouded by the changes in fluorescence spectrum which can result from the changed hydrophobicity of the immediate environment of tryptophans, and by the generation of other lipid fluorophores whose spectra overlap (Kontush *et al.* 1995). However, it seems fair to conclude from these data that tryptophan is consumed from the early stages of LDL oxidation in a variety of systems. Protein carbonyls may be formed (Matsugo *et al.* 1995), and similarly, non-enzymic protein fragmentation occurs (Schuh *et al.* 1978; Fong *et al.* 1987; Bedwell *et al.* 1989; Hunt *et al.* 1994; Noguchi and Niki 1994). ApoB fragments can also be detected in plasma of atherosclerotic patients (Lecomte *et al.* 1993). Particularly during HOCl oxidation, LDL may conversely become aggregated through changes in the lysine groups (Hazell *et al.* 1994) and aggregated LDL produced by this or other means is an effective donor of large quantities of lipid to macrophage cells (Suits *et al.* 1989). Haemoglobin may push other per-oxidative pathways to similar effects, via cross-linking of protein radicals (Miller *et al.* 1996). There are some indications that tyrosyl or tryptophanyl residues, especially if external to the LDL particle, may initiate LDL lipid peroxidation (Savenkova *et al.* 1994; Giessauf *et al.* 1995).

It has been conventional to equate the changes in relative electrophoretic mobility of the LDL particle with protein oxidation, but as pointed out already, the addition of aldehydes to the lysine-free amino group is an indirect modification due to lipid oxidation, not a direct oxidation, and yet appears to be the major cause of the changed charge on the particle, and hence the changed migration. Such an interpretation is thus not adequate.

Only very recently has data begun to be gathered as to the oxidation of apoB protein, as judged by specific oxidation products. We have defined the production of hydroxides, DOPA, and other tyrosine derivatives during oxidation by γ-radiolysis in the presence of oxygen, following our earlier work on protein fragmentation using these defined radical systems. These species are produced even at low radiation doses (i.e. low radical fluxes), and are present at very low levels in freshly isolated LDL. While LDL may inevitably be subject to slight oxidation during isolation, we have also been able to detect the same range of species in fresh human plasma which was carefully protected against oxidation by antioxidants during the brief extraction procedures. These moieties are thus intrinsic, and there is more DOPA per mole of tyrosine, than hydroxide per mole of parent amino acid, in agreement with previous discussions.

Kinetic studies using metal-ion-catalysed or peroxyl-radical-induced oxidation, or cell-mediated oxidation, have yet to be published, though Heinecke has shown some profiles of di-tyrosine formation which are congruent with the data just discussed. More detailed studies of two-electron oxidation by hypochlorite have also been published (Hazell and Stocker 1993; Hazell *et al.* 1994). These indicate that, unlike the radical systems discussed above, hypochlorite is selective for the protein moiety of LDL, and hardly oxidizes the lipid until protein oxidation has already occurred to a very significant extent; some conflicting data does, however, exist (Panasenko *et al.* 1994). Lysine, tryptophan, cysteine, and methionine are consumed stoichiometrically when HOCl is supplied in bolus form; this results in chloramine formation, and protein carbonyls from their subsequent decay. Cell-mediated oxidation through hypochlorite may be an important (at least initially), non-radical mechanism of protein oxidation in plaque, as also indicated by the convincing detection of hypochlorite-modified proteins; however, the quantitative importance of this route is unclear, in view of the relative lack of 3-chlorotyrosine (judged by the chemical determinations) in plaque.

When we consider cell-mediated oxidation further, we have to take into account that the handling of LDL (or, for that matter, any protein) is not simply an extracellular matter. Does oxidation, as well as proteolysis, proceed intracellularly? The vacuolar compartment, of endosomes, Golgi, and lysosomes is no doubt normally protected against oxidant generation, for example by preventing the availability of free transition metal ions. These compartments are also endowed with a range of antioxidants. However, the uptake of extracellular components from an intima in which metal ion supply might already be exaggerated presents an unusual challenge to the vacuolar system, and some evidence (Brunk *et al.* 1992) suggests that intralysosomal oxidative events might be important. Iron ions may also be present in increased quantities in the intralysosomal sites of foam macrophages (Yuan *et al.* 1996). The impact of this may be to enhance cell-mediated LDL oxidation by releasing iron ions from the cells, since such an effect can be observed with macrophages which have engulfed damaged erythrocytes (Yuan *et al.* 1996). This may perhaps relate to the fact that oxidized LDL (oxLDL)-loaded macrophages oxidize fresh LDL more effectively than unloaded cells, or cells loaded with unoxidized lipid (Bolton *et al.* 1994), in that these oxLDL-loaded cells may also mobilize more significant amounts of intracellular iron ions.

However, the difficulty of intralysosomal hydrolysis of oxidized apoB and other proteins has already been discussed. Thus, it is to be expected that foam cells in plaque will not only contain oxidized lipids, as has already been well demonstrated, but also oxidized proteins, which has yet to be properly studied. How the intracellular and extracellular pools of these proteins relate is not yet clear. But the intracellular pool will probably feed the extracellular when cells die, and, furthermore, exocytosis of lysosomal and other vacuolar components is well known.

Plausible mechanisms for the generation of oxidized proteins in the intima, and for the establishment of significant intra- and extracellular pools thus exist. What are the consequences of their presence? Again we scratch the boundaries of present knowledge, and can only postulate that the reactive species present on the protein molecules may contribute to secondary damage, while the presence of relatively large amounts of 'stored', oxidized protein may perturb normal tissue metabolism. The intracellular pool may influence membrane flow through the cells (Bolton *et al.* 1997), with consequent changes in secretion, intra-, and extracellular degradation control, and so on. The extracellular pool may be a component of the mechanisms which enhance smooth muscle cell growth (Bjorkerud and Bjorkerud 1996), trigger mediator production from the participant cells (Lipton *et al.* 1995; Schackelford *et al.* 1995), and further the development of the atherosclerotic tissue (Ares *et al.* 1995; reviewed: Navab *et al.* 1995). For example, oxidized proteins, like many other denatured proteins, are often chemotactic for several cell types, and they also may be present at sites through which cell migration is facilitated because the normally resistant extracellular matrix components are lacking or displaced. At later stages of the disease these proteins may also contribute toxic actions on the cells, by virtue either of their radical generating capacities, or through hydrophobic binding and interference with cell-surface homeostasis. Of the plethora of actions of 'minimally modified' LDL (Parhami *et al.* 1993), or even of LDL subject to defined degrees of oxidation, it is very unclear which can be attributed to lipid or to protein components, and which involve both (Hamilton *et al.* 1995)).

In discussing the second disease to be considered here, Alzheimer's, such toxic roles as we have just mentioned are often foregrounded (reviewed: Mattson 1994; Cummings 1995). In this case there has been a particular emphasis on protein, as opposed to lipid, oxidation (Smith, C. D. *et al.* 1992*a*) because of the central importance of amyloid β-protein, which seems to accumulate in diseased brains, and to form part of the neurofibrillary tangles which characterize its progression morphologically. Aggregation of this protein, which may occur through oxidation, is involved (Dyrks *et al.* 1993). However, lipid oxidation is also believed to be elevated in the brain Alzheimer's, and it has been argued the 4-hydroxynonenal in particular may be important in cytoskeletal damage during its progression, largely by protein cross-linking (Montine *et al.* 1996). Mitochondrial dysfunction in the brains of Alzheimer's patients and other brain diseases has also been claimed as a likely source of enhanced radical flux critical to disease progression (Dykens 1994).

Early evidence from Carney and colleagues indicated that direct protein oxidation products are more pronounced in the brains of Alzheimer's patients than normal people, as judged by protein carbonyls and loss of activity of two enzymes which (like most) can be oxidatively inactivated, glutamine synthetase and creatine kinase (Smith *et al.* 1991; see also Le Prince *et al.* 1995). Subsequent work has refined and extended this data, showing that there is considerable regional specificity to the accumulation of oxidation products, the membrane protein alterations detected by the MAL-6 spin probe (Hensley *et al.* 1994*a*), and the loss of enzyme activities

(Carney *et al.* 1994; Hensley *et al.* 1995*c*). The product distribution, such as carbonyls detected immunohistochemically (Smith *et al.* 1996), corresponds well with disease histochemistry of senile plaques and neurofibrillary tangles. There is not always a complete parallel between the parameters of protein oxidation and loss of enzyme activity. In view of the heterogeneity of reaction mechanisms which may contribute to these various consequences of protein oxidation such a specificity is, perhaps, not surprising. Glycation and glycoxidation products are also accumulated in Alzheimer's brains (Smith *et al.* 1994; Yan, S. D. *et al.* 1995). Other evidence has suggested a parallel between regional accumulation of protein oxidation products in animal brains and specific cognitive defects (Forster *et al.* 1996). We have already discussed, in the section on ageing, the possibility that the spin trap PBN retards protein oxidation product accumulation, and improves cognitive function in gerbils and other species (Carney *et al.* 1991; Floyd and Carney 1992)). We have also discussed brain ischemia/reperfusion damage in section 5.3.1.

What is the role of protein oxidation and amyloid in particular? Amyloid β-protein has for some time been observed to be cytotoxic, and to induce oxidative damage in certain target cells of the brain (Behl *et al.* 1994; Manelli and Puttfarcken 1995; Puttfarcken *et al.* 1996), but also in other tissues such as the eye (Frederikse *et al.* 1996) and vasculature (Thomas *et al.* 1996). A synthetic catalytic antioxidant has been found to protect hippocampal cultures against amyloid β-protein (Bruce *et al.* 1996), and lazaroids are also effective (Richardson *et al.* 1996). In addition, C2-ceramide can protect hippocampal neurons against this attack, possibly by inducing antioxidant defences (Behl *et al.* 1995; Sagara *et al.* 1996); it is a known trigger of NF-κB, which may play a role in such defence (Barger and Mattson 1996; Goodman and Mattson 1996), and of NO release from microglia (Goodwin *et al.* 1995).

The mechanism of amyloid β-protein toxicity may also involve a conventional receptor (or at least trigger) mechanism, but on the other hand it has been claimed in a remarkable group of papers that amyloid β-protein *itself* can generate radicals which could be spin trapped with PBN (Butterfield *et al.* 1994*b*; Hensley *et al.* 1994*b*, 1995*b*), though freshly dissolved samples were inactive (Harris *et al.* 1995*b*). The radicals could inactivate glutamine synthetase and creatine kinase, and cause salicylate hydroxylation (Hensley *et al.* 1994*b*). Later work showed that there is significant inter-preparation variation in the peptide samples, and that some are poorer at radical generation and glutamine synthetase inactivation than those described initially (Hensley *et al.* 1995*a*). It is, however, likely that these claims for direct radical generation by the protein itself are artefactual, consequent on contaminants in some of the preparations studied. This conclusion is based on the fact that the published EPR spectra lack the usual β-hydrogen coupling that should be present for spin adducts formed from the spin trap PBN. The authors' assertion that this coupling is not observed as a result of the large size, and hence restricted rotation, of the spin adduct is unlikely to be correct, as it has been shown that such hindered rotation results in a high degree of anisotropy of the nitroxide nitrogen coupling which was *not* observed; the published spectra are almost completely isotropic in nature, and thus likely to be due to low-molecular-weight species. Iron ions (or other pseudo Fenton catalysts) may well facilitate the formation of such species (Schubert and Chevion 1995), and be present in variable quantities in the different preparations. This may relate to the otherwise surprising enhancement of amyloid toxicity by the addition of exogenous glutamine synthetase (Aksenov *et al.* 1995). Others have shown differences between peptides 'aged' *in vitro* (i.e. stored in solution) for various periods, and demonstrated that the methionine at position 35 in the peptide is not essential for its toxic actions (Manelli and Puttfarcken 1995). The amyloid precursor protein also appears to possess a reductive residue, which might induce a radical flux via metal-ion reduction (Multhaup *et al.* 1996). Amyloid-induced radical fluxes are also claimed to inhibit astrocyte glutamate transport (Harris *et al.* 1995a) and ion-motive ATPases (Mark *et al.* 1995). If these fluxes are intrinsic to the protein, the mechanisms involved will require a substantial revising of, and/or addition to, the mechanisms of protein oxidation discussed earlier.

Whether or not amyloid β-protein is a radical-generating machine in and of itself, in the case of the observed mechanisms of progression of Alzheimer's, it is somewhat easier than with atherosclerosis to envisage roles for radical metabolism (Benzi and Moretti 1995), and specifically protein oxidation and its intermediates. They may contribute to the cross-linking and aggregation mechanisms of tangle formation, and could contribute to the cytotoxic signals which influence the metabolism of brain cells, as modelled *in vitro* with the studies of PC12 cultures. Radical-mediated damage to protein ion-transporters, leading to alterations of neurotransmission as well as to lytic events, may well be important (Pellmar 1995). Besides these specific mechanisms, a range of the other postulated damaging mechanisms we have discussed earlier may also contribute.

The question inevitably arises how such protein oxidative events might be controlled, and whether prevention of their occurrence would restrict age-related disease. These are the questions to which we turn in the final chapter.

6 Future directions in the study of protein oxidation

It should be obvious from the preceding five chapters that though considerable advances have been made over the last 90 years, there are still many important gaps in our understanding of the mechanisms and consequences of radical-induced protein oxidation. Some of the more important of these, at least in the view of the authors, are summarized briefly below, and are arranged in the same order as the chapters from which they arose. Thus, our initial discussion is at a molecular/mechanistic level, before progressing on to questions that still remain at the functional and physiological/pathological levels.

6.1 Some key issues in the study of the chemistry of protein oxidation

Despite considerable advances in our appreciation of the mechanisms of radical attack on individual amino acids and small peptides, we are still lacking precise knowledge of the products that are obtained in several conditions, and the processes by which these arise. The relative lack of progress in the application of existing knowledge to peptides and proteins, means that we do not understand many issues:

1. What factors control the selectivity of attack of radicals on proteins and particularly, the effects of accessibility and 3-D structure on the radical processes that have been elucidated with individual amino acids? There is still controversy as to the conditions under which attack on proteins is selective, and the reasons why it is selective. This is true even of the most extensively studied radicals, such as HO·, though some progress has been made with regard to both site-specific damage, as a result of metal ion binding, and the stability of the various possible initial radicals.

2. We have not yet defined the quantitative importance of the various pathways which have been elucidated for the fragmentation of the backbone of proteins, and even whether those pathways which have been suggested

are the only operative mechanisms. There is also a dearth of information as to what factors control these reactions.

3. Though a number of pathways have been elucidated which give rise to protein cross-links (either inter- or intramolecular), there are still significant numbers of cross-linked products which do not belong to these categories, and hence there must be a number of additional processes remaining to be defined.

4. The extent and significance of protein chain reactions and individual radical transfer pathways within a protein remain uncertain. Despite the considerable amount of data that has been obtained, particularly on transfer between various aromatic residues, thiols, and sulfides, there is obviously still much to be learnt, as it is difficult to account for the observed chain lengths and quantities of amino acids destroyed under any conditions on the basis of these aromatic and thiol/sulfide transfer processes alone. The realization that alkoxyl as well as peroxyl radicals are major players, and the recent information on the reactions that these species undergo (see, for example, Scheme 2.8), suggests that progress can be made relatively rapidly in this area. The occurrence of such processes may account for some of the problems and diverse opinions in the interpretation of data obtained on the selectivity of radical attack on proteins and peptides, and the methods by which such reactions are analysed. Thus, the discrepancy between some EPR data, particularly that obtained at low temperatures with solid samples, which suggests that radical attack can be highly selective, and that obtained from analysis of amino acid loss, may depend on the extent of radical transfer reactions under the various conditions employed.

5. The transfer of damage between protein radicals and other biological targets, including other undamaged protein molecules, remains a poorly understood area. There are a few well characterized examples present in the literature, but these are generally concerned with highly specific processes, such as electron transfer between proteins which form part of an electron transport chain. There are, however, encouraging signs from a number of recent publications and the work in progress in a number of laboratories, that the more general problem of understanding the reactions of, for example, generic protein-derived, carbon-centred, alkoxyl and peroxyl radicals with other proteins, lipids, DNA, and complex carbohydrates is being addressed.

6.2 Consequences of protein oxidation for molecular function

At a functional, molecular level the field is somewhat more advanced, but some areas need much further study. Though it is now fairly well understood what types of damage can cause functional inactivation, at least at a gross level (e.g. what amino acid damage can cause loss of enzyme activity), the more subtle, structural effects are more poorly understood. It is still unclear what particular chemical modifications can result in unfolding or alteration of a protein structure, and which are essentially harmless events. It is likely that there will not be a general answer to this point, as each individual protein will have its own idiosyncrasies, but it should be possible, in due course, to outline, at least in general terms, what types of lesion are likely to be deleterious. For example, conversion of highly hydrophobic side chains present in the interior of a protein to significantly more hydrophilic ones, such as tyrosine to 3-nitrotyrosine, is likely to be deleterious, while conversions of external/surface amino acids to hydroxides may well not be.

It is also still unclear where the boundary lies, with regard to both the extent and type of processes, between reversible and irreversible damage. We know, for example, that oxidation of methionine to methionine sulfoxide occurs in a number of proteins subjected to radical attack, and that this lesion can be enzymatically repaired. It is, however, unclear as to whether this is a significant pathway *in vivo*, and under what circumstances. Such repair may make biological sense in the case of long-lived proteins (such as the crystallin proteins of the eye, where protein syntheis and turnover are extremely low), but it may not be energetically worthwhile in other cases. The situation with thiol oxidation is better understood, at least in some cases, but our understanding of possible repair processes with other lesions is very poor.

Similarly, we do not yet fully understand whether unfolding is a reversible process, to what extent this occurs, and again where the boundary lies between reversible and irreversible events. This problem is more likely to be resolved initially at a gross level than at a molecular level, as the latter will require an understanding of the effects of a large number of different lesions, and will probably be protein specific. This aspect is, therefore, unlikely to be readily answered.

6.3 Research issues concerning the influence of protein oxidation on cellular functions

It is well established that incorporation of amino acid analogues or errors in protein synthesis bring into play a number of regulatory and recovery mechanisms, designed either to refold correctly, or to remove, the abnormal proteins. Nevertheless, some abnormal proteins are transported to unusual sites, and may establish significant pools there, as well as being degraded there. The degree to which such mechanisms apply to oxidized proteins is unclear. For example, does the oxidation, inactivation, and unfolding of a cytosolic protein normally lead to attempts to refold and reactivate it? Or is it usually immediately degraded like many unfolded proteins? If the latter, is there selective transport to the proteasome or to the lysosomal system, as is known for some categories of proteins, such as certain complexed antigens or serum-regulated proteins, respectively.

The whole issue of recognition of oxidized proteins by chaperones, other proteins, membrane receptors, and proteinases has barely been studied. Such information will be necessary to appreciate what can cause deranged subcellular transport of oxidized proteins. Conversely, it is already clear that oxidized proteins in some cases, and especially after extensive oxidation, may be poorly degraded (as in the case of endocytosed oxidized proteins being poorly degraded in lysosomes). What are the molecular features which dictate this resistance? We have already pointed to the likelihood that oxidized amino acids released by degradation of oxidized proteins may in some cases be reincorporated by protein synthesis, and hence lead to reformation of oxidized proteins without further radical attack. The metabolic consequences of this can only be appreciated by quantitative and kinetic studies.

There may be important differences between the handling of extracellular, oxidized proteins and those generated endogenously in cells. Membrane binding, and possibly receptor recognition, may be relevant to both, but the range and nature of the receptors and enzymes which can act outside cells, at cell surfaces, and on intracellular membranes, are distinct. Furthermore, specialized cells, such as the leukocytes, may have specific roles in relation to extracellular, oxidized proteins, including that of releasing them from macromolecular aggregates, such as cartilage, so that they can be internalized and handled by cells.

The reactive intermediates of protein oxidation, such as the hydroperoxides and DOPA we have defined, may generate further damage to proteins and other molecules unless they are contained. Thus the issue of detoxification is important, and the limited evidence, for example, that protein hydroperoxides can be reduced at cell surfaces, need much further elaboration. For example, is this a harmless process, or are radicals a by-product? What are the enzymatic or electron-transport machineries involved? Again, there may be specialised roles for leukocytes.

6.4 Is protein oxidation important to the organism?

The preceding issues lead directly into the central biological question which is still generally unresolved: does the formation of oxidized proteins have a significant physiological or pathological impact, or is it a secondary phenomenon? Many arguments have been raised earlier in the book to indicate that it may be of functional, physiological significance, and that in some pathologies it is not solely a secondary consequence. However, the validity of these arguments will only be firmly established by direct perturbation studies, in which a stimulation or inhibition of protein oxidation, independent of other oxidative processes, is achieved, and its effects on physiology and pathology determined. The action of a highly selective protein-oxidant, or the use of oxidized amino acids and their incorporation into proteins by biosynthesis, would be possible approaches to the stimulation of protein oxidation, or at least the enlargement of the supply of oxidized proteins. The action of a highly selective inhibitor of protein oxidation would be the desirable converse approach.

6.5 Is it possible to achieve selective inhibition of protein oxidation?

From the preceding discussion we would predict that the selective inhibition of protein oxidation might ameliorate several pathologies, and might be a means of controlling some physiological processes in which protein oxidation is central. We have also noted that such a selective inhibition would be one of the most valuable ways of rigorously testing the proposition that protein oxidation is important in these processes. Thus, it is very desirable that future research address the possibility of selective antioxidation of proteins.

Given the importance of protein oxidation in physiology and pathology discussed above, it is perhaps surprising that there are, as yet, few reports on protein antioxidation, at least when compared with the vast literature on lipid antioxidation. However, the mechanisms of protein oxidation are more complex than those of lipid (per)oxidation, and so protein antioxidation is also likely to be more complex than lipid antioxidation.

As mentioned above, biological systems contain several layers of antioxidant defences that act at the level of prevention of formation of primary radicals, the scavenging of these oxidants, and the repair and/or removal of oxidized moieties (and hence inhibition of possible secondary events). Given the catalytic role transition metal ions play in both the initiation and propagation of protein oxidation, their sequestration in redox-inactive forms, principally by copper and iron transport and storage proteins, is of great importance for protein antioxidation, and it will be interesting to assess whether there are alterations in the prevalence of protein oxidation in diseases involving altered metal ion transport and storage.

Among enzymic protein antioxidants, the roles of methionine sulfoxide reductase and disulfide isomerase have been mentioned already. Like the latter, thioredoxin plus thioredoxin reductase, can reduce protein disulfides, including those formed in the thiol-specific antioxidant enzyme (TSA) upon reduction of alkyl hydroperoxides (Chae *et al.* 1994). The S–S -----> SH reducing activity of thioredoxin is thought to be responsible for the involvement of the enzyme in the regulation of redox-sensitive transcription factors. In addition, thioredoxin reductase and thioredoxin have alkyl hydroperoxide reductase activity, and are efficient electron donors to plasma glutathione peroxidase (Bjornstedt *et al.* 1995). It is not known whether this reductase can act on protein hydroperoxides, though it is clear the glutathione peroxidase and human plasma components can (Fu *et al.* 1995a). As discussed above, TSA also protects proteins against thiyl-radical-induced inactivation (Yim *et al.* 1994), though it is currently not known whether thiyl radicals on proteins are substrates for TSA.

Regarding non-proteinaceous antioxidants for proteins, several important aspects need to be considered. First, aliphatic amino acids in proteins are less reactive than lipids containing bisallylic hydrogens, so that reactive radical oxidants (HO·, RO·) are of greater relevance to protein than lipid (per)oxidation. Since the differences in rate constants for reaction of a radical with its targets decrease with increasing reactivity of the radical, it follows that the conventional scavenging antioxidants (α-tocopherol, ascorbate, urate, etc.) are less likely to offer specific protection to proteins than lipids.

Accessibility of a protein radical to a potential antioxidant is also probably a major factor, particularly with regard to the core of proteins. Unlike lipid systems, where there is very rapid diffusion of antioxidants such as α-tocopherol throughout the lipid phase, diffusion of antioxidant molecules within a protein structure is likely to be poor, at best, especially with globular proteins. Thus, chain reactions within a globular protein molecule are probably very difficult to interrupt, and direct reaction with an antioxidant is only likely to occur with a radical present on the protein surface. As many of the 'sinks' for radicals, such as disulfide groups and aromatic rings (Trp, Tyr, etc.), are usually found buried within a protein core, repair of such sinks is likely to be slow. Such repair probably does occur to some degree, since long-range transfer of oxidizing and reducing equivalents is known (see, for example, Chapter 2).

Second, the chain reaction of lipid peroxidation is probably the result of the predominant presence of a single chain-carrying species. It has been argued that, at least in lipid emulsions including lipoproteins, and in the absence of co-antioxidants such as ascorbate or ubiquinol, the α-tocopheroxyl radical is the likely chain carrier, as long as vitamin E is present (Neuzil *et al.* 1997), whereas after tocopherol depletion, lipid peroxyl radicals become the chain-carrying species. Thus, an antioxidant for lipids can focus on the elimination of a single reactant, independent of the nature of the radical initiating the peroxidation process. It is not surprising then that certain individual antioxidants can *strongly inhibit* lipid peroxidation induced by a wide variety of different radical oxidants (Neuzil *et al.* 1997). In contrast, there are almost certainly several chain-carrying species during radical-induced protein (per)oxidation, and many competing or complementary pathways (cf. the discovery that there appear to be several different routes which lead to backbone cleavage (Davies 1996)), such that individual antioxidants may perhaps be expected only to *attenuate* particular reactions, and not the overall process.

One feature of the major involvement of alkoxyl, as well as peroxyl, radicals in protein oxidation is that repair of the former seemingly does not occur, while there is a reasonable likelihood of chain reactions involving protein peroxyl radicals giving rise to a modified amino acid. If the result is a hydroperoxide, it may be able (like lipid hydroperoxides) to initiate further damage. Metal ions are probably more important in protein oxidation than lipid, because they are not essential for propagation of lipid peroxidation chains, but may be for protein. Thus, the significance of metal-ion-induced secondary radical initiation is probably much greater for proteins. On the other hand, the apparently more substantial role of the alkoxyl radicals in protein peroxidation than in lipid may offer at least a selective target for inhibition of protein, rather than lipid, oxidation. In this case, the alkoxyl radical would react without initiating further protein radicals, and be detoxified to an alcohol with the result that the amino acid on which it was present would be modified, but also be incapable of initiating further damage. It is not clear what the direct consequence of such alcohol formation would be (e.g. unfolding, or recognition by proteinases?), though it is unlikely that the products would be significantly toxic at the levels at which they are likely to be generated *in vivo*.

The effect of chain-breaking antioxidants is also likely to be much less significant when the chain lengths are short, as is observed in protein oxidation, compared to that of lipid oxidation. Thus, removal of one chain-carrying species in lipid oxidation may result in the sparing of hundreds of lipid molecules, whereas in protein oxidation, where the chain lengths are < 15, the number of molecules spared is smaller.

6.6 Selective prevention of intermolecular reaction of radicals and other products of protein oxidation?

We have noted that certain components of oxidized proteins may inflict damage on other biomolecules, for example initiating lipid peroxidation or damaging DNA. Thus the question arises whether the selective inhibition of protein oxidation per se, discussed in the preceding section, is the only approach to controlling or restricting such intermolecular damage, which would again be desirable in theory. For example, control of metal-ion availability might be a means of limiting the action of protein-catechol-quinone systems such as DOPA, and thereby enhancing the likelihood of their detoxification. However, most of the approaches one can readily envisage are either those appropriate to restricting radical reactions generally (as in the case of controlling metal-ion availability), or are congruent with those discussed as possible means of controlling protein oxidation itself. If novel approaches to controlling intermolecule reaction of oxidized proteins can be developed, this may again be therapeutically, as well as experimentally, valuable and informative.

In this context it can be noted that there have been occasional claims that amino acids or peptides can function as general radical protectants. Most recently, the simple peptide melatonin has been so promoted (Reiter 1995a, b). Melatonin, a pineal hormone, clearly has important physiological roles. However, the claims that it is 'antioxidant' seem to be based on inappropriate comparisons, for example with molecules like tocopherol, undertaken in conditions in which the latter is not readily accessible to the oxidants studied. Like any peptide, it is quite a good hydroxyl radical scavenger, but the available evidence, if carefully assessed, does not suggest that it is exceptional.

6.7 Does retardation of age-related disease require inhibition of protein oxidation and/or removal of oxidized proteins?

The ultimate objective of studies of protein oxidation in biology must be therapeutic. The burden of this book, while critically assessing the available literature, has been that protein oxidation must perturb biological function, and that it very probably does contribute to pathologies, particularly age-related pathologies such as neurodegenerative and vascular diseases, as well as to ageing per se.

We therefore envisage that knowledge which eventually allows us to control protein oxidation will also lead to improved therapies. Indeed, it is likely that without direct or indirect control of protein oxidation, age-related diseases will not be overcome. Only considerable and intense future study will establish whether this brave prediction has force. Our main hope is that this effort will be undertaken, and that the ideas we have analysed and proposed in this book will contribute modestly to its success.

References

Abate, C., Baker, S.J., Lees, M.S., Anderson, C.W., Marshak, D.R., and Curran, T. (1993). Dimerization and DNA binding alter phosphorylation of Fos and Jun. *Proceedings of the National Academy of Science of the United States of America*, **90**, 6766–6770.

Abe, M.K., Chao, T.S., Solway, J., Rosner, M.R., and Hershenson, M.B. (1994). Hydrogen peroxide stimulates mitogen-activated protein kinase in bovine tracheal myocytes: implications for human airway disease. *American Journal of Respiratory and Cellular Molecular Biology*, **11**, 577–585.

Abeliovich, H., and Shlomai, J. (1995). Reversible oxidative aggregation obstructs specific proteolytic cleavage of glutathione S-transferase fusion proteins. *Analytical Biochemistry*, **228**, 351–354.

Abell, P.I. (1973). Addition to multiple bonds. In *Free Radicals*, (ed. J.K. Kochi), pp. 63–112. John Wiley and Sons, New York.

Aberhart, D.J. (1988). Separation by high-performance liquid chromatography of alpha- and beta-amino acids: application to assays of lysine 2,3-aminomutase and leucine 2,3-aminomutase. *Analytical Biochemistry*, **169**, 350–355.

Abeyama, K., Kawano, K., Nakajima, T., Takasaki, I., Kitajima, I., and Maruyama, I. (1995). Interleukin 6 mediated differentiation and rescue of cell redox in PC12 cells exposed to ionizing radiation. *FEBS Letters*, **364**, 298–300.

Abramovitch, S., and Rabani, J. (1976). Pulse radiolytic investigations of peroxy radicals in aqueous solutions of acetate and glycine. *Journal of Physical Chemistry*, **80**, 1562–1565.

Abuja, P.M., and Esterbauer, H. (1995). Simulation of lipid peroxidation in low-density lipoprotein by a basic 'skeleton' of reactions. *Chemical Research in Toxicology*, **8**, 753–763.

Adachi, O., Matsushita, K., and Ameyama, M. (1992). Biochemistry and physiology of pyrroloquinoline quinone and quinoprotein dehydrogenases. *Journal of Nutritional Science and Vitaminology Tokyo*, **38**, 224–227.

Adachi, O., Okamoto, K., Shinagawa, E., Matsushita, K., and Ameyama, M. (1988). Adduct formation of pyrroloquinoline quinone and amino acid. *Biofactors*, **1**, 251–254.

Adamic, K., Howard, J.A., and Ingold, K.U. (1969). Absolute rate constants for hydrocarbon autoxidation. XVI. Reactions of peroxy radicals at low temperatures. *Canadian Journal of Chemistry*, **47**, 3803–3808.

Adams, G.E. (1972). Radiation mechanisms in radiation biology. *Advances in Radiation Chemistry*, **3**, 125–208.

Adams, G.E., and Redpath, J.L. (1974). Selective free-radical reactions with proteins and enzymes: pulse radiolysis and inactivation studies on papain. *International Journal of Radiation Biology and Related Studies on Physical Chemistry and Medicine*, **25**, 129–138.

Adams, G.E., and Willson, R.L. (1969). Pulse radiolysis studies on the oxidation of organic radicals in aqueous solution. *Transactions of the Faraday Society*, **65**, 2981–2987.

Adams, G.E., McNaughton, G.S., and Michael, B.D. (1967). The pulse radiolysis of sulphur compounds. Part 1. Cysteamine and cystamine. In *The Chemistry of Ionization and Excitation*, (ed. G.R.A. Johnson and G. Scholes), pp. 281–293. Taylor and Francis, London.

Adams, G.E., McNaughton, G.S., and Michael, B.D. (1968). Pulse radiolysis of sulphur compounds. Part 2. Free radical 'repair' by hydrogen transfer from sulphydryl compounds. *Transactions of the Faraday Society*, **64**, 902–910.

Adams, G.E., Armstrong, R.C., Charlesby, A., Michael, B.D., and Willson, R.L. (1969a). Pulse radiolysis of sulphur compounds. Part 3. Repair by hydrogen transfer of a macromolecule irradiated in aqueous solution. *Transactions of the Faraday Society*, **65**, 732–742.

Adams, G.E., Willson, R.L., Aldrich, J.E., and Cundall, R.B. (1969b). On the mechanism of the radiation-induced inactivation of lysozyme in dilute aqueous solution. *International Journal of Radiation Biology and Related Studies on Physical Chemistry and Medicine*, **16**, 333–342.

Adams, G.E., Aldrich, J.E., Bisby, R.H., Cundall, R.B., Redpath, J.L., and Willson, R.L. (1972a). Selective free radical reactions with proteins and enzymes: reactions of inorganic radical anions with amino acids. *Radiation Research*, **49**, 278–289.

Adams, G.E., Bisby, R.H., Cundall, R.B., Redpath, J.L., and Willson, R.L. (1972b). Selective free radical reactions with proteins and enzymes: the inactivation of ribonuclease. *Radiation Research*, **49**, 290–299.

Adams, G.E., Baverstock, K.F., Cundall, R.B., and Redpath, J.L. (1973). Radiation effects on α-chymotrypsin in aqueous solution: pulse radiolysis and inactivation studies. *Radiation Research*, **54**, 375–387.

Adams, G.E., Posener, M.L., Bisby, R.H., Cundall, R.B., and Key, J.R. (1979). Free radical reactions with proteins and enzymes: the inactivation of pepsin. *International Journal of Radiation Biology and Related Studies on Physical Chemistry and Medicine*, **35**, 497–507.

Adamska, I., Kloppstech, K., and Ohad, I. (1992). UV light stress induces the synthesis of the early light-inducible protein and prevents its degradation. *Journal of Biological Chemistry*, **267**, 24732–24737.

Adamska, I., Kloppstech, K., and Ohad, I. (1993). Early light-inducible protein in pea is stable during light stress but is degraded during recovery at low light intensity. *Journal of Biological Chemistry*, **268**, 5438–5444.

Adeniyi, Jones, S.K., and Karnovsky, M.L. (1981). Oxidative decarboxylation of free and peptide-linked amino acids in phagocytizing guinea pig granulocytes. *Journal of Clinical Investigation*, **68**, 365–373.

Adhikari, S., and Gopinathan, C. (1996). Oxidation reactions of a bovine serum albumin-bilirubin complex. A pulse radiolysis study. *International Journal of Radiation Biology and Related Studies in Physics, Chemistry and Medicine*, **69**, 89–98.

Adhikari, H.R., and Tappel, A.L. (1975). Letter: Flourescent products from irradiated amino acids and proteins. *Radiation Research*, **61**, 177–183.

Aeschbach, R., Amado, R., and Neukom, H. (1976). Formation of dityrosine cross-links in proteins by oxidation of tyrosine residues. *Biochimica et Biophysica Acta*, **439**, 292–301.

Afonso, S.G., Chinarro, S., Enriquez, d.S.R., and Batlle, A.M. (1994). How the atmosphere and the presence of substrate affect the photo and non-photo-inactivation of heme enzymes by uroporphyrin I. *International Journal of Biochemistry*, **26**, 259–262.

Aft, R.L., and Mueller, G.C. (1984). Hemin-mediated oxidative degradation of proteins. *Journal of Biological Chemistry*, **259**, 301–305.

Agarwal, S., and Sohal, R.S. (1993). Relationship between aging and susceptibility to protein oxidative damage. *Biochemical and Biophysical Research Communications*, **194**, 1203–1206.

Agarwal, S., and Sohal, R.S. (1994a). Aging and proteolysis of oxidized proteins. *Archives of Biochemistry and Biophysics*, **309**, 24–28.

Agarwal, S., and Sohal, R.S. (1994b). DNA oxidative damage and life expectancy in houseflies. *Proceedings of the National Academy of Science of the United States of America*, **91**, 12332–12335.

Agrup, G., Hansson, C., Rorsman, H., Rosengren, A.M., and Rosengren, E. (1978). Free and bound 5-S-cysteinylDOPA and DOPA in human malignant melanomas. *Acta Dermatologica Venereologica*, **58**, 270–272.

Aguirre, J., and Hansberg, W. (1986). Oxidation of *Neurospora crassa* glutamine synthetase. *Journal of Bacteriology*, **166**, 1040–1045.

Aguirre, J., Rodriguez, R., and Hansberg, W. (1989). Oxidation of Neurospora crassa NADP-specific glutamate dehydrogenase by activated oxygen species. *Journal of Bacteriology*, **171**, 6243–6250.

Ahlskog, J.E., Uitti, R.J., Low, P.A., Tyce, G.M., Nickander, K.K., Petersen, R.C., et al. (1995). No evidence for systemic oxidant stress in Parkinson's or Alzheimer's disease. *Movement Disorders*, **10**, 566–573.

Ahmad, S. (1995). Oxidative stress from environmental pollutants. *Archives of Insect Biochemistry and Physiology*, **29**, 135–157.

Ahmed, M.S., Ainley, K., Parish, J.H., and Hadi, S.M. (1994). Free radical-induced fragmentation of proteins by quercetin. *Carcinogenesis*, **15**, 1627–1630.

Ahn, B., Rhee, S.G., and Stadtman, E.R. (1987). Use of fluorescein hydrazide and fluorescein thiosemicarbazide reagents for the fluorometric determination of protein carbonyl groups and for the detection of oxidized protein on poly-acrylamide gels. *Analytical Biochemistry*, **161**, 245–257.

Aizenman, E., Boeckman, F.A., and Rosenberg, P.A. (1992). Glutathione prevents 2,4,5-trihydroxyphenylalanine excitotoxicity by maintaining it in a reduced, non-active form. *Neuroscience Letters*, **144**, 233–236.

Aizenman, E., White, W.F., Loring, R.H., and Rosenberg, P.A. (1990). A 3,4-dihydroxyphenylalanine oxidation product is a non-N-methyl-D-aspartate gluta-matergic agonist in rat cortical neurons. *Neuroscience Letters*, **116**, 168–171.

Akaike, T., Noguchi, Y., Ijiri, S., Setoguchi, K., Suga, M., Zheng, Y.M., et al. (1996). Pathogenesis of influenza virus-induced pneumonia: involvement of both nitric oxide and oxygen radicals. *Proceedings of the National Academy of Science of the United States of America*, **93**, 2448–2453.

Aksenov, M., Aksenova, M.V., Harris, M.E., Hensley, K., Butterfield, D.A., and Carney, J.M. (1995). Enhancement of beta-amyloid peptide A beta(1-40)-mediated neurotoxicity by glutamine synthetase. *Journal of Neurochemistry*, **65**, 1899–1902.

Al-Massad, F.K., Kadir, F.H., and Moore, G.R. (1992). Animal ferritin and bacterioferritin contain quinones. *Biochemical Journal*, **283**, 177–180.

Alayash, A.I., Ryan, B.A., and Fratantoni, J.C. (1993). Oxidation reactions of human, opossum (*Didelphis virginiana*) and spot (*Leiostomus xanthurus*) hemoglobins: a search for a correlation with some structural-functional proper-ties. *Comparative Biochemistry and Physiology B*, **106**, 427–432.

Albrich, J.M., McCarthy, C.A., and Hurst, J.K. (1981). Biological reactivity of hypochlorous acid: implications for microbicidal mechanisms of leukocyte myeloperoxidase. *Proceedings of the National Academy of Science of the United States of America*, **78**, 210–214.

Aldrich, J.E., Cundall, R.B., Adams, G.E., and Willson, R.L. (1969). Identification of essential residues in lysozyme: a pulse radiolysis method. *Nature*, **221**, 1049–1050.

Alexander, P., Fox, M., Stacey, K.A., and Rosen, D. (1956). Comparison of some direct and indirect effects of ionising radiation in proteins. *Nature*, **178**, 846–849.

Alican, I., Coskun, T., Corak, A., Yegen, B.C., Oktay, S., and Kurtel, H. (1995). Role of neutrophils in indomethacin-induced gastric mucosal lesions in rats. *Inflammation Research*, **44**, 164–168.

Allen, R.G., Oberley, L.W., Elwell, J.H., and Sohal, R.S. (1991). Developmental patterns in the antioxidant defenses of the housefly, *Musca domestica*. *Journal of Cellular Physiology*, **146**, 270–276.

Alleva, R., Tomasetti, M., Battino, M., Curatola, G., Littarru, G.P., and Folkers, K. (1995). The roles of coenzyme Q10 and vitamin E on the peroxidation of human low density lipoprotein subfractions. *Proceedings of the National Academy of Science of the United States of America*, **92**, 9388–9391.

Alonso, E., and Rubio, V. (1987). Inactivation of mitochondrial carbamoyl phosphate synthetase induced by ascorbate, oxygen, and Fe^{3+} in the presence of acetylglutamate: protection by ATP and HCO_3^- and lack of inactivation of ornithine transcarbamylase. *Archives of Biochemistry and Biophysics*, **258**, 342–350.

Altman, S.A., Zastawny, T.H., Randers, E.L., Cacciuttolo, M.A., Akman, S.A., Dizdaroglu, M., *et al.* (1995). Formation of DNA-protein cross-links in cultured mammalian cells upon treatment with iron ions. *Free Radical Biology and Medicine*, **19**, 897–902.

Alvarado, A., Butterfield, D.A., and Hennig, B. (1994). Disruption of endothelial barrier function: relationship to fluidity of membrane extracellular lamella. *International Journal of Biochemistry*, **26**, 575–581.

Alvarez, B., Rubbo, H., Kirk, M., Barnes, S., Freeman, B.A., and Radi, R. (1996). Peroxynitrite-dependent tryptophan nitration. *Chemical Research in Toxicology*, **9**, 390–396.

Amato, R., Aeschbach, R., and Neukom, H. (1984). Dityrosine: *In vitro* production and characterisation. *Methods in Enzymology*, **107**, 377–388.

Ambe, K.S., and Tappel, A.L. (1961). Oxidative damage to amino acids, peptides, and proteins by radiations. *Journal of Food Science*, **26**, 448–451.

Ambe, K.S., Kumta, U.S., and Tappel, A.L. (1961). Radiation damage to cytochrome *c* and hemoglobin. *Radiation Research*, **15**, 709–719.

Ames, B.N., and Shigenaga, M.K. (1992). Oxidants are a major contributor to aging. *Annals of the New York Academy of Science*, **663**, 85–96.

Ames, B.N., Shigenaga, M.K., and Hagen, T.M. (1993). Oxidants, antioxidants, and the degenerative diseases of aging. *Proceedings of the National Academy of Science of the United States of America*, **90**, 7915–7922.

Ames, B.N., Shigenaga, M.K., and Hagen, T.M. (1995). Mitochondrial decay in aging. *Biochimica et Biophysica Acta*, **1271**, 165–170.

Amici, A., Levine, R.L., Tsai, L., and Stadtman, E.R. (1989). Conversion of amino acid residues in proteins and amino acid homopolymers to carbonyl derivatives by metal-catalyzed oxidation reactions. *Journal of Biological Chemistry*, **264**, 3341–3346.

Amiconi, G., Ascoli, F., Concetti, A., Matarese, M., Verzili, D., and Brunori, M. (1985). Determination of methionine sulfoxide in proteins: comparison of a gas-chromatographic and electrophoretic method. *Journal of Biochemical and Biophysical Methods*, **11**, 241–249.

Andersen, H.J., Chen, H., Pellett, L.J., and Tappel, A.L. (1993). Ferrous-iron-induced oxidation in chicken liver slices as measured by hemichrome formation and thiobarbituric acid-reactive substances: effects of dietary vitamin E and beta-carotene. *Free Radical Biology and Medicine*, **15**, 37–48.

Andersen, H.J., Pellett, L., and Tappel, A.L. (1994). Hemichrome formation, lipid peroxidation, enzyme inactivation and protein degradation as indexes of oxidative damage in homogenates of chicken kidney and liver. *Chemico-Biological Interactions*, **93**, 155–169.

Andersen, S.O. (1972). 3-Chlorotyrosine in insect cuticular proteins. *Acta Chimica Scandinavia*, **26**, 3097–3100.

Anderson, C.H., and Holwerda, R.A. (1985). Mechanistic flexibility in the reduction of copper(II) complexes of aliphatic polyamines by mercapto amino acids. *Journal of Inorganic Biochemistry*, **23**, 29–41.

Anderson, M.T., Staal, F.J., Gitler, C., Herzenberg, L.A., and Herzenberg, L.A. (1994). Separation of oxidant-initiated and redox-regulated steps in the NF-kappa B signal transduction pathway. *Proceedings of the National Academy of Science of the United States of America*, **91**, 11527–11531.

Anderson, R.F., Patel, K.B., and Adams, G.E. (1977). Critical residues in D-amino acid oxidase. A pulse-radiolysis and inactivation study. *International Journal of Radiation Biology and Related Studies in Physics, Chemistry and Medicine*, **32**, 523–531.

Anderson, R.S. (1954). A delayed effect of X-rays on pepsin. *British Journal of Radiology*, **27**, 56–61.

Ando, M., and Tappel, A.L. (1985*a*). Methyl ethyl ketone peroxide damage to cytochrome P-450 peroxidase activities. *Toxicology and Applied Pharmacology*, **81**, 517–524.

Ando, M., and Tappel, A.L. (1985*b*). Effect of dietary vitamin E on methyl ethyl ketone peroxide damage to microsomal cytochrome P-450 peroxidase. *Chemico-Biological Interactions*, **55**, 317–326.

Androes, G.M., Gloria, H.R., and Reinisch, R.F. (1972). Concerning the production of free radicals in proteins by ultraviolet light. *Photochemistry and Photobiology*, **15**, 375–393.

Aniya, Y., and Anders, M.W. (1992). Activation of rat liver microsomal glutathione S-transferase by hydrogen peroxide: role for protein-dimer formation. *Archives of Biochemistry and Biophysics*, **296**, 611–616.

Anthony, C. (1992). The structure of bacterial quinoprotein dehydrogenases. *International Journal of Biochemistry*, **24**, 29–39.

Anthony, C., Ghosh, M., and Blake, C.C. (1994). The structure and function of methanol dehydrogenase and related quinoproteins containing pyrrolo-quinoline quinone. *Biochemical Journal*, **304**, 665–674.

Antonini, E., and Brunori, M. (1971). *Hemoglobin and Myoglobin in Their Reactions with Ligands*. North-Holland Pub. Co., Amsterdam and London.

Antosiewicz, J., Popinigis, J., Wozniak, M., Damiani, E., Carloni, P., and Greci, L. (1995). Effects of indolinic and quinolinic aminoxyls on protein and lipid peroxidation of rat liver microsomes. *Free Radical Biology and Medicine*, **18**, 913–917.

Aoki, Y., Yanagisawa, Y., Yazaki, K., Oguchi, H., Kiyosawa, K., and Furuta, S. (1992). Protective effect of vitamin E supplementation on increased thermal stability of collagen in diabetic rats. *Diabetologia*, **35**, 913–916.

Apffel, A., Fischer, S., Goldberg, G., Goodley, P.C., and Kuhlmann, F.E. (1995). Enhanced sensitivity for peptide mapping with electrospray liquid chromatography-mass spectrometry in the presence of signal suppression due to trifluoroacetic acid-containing mobile phases. *Journal of Chromatography A*, **712**, 177–190.

Archakov, A.I., and Mokhosoev, I.M. (1989). Modification of proteins by active oxygen and their degradation. *Biokhimica*, **54**, 179–186.

Arduini, A., Eddy, L., and Hochstein, P. (1990). Detection of ferryl myoglobin in the isolated ischemic rat heart. *Free Radical Biology and Medicine*, **9**, 511–513.

Ares, M.P., Kallin, B., Eriksson, P., and Nilsson, J. (1995). Oxidized LDL induces transcription factor activator protein-1 but inhibits activation of nuclear factor-kappa B in human vascular smooth muscle cells. *Arteriosclerosis Thrombosis and Vascular Biology*, **15**, 1584–1590.

Arizono, K., Kagawa, S., Hamada, H., and Ariyoshi, T. (1995). Nitric oxide mediated metallothionein induction by lipopolysaccharide. *Research Communications in Molecular Pathology and Pharmacology*, **90**, 49–58.

Armstrong, A.P., Franklin, A.A., Uittenbogaard, M.N., Giebler, H.A., and Nyborg, J.K. (1993). Pleiotropic effect of the human T-cell leukemia virus Tax protein on the DNA binding activity of eukaryotic transcription factors. *Proceedings of the National Academy of Science of the United States of America*, **90**, 7303–7307.

Armstrong, D.A. (1990). Applications of pulse radiolysis for the study of short-lived sulphur species. In *Sulfur-Centered Reactive Intermediates in Chemistry and Biology*, (ed. C. Chatgilialoglu and K.-D. Asmus), pp. 121–134. Plenum Press, New York.

Armstrong, D.A., and Wilkening, V.G. (1964). Effects of pH in the γ-radiolysis of aqueous solution of cysteine and methyl mercaptan. *Canadian Journal of Chemistry*, **42**, 2631–2635.

Armstrong, D.A., Rauk, A., and Yu, D. (1995). Solution thermochemistry of the radicals of glycine. *Journal of the Chemical Society Perkin Transactions 2*, 553–560.

Armstrong, R.C., and Swallow, A.J. (1969). Pulse- and gamma-radiolysis of aqueous solutions of tryptophan. *Radiation Research*, **40**, 563–579.

Armstrong, S.G., and Dean, R.T. (1995). A sensitive fluorometric assay for protein-bound DOPA and related products of radical-mediated protein oxidation. *Redox Report*, **1**, 291–298.

Armstrong, W.A., and Humphreys, W.G. (1967). Amino acid radicals produced chemically in aqueous solutions. Electron spin resonance spectra and relation to radiolysis products. *Canadian Journal of Chemistry*, **45**, 2589–2597.

Arnow, L.E. (1935). Physicochemical effects produced by the irradiation of crystalline egg albumin solutions with alpha-particles. *Journal of Biological Chemistry*, **110**, 43–59.

Arnow, L.E. (1936). Effects produced by the irradiation of proteins and amino acids. *Physiological Reviews*, **16**, 671–685.

Aronson, R.B., Sinex, F.M., Franzblau, C., and Van, S.D. (1967). The oxidation of protein-bound hydroxylysine by periodate. *Journal of Biological Chemistry*, **242**, 809–812.

Arroyo, C.M., Kramer, J.H., Dickens, B.F., and Weglicki, W.B. (1987*a*). Identification of free radicals in myocardial ischemia/reperfusion by spin trapping with the nitrone DMPO. *FEBS Letters.*, **221**, 101–104.

Arroyo, C.M., Kramer, J.H., Leiboff, R.H., Mergner, G.W., Dickens, B.F., and Weglicki, W.B. (1987*b*). Spin trapping of oxygen and carbon-centred free radicals in ischemic canine myocardium. *Free Radical Biology and Medicine*, **3**, 313–316.

Aruoma, O.I., and Halliwell, B. (1989). Inactivation of alpha-1-antiproteinase by hydroxyl radicals. The effect of uric acid. *FEBS Letters*, **244**, 76–80.

Asmus, K.-D. (1979). Stabilization of oxidised sulfur centers in organic sulfides. Radical cations and odd electron sulfur-sulfur bonds. *Accounts of Chemical Research*, **12**, 436–442.

Asmus, K.-D., Mockel, H., Henglein, A. (1973). Pulse radiolytic study of the site of OH· radical attack on aliphatic alcohols in aqueous solution. *Journal of Physical Chemistry*, **77**, 1218–1221.

Asquith, R.S., and Carthew, P. (1972). The preparation and subsequent identification of a dehydroalanyl peptide from alkali-treated oxidised glutathione. *Biochimica et Biophysica Acta*, **285**, 346–351.

Atassi, M.Z. (1968). Immunochemistry of sperm whale myoglobin. 3. Modification of the three tyrosine residues and their role in the conformation and differentiation of their roles in the antigenic reactivity. *Biochemistry*, **7**, 3078–3085.

Atherton, N.M. (1993). *Principles of Electron Spin Resonance*. Prentice-Hall, New York.

Atkins, H.L., Bennett-Corniea, W., and Garrison, W.M. (1967). The radiation-induced oxidation of peptides in aqueous solutions. *Journal of Physical Chemistry*, **71**, 772–774.

Ator, M.A., and Ortiz de Montellano, P.R. (1987). Protein control of prosthetic heme reactivity. Reaction of substrates with the heme edge of horseradish peroxidase. *Journal of Biological Chemistry*, **262**, 1542–1551.

Ator, M.A., David, S.K., and Ortiz de Montellano, P.R. (1987). Structure and catalytic mechanism of horseradish peroxidase. Regiospecific meso alkylation of the prosthetic heme group by alkylhydrazines. *Journal of Biological Chemistry*, **262**, 14954–14960.

Aubailly, M., Salmon, S., Haigle, J., Bazin, J.C., Maziere, J.C., and Santus, R. (1994). Peroxidation of model lipoprotein solutions sensitized by photoreduction of ferritin by 365 nm radiation. *Journal of Photochemistry and Photobiology*, **26**, 185–191.

Augenstine, L.G. (1962). The effects of ionising radiation on enzymes. *Advances in Enzymology*, **XXIV**, 359–413.

Aune, T.M., and Thomas, E.L. (1977). Accumulation of hypothiocyanite ion during peroxidase-catalyzed oxidation of thiocyanate ion. *European Journal of Biochemistry*, **80**, 209–214.

Aune, T.M., and Thomas, E.L. (1978). Oxidation of protein sulfhydryls by products of peroxidase-catalyzed oxidation of thiocyanate ion. *Biochemistry*, **17**, 1005–1010.

Aune, T.M., Thomas, E.L., and Morrison, M. (1977). Lactoperoxidase-catalyzed incorporation of thiocyanate ion into a protein substrate. *Biochemistry*, **16**, 4611–4615.

Aupeix, K., Toti, F., Satta, N., Bischoff, P., and Freyssinet, J.M. (1996). Oxysterols induce membrane procoagulant activity in monocytic THP-1 cells. *Biochemical Journal*, **314**, 1027–1033.

Aust, S.D. (1995). Ferritin as a source of iron and protection from iron-induced toxicities. *Toxicology Letters*, **83**, 941–944.

Avdulov, N.A., Chochina, S.V., Daragan, V.A., Schroeder, F., Mayo, K.H., and Wood, W.G. (1996). Direct binding of ethanol to bovine serum albumin: a fluorescent and 13C NMR multiplet relaxation study. *Biochemistry*, **35**, 340–347.

Avezoux, A., Goodwin, M.G., and Anthony, C. (1995). The role of the novel disulphide ring in the active site of the quinoprotein methanol dehydrogenase from *Methylobacterium extorquens*. *Biochemical Journal*, **307**, 735–741.

Ayala, A., and Cutler, R.G. (1996*a*). Comparison of 5-hydroxy-2-amino valeric acid with carbonyl group content as a marker of oxidized protein in human and mouse liver tissues. *Free Radical Biology and Medicine*, **21**, 551–558.

Ayala, A., and Cutler, R.G. (1996*b*). The utilization of 5-hydroxyl-2-amino valeric acid as a specific marker of oxidized arginine and proline residues in proteins. *Free Radical Biology and Medicine*, **21**, 65–80.

Ayene, I.S., Dodia, C., and Fisher, A.B. (1992). Role of oxygen in oxidation of lipid and protein during ischemia/reperfusion in isolated perfused rat lung. *Archives of Biochemistry and Biophysics*, **296**, 183–189.

Ayene, I.S., al Mehdi, M.A., and Fisher, A.B. (1993). Inhibition of lung tissue oxidation during ischemia/reperfusion by 2-mercaptopropionylglycine. *Archives of Biochemistry and Biophysics*, **303**, 307–312.

Azzi, A., Boscoboinik, D., Marilley, D., Ozer, N.K., Stauble, B., and Tasinato, A. (1995). Vitamin E: a sensor and an information transducer of the cell oxidation state. *American Journal of Clinical Nutrition*, **62 (Suppl. 6)**, 1337S–1346S.

Babiy, A.V., Gebicki, J.M., and Sullivan, D.R. (1990). Vitamin E content and low density lipoprotein oxidizability induced by free radicals. *Atherosclerosis*, **81**, 175–182.

Babiy, A.V., Gebicki, J.M., Sullivan, D.R., and Willey, K. (1992). Increased oxidizability of plasma lipoproteins in diabetic patients can be decreased by probucol therapy and is not due to glycation. *Biochemical Pharmacology*, **43**, 995–1000.

Babu, K.S., Yeo, T.C., Martin, W.L., Duron, M.R., Rogers, R.D., and Goldstein, A.H. (1995). Cloning of a mineral phosphate-solubilizing gene from *Pseudomonas cepacia*. *Applied Environmental Microbiology*, **61**, 972–978.

Bagasra, O., Michaels, F.H., Zheng, Y.M., Bobroski, L.E., Spitsin, S.V., Fu, Z.F., *et al.* (1995). Activation of the inducible form of nitric oxide synthase in the brains of patients with multiple sclerosis. *Proceedings of the National Academy of Science of the United States of America*, **92**, 12041–12045.

Bagguley, D.M.S., and Griffiths, J.H.E. (1947). Paramagnetic resonance and magnetic energy levels in chrome alum. *Nature (London)*, **160**, 532–533.

Baker, J.E., Kalyanaraman, B. (1989). Ischemia-induced changes in myocardial paramagnetic metabolites: implications for intracellular oxy-radical generation. *FEBS Letters*, **244**, 311–314.

Baker, J.E., Felix, C.C., Olinger, G.N., Kalyanaraman, B. (1988). Myocardial ischemia and reperfusion: direct evidence for free radical generation by electron spin resonance spectroscopy. *Proceedings of the National Academy of Science of the United States of America*, **85**, 2786–2789.

Baker, M.Z., Badiello, R., Tamba, M., Quintiliani, M., and Gorin, G. (1982). Pulse radiolytic study of hydrogen transfer from glutathione to organic radicals. *International Journal of Radiation Biology and Related Studies on Physical Chemistry and Medicine*, **41**, 595–602.

Baker, R.W.R. (1947). Studies on the reaction between sodium hypochlorite and proteins. 1. Physico-chemical study of the course of the reaction. *Biochemical Journal*, **41**, 337–342.

Balakrishnan, I., and Reddy, M.P. (1970). Mechanism of reaction of hydroxyl radicals with benzene in the γ radiolysis of the aerated aqueous benzene system. *Journal of Physical Chemistry*, **74**, 850–855.

Balasubramanian, D., Du, X., and Zigler, J.J. (1990). The reaction of singlet oxygen with proteins, with special reference to crystallins. *Photochemistry and Photobiology*, **52**, 761–768.

Balasubramanian, P.N., Lindsay Smith, J.R., Davies, M.J., Kaaret, T.W., and Bruice, T.C. (1989). Dynamics of reaction of (*meso*-tetrakis(2.6-dimethyl-3-sulfonatophenyl)porphinato)-iron(III) hydrate with *tert*-butyl hydroperoxide in aqueous solution. 2. Establishment of a mechanism that involves homolytic O–O bond breaking and one-electron oxication of the iron(III) porphyrin. *Journal of the American Chemical Society*, **111**, 1477–1483.

Ballard, F.J., and Hopgood, M.F. (1976). Inactivation of phosphoenolpyruvate carboxykinase (GTP) by liver extracts. *Biochemical Journal*, **154**, 717–724.

Bamezai, S., Banez, M.A., and Breslow, E. (1990). Structural and functional changes associated with modification of the ubiquitin methionine. *Biochemistry*, **29**, 5389–5396.

Banerjee, S.K., and Mudd, J.B. (1992). Reaction of ozone with glycophorin in solution and in lipid vesicles. *Archives of Biochemistry and Biophysics*, **295**, 84–89.

Banfi, P., Parolini, O., Lanzi, C., and Gambetta, R.A. (1992). Lipid peroxidation, phosphoinositide turnover and protein kinase C activation in human platelets treated with anthracyclines and their complexes with Fe(III). *Biochemical Pharmacology*, **43**, 1521–1527.

Bansal, K.M., and Sellers, R.M. (1975). Polarographic and optical pulse radiolysis study of the radicals formed by OH attack on imidazole and related compounds in aqueous solutions. *Journal of Physical Chemistry*, **79**, 1775–1780.

Barae, G., and Roseman, R. (1946). Plasma proteins as antioxidant of bilirubin, and a hypothesis on the structure of the plasma albumin-bilirubin complex. *Journal of the Washington Academy of Science*, **36**, 296–301.

Barchowsky, A., Munro, S.R., Morana, S.J., Vincenti, M.P., and Treadwell, M. (1995). Oxidant-sensitive and phosphorylation-dependent activation of NF-kappa B and AP-1 in endothelial cells. *American Journal of Physiology*, **269**, L829–L836.

Barger, S.W., and Mattson, M.P. (1996). Participation of gene expression in the protection against amyloid beta-peptide toxicity by the beta-amyloid precursor protein. *Annals of the New York Academy of Science*, **777**, 303–309.

Barja, G., Lopez, T.M., Perez, C.R., Rojas, C., Cadenas, S., Prat, J., et al. (1994). Dietary vitamin C decreases endogenous protein oxidative damage, malondialdehyde, and lipid peroxidation and maintains fatty acid unsaturation in the guinea pig liver. *Free Radical Biology and Medicine*, **17**, 105–115.

Barr, D.P., Gunther, M.R., Deterding, L.J., Tomer, K.B., Mason, R.P. (1996). ESR spin-trapping of a protein-derived tyrosyl radical from the reaction of cytochrome *c* with hydrogen peroxide. *Journal of Biological Chemistry*, **271**, 15498–15503.

Barron, E.S.G., and Talmage, P. (1952). Studies on the mechanism of action of ionizing radiations. VIII. Effect of hydrogen peroxide on cell metabolism, enzymes, and proteins. *Archives of Biochemistry and Biophysics*, **41**, 188–202.

Barron, E.S.G., Ambrose, J., and Johnson, P. (1955). Studies on the mechanism of action of ionizing radiations. XIII. The effect of X-irradiation on some physicochemical properties of amino acids and proteins. *Radiation Research*, **2**, 145–158.

Bartlett, P.D., and Guaraldi, G. (1967). Di-*t*-butyl trioxide and di-*t*-butyl tetroxide. *Journal of the American Chemical Society*, **1967**, 4799–4801.

Bartnicki, E.W., Belser, N.O., and Castro, C.E. (1978). Oxidation of heme proteins by alkyl halides: a probe for axial inner sphere redox capacity in solution and in whole cells. *Biochemistry*, **17**, 5582–5586.

Barton, D.H.R., Doller, D. (1992). The selective functionalization of saturated hydrocarbons: Gif chemistry. *Accounts of Chemical Research*, **25**, 504–512.

Barton, J.P., and Packer, J.E. (1970). The radiolysis of oxygenated cysteine solutions at neutral pH. The role of $RSSR^-$ and O_2^-. *International Journal of Radiation and Physical Chemistry*, **2**, 159–166.

Bartosz, G., Gaczynska, M., Retelewska, W., Grzelinska, E., and Rosin, J. (1990). Hyperthermia, unlike ionizing radiation and chemical oxidative stress, does not stimulate proteolysis in erythrocytes. *International Journal of Biochemistry*, **22**, 25–30.

Bartosz, G., Kedziora, J., and Retelewska, W. (1991). Decreased oxidant-induced proteolysis in erythrocytes with enhanced antioxidative defence enzymes due to Down's syndrome. *Clinica Chimica Acta*, **198**, 239–243.

Basiuk, V.A., Gromovoy, T.Y., Chuiko, A.A., Soloschonik, V.A., and Kukhar, V.P. (1992). A novel approach to the synthesis of symmetric optically active 2,5-Dioxopiperazines. *Synthesis*, 449–451.

Basu, A., Williams, K.R., and Modak, M.J. (1987). Ferrate oxidation of *Escherichia coli* DNA polymerase-I. Identification of a methionine residue that is essential for DNA binding. *Journal of Biological Chemistry*, **262**, 9601–9607.

Bateman, R.C., Youngblood, W.W., Busby, W.H., and Kizer, J.S. (1985). Nonenzymic peptide amidation. Implication for a novel enzyme mechanism. *Journal of Biological Chemistry*, **260**, 9088–9091.

Bates, E.J., Harper, G.S., Lowther, D.A., and Preston, B.N. (1984). Effect of oxygen-derived reactive species on cartilage proteoglycan-hyaluronate aggregates. *Biochemistry International*, **8**, 629–637.

Battistuzzi, G., Borsari, M., Dallari, D., Ferretti, S., and Sola, M. (1995). Cyclic voltammetry and 1H-NMR of *Rhodopseudomonas palustris* cytochrome *c*2. Probing surface charges through anion-binding studies. *European Journal of Biochemistry*, **233**, 335–339.

Bauminger, E.R., Harrison, P.M., Hechel, D., Hodson, N.W., Nowik, I., Treffry, A., *et al.* (1993). Iron (II) oxidation and early intermediates of iron-core formation in recombinant human H-chain ferritin. *Biochemical Journal*, **296**, 709–719.

Baverstock, K., Cundall, R.B., Adams, G.E., and Redpath, J.L. (1974). Selective free radical reactions with proteins and enzymes: the inactivation of alpha-chymotrypsin. *International Journal of Radiation Biology and Related Studies on Physical Chemistry and Medicine*, **26**, 39–46.

Baynes, J.W. (1991). Role of oxidative stress in development of complications in diabetes. *Diabetes*, **40**, 405–412.

Baynes, J.W. (1996a). Reactive oxygen in the aetiology and complications of diabetes. In *Drugs, Diet and Disease, Vol.2 Mechanistic Approaches to Diabetes.*, (ed. C. Ioannides), pp. 201–240. Pergamon, London.

Baynes, J.W. (1996b). The role of oxidation in the Maillard reaction in vivo. In *The Maillard Reaction: Consequences for the Chemical and Life Scienceences*, (ed. R. Ikan), pp. 55–72. Wiley, New York.

Beal, M.F., Ferrante, R.J., Henshaw, R., Matthews, R.T., Chan, P.H., Kowall, N.W., *et al.* (1995). 3-Nitropropionic acid neurotoxicity is attenuated in copper/zinc superoxide dismutase transgenic mice. *Journal of Neurochemistry*, **65**, 919–922.

Bechtold, M.M., Gee, D.L., Bruenner, U., and Tappel, A.L. (1982). Carbon tetrachloride-mediated expiration of pentane and chloroform by the intact rat: the effects of pretreatment with diethyl maleate, SKF-525A and phenobarbital. *Toxicology Letters*, **11**, 165–171.

Becker, D., Swarts, S., Champagne, M., and Sevilla, M.D. (1988). An ESR investigation of the reactions of glutathione, cysteine and penicillamine thiyl radicals: competitive formation of RSO·, R·, RSSR⁻., and RSS· *International Journal of Radiation Biology*, **53**, 767–786.

Becker, M.M., and Wang, J.C. (1984). Use of light for footprinting DNA *in vivo*. *Nature*, **309**, 682–687.

Beckman, J.S., Ye, Y.Z., Anderson, P.G., Chen, J., Accavitti, M.A., Tarpey, M.M., *et al.* (1994). Extensive nitration of protein tyrosines in human atherosclerosis detected by immunohistochemistry. *Biological Chemistry, Hoppe-Seyler*, **375**, 81–88.

Bedwell, S., Dean, R.T., and Jessup, W. (1989). The action of defined oxygen-centred free radicals on human low-density lipoprotein. *Biochemical Journal*, **262**, 707–712.

Behl, C., Davis, J.B., Lesley, R., and Schubert, D. (1994). Hydrogen peroxide mediates amyloid beta protein toxicity. *Cell*, **77**, 817–827.

Behl, C., Widmann, M., Trapp, T., and Holsboer, F. (1995). 17-Beta estradiol protects neurons from oxidative stress-induced cell death in vitro. *Biochemical and Biophysical Research Communications*, **216**, 473–482.

Behravan, G., Sen, S., Rova, U., Thelander, L., Eckstein, F., and Graslund, A. (1995). Formation of a free radical of the sulfenylimine type in the mouse ribonucleotide reductase reaction with 2'-azido-2'-deoxycytidine 5'-diphosphate. *Biochimica et Biophysica Acta*, **1264**, 323–329.

Behrens, G., and Koltzenburg, G. (1985). Elimination of ammonium ion from the α-hydroxyalkyl radicals of serine and threonine in aqueous solution and the difference in the reaction mechanism. *Zeitschrift fur Naturforschung: C Biosciences*, **40C**, 785–797.

Bell, S.H., Dickson, D.P., Rieder, R., Cammack, R., Patil, D.S., Hall, D.O., *et al.* (1984). Spectroscopic studies of the nature of the iron clusters in the soluble hydrogenase from *Desulfovibrio desulfuricans* (strain Norway 4). *European Journal of Biochemistry*, **145**, 645–651.

Bellary, S.S., Anderson, K.W., Arden, W.A., and Butterfield, D.A. (1994). Effect of lipopolysaccharide on the physical conformation of the erythrocyte cytoskeletal proteins. *Life Science*, **56**, 91–98.

Ben, H.E., Dubbelman, T.M., and Van, S.J. (1991). The effect of fluoride on binding and photodynamic action of phthalocyanines with proteins. *Photochemistry and Photobiology*, **54**, 703–707.

Ben, H.E., Dubbelman, T.M., and Van, S.J. (1992a). Effect of fluoride on inhibition of plasma membrane functions in Chinese hamster ovary cells photosensitized by aluminum phthalocyanine. *Radiation Research*, **131**, 47–52.

Ben, H.E., Hoeben, R.C., Van, O.H., Dubbelman, T.M., and Van, S.J. (1992b). Photodynamic inactivation of retroviruses by phthalocyanines: the effects of sulphonation, metal ligand and fluoride. *Photochemistry and Photobiology B*, **13**, 145–152.

Ben, S.D., Zuk, R., and Glinka, Y. (1995). Dopamine neurotoxicity: inhibition of mitochondrial respiration. *Journal of Neurochemistry*, **64**, 718–723.

Benavente, M.G., and Truscott, R.J. (1991). Modification of proteins by 3-hydroxyanthranilic acid: the role of lysine residues. *Archives of Biochemistry and Biophysics*, **290**, 451–457.

Bender, C.J., Sahlin, M., Babcock, G.T., Barry, B.A., Chandrashekar, T.K., Salowe, S.P., *et al.* (1989). An ENDOR study of the tyrosyl free radical in ribonucleotide reductase from *Escherichia coli*. *Journal of the American Chemical Society*, **111**, 8076–8083.

Bennett, J.E. (1990). Kinetic electron paramagnetic resonance study of the reactions of *t*-butylperoxyl radicals in aqueous solution. *Journal of the Chemical Society, Faraday Transactions*, **86**, 3247–3252.

Bennett, J.E., Brown, D.M., Mile, B. (1970). Studies by electron spin resonance of the reactions of alkylperoxy radicals. Part 2. Equilibrium between alkyl-peroxy radicals and tetroxide molecules. *Transactions of the Faraday Society*, **66**, 397–405.

Benning, M.M., Meyer, T.E., Rayment, I., and Holden, H.M. (1994). Molecular structure of the oxidized high-potential iron-sulfur protein isolated from *Ectothiorhodospira vacuolata*. *Biochemistry*, **33**, 2476–2483.

Bensasson, R.V., Land, E.J., and Truscott, T.G. (1983). *Pulse Radiolysis and Flash Photolysis: Contributions to the Chemistry of Biology and Medicine*. Pergamon Press, Oxford.

Bensasson, R.V., Land, E.J., and Truscott, T.G. (1993). *Excited States and Free Radicals in Biology and Medicine*. Oxford University Press, Oxford.

Bent, D.V., and Hayon, E. (1975). Excited state chemistry of aromatic amino acids and related peptides. II. Phenylalanine. *Journal of Physical Chemistry*, **97**, 2606–2612.

Benzi, G., and Moretti, A. (1995). Are reactive oxygen species involved in Alzheimer's disease? *Neurobiological Aging*, **16**, 661–674.

Berberich, I., Shu, G.L., and Clark, E.A. (1994). Cross-linking CD40 on B cells rapidly activates nuclear factor-kappa B. *Journal of Immunology*, **153**, 4357–4366.

Berdnikov, V.M., Bazhin, N.M., Federov, V.K., and Polyakov, O.V. (1972). Isomerization of the ethoxyl radical to the α-hydroxyethyl radical in aqueous solution. *Kinetica Katalika (English Translation)*, **13**, 986–987.

Berghuis, A.M., and Brayer, G.D. (1992). Oxidation state-dependent conformational changes in cytochrome *c*. *Journal of Molecular Biology*, **223**, 959–976.

Berlett, B.S., Chock, P.B., Yim, M.B., and Stadtman, E.R. (1990). Manganese(II) catalyzes the bicarbonate-dependent oxidation of amino acids by hydrogen peroxide and the amino acid-facilitated dismutation of hydrogen peroxide. *Proceedings of the National Academy of Science of the United States of America*, **87**, 389–393.

Berlett, B.S., Levine, R.L., and Stadtman, E.R. (1996). Comparison of the effects of ozone on the modification of amino acid residues in glutamine synthetase and bovine serum albumin. *Journal of Biological Chemistry*, **271**, 4177–4182.

Bernatek, E., Ledaal, T., and Åsen, S. (1964). Ozonolysis of acetylene-dicarboxylic acid. *Acta Chimica Scandinavia*, **18**, 1317–1318.

Bernier, M., Hearse, D.J., and Manning, A.S. (1986). Reperfusion-induced arrhythmias and oxygen-derived free radicals. Studies with 'anti-free radical' interventions and a free radical-generating system in the isolated perfused rat heart. *Circulation Research*, **58**, 331–340.

Bernier, M., Manning, A.S., and Hearse, D.J. (1989). Reperfusion arrhythmias: dose-related protection by anti-free radical interventions. *American Journal of Physiology*, **256**, H1344–H1352.

Bernier, M., Kusama, Y., Borgers, M., Ver, D.L., Valdes, A.O., Neckers, D.C., *et al.* (1991). Pharmacological studies of arrhythmias induced by rose bengal photoactivation. *Free Radical Biology and Medicine*, **10**, 287–296.

Bernofsky, C. (1991). Nucleotide chloramines and neutrophil-mediated cytotoxicity. *FASEB Journal*, **5**, 295–300.

Berthomieu, C., and Boussac, A. (1995). Histidine oxidation in the S2 to S3 transition probed by FTIR difference spectroscopy in the Ca^{2+}-depleted photosystem II: comparison with histidine radicals generated by UV irradiation. *Biochemistry*, **34**, 1541–1548.

Bertini, I., Capozzi, F., Luchinat, C., and Piccioli, M. (1993). ^{1}H-NMR investigation of oxidized and reduced high-potential iron-sulfur protein from *Rhodopseudomonas globiformis*. *European Journal of Biochemistry*, **212**, 69–78.

Bertini, I., Dikiy, A., Kastrau, D.H., Luchinat, C., and Sompornpisut, P. (1995). Three-dimensional solution structure of the oxidized high potential iron-sulfur protein from *Chromatium vinosum* through NMR. Comparative analysis with the solution structure of the reduced species. *Biochemistry*, **34**, 9851–9858.

Bevilotti, V. (1945). Biological action of radioactive substances. III. Influence of uranium acetate on the activity of the proteolytic ferment of the pancreas. *Bolletino Societa Italiana Biologia Sperimentale*, **20**, 128–129.

Bezrukova, A.G., and Ostashevsky, I. (1977). Gamma-irradiated chymotrypsin-like proteins. I. Structural changes. *International Journal of Radiation Biology and Related Studies on Physical Chemistry and Medicine*, **31**, 131–144.

Bhatnagar, A. (1994). Biochemical mechanism of irreversible cell injury caused by free radical-initiated reactions. *Molecular and Cellular Biochemistry*, **137**, 9–16.

Bhattacharyya, A., Tollin, G., McIntire, W., and Singer, T.P. (1985). Laser-flash-photolysis studies of *p*-cresol methylhydroxylase. Electron-transfer properties of the flavin and haem components. *Biochemical Journal*, **228**, 337–345.

Bhuyan, K.C., Bhuyan, D.K., and Podos, S.M. (1991). Free radical enhancer xenobiotic is an inducer of cataract in rabbit. *Free Radical Research Communications*, **2**, 609–620.

Biaglow, J.E., Varnes, M.E., Epp, E.R., Clark, E.P., Tuttle, S.W., and Held, K.D. (1989). Role of glutathione in the aerobic radiation response. *International Journal of Radiation Oncology and Biological Physiology*, **16**, 1311–1314.

Bicout, D.J., Field, M.J., Gouet, P., and Jouve, H.M. (1995). Simulations of electron transfer in the NADPH-bound catalase from *Proteus mirabilis PR*. *Biochimica et Biophysica Acta*, **1252**, 172–176.

Bidlack, W.R., and Tappel, A.L. (1972). A proposed mechanism for the TPNH enzymatic lipid peroxidizing system of rat liver microsomes. *Lipids*, **7**, 564–565.

Bidlack, W.R., and Tappel, A.L. (1973). Damage to microsomal membrane by lipid peroxidation. *Lipids*, **8**, 177–182.

Bielski, B.H.J., and Richter, H.W. (1977). A study of the superoxide radical chemistry by stopped-flow radiolysis and radiation induced oxygen consumption. *Journal of the American Chemical Society*, **99**, 3019–3023.

Bielski, B.H.J., Cabelli, D.E., Arudi, R.L., and Ross, A.B. (1985). Reactivity of HO_2/O_2^- Radicals in aqueous solution. *Journal of Physical Chemistry Reference Data*, **14**, 1041–1100.

Bietz, J.A., and Sandford, P.A. (1971). Reaction of sodium hypochlorite with amines and amides: automation of the method. *Analytical Biochemistry*, **44**, 122–133.

Bisby, R.H., Cundall, R.B., Movassaghi, S., Adams, G.E., Posener, M.L., and Wardman, P. (1982). Selective free radical reactions with proteins and enzymes: a reversible equilibrium in the reaction of (SCN)2 radical with lysozyme. *International Journal of Radiation Biology and Related Studies on Physical Chemistry and Medicine*, **42**, 163–171.

Bisby, R.H., Ahmed, S., and Cundall, R.B. (1984). Repair of amino acid radicals by a vitamin E analogue. *Biochemical and Biophysical Research Communications*, **119**, 245–251.

Bjork, I., and Nordling, K. (1979). Evidence by chemical modification for the involvement of one or more tryptophanyl residues of bovine antithrombin in the binding of high-affinity heparin. *European Journal of Biochemistry*, **102**, 497–502.

Bjorkerud, B., and Bjorkerud, S. (1996). Contrary effects of lightly and strongly oxidized LDL with potent promotion of growth versus apoptosis on arterial smooth muscle cells, macrophages, and fibroblasts. *Arteriosclerosis Thrombosis and Vascular Biology*, **16**, 416–424.

Bjornstedt, M., Hamberg, M., Kumar, S., Sue, J., and Homgren, A. (1995). Human thioredoxin reductase directly reduces lipid hydroperoxides by NADPH and selenocystine strongly stimulates the reaction via catalytically generated selenols. *Journal of Biological Chemistry*, **270**, 11761–11764.

Blackburn, N.J., Hasnain, S.S., Pettingill, T.M., and Strange, R.W. (1991). Copper K-extended X-ray absorption fine structure studies of oxidized and reduced dopamine beta-hydroxylase. Confirmation of a sulfur ligand to copper(I) in the reduced enzyme. *Journal of Biological Chemistry*, **266**, 23120–23127.

Blake, C.C., Ghosh, M., Harlos, K., Avezoux, A., and Anthony, C. (1994). The active site of methanol dehydrogenase contains a disulphide bridge between adjacent cysteine residues. *Nature (Structural Biology)*, **1**, 102–105.

Blake, D.R., Winyard, P.G., and Marok, R. (1994). The contribution of hypoxia-reperfusion injury to inflammatory synovitis: the influence of reactive oxygen intermediates on the transcriptional control of inflammation. *Annals of the New York Academy of Science*, **723**, 308–317.

Blake, P.R., Park, J.B., Bryant, F.O., Aono, S., Magnuson, J.K., Eccleston, E., *et al.* (1991). Determinants of protein hyperthermostability: purification and amino acid sequence of rubredoxin from the hyperthermophilic archaebacterium *Pyrococcus furiosus* and secondary structure of the zinc adduct by NMR. *Biochemistry*, **30**, 10885–10895.

Blakeman, D.P., Ryan, T.P., Jolly, R.A., and Petry, T.W. (1995). Diquat-dependent protein carbonyl formation. Identification of lipid-dependent and lipid-independent pathways. *Biochemical Pharmacology*, **50**, 929–935.

Blanchard, L., Marion, D., Pollock, B., Voordouw, G., Wall, J., Bruschi, M., *et al.* (1993). Overexpression of *Desulfovibrio vulgaris Hildenborough* cytochrome *c*553 in *Desulfovibrio desulfuricans* G200. Evidence of conformational heterogeneity in the oxidized protein by NMR. *European Journal of Biochemistry*, **218**, 293–301.

Blasig, I.E., Ebert, B., and Lowe, H. (1986). Identification of free radicals trapped during myocardial ischemia *in vitro* by ESR. *Studia Biophysica*, **116**, 35–42.

Blumberg, W.E., Peisach, J., Eisenberger, P., and Fee, J.A. (1978). Superoxide dismutase, a study of the electronic properties of the copper and zinc by X-ray absorption spectroscopy. *Biochemistry*, **17**, 1842–1846.

Bobrowski, K., and Holcman, J. (1987). Formation of three-electron bonds in one-electron oxidized methionine dipeptides: a pulse radiolytic study. *International Journal of Radiation Biology and Related Studies on Physical Chemistry and Medicine*, **52**, 139–144.

Bobrowski, K., Wierzchowski, K.L., Holcman, J., and Ciurak, M. (1990). Intramolecular electron transfer in peptides containing methionine, tryptophan and tyrosine: a pulse radiolysis study. *International Journal of Radiation Biology and Related Studies on Physical Chemistry and Medicine*, **57**, 919–932.

Bobrowski, K., Schöneich, C., Holcman, J., and Asmus, K.-D. (1991). OH radical induced decarboxylation of methionine-containing peptides. Influence of peptide sequence and net charge. *Journal of the Chemical Society Perkin Transactions*, **2**, 353–362.

Bogaert, Y.E., Rosenthal, R.E., and Fiskum, G. (1994). Postischemic inhibition of cerebral cortex pyruvate dehydrogenase. *Free Radical Biology and Medicine*, **16**, 811–820.

Boger, D.L., Colletti, S.L., Teramoto, S., Ramsey, T.M., and Zhou, J. (1995). Synthesis of key analogs of bleomycin A2 that permit a systematic evaluation of the linker region: identification of an exceptionally prominent role for the L-threonine substituent. *Bioorganic Medicine and Chemistry*, **3**, 1281–1295.

Boguta, G., and Dancewicz, A.M. (1981). Radiation-induced dimerization of tyrosine and glycyltyrosine in aqueous solutions. *International Journal of Radiation Biology and Related Studies on Physical Chemistry and Medicine*, **39**, 163–174.

Boguta, G., and Dancewicz, A.M. (1982). Radiolytic dimerization of tyrosine in alkaline solutions of poly-L-tyrosine, glycyl-L-tyrosine and tyrosine. *Radiation and Physical Chemistry*, **20**, 359–363.

Boguta, G., and Dancewicz, A.M. (1983). Radiolytic and enzymatic dimerization of tyrosyl residues in insulin, ribonuclease, papain and collagen. *International Journal of Radiation Biology and Related Studies on Physical Chemistry and Medicine*, **43**, 249–265.

Boiteux, S., Gajewski, E., Laval, J., and Dizdaroglu, M. (1992). Substrate specificity of the *Escherichia coli* Fpg protein (formamidopyrimidine-DNA glycosylase): excision of purine lesions in DNA produced by ionizing radiation or photosensitization. *Biochemistry*, **31**, 106–110.

Boldyrev, A.A., Bulygina, E.R., Volynskaia, E.A., Kurella, E.G., and Tiulina, O.V. (1995). The effect of hydrogen peroxide and hypochlorite on brain Na,K-ATPase activity. *Biokhimica*, **60**, 1688–1696.

Bolewska, K., Krowarsch, D., Otlewski, J., Jaroszewski, L., and Bierzynski, A. (1995). Synthesis, cloning and expression in *Escherichia coli* of a gene coding for the Met8⟶Leu CMTI I—a representative of the squash inhibitors of serine proteinases. *FEBS Letters*, **377**, 172–174.

Blake, P.R., Park, J.B., Bryant, F.O., Aono, S., Magnuson, J.K., Eccleston, E., *et al.* (1991). Determinants of protein hyperthermostability: purification and amino acid sequence of rubredoxin from the hyperthermophilic archaebacterium Pyrococcus furiosus and secondary structure of the zinc adduct by NMR. *Biochemistry*, **30**, 10885–10895.

Bolli, R., Patel, B.S., Jeroudi, M.O., Lai, E.K., and McCay, P.B. (1988). Demonstration of free radical generation in 'stunned' myocardium of intact dogs with the use of the spin trap α-phenyl *N-tert*-butyl nitrone. *Journal of Clinical Investigation*, **82**, 476–485.

Bolton, E.J., Jessup, W., Stanley, K.K., and Dean, R.T. (1994). Enhanced LDL oxidation by murine macrophage foam cells and their failure to secrete nitric oxide. *Atherosclerosis*, **106**, 213–223.

Bolton, E.J., Jessup, W., Stanley, K.K., and Dean, R.T. (1997). Loading with oxidised low density lipoprotein alters endocytic and secretory activities of murine macrophages. *Biochimica et Biophysica Acta*, **1356**, 12–22.

Bolwell, G.P., Butt, V.S., Davies, D.R., and Zimmerlin, A. (1995). The origin of the oxidative burst in plants. *Free Radical Research*, **23**, 517–532.

Bongarzone, E.R., Soto, E.F., and Pasquini, J.M. (1995a). Increased susceptibility to degradation by trypsin and subtilisin of *in vitro* peroxidized myelin proteins. *Neurochemistry Research*, **20**, 421–426.

Bongarzone, E.R., Pasquini, J.M., and Soto, E.F. (1995b). Oxidative damage to proteins and lipids of CNS myelin produced by *in vitro* generated reactive oxygen species. *Journal of Neuroscience Research*, **41**, 213–221.

Bonifacic, M., Mockel, H., Bahneman, D., and Amus, K.-D. (1975). Formation of positive ions and other promary species in the oxidation of sulphides by hydroxyl radicals. *Journal of the Chemical Society, Perkin Transactions*, **2**, 675–685.

Bonnes, T.D., Guerin, M.C., Torreilles, J., Ceballos, P.I., and de Paulet, A.C. (1993). 4-Hydroxynonenal content lower in brains of 25 month old transgenic mice carrying the human CuZn superoxide dismutase gene than in brains of their non-transgenic littermates. *Journal of Lipid Mediators*, **8**, 111–120.

Bonomo, R.P., Marchelli, R., and Tabbi, G. (1995). Study of H_2O_2 interaction with copper(II) complexes with diamino-diamide type ligands, diastereoisomeric dipeptides, and tripeptides. *Journal of Inorganic Biochemistry*, **60**, 205–218.

Blake, P.R., Park, J.B., Bryant, F.O., Aono, S., Magnuson, J.K., Eccleston, E., *et al.* (1991). Determinants of protein hyperthermostability: purification and amino acid sequence of rubredoxin from the hyperthermophilic archaebacterium Pyrococcus furiosus and secondary structure of the zinc adduct by NMR. *Biochemistry*, **30**, 10885–10895.

Booker, S., Licht, S., Broderick, J., and Stubbe, J. (1994). Coenzyme B12-dependent ribonucleotide reductase: evidence for the participation of five cysteine residues in ribonucleotide reduction. *Biochemistry*, **33**, 12676–12685.

Borden, K.L., and Richards, F.M. (1990). Folding of the reduced form of the thioredoxin from bacteriophage T4. *Biochemistry*, **29**, 8207–8210.

Borg, D. (1965). Transient free radical forms of hormones: EPR spectra from iodothyronines, indoles, estrogens and insulin. *Proceedings of the National Academy of Science of the United States of America*, **53**, 829–836.

Borg, D., and Elmore Jr., J. (1967). Evidence for restricted molecular conformation and for hindered rotation of side chain groups from E.P.R. of labile free radicals. In *Magnetic Resonance in Biological Systems*, (ed. A. Ehrenberg and V. Malmstrom), pp. 341–349. Pergamon Press, Oxford.

Borovyagin, V.L., Muronov, A.F., Rumyantseva, V.D., Tarachovsky, Y.S., and Vasilenko, I.A. (1984). Model membrane morphology and crosslinking of oxidized lipids with proteins. *Journal of Ultrastructure Research*, **89**, 261–273.

Bors, W., Tait, D., Michel, C., Saran, M., and Erben-Russ, M. (1984). Reactions of alkoxy radicals in aqueous solution. *Israel Journal of Chemistry*, **24**, 17–24.

Bors, W., Czapski, G., and Saran, M. (1991). An expanded function for superoxide dismutase. *Free Radical Research Communications*, **1**, 411–417.

Boschmann, M., Frenz, U., Noack, R., Aust, L., and Murphy, C.M. (1994). Energy metabolism and metabolite patterns of rats after application of dexfenfluramine. *International Journal of Obesity Related Metabolism Disorders*, **18**, 235–242.

Bothe, E., and Schulte-Frohlinde, D. (1978). The bimolecular decay of the α-hydroxymethylperoxyl radicals in aqueous solution. *Zeitschrift für Naturforschung*, **33b**, 786–788.

Bothe, E., Behrens, G., and Schulte-Frohlinde, D. (1977). Mechanism of the first order decay of 2-hydroxypropyl-2-peroxyl radicals and $O_2 \cdot^-$ formation in aqueous solution. *Zeitschrift für Naturforschung*, **32b**, 886–889.

Bothe, E., Schuchmann, M.N., Schulte-Frohlinde, D., and von Sonntag, C. (1978). $HO_2 \cdot$ elimination from α-hydroxyalkylperoxyl radicals in aqueous solution. *Photochemistry and Photobiology*, **28**, 639–644.

Boudier, C., and Bieth, J.G. (1994). Oxidized mucus proteinase inhibitor: a fairly potent neutrophil elastase inhibitor. *Biochemical Journal*, **303**, 61–68.

Bourguignon, J., Merand, V., Rawsthorne, S., Forest, E., and Douce, R. (1996). Glycine decarboxylase and pyruvate dehydrogenase complexes share the same dihydrolipoamide dehydrogenase in pea leaf mitochondria: evidence from mass spectrometry and primary-structure analysis. *Biochemical Journal*, **313**, 229–234.

Boussac, A., and Rutherford, A.W. (1994). Electron transfer events in chloride-depleted photosystem II. *Journal of Biological Chemistry*, **269**, 12462–12467.

Boutelje, J., Karlstrom, A.R., Hartmanis, M.G., Holmgren, E., Sjogren, A., and Levine, R.L. (1990). Human immunodeficiency viral protease is catalytically active as a fusion protein: characterization of the fusion and native enzymes produced in *Escherichia coli*. *Archives of Biochemistry and Biophysics*, **283**, 141–149.

Bouthier, d.l.T.C., Kaltoum, H., Portemer, C., Confalonieri, F., Huber, R., and Duguet, M. (1995). Cloning and sequencing of the gene coding for topoisomerase I from the extremely thermophilic eubacterium, *Thermotoga maritima*. *Biochimica et Biophysica Acta*, **1264**, 279–283.

Bowling, A.C., and Beal, M.F. (1995). Bioenergetic and oxidative stress in neurodegenerative diseases. *Life Science*, **56**, 1151–1171.

Bowling, A.C., Schulz, J.B., Brown, R.J., and Beal, M.F. (1993). Superoxide dismutase activity, oxidative damage, and mitochondrial energy metabolism in familial and sporadic amyotrophic lateral sclerosis. *Journal of Neurochemistry*, **61**, 2322–2325.

Bowman, N.J., Hay, M.P., and Love, S.G. (1988). Regioselective chlorination of valine derivatives. *Journal of the Chemical Society Perkin Transactions*, **1**, 259–264.

Bowry, V.W., Stanley, K.K., and Stocker, R. (1992a). High density lipoprotein is the major carrier of lipid hydroperoxides in human blood plasma from fasting donors. *Proceedings of the National Academy of Science of the United States of America*, **89**, 10316–10320.

Bowry, V.W., Ingold, K.U., and Stocker, R. (1992b). Vitamin E in human low-density lipoprotein. When and how this antioxidant becomes a pro-oxidant. *Biochemical Journal*, **288**, 341–344.

Bowry, V.W., Mohr, D., Cleary, J., and Stocker, R. (1995). Prevention of tocopherol-mediated peroxidation in ubiquinol-10-free human low density lipoprotein. *Journal of Biological Chemistry*, **270**, 5756–5763.

Box, H., Freund, H., and Lilga, K.T. (1961). Radiation-induced paramagnetism in some simple peptides. In *Free Radicals in Biological Systems*, (ed. M. Blois), pp. 239–248. Academic Press, New York.

Box, H.C., Lilga, K.T., and Potienko, G. (1977). ^{13}C nuclear magnetic resonance studies of radiation damage: radiation-induced degradation of glycine. *Proceedings of the National Academy of Science of the United States of America*, **74**, 2394–2396.

Brabec, V., and Mornstein, V. (1980). Electrochemical behaviour of proteins at graphite electrodes. I. Electrooxidation of proteins as a new probe of protein structure and reactions. *Biochimica et Biophysica Acta*, **625**, 43–50.

Bray, M.R., Carriere, A.D., and Clarke, A.J. (1994). Quantitation of tryptophan and tyrosine residues in proteins by fourth-derivative spectroscopy. *Analytical Biochemistry*, **221**, 278–284.

Breinl, F., and Baudisch, O. (1907). The action of hydrogen peroxide on keratin. *Hoppe-Seyler's Zeitschrift für Physiologische Chemie*, **52**, 158–169.

Brennan, S.O., Shaw, J., Allen, J., and George, P.M. (1992). Beta 141 Leu is not deleted in the unstable haemoglobin Atlanta-Coventry but is replaced by a novel amino acid of mass 129 daltons. *British Journal of Haematology*, **81**, 99–103.

Brennan, S.O., Shaw, J.G., George, P.M., and Huisman, T.H. (1993). Posttranslational modification of beta 141 Leu associated with the beta 75(E19)Leu⟶Pro mutation in Hb Atlanta. *Hemoglobin*, **17**, 1–7.

Bresler, H.S., Burek, C.L., and Rose, N.R. (1990). Autoantigenic determinants on human thyroglobulin. I. Determinant specificities of murine monoclonal antibodies. *Clinical Immunology and Immunopathology*, **54**, 64–75.

Breslow, E., Chauhan, Y., Daniel, R., and Tate, S. (1986). Role of methionine-1 in ubiquitin conformation and activity. *Biochemical and Biophysical Research Communications*, **138**, 437–444.

Breton, J., Berks, B.C., Reilly, A., Thomson, A.J., Ferguson, S.J., and Richardson, D.J. (1994). Characterization of the paramagnetic iron-containing redox centres of *Thiosphaera pantotropha* periplasmic nitrate reductase. *FEBS Letters*, **345**, 76–80.

Brett, J., Schmidt, A.M., Yan, S.D., Zou, Y.S., Weidman, E., Pinsky, D., *et al.* (1993). Survey of the distribution of a newly characterized receptor for advanced glycation end products in tissues. *American Journal of Pathology*, **143**, 1699–1712.

Bridges, R.B., Wyatt, R.J., and Rehm, S.R. (1985). Effect of smoking on peripheral blood leukocytes and serum antiproteases. *European Journal of Respiratory Disorders Supplement*, **139**, 24–33.

Brigelius, R., Muckel, C., Akerboom, T.P., and Sies, H. (1983). Identification and quantitation of glutathione in hepatic protein mixed disulfides and its relationship to glutathione disulfide. *Biochemical Pharmacology*, **32**, 2529–2534.

Brigl, P., Held, R., and Hartung, K. (1928). *Hoppe Seyler's Zeitschrift fur Physiologische Chemie*, **173**, 129.

Brocks, D.R., Dennis, M.J., and Schaefer, W.H. (1995). A liquid chromatographic assay for the stereospecific quantitative analysis of halofantrine in human plasma. *Journal of Pharmacological Biomedicine Annals*, **13**, 911–918.

Brodskaya, G.A., and Sharpatyi, V.A. (1967). Radiolysis of aqueous solutions of phenylalanine. *Russian Journal of Physical Chemistry (English Translation)*, **41**, 583–586.

Brooks, H.B., and Davidson, V.L. (1993). A method for extracting rate constants from initial rates of stopped-flow kinetic data: application to a physiological electron-transfer reaction. *Biochemical Journal*, **294**, 211–213.

Brooks, H.B., and Davidson, V.L. (1994). Kinetic and thermodynamic analysis of a physiologic intermolecular electron-transfer reaction between methylamine dehydrogenase and amicyanin. *Biochemistry*, **33**, 5696–5701.

Brooks, H.B., Jones, L.H., and Davidson, V.L. (1993). Deuterium kinetic isotope effect and stopped-flow kinetic studies of the quinoprotein methylamine dehydrogenase. *Biochemistry*, **32**, 2725–2729.

Brot, N., Weissbach, L., Werth, J., and Weissbach, H. (1981). Enzymatic reduction of protein-bound methionine sulfoxide. *Proceedings of the National Academy of Science of the United States of America*, **78**, 2155–2158.

Brot, N., Rahman, M.A., Moskovitz, J., and Weissbach, H. (1995). *Escherichia coli* peptide methionine sulfoxide reductase: cloning, high expression, and purification. *Methods in Enzymology*, **251**, 462–470.

Brown, D.E., McGuirl, M.A., Dooley, D.M., Janes, S.M., Mu, D., and Klinman, J.P. (1991). The organic functional group in copper-containing amine oxidases. Resonance Raman spectra are consistent with the presence of topa quinone (6-hydroxydopa quinone) in the active site. *Journal of Biological Chemistry*, **266**, 4049–4051.

Brown, D.M., Upcroft, J.A., and Upcroft, P. (1995). Free radical detoxification in Giardia duodenalis. *Molecular and Biochemical Parasitology*, **72**, 47–56.

Brown, K.C., Yang, S.H., and Kodadek, T. (1995). Highly specific oxidative cross-linking of proteins mediated by a nickel-peptide complex. *Biochemistry*, **34**, 4733–4739.

Brown, R.K., and Kelly, F.J. (1994). Evidence for increased oxidative damage in patients with cystic fibrosis. *Pediatric Research*, **36**, 487–493.

Bruce, A.J., and Baudry, M. (1995). Oxygen free radicals in rat limbic structures after kainate-induced seizures. *Free Radical Biology and Medicine*, **18**, 993–1002.

Bruce, A.J., Malfroy, B., and Baudry, M. (1996). Beta-amyloid toxicity in organotypic hippocampal cultures: protection by EUK-8, a synthetic catalytic free radical scavenger. *Proceedings of the National Academy of Science of the United States of America*, **93**, 2312–2316.

Bruenner, B.A., Jones, A.D., and German, J.B. (1995). Direct characterization of protein adducts of the lipid peroxidation product 4-hydroxy-2-nonenal using electrospray mass spectrometry. *Chemical Research Toxicology*, **8**, 552–559.

Brumell, J.H., Burkhardt, A.L., Bolen, J.B., and Grinstein, S. (1996). Endogenous reactive oxygen intermediates activate tyrosine kinases in human neutrophils. *Journal of Biological Chemistry*, **271**, 1455–1461.

Brune, B., and Lapetina, E.G. (1995). Protein thiol modification of glyceraldehyde-3-phosphate dehydrogenase as a target for nitric oxide signaling. *Genetic Engineering (New York)*, **17**, 149–164.

Brune, B., Mohr, S., and Messmer, U.K. (1996). Protein thiol modification and apoptotic cell death as cGMP-independent nitric oxide (NO) signaling pathways. *Review of Physiological and Biochemical Pharmacology*, **127**, 1–30.

Brunk, U.T., Jones, C.B., and Sohal, R.S. (1992). A novel hypothesis of lipofuscinogenesis and cellular aging based on interactions between oxidative stress and autophagocytosis. *Mutation Research*, **275**, 395–403.

Brunner, H., and Brunner, A. (1973). Fractionation of tyrosine-rich proteins from oxidized wool by ion-exchange chromatography and preparative electrophoresis. *European Journal of Biochemistry*, **32**, 350–355.

Brush, E.J., Lipsett, K.A., and Kozarich, J.W. (1988). Inactivation of *Escherichia coli* pyruvate formate-lyase by hypophosphite: evidence for a rate-limiting phosphorus-hydrogen bond cleavage. *Biochemistry*, **27**, 2217–2222.

Buchanan, J.H. (1977). A cystine-rich protein fraction from oxidized alpha-keratin. *Biochemical Journal*, **167**, 489–491.

Buettner, G.R. (1987). The reaction of superoxide, formate radical, and hydrated electron with transferrin and its model compound, Fe(III)-ethylenediamine-N, N'-bis[2-(2-hydroxyphenyl)acetic acid] as studied by pulse radiolysis. *Journal of Biological Chemistry*, **262**, 11995–11998.

Buffinton, G.D., Christen, S., Peterhans, E., and Stocker, R. (1992). Oxidative stress in lungs of mice infected with influenza A virus. *Free Radical Research Communications*, **16**, 99–110.

Buley, A.L., Norman, R.O.C., and Pritchett, R.J. (1966). Electron spin resonance studies of oxidation. Part VIII. Elimination reactions of some hydroxyalkyl radicals. *Journal of the Chemical Society (B)*, 849–852.

Bump, E.A., and Brown, J.M. (1990). Role of glutathione in the radiation response of mammalian cells *in vitro* and *in vivo*. *Pharmacology and Theraputics*, **47**, 117–136.

Burcham, P.C., and Kuhan, Y.T. (1996). Introduction of carbonyl groups into proteins by the lipid peroxidation product, malondialdehyde. *Biochemical and Biophysical Research Communications*, **220**, 996–1001.

Burgess, V.A., and Easton, C.J. (1987). Selective γ-hydrogen atom abstraction in reactions of N-acetylaminoacids and N-alkylacetamides with titanous ion and hydrogen peroxide. *Tetrahedron Letters*, **28**, 2747–2750.

Burgess, V.A., Easton, C.J., and Hay, M.P. (1989). Selective reaction of glycine residues in hydrogen atom transfer from amino acid derivatives. *Journal of the American Chemical Society*, **111**, 1047–1052.

Burk, R.F. (1983). Glutathione-dependent protection by rat liver microsomal protein against lipid peroxidation. *Biochimica et Biophysica Acta*, **757**, 21–28.

Burleson, J.L., Peyton, G.R., and Glaze, W.H. (1978). Chlorinated tyrosine in municipal waste treatment plant products after superchlorination. *Bulletin of Environmental and Contamination Toxicology*, **19**, 724–728.

Burnap, R.L., Qian, M., and Pierce, C. (1996). The manganese stabilizing protein of photosystem II modifies the *in vivo* deactivation and photoactivation kinetics of the H_2O oxidation complex in *Synechocystis* sp. PCC6803. *Biochemistry*, **35**, 874–882.

Burness, A.T., Pardoe, I.U., and Allaway, G.P. (1986). Aggregation of encephalomyocarditis virus induced by radio-iodination. *Journal of Virological Methods*, **14**, 167–176.

Burton, N.P., Williams, T.D., and Norris, P.R. (1995). A potential anti-oxidant protein in a ferrous iron-oxidizing *Sulfolobus* species. *FEMS Microbiology Letters*, **134**, 91–95.

Busch, A.E., Waldegger, S., Herzer, T., Raber, G., Gulbins, E., Takumi, T., *et al.* (1995). Molecular basis of IsK protein regulation by oxidation or chelation. *Journal of Biological Chemistry*, **270**, 3638–3641.

Busciglio, J., and Yankner, B.A. (1995). Apoptosis and increased generation of reactive oxygen species in Down's syndrome neurons *in vitro*. *Nature*, **378**, 776–779.

Busconi, L., and Michel, T. (1995). Recombinant endothelial nitric oxide synthase: post-translational modifications in a baculovirus expression system. *Molecular Pharmacology*, **47**, 655–659.

Busse, M., and Vaupel, P. (1996). Accumulation of purine catabolites in solid tumors exposed to therapeutic hyperthermia. *Experienta*, **52**, 469–473.

Butler, J.A.V., and Robins, A.B. (1960). Effect of oxygen on the inactivation of trypsin by ionizing radiation. *Nature*, **186**, 697–698.

Butler, J., Land, E.J., Prutz, W.A., and Swallow, A.J. (1982). Charge transfer between tryptophan and tyrosine in proteins. *Biochimica et Biophysica Acta*, **705**, 150–162.

Butler, J., Land, E.J., Swallow, A.J., and Prutz, W. (1984). The azide radical and its reaction with tryptophan and tyrosine. *Radiation and Physical Chemistry*, **23**, 265–270.

Butterfield, D.A., and Lee, J. (1994). Active site structure and stability of the thiol protease papain studied by electron paramagnetic resonance employing a methanethiosulfonate spin label. *Archives of Biochemistry and Biophysics*, **310**, 167–171.

Butterfield, D.A., Schneider, A.M., and Rangachari, A. (1991). Electron paramagnetic resonance studies of the effects of tri-n-butyltin on the physical state of proteins and lipids in erythrocyte membranes (letter). *Chemical Research in Toxicology*, **4**, 141–143.

Butterfield, D.A., Hall, N.C., and Cross, S.J. (1993). Effects of beta-(N-methylamino)-L-alanine on cytoskeletal proteins of erythrocyte membranes. *Chemical Research in Toxicology*, **6**, 417–420.

Butterfield, D.A., Trad, C.H., and Hall, N.C. (1994a). Effects of dehydroabietic acid on the physical state of cytoskeletal proteins and the lipid bilayer of erythrocyte membranes. *Biochimica et Biophysica Acta*, **1192**, 185–189.

Butterfield, D.A., Hensley, K., Harris, M., Mattson, M., and Carney, J. (1994b). beta-Amyloid peptide free radical fragments initiate synaptosomal lipoperoxidation in a sequence-specific fashion: implications to Alzheimer's disease. *Biochemical and Biophysical Research Communications*, **200**, 710–715.

Butterfield, D.A., Sun, B., Bellary, S., Arden, W.A., and Anderson, K.W. (1994c). Effect of endotoxin on lipid order and motion in erythrocyte membranes. *Biochimica et Biophysica Acta*, **1225**, 231–234.

Buttery, L.D., Springall, D.R., Chester, A.H., Evans, T.J., Standfield, E.N., Parums, D.V., *et al.* (1996). Inducible nitric oxide synthase is present within human atherosclerotic lesions and promotes the formation and activity of peroxynitrite. *Laboratory Investigations*, **75**, 77–85.

Buxton, G.V., Greeenstock, C.L., Helman, W.P., Ross, A.B. (1988). Critical review of rate constants for reactions of hydrated electrons, hydrogen atoms and hydroxyl radicals ($\cdot OH/\cdot O^-$) in aqueous solution. *Journal of Physical Chemistry Reference Data*, **17**, 513–886.

Cabiscol, E., and Levine, R.L. (1995). Carbonic anhydrase III. Oxidative modification *in vivo* and loss of phosphatase activity during aging. *Journal of Biological Chemistry*, **270**, 14742–14747.

Cabiscol, E., and Levine, R.L. (1996). The phosphatase activity of carbonic anhydrase III is reversibly regulated by glutathiolation. *Proceedings of the National Academy of Science of the United States of America*, **93**, 4170–4174.

Cadenas, S., Rojas, C., Perez, C.R., Lopez, T.M., and Barja, G. (1994). Effect of dietary vitamin C and catalase inhibition of antioxidants and molecular markers of oxidative damage in guinea pigs. *Free Radical Research*, **21**, 109–118.

Cai, D., and Klinman, J.P. (1994). Copper amine oxidase: heterologous expression, purification, and characterization of an active enzyme in *Saccharomyces cerevisiae*. *Biochemistry*, **33**, 7647–7653.

Caira, F., Cherkaoui, M.M., Hoefler, G., and Latruffe, N. (1996). Cloning and tissue expression of two cDNAs encoding the peroxisomal 2-enoyl-CoA hydratase/3-hydroxyacyl-CoA dehydrogenase in the guinea pig liver. *FEBS Letters*, **378**, 57–60.

Calabrese, L., and Carbonaro, M. (1986). An e.p.r. study of the non-equivalence of the copper sites of caeruloplasmin. *Biochemical Journal*, **238**, 291–295.

Caldwell, K.A., and Tappel, A.L. (1965). Acceleration of sulfhydryl oxidations by selenocystine. *Archives of Biochemistry and Biophysics*, **112**, 196–200.

Caldwell, K.A., and Tappel, A.L. (1968a). Decomposition of hydrogen peroxide by disulfo- and diselenodicarboxylic acids. *Archives of Biochemistry and Biophysics*, **127**, 259–262.

Caldwell, K.A., and Tappel, A.L. (1968b). Separation by gas-liquid chromatography of silylated derivatives of some sulfo- and selenoamino acids and their oxidation products. *Journal of Chromatography*, **32**, 635–640.

Calzi, M.L., Raviolo, C., Ghibaudi, E., de Gioia, L., Salmona, M., Cazzaniga, G., *et al.* (1995). Purification, cDNA cloning, and tissue distribution of bovine liver aldehyde oxidase. *Journal of Biological Chemistry*, **270**, 31037–31045.

Cammack, R., Kovacs, K.L., McCracken, J., and Peisach, J. (1989a). Spectroscopic characterization of the nickel and iron-sulphur clusters of hydrogenase from the purple photosynthetic bacterium *Thiocapsa roseopersicina*. 2. Electron spin-echo spectroscopy. *European Journal of Biochemistry*, **182**, 363–366.

Cammack, R., Bagyinka, C., and Kovacs, K.L. (1989*b*). Spectroscopic characterization of the nickel and iron-sulphur clusters of hydrogenase from the purple photosynthetic bacterium Thiocapsa roseopersicina. 1. Electron spin resonance spectroscopy. *European Journal of Biochemistry*, **182**, 357–362.

Campbell, K.S., Bedzyk, W.D., and Cambier, J.C. (1995). Manipulation of B cell antigen receptor tyrosine phosphorylation using aluminum fluoride and sodium orthovanadate. *Molecular Immunology*, **32**, 1283–1294.

Candeias, L.P., Patel, K.B., Stratford, M.R., and Wardman, P. (1993). Free hydroxyl radicals are formed on reaction between the neutrophil-derived species superoxide anion and hypochlorous acid. *FEBS Letters*, **333**, 151–153.

Candeias, L.P., Stratford, M.R., and Wardman, P. (1994). Formation of hydroxyl radicals on reaction of hypochlorous acid with ferrocyanide, a model iron(II) complex. *Free Radical Research*, **20**, 241–249.

Cantoni, O., Sestili, P., Cattabeni, F., Bellomo, G., Pou, S., Cohen, M., *et al.* (1989). Calcium chelator Quin 2 prevents hydrogen-peroxide-induced DNA breakage and cytotoxicity. *European Journal of Biochemistry*, **182**, 209–212.

Cao, G., and Cutler, R.G. (1995*a*). Protein oxidation and aging. II. Difficulties in measuring alkaline protease activity in tissues using the fluorescamine procedure. *Archives of Biochemistry and Biophysics*, **320**, 195–201.

Cao, G., and Cutler, R.G. (1995*b*). Protein oxidation and aging. I. Difficulties in measuring reactive protein carbonyls in tissues using 2,4-dinitrophenylhydrazine. *Archives of Biochemistry and Biophysics*, **320**, 106–114.

Capony, J.P., and Pechere, J.F. (1973). The primary structure of the major parvalbumin from hake muscle. Tryptic peptides derived from the S-sulfo and the performic-acid-oxidized proteins. *European Journal of Biochemistry*, 32, 88–96.

Cappiello, M., Voltarelli, M., Giannessi, M., Cecconi, I., Camici, G., Manao, G., *et al.* (1994). Glutathione dependent modification of bovine lens aldose reductase. *Experimental Eye Research*, **58**, 491–501.

Caputo, A., and Dose, K. (1957). On the direct action of Rontgen rays on proteins, peptides and amino acids. I. Investigations on proteins: irradiation of lysozyme. *Zeitschrift fur Naturforschung*, **12b**, 172–180.

Carceller, E., Merlos, M., Giral, M., Balsa, D., Garcia, R.J., and Forn, J. (1996). Design, synthesis, and structure-activity relationship studies of novel 1-[(1-acyl-4-piperidyl)methyl]-1H-2- methylimidazo[4,5-c]pyridine derivatives as potent, orally active platelet-activating factor antagonists. *Journal of Medicinal Chemistry*, **39**, 487–493.

Cardenas, A.M., Cortes, M.P., Fernandez, E., and Pena, W. (1992). Lipid peroxidation and loss of potassium from red blood cells produced by phototoxic quinolones. *Toxicology*, **72**, 145–151.

Carmichael, P.L., and Hipkiss, A.R. (1991). Differences in susceptibility between crystallins and non-lenticular proteins to copper and H_2O_2-mediated peptide bond cleavage. *Free Radical Research Communications*, **15**, 101–110.

Carmine, T.C., Evans, P., Bruchelt, G., Evans, R., Handgretinger, R., Niethammer, D., *et al.* (1995). Presence of iron catalytic for free radical reactions in patients undergoing chemotherapy: implications for therapeutic management. *Cancer Letters*, **94**, 219–226.

Carney, J.M., and Floyd, R.A. (1991). Protection against oxidative damage to CNS by alpha-phenyl-tert-butyl nitrone (PBN) and other spin-trapping agents: a novel series of nonlipid free radical scavengers. *Journal of Molecular Neuroscience*, **3**, 47–57.

Carney, J.M., Starke, R.P., Oliver, C.N., Landum, R.W., Cheng, M.S., Wu, J.F., et al. (1991). Reversal of age-related increase in brain protein oxidation, decrease in enzyme activity, and loss in temporal and spatial memory by chronic administration of the spin-trapping compound N-tert-butyl-alpha-phenylnitrone. *Proceedings of the National Academy of Science of the United States of America,* **88**, 3633–3636.

Carney, J.M., Smith, C.D., Carney, A.M., and Butterfield, D.A. (1994). Aging- and oxygen-induced modifications in brain biochemistry and behavior. *Annals of the New York Academy of Science,* **738**, 44–53.

Carrington, A., and McLauchlan, A.D. (1979) *Introduction to Magnetic Resonance.* Chapman and Hall, London.

Carter, C.J., Kraut, J., Freer, S.T., and Alden, R.A. (1974). Comparison of oxidation-reduction site geometries in oxidized and reduced *Chromatium* high potential iron protein and oxidized *Peptococcus aerogenes* ferredoxin. *Journal of Biological Chemistry,* **249**, 6339–6346.

Carter, D.C., Melis, K.A., O'Donnell, S.E., Burgess, B.K., Furey, W.J., Wang, B.C., et al. (1985). Crystal structure of Azotobacter cytochrome c5 at 2.5 A resolution. *Journal of Molecular Biology,* **184**, 279–295.

Carter, S.R., McGuirl, M.A., Brown, D.E., and Dooley, D.M. (1994). Purification and active-site characterization of equine plasma amine oxidase. *Journal of Inorganic Biochemistry,* **56**, 127–141.

Carubelli, R., Schneider, J.J., Pye, Q.N., and Floyd, R.A. (1995). Cytotoxic effects of autoxidative glycation. *Free Radical Biology and Medicine,* **18**, 265–269.

Casamayor, A., Aldea, M., Casas, C., Herrero, E., Gamo, F.J., Lafuente, M.J., et al. (1995). DNA sequence analysis of a 13 kbp fragment of the left arm of yeast chromosome XV containing seven new open reading frames. *Yeast,* **11**, 1281–1288.

Casini, A.F., Maellaro, E., Pompella, A., Ferrali, M., and Comporti, M. (1987). Lipid peroxidation, protein thiols and calcium homeostasis in bromobenzene-induced liver damage. *Biochemical Pharmacology,* **36**, 3689–3695.

Castedo, M., Macho, A., Zamzami, N., Hirsch, T., Marchetti, P., Uriel, J., et al. (1995). Mitochondrial perturbations define lymphocytes undergoing apoptotic depletion *in vivo. European Journal of Immunology,* **25**, 3277–3284.

Castellani, R., Smith, M.A., Richey, P.L., Kalaria, R., Gambetti, P., and Perry, G. (1995). Evidence for oxidative stress in Pick disease and corticobasal degeneration. *Brain Research,* **696**, 268–271.

Castilho, R.F., Meinicke, A.R., Almeida, A.M., Hermes, L.M., and Vercesi, A.E. (1994). Oxidative damage of mitochondria induced by Fe(II)citrate is potentiated by $Ca2+$ and includes lipid peroxidation and alterations in membrane proteins. *Archives of Biochemistry and Biophysics,* **308**, 158–163.

Castro, O.S., and Covarrubias, L. (1996). Role of retinoic acid and oxidative stress in embryonic stem cell death and neuronal differentiation. *FEBS Letters,* **381**, 93–97.

Castro, S.L., Sved, A.F., and Zigmond, M.J. (1996). Increased neostriatal tyrosine hydroxylation during stress: role of extracellular dopamine and excitatory amino acids. *Journal of Neurochemistry,* **66**, 824–833.

Catalano, C.E., Choe, Y.S., and Ortiz de Montellano, P.R. (1989). Reactions of the protein radical in peroxide-treated myoglobin. *Journal of Biological Chemistry,* **264**, 10534–10541.

Catterall, H., Davies, M.J., and Gilbert, B.C. (1992). An EPR study of the transfer of radical-induced damage from the base to sugar in nucleic acid components:

relevance to the occurrence of strand breaks. *Journal of the Chemical Society, Perkin Transactions*, **2**, 1379–1385.

Catterall, H., Davies, M.J., Gilbert, B.C., and Polack, N.P. (1993). EPR spin-trapping studies of the reaction of the hydroxyl radical with pyrimidine nucleobases, nucleosides and nucleotides, polynucleotides, and RNA. Direct evidence for sites of initial attack and for strand breakage. *Journal of the Chemical Society, Perkin Transactions*, **2**, 2039–2047.

Cayota, A., Vuillier, F., Gonzalez, G., and Dighiero, G. (1996). *In vitro* antioxidant treatment recovers proliferative responses of anergic CD4+ lymphocytes from human immunodeficiency virus-infected individuals. *Blood*, **87**, 4746–4753.

Cefalu, W.T., Bell-Farrow, A.D., Wang, Z.Q., Sonntag, W.E., Fu, M.-X., Baynes, J.W., *et al.* (1995). Caloric restriction decreases age-dependent accumulation of the glycoxidation products, N^{ε}-(carboyxmethyl)lysine and pentosidine, in rat skin collagen. *Journal of Gerontology*, **50A**, 8337–8341.

Cervera, J., and Levine, R.L. (1988). Modulation of the hydrophobicity of glutamine synthetase by mixed-function oxidation. *FASEB Journal*, **2**, 2591–2595.

Cha, J.H., Dure, L.I., Sakurai, S.Y., Penney, J.B., and Young, A.B. (1991). 2,4,5-Trihydroxyphenylalanine (6-hydroxy-dopa) displaces [3H]AMPA binding in rat striatum. *Neuroscience Letters*, **132**, 55–58.

Chace, K.V., Carubelli, R., and Nordqvist, R.E. (1991). The role of non-enzymatic glycosylation, transition metals, and free radicals in the formation of collagen aggregates. *Archives of Biochemistry and Biophysics*, **288**, 473–480.

Chacko, G.K. (1985). Modification of human high density lipoprotein (HDL3) with tetranitromethane and the effect on its binding to isolated rat liver plasma membranes. *Journal of Lipid Research*, **26**, 745–754.

Chae, H.Z., Chung, S.J., and Rhee, S.G. (1994). Thioredoxin-dependent peroxide reductase from yeast. *Journal of Biological Chemistry*, **269**, 27670–27678.

Chai, J.G., Okamoto, M., Bando, T., Nagasawa, H., Hisaeda, H., Sakai, T., *et al.* (1995). Dissociation between the mitogenic effect and antitumor activity of seed extract from *Aeginetia indica* L. *Immunopharmacology*, **30**, 209–215.

Chai, Y.C., Jung, C.H., Lii, C.K., Ashraf, S.S., Hendrich, S., Wolf, B., *et al.* (1991). Identification of an abundant S-thiolated rat liver protein as carbonic anhydrase III; characterization of S-thiolation and dethiolation reactions. *Archives of Biochemistry and Biophysics*, **284**, 270–278.

Chai, Y.C., Ashraf, S.S., Rokutan, K., Johnston, R.J., and Thomas, J.A. (1994*a*). S-thiolation of individual human neutrophil proteins including actin by stimulation of the respiratory burst: evidence against a role for glutathione disulfide. *Archives of Biochemistry and Biophysics*, **310**, 273–281.

Chai, Y.C., Hendrich, S., and Thomas, J.A. (1994*b*). Protein S-thiolation in hepatocytes stimulated by *t*-butyl hydroperoxide, menadione, and neutrophils. *Archives of Biochemistry and Biophysics*, **310**, 264–272.

Chait, A., and Heinecke, J.W. (1994). Lipoprotein modification: cellular mechanisms. *Current Opinion in Lipidology*, **5**, 365–370.

Chakrabarti, S., Kumar, S., and Shankar, R. (1986). Reserpine inhibition of lipid peroxidation and protein phosphorylation in rat brain. *Biochemical Pharmacology*, **35**, 1611–1613.

Chakrabartty, S.K. (1978). Alkaline hypohalite oxidations. In *Oxidation in Organic Chemistry, Part C*, (ed. W.S. Trahanovsky), pp. 343–370. Academic Press, New York.

Chambers, D.J., Braimbridge, M.V., and Hearse, D.J. (1987*ₓa*). Free radicals and cardioplegia: the absence of an additive effect with allopurinol pretreatment and the use of antioxidant enzymes in the rat. *European Journal of Cardiothoracic Surgery*, **1**, 80–90.

Chambers, D.J., Braimbridge, M.V., and Hearse, D.J. (1987*b*). Free radicals and cardioplegia. Free radical scavengers improve postischemic function of rat myocardium. *European Journal of Cardiothoracic Surgery*, **1**, 37–45.

Chambers, D.J., Braimbridge, M.V., and Hearse, D.J. (1987*c*). Free radicals and cardioplegia: allopurinol and oxypurinol reduce myocardial injury following ischemic arrest. *Annals of Thoracic Surgery*, **44**, 291–297.

Chambers, D.J., Astras, G., Takahashi, A., Manning, A.S., Braimbridge, M.V., and Hearse, D.J. (1989). Free radicals and cardioplegia: organic anti-oxidants as additives to the St Thomas' Hospital cardioplegic solution. *Cardiovascular Research*, **23**, 351–358.

Chambers, D.J., Takahashi, A., Humphrey, S.M., Harvey, D.M., and Hearse, D.J. (1992). Allopurinol-enhanced myocardial protection does not involve xanthine oxidase inhibition or purine salvage. *Basic Research in Cardiology*, **87**, 227–238.

Chan, H.T., and Anthony, C. (1991). The interaction of methanol dehydrogenase and cytochrome cL in the acidophilic methylotroph *Acetobacter methanolicus*. *Biochemical Journal*, **280**, 139–146.

Chan, H.W.-S. (1987). *Autoxidation of Unsaturated Lipids*. Academic Press, London.

Chan, P.C., Bielski, B.H.J. (1973). Pulse radiolysis study of optical absorption and kinetic properties of dithiothreitol free radical. *Journal of the American Chemical Society*, **95**, 5504–5508.

Chance, M., Powers, L., Kumar, C., and Chance, B. (1986). X-ray absorption studies of myoglobin peroxide reveal functional differences between globins and heme enzymes. *Biochemistry*, **25**, 1259–1265.

Chang, H.W., and Bock, E. (1980). Pitfalls in the use of commercial non-ionic detergents for the solubilization of integral membrane proteins: sulfhydryl oxidizing contaminants and their elimination. *Analytical Biochemistry*, **104**, 112–117.

Chanoki, M., Ishii, M., Kobayashi, H., Fushida, H., Yashiro, N., Hamada, T., et al. (1995). Increased expression of lysyl oxidase in skin with scleroderma. *British Journal of Dermatology*, **133**, 710–715.

Chapman, M.L., Rubin, B.R., and Gracy, R.W. (1989). Increased carbonyl content of proteins in synovial fluid from patients with rheumatoid arthritis. *Journal of Rheumatology*, **16**, 15–18.

Charlesworth, M., Farrall, L., Stokes, T., and Tunrbull, D. (1989). *Life Among the Scientists*. Oxford University Press, Melbourne.

Charrier, B., Coronado, C., Kondorosi, A., and Ratet, P. (1995). Molecular characterization and expression of alfalfa (*Medicago sativa L.*) flavanone-3-hydroxylase and dihydroflavonol-4-reductase encoding genes. *Plant Molecular Biology*, **29**, 773–786.

Chauvet, M.T., Chauvet, J., and Acher, R. (1987). Guinea pig MSEL-neurophysin. Sequence comparison of eight mammalian MSEL-neurophysins. *International Journal of Peptide and Protein Research*, **30**, 676–682.

Royal Society of Chemistry (1973–1997) *Electron Spin Resonance: Specialist Periodical Reports vols. 1–15*. Royal Society of Chemistry, Cambridge.

Chen, C., and Loo, G. (1995). Cigarette smoke extract inhibits oxidative modification of low density lipoprotein. *Atherosclerosis*, **112**, 177–185.

Chen, H., and Tappel, A.L. (1993). Protection of heme proteins by vitamin E, selenium, and beta-carotene against oxidative damage in rat heart, kidney, lung and spleen. *Free Radical Research Communications*, **19**, 183–190.

Chen, H., and Tappel, A.L. (1994). Protection by vitamin E selenium, trolox C, ascorbic acid palmitate, acetylcysteine, coenzyme Q, beta-carotene, canthaxanthin, and (+)-catechin against oxidative damage to liver slices measured by oxidized heme proteins. *Free Radical Biology and Medicine*, **16**, 437–444.

Chen, H., and Tappel, A.L. (1995a). Protection of vitamin E, selenium, trolox C, ascorbic acid palmitate, acetylcysteine, coenzyme Q0, coenzyme Q10, beta-carotene, canthaxanthin, and (+)-catechin against oxidative damage to rat blood and tissues *in vivo*. *Free Radical Biology and Medicine*, **18**, 949–953.

Chen, H., and Tappel, A.L. (1995b). Vitamin E, selenium, trolox C, ascorbic acid palmitate, acetylcysteine, coenzyme Q, beta-carotene, canthaxanthin, and (+)-catechin protect against oxidative damage to kidney, heart, lung and spleen. *Free Radical Research*, **22**, 177–186.

Chen, H., Pellett, L.J., Andersen, H.J., and Tappel, A.L. (1993a). Protection by vitamin E, selenium, and beta-carotene against oxidative damage in rat liver slices and homogenate. *Free Radical Biology and Medicine*, **14**, 473–482.

Chen, H., Tappel, A.L., and Boyle, R.C. (1993b). Oxidation of heme proteins as a measure of oxidative damage to liver tissue slices. *Free Radical Biology and Medicine*, **14**, 509–517.

Chen, J.G., Woltman, S.J., and Weber, S.G. (1995). Sensitivity and selectivity of the electrochemical detection of the copper(II) complexes of bioactive peptides, and comparison to model studies by rotating ring-disc electrode. *Journal of Chromatography A*, **691**, 301–315.

Chen, J.Y., Chang, W.C., Chang, T., Chang, W.C., Liu, M.Y., Payne, W.J., *et al.* (1996). Cloning, characterization, and expression of the nitric oxide-generating nitrite reductase and of the blue copper protein genes of *Achromobacter cycloclastes*. *Biochemical and Biophysical Research Communications*, **219**, 423–428.

Chen, L., Durley, R., Poliks, B.J., Hamada, K., Chen, Z., Mathews, F.S., *et al.* (1992). Crystal structure of an electron-transfer complex between methylamine dehydrogenase and amicyanin. *Biochemistry*, **31**, 4959–4964.

Chen, L., Mathews, F.S., Davidson, V.L., Tegoni, M., Rivetti, C., and Rossi, G.L. (1993). Preliminary crystal structure studies of a ternary electron transfer complex between a quinoprotein, a blue copper protein, and a *c*-type cytochrome. *Protein Science*, **2**, 147–154.

Chen, L., Durley, R.C., Mathews, F.S., and Davidson, V.L. (1994). Structure of an electron transfer complex: methylamine dehydrogenase, amicyanin, and cytochrome *c*551i. *Science*, **264**, 86–90.

Chen, L.Y., Mathews, F.S., Davidson, V.L., Huizinga, E.G., Vellieux, F.M., Duine, J.A., *et al.* (1991). Crystallographic investigations of the tryptophan-derived cofactor in the quinoprotein methylamine dehydrogenase. *FEBS Letters*, **287**, 163–166.

Chen, P., Wiesler, D., Chmelik, J., and Novotny, M. (1996). Substituted 2-hydroxy-1,2-dihydropyrrol-3-ones : fluorescent markers pertaining to oxidative stress and aging. *Chemical Research in Toxicology*, **9**, 970–979.

Chen, Q., Fischer, A., Reagan, J.D., Yan, L.J., and Ames, B.N. (1995). Oxidative DNA damage and senescence of human diploid fibroblast cells. *Proceedings of the National Academy of Science of the United States of America*, **92**, 4337–4341.

Chen, Q.M., Smyth, D.D., McKenzie, J.K., Glavin, G.B., Gu, J.G., Geiger, J.D., *et al.* (1994). Chlorotyrosine exerts renal effects and antagonizes renal and gastric responses to atrial natriuretic peptide. *Journal of Pharmacology and Experimental Therapeutics*, **269**, 709–716.

Chen, S., Morimoto, S., Tamatani, M., Fukuo, K., Nakahashi, T., Nishibe, A., *et al.* (1996). Calcitonin prevents CCl4-induced hydroperoxide generation and cytotoxicity possibly through C1b receptor in rat hepatocytes. *Biochemical and Biophysical Research Communications*, **218**, 865–871.

Chen, Y.N., Bienkowski, M.J., and Marnett, L.J. (1987). Controlled tryptic digestion of prostaglandin H synthase. Characterization of protein fragments and enhanced rate of proteolysis of oxidatively inactivated enzyme. *Journal of Biological Chemistry*, **262**, 16892–16899.

Cheng, H., Westler, W.M., Xia, B., Oh, B.H., and Markley, J.L. (1995). Protein expression, selective isotopic labeling, and analysis of hyperfine-shifted NMR signals of Anabaena 7120 vegetative [2Fe-2S]ferredoxin. *Archives of Biochemistry and Biophysics*, **316**, 619–634.

Cheng, R.Z., Uchida, K., and Kawakishi, S. (1992). Selective oxidation of histidine residues in proteins or peptides through the copper(II)-catalysed autoxidation of glucosone. *Biochemical Journal*, **285**, 667–671.

Chentanez, T., Patradilok, P., Glinsukon, T., and Piyachaturawat, P. (1988). Effects of cortisol pretreatment on the acute hepatotoxicity of aflatoxin B1. *Toxicology Letters*, **42**, 237–248.

Chentsova, T.V., and Kravchenko, N.A. (1978). Mobility on peptide maps of peptides obtained by tryptic hydrolysis of lysozyme oxidized at the S-S-bonds. *Biokhimica*, **43**, 1977–1982.

Cherian, M., and Abraham, E.C. (1995). Decreased molecular chaperone property of alpha-crystallins due to posttranslational modifications. *Biochemical and Biophysical Research Communications*, **208**, 675–679.

Cherry, P.D., and Wolin, M.S. (1989). Ascorbate activates soluble guanylate cyclase via H_2O_2-metabolism by catalase. *Free Radical Biology and Medicine*, **7**, 485–490.

Chevalier, M., Lin, E.C., and Levine, R.L. (1990). Hydrogen peroxide mediates the oxidative inactivation of enzymes following the switch from anaerobic to aerobic metabolism in *Klebsiella pneumoniae*. *Journal of Biological Chemistry*, **265**, 40–46.

Chevion, M. (1988). A site-specific mechanism for free radical induced biological damage: the essential role of redox-active transition metals. *Free Radical Biology and Medicine*, **5**, 27–37.

Chevion, M., Jiang, Y., Har, E.R., Berenshtein, E., Uretzky, G., and Kitrossky, N. (1993). Copper and iron are mobilized following myocardial ischemia: possible predictive criteria for tissue injury. *Proceedings of the National Academy of Science of the United States of America*, **90**, 1102–1106.

Chio, K.S., and Tappel, A.L. (1969*a*). Inactivation of ribonuclease and other enzymes by peroxidizing lipids and by malonaldehyde. *Biochemistry*, **8**, 2827–2832.

Chio, K.S., and Tappel, A.L. (1969*b*). Synthesis and characterization of the fluorescent products derived from malonaldehyde and amino acids. *Biochemistry*, **8**, 2821–2826.

Chiou, S.-H. (1983). DNA- and Protein-scission activities of ascorbate in the presence of copper ion and a copper-peptide complex. *Journal of Biochemistry*, **94**, 1259–1267.

Chipens, G.I., Balodis, I., and Gnilomedova, L.E. (1991). Polarity and hydropathic properties of natural amino acids. *Ukrainskii Biokhimichiskii Zhurnal*, **63**, 20–29.

Choe, Y.S., Rao, S.I., and Ortiz, d.M.P. (1994). Requirement of a second oxidation equivalent for ferryl oxygen transfer to styrene in the epoxidation catalyzed by myoglobin-H_2O_2. *Archives of Biochemistry and Biophysics*, **314**, 126–131.

Choi, H.S., and Moore, D.D. (1993). Induction of c-fos and c-jun gene expression by phenolic antioxidants. *Molecular Endocrinology*, **7**, 1596–1602.

Choi, Y.H., Matsuzaki, R., Fukui, T., Shimizu, E., Yorifuji, T., Sato, H., *et al.* (1995). Copper/topa quinone-containing histamine oxidase from *Arthrobacter globiformis*. Molecular cloning and sequencing, overproduction of precursor enzyme, and generation of topa quinone cofactor. *Journal of Biological Chemistry*, **270**, 4712–4720.

Chokekijchai, S., Shirasaka, T., Weinstein, J.N., and Mitsuya, H. (1995). *In vitro* anti-HIV-1 activity of HIV protease inhibitor KNI-272 in resting and activated cells: implications for its combined use with AZT or ddI. *Antiviral Research*, **28**, 25–38.

Choughuley, A.S., Subbaraman, A.S., Kazi, Z.A., and Chadha, M.S. (1975). Transformation of some hydroxy amino acids to other amino acids. *Origins of Life*, **6**, 527–535.

Chow, C.K., and Tappel, A.L. (1972). An enzymatic protective mechanism against lipid peroxidation damage to lungs of ozone-exposed rats. *Lipids*, **7**, 518–524.

Chow, C.K., and Tappel, A.L. (1973). Activities of pentose shunt and glycolytic enzymes in lungs of ozone-exposed rats. *Archives of Environmental Health*, **26**, 205–208.

Chow, C.K., Reddy, K., and Tappel, A.L. (1973). Effect of dietary vitamin E on the activities of the glutathione peroxidase system in rat tissues. *Journal of Nutrition*, **103**, 618–624.

Chowdhury, S.K., Eshraghi, J., Wolfe, H., Forde, D., Hlavac, A.G., and Johnston, D. (1995). Mass spectrometric identification of amino acid transformations during oxidation of peptides and proteins: modifications of methionine and tyrosine. *Analytical Chemistry*, **67**, 390–398.

Christen, S., and Stocker, R. (1992). Simultaneous determination of 3-hydroxy-anthranilic and cinnabarinic acid by high-performance liquid chromatography with photometric or electrochemical detection. *Analytical Biochemistry*, **200**, 273–279.

Christen, S., Peterhans, E., and Stocker, R. (1990). Antioxidant activities of some tryptophan metabolites: possible implication for inflammatory diseases. *Proceedings of the National Academy of Science of the United States of America*, **87**, 2506–2510.

Christen, S., Southwell, K.P., and Stocker, R. (1992). Oxidation of 3-hydroxy-anthranilic acid to the phenoxazinone cinnabarinic acid by peroxyl radicals and by compound I of peroxidases or catalase. *Biochemistry*, **31**, 8090–8097.

Christen, S., Thomas, S.R., Garner, B., and Stocker, R. (1994). Inhibition by interferon-gamma of human mononuclear cell-mediated low density lipoprotein oxidation. Participation of tryptophan metabolism along the kynurenine pathway. *Journal of Clinical Investigation*, **93**, 2149–2158.

Christensen, H.E., Ulstrup, J., and Sykes, A.G. (1990). Effects of NO_2-modification of Tyr83 on the reactivity of spinach plastocyanin with inorganic redox partners $[Fe(CN)_6]^{3-/4-}$ and $[Co(phen)_3]^{3+/2+}$. *Biochimica et Biophysica Acta*, **1039**, 94–102.

Christison, J., Sies, H., and Stocker, R. (1994). Human blood cells support the reduction of low-density-lipoprotein-associated cholesteryl ester hydroperoxides by albumin-bound ebselen. *Biochemical Journal*, **304**, 341–345.

Christison, J., Karjalainen, A., Brauman, J., Bygrave, F., and Stocker, R. (1996). Rapid reduction and removal of HDL- but not LDL-associated cholesteryl ester hydroperoxides by rat liver perfused *in situ*. *Biochemical Journal*, **314**, 739–742.

Chrysochoos, J. (1968). Pulse radiolysis of phenylalanine and tyrosine. *Radiation Research*, **33**, 465–479.

Chung, M.H., Kesner, L., and Chan, P.C. (1984). Degradation of articular cartilage by copper and hydrogen peroxide. *Agents and Actions*, **15**, 328–335.

Chupin, V., Leenhouts, J.M., de Kroon, A.I., and de Kruijff, B. (1996). Secondary structure and topology of a mitochondrial presequence peptide associated with negatively charged micelles. A 2D H-NMR study. *Biochemistry*, **35**, 3141–3146.

Cini, M., and Moretti, A. (1995). Studies on lipid peroxidation and protein oxidation in the aging brain. *Neurobiology of Aging*, **16**, 53–57.

Clapp, P.A., Davies, M.J., French, M.S., and Gilbert, B.C. (1994). The bactericidal action of peroxides; an E.P.R. spin-trapping study. *Free Radical Research*, **21**, 147–167.

Clark, A.V., and Tannenbaum, S.R. (1970). Isolation and characterization of pigments from protein-carbon browning systems. Isolation, purification, and properties. *Journal of Agricultural and Food Chemistry*, **18**, 891–894.

Clark, R.A., Stone, P.J., El Hag, A., Calore, J.D., and Franzblau, C. (1981). Myeloperoxidase-catalyzed inactivation of α_1-protease inhibitor by human neutrophils. *Journal of Biological Chemistry*, **256**, 3348–3353.

Clayson, E.T., Kelly, S.A., and Meier, H.L. (1993). Effects of specific inhibitors of cellular functions on sulfur mustard-induced cell death. *Cellular and Biological Toxicology*, **9**, 165–175.

Clement, J.R., Lin, W.S., and Armstrong, D.A. (1977). Changes in optical density, amino acid composition, and fluorescence of papain inactivated by hydroxyl radicals and hydrogen peroxide. *Radiation Research*, **72**, 427–439.

Clement, M.V., and Stamenkovic, I. (1996). Superoxide anion is a natural inhibitor of FAS-mediated cell death. *EMBO Journal*, **15**, 216–225.

Climent, I., and Levine, R.L. (1991). Oxidation of the active site of glutamine synthetase: conversion of arginine-344 to gamma-glutamyl semialdehyde. *Archives of Biochemistry and Biophysics*, **289**, 371–375.

Climent, I., Tsai, L., and Levine, R.L. (1989). Derivatization of gamma-glutamyl semialdehyde residues in oxidized proteins by fluoresceinamine. *Analytical Biochemistry*, **182**, 226–232.

Clot, P., Bellomo, G., Tabone, M., Arico, S., and Albano, E. (1995). Detection of antibodies against proteins modified by hydroxyethyl free radicals in patients with alcoholic cirrhosis. *Gastroenterology*, **108**, 201–207.

Coetzee, W.A., Ichikawa, H., and Hearse, D.J. (1994). Oxidant stress inhibits Na-Ca-exchange current in cardiac myocytes: mediation by sulfhydryl groups? *American Journal of Physiology*, **266**, K909–K919.

Cohen, S.G., and Ojanpera, S. (1975). Letter: Photooxidation of methionine and related compounds. *Journal of the American Chemical Society*, **97**, 5633–5634.

Cohn, J.A., Tsai, L., Friguet, B., and Szweda, L.I. (1996). Chemical characterization of a protein-4-hydroxy-2-nonenal cross-link: immunochemical detection in mitochondria exposed to oxidative stress. *Archives of Biochemistry and Biophysics*, **328**, 158–164.

Collis, C.S., Davies, M.J., and Rice, E.C. (1993). Comparison of N-methyl hexanoylhydroxamic acid, a novel antioxidant, with desferrioxamine and N-acetyl cysteine against reperfusion-induced dysfunctions in isolated rat heart. *Journal of Cardiovascular Pharmacology*, **22**, 336–342.

Colombo, B.M., Klimaschewski, L., and Heym, C. (1996). Immunohistochemical heterogeneity of nerve cells in the human adrenal gland with special reference to substance P. *Journal of Histochemistry and Cytochemistry*, **44**, 369–375.

Colomer, V., Kicska, G.A., and Rindler, M.J. (1996). Secretory granule content proteins and the luminal domains of granule membrane proteins aggregate *in vitro* at mildly acidic pH. *Journal of Biological Chemistry*, **271**, 48–55.

Combrisson, J., and Uebersfield, J. (1954). Magnétisme. Détection de la résonance paramagnétique dans certaines substances organiques irradiées. *Compte Rendus Academy Science (Paris)*, **238**, 1397–1398.

Conconi, M., Szweda, L.I., Levine, R.L., Stadtman, E.R., and Friguet, B. (1996). Age-related decline of rat liver multicatalytic proteinase activity and protection from oxidative inactivation by heat-shock protein 90. *Archives of Biochemistry and Biophysics*, **331**, 232–240.

Cooksey, C.J., Land, E.J., Ramsden, C.A., and Riley, P.A. (1995). Tyrosinase-mediated cytotoxicity of 4-substituted phenols: quantitative structure-thiol-reactivity relationships of the derived o-quinones. *Anticancer Drug Research*, **10**, 119–129.

Cooper, B., Creeth, M., and Donald, A.S.R. (1985). Studies of the limited degradation of mucus glycoproteins. The mechanism of the peroxide reaction. *Biochemical Journal*, **228**, 615–626.

Cooper, C.E., Green, E.S., Rice, E.C., Davies, M.J., and Wrigglesworth, J.M. (1994). A hydrogen-donating monohydroxamate scavenges ferryl myoglobin radicals. *Free Radical Research*, **20**, 219–227.

Cooper, R.A., Knowles, P.F., Brown, D.E., McGuirl, M.A., and Dooley, D.M. (1992). Evidence for copper and 3,4,6-trihydroxyphenylalanine quinone cofactors in an amine oxidase from the gram-negative bacterium *Escherichia coli K-12*. *Biochemical Journal*, **288**, 337–340.

Copeland, E.S., Sanner, T., and Pihl, A. (1968). Role of intermolecular reactions in the formation of secondary radicals in proteins irradiated in the dry state. *Radiation Research*, **35**, 437–450.

Copley, S.D., Frank, E., Kirsch, W.M., and Koch, T.H. (1992). Detection and possible origins of aminomalonic acid in protein hydrolysates. *Analytical Biochemistry*, **201**, 152–157.

Corey, E.J., Mehrotra, M.M., and Khan, A.U. (1987). Antiarthritic gold compounds effectively quench electronically excited singlet oxygen. *Science*, **236**, 68–69.

Corin, A.F., and Gould, I.R. (1989). Photo-induced electron ejection from the reduced copper of *Pseudomonas aeruginosa azurin*. *Photochemistry and Photobiology*, **50**, 413–418.

Cortazzo, M., and Schor, N.F. (1996). Potentiation of enediyne-induced apoptosis and differentiation by Bcl-2. *Cancer Research*, **56**, 1199–1203.

Costa, M., Salnikow, K., Cosentino, S., Klein, C.B., Huang, X., and Zhuang, Z. (1994). Molecular mechanisms of nickel carcinogenesis. *Environmental Health Perspectives*, **3**, 127–130.

Costabel, U., Maier, K., Teschler, H., and Wang, Y.M. (1992). Local immune components in chronic obstructive pulmonary disease. *Respiration*, **1**, 17–19.

Cotgreave, I.A., and Moldeus, P. (1986). Methodologies for the application of monobromobimane to the simultaneous analysis of soluble and protein thiol components of biological systems. *Journal of Biochemical and Biophysical Methods*, **13**, 231–249.

Courgeon, A.M., Maingourd, M., Maisonhaute, C., Montmory, C., Rollet, E., Tanguay, R.M., *et al.* (1993). Effect of hydrogen peroxide on cytoskeletal proteins of *Drosophila* cells: comparison with heat shock and other stresses. *Experimental Cell Research*, **204**, 30–37.

Couser, W.G. (1990). Mediation of immune glomerular injury. *Journal of the American Society of Nephrology*, **1**, 13–29.

Coux, P., Tanaka, K., and Goldberg, A.L. (1996). Structure and functions of the 20S and 26S proteasomes. *Annual Reviews of Biochemistry*, **65**, 801–847.

Cozier, G.E., Giles, I.G., and Anthony, C. (1995). The structure of the quinoprotein alcohol dehydrogenase of *Acetobacter aceti* modelled on that of methanol dehydrogenase from *Methylobacterium extorquens*. *Biochemical Journal*, **308**, 375–379.

Craggs, J., Kirk, S.H., and Ahmad, S.I. (1994). Synergistic action of near-UV and phenylalanine, tyrosine or tryptophan on the inactivation of phage T7: role of superoxide radicals and hydrogen peroxide. *Journal of Photochemistry and Photobiology B*, **24**, 123–128.

Cramer, R., Soranzo, M.R., and Patriarca, P. (1981). Evidence that eosinophils catalyze the bromide-dependent decarboxylation of amino acids. *Blood*, **58**, 1112–1118.

Crawford, D.L., Yu, T.C., and Sinnhuber, R.O. (1967). Reaction of malonaldehyde with protein. *Journal of Food Science*, **32**, 332–335.

Crawford, D.R., and Davies, K.J.A. (1994). Adaptive response and oxidative stress. *Environmental Health Perspectives*, **10**, 25–28.

Crawford, D.R., Edbauer, N.C., Lowry, C.V., Salmon, S.L., Kim, Y.K., Davies, J.M., *et al.* (1994). Assessing gene expression during oxidative stress. *Methods in Enzymology*, **234**, 175–217.

Crawford, D.R., Schools, G.P., Salmon, S.L., and Davies, K.J. (1996). Hydrogen peroxide induces the expression of adapt15, a novel RNA associated with polysomes in hamster HA-1 cells. *Archives of Biochemistry and Biophysics*, **325**, 256–264.

Crawford, G.R., and Wright, P.J. (1987). Characterization of novel viral polyproteins detected in cells infected by the flavivirus Kunjin and radiolabelled in the presence of the leucine analogue hydroxyleucine. *Journal of General Virology*, **68**, 365–376.

Crawford, R.M.M., Linsday, D.A., Walton, J.C., and Wollenweber-Ratzer, B. (1994). Towards the characterization of radicals formed in rhizomes of *Iris germanica*. *Phytochemistry*, **37j**, 979–985.

Creed, D. (1984*a*). The photophysics and photochemistry of the near-UV absorbing amino acids. II. Tyrosine and its simple derivatives. *Photochemistry and Photobiology*, **39**, 363–375.

Creed, D. (1984*b*). The photophysics and photochemistry of the near-UV absorbing amino acids. III. Cystine and its simple derivatives. *Photochemistry and Photobiology.*, **39**, 577–583.

Creed, D. (1984*c*). The photophysics and photochemistry of the near-UV absorbing amino acids. I. Tryptophan and its simple derivatives. *Photochemistry and Photobiology*, **39**, 537–562.

Creeth, J.M., Cooper, B., Donald, A.S.R., and Clamp, J.R. (1983). Studies on the limited degradation of mucus glycoproteins: the effect of dilute hydrogen peroxide. *Biochemical Journal*, **211**, 323–332.

Croft, S., Gilbert, B.C., Smith, J.R., and Whitwood, A.C. (1992). An E.S.R. investigation of the reactive intermediate generated in the reaction between FeII and H_2O_2 in aqueous solution. Direct evidence for the formation of the hydroxyl radical. *Free Radical Research Communications*, **17**, 21–39.

Cross, C.E., Forte, T., Stocker, R., Louie, S., Yamamoto, Y., Ames, B.N., *et al.* (1990). Oxidative stress and abnormal cholesterol metabolism in patients with adult respiratory distress syndrome. *Journal of Laboratory and Clinical Medicine,* **115**, 396–404.

Cross, C.E., Reznick, A.Z., Packer, L., Davis, P.A., Suzuki, Y.J., and Halliwell, B. (1992). Oxidative damage to human plasma proteins by ozone. *Free Radical Research Communications,* **15**, 347–352.

Cross, C.E., O'Neill, C.A., Reznick, A.Z., Hu, M.L., Marcocci, L., Packer, L., *et al.* (1993). Cigarette smoke oxidation of human plasma constituents. *Annals of the New York Academy of Science,* **686**, 72–89.

Crowther, J.A., and Liebmann, H. (1939). An effect of gamma-radiation on egg albumin. *Nature,* **143**, 598.

Cucurou, C., Battioni, J.P., Daniel, R., and Mansuy, D. (1991*a*). Peroxidase-like activity of lipoxygenases: different substrate specificity of potato 5-lipoxygenase and soybean 15-lipoxygenase and particular affinity of vitamin E derivatives for the 5-lipoxygenase. *Biochimica et Biophysica Acta,* **1081**, 99–105.

Cucurou, C., Battioni, J.P., Thang, D.C., Nam, N.H., and Mansuy, D. (1991*b*). Mechanisms of inactivation of lipoxygenases by phenidone and BW755C. *Biochemistry,* **30**, 8964–8970.

Cudina, I., and Josimovic, L. (1987). The effect of oxygen on the radiolysis of tyrosine in aqueous solution. *Radiation Research,* **109**, 206.

Cuervo, A.M., Knecht, E., Terlecky, S.R., and Dice, J.F. (1995). Activation of a selective pathway of lysosomal proteolysis in rat liver by prolonged starvation. *American Journal of Physiology,* **269**, C1200–C1208.

Cummerow, R.L., and Halliday, D. (1946). Paramagnetic losses in two manganous salts. *Physiology Reviews,* **70**, 433.

Cummings, J.L. (1995). Lewy body diseases with dementia: pathophysiology and treatment. *Brain Cognition,* **28**, 266–280.

Cynshi, O., Saitoh, M., Cynshi, F., Tanemura, M., Hata, S., and Nakano, M. (1990). Anti-oxidative profile of lobenzarit disodium (CCA). *Biochemical Pharmacology,* **40**, 2117–2122.

Czapski, G., and Ilan, Y.A. (1978). On the generation of the hydroxylating agent from superoxide radical. Can the Haber-Weiss reaction be the source of ·OH radicals? *Photochemistry and Photobiology,* **28**, 6561–6653.

D'Arcy, J.B., and Sevilla, M. (1979). An electron spin resonance study of electron reactions with peptides: competitive mechanisms. Deamination *vs* protonation. *Radiation Physics and Chemistry,* **13**, 119–126.

D'Costa, E.J., Higgins, I.J., and Turner, A.P. (1986). Quinoprotein glucose dehydrogenase and its application in an amperometric glucose sensor. *Biosensors,* **2**, 71–87.

D'Ettorre, C., and Levine, R.L. (1994). Reactivity of cysteine-67 of the human immunodeficiency virus-1 protease: studies on a peptide spanning residues 59 to 75. *Archives of Biochemistry and Biophysics,* **313**, 71–76.

Dabbagh, A.J., and Frei, B. (1995). Human suction blister interstitial fluid prevents metal ion-dependent oxidation of low density lipoprotein by macrophages and in cell-free systems. *Journal of Clinical Investigation,* **96**, 1958–1966.

Dabbagh, A.J., Mannion, T., Lynch, S.M., and Frei, B. (1994). The effect of iron overload on rat plasma and liver oxidant status *in vivo*. *Biochemical Journal,* **300**, 799–803.

Dai, Z., and An, G. (1995). Induction of nopaline synthase promoter activity by H_2O_2 has no direct correlation with salicylic acid. *Plant Physiology,* **109**, 1191–1197.

Dain, A., Kerkut, G.A., Smith, R.C., Munday, K.A., and Wilmshurst, T.H. (1964). The interaction of free radicals in protein and melanin. *Experientia*, **20**, 76–78.

Dainton, F.S., and Peterson, D.B. (1962). Forms of H and OH produced in the radiolysis of aqueous solutions. *Proceedings of the National Academy of Science of the United States of America Royal Society (London) A*, **267**, 443–463.

Dakin, H.D. (1906). The oxidation of amido-acids with the production of substances of biological importance. *Journal of Biological Chemistry*, **1**, 171–176.

Dakin, H.D. (1908a). The oxidation of leucine, α-amido-isovaleric acid and of α-amido-*n*-valeric acid with hydrogen peroxide. *Journal of Biological Chemistry*, **4**, 63–76.

Dakin, H.D. (1908b). Note on the oxidation of glutamic acid by means of hydrogen peroxide. *Journal of Biological Chemistry*, **5**, 409–411.

Dakin, H.D. (1909). The fate of inactive tyrosine in the animal body together with some obervations upon the detection of tyrosine and its derivatives in the urine. *Journal of Biological Chemistry*, **8**, 25–33.

Dakin, H.D. (1917). Behaviour of hypochlorites on IV injection and their action on blood serum. *British Medical Journal*, **1**, 852–854.

Dakin, H.D. (1919). Amino acids. II. Hydroxyglutamic acid. *Biochemical Journal*, **13**, 398–429.

Dakin, H.D. (1922a) *Oxidations and Reductions in the Animal Body*. Longmans Green and Co., New York.

Dakin, H.D. (1922b). The resolution of hydroxy-aspartic acid into optically active forms. *Journal of Biological Chemistry*, **50**, 403–411.

Dakin, H.D. (1944). Hydroxyleucines. *Journal of Biological Chemistry*, **154**, 549–555.

Dakin, H.D. (1946). γ-methyl-proline. *Journal of Biological Chemistry*, **164**, 615–620.

Dakin, H.D., and Carlisle, H.G.J. (1916). Report on the use of sodium hypochlorite prepared by the electrolysis of sea water for disinfecting and antiseptic purposes on HMHS 'Aquitania'. *Journal of the Royal Army Medical Corps*, **26**, 209–227.

Dakin, H.D., Cohen, J.B., and Kenyon, J. (1916a). Studies on antiseptics. II. 'Chloramine', its preparation, properties and use. *British Medical Journal*, **1**, 160–162.

Dakin, H.D., Cohen, J.B., Daufresne, M., and Kenyon, J. (1916b). Antiseptic action of substances of the chloroamine group. *Proceedings of the Royal Society of London B*, **89**, 233–251.

Dale, W.M. (1940). The effect of X-rays on enzymes. *Biochemical Journal*, **34**, 1367–1373.

Dale, W.M., and Russell, C. (1956). A study of irradiation of catalase in the presence of cysteine, cystine and glutathione. *Biochemical Journal*, **62**, 50–57.

Dale, W.M., Davies, J.V., and Gilbert, C.W. (1949). The kinetics and specificities of deamination of nitrogenous compounds by X-radiation. *Biochemical Journal*, **45**, 93–99.

DalleDonne, I., Milzani, A., and Colombo, R. (1995). H_2O_2-treated actin: assembly and polymer interactions with cross-linking proteins. *Biophysical Journal*, **69**, 2710–2719.

Dalton, D.A., Langeberg, L., and Robbins, M. (1992). Purification and characterization of monodehydroascorbate reductase from soybean root nodules. *Archives of Biochemistry and Biophysics*, **292**, 281–286.

Danen, W.C., and Neugebauer, F.A. (1975). Aminyl Free Radicals. *Angewandte Chemie International. (Edition in English)*, **14**, 783–789.

Darskus, R.L. (1971). Rapid staining of proteins and peptides in starch gels by chlorination. *Journal of Chromatography*, **55**, 424–425.

Das, S., and von Sonntag, C. (1986). Oxidation of trimethylamine by OH radicals in aqueous solution as studied by pulse radiolysis, ESR and product analysis. Reactions of the alkyl-amino radical cation, the aminoalkyl radical and the protonated aminoalkyl radical. *Zeitschrift für Naturforschung*, **41b**, 505–513.

Das, S., Mieden, O.J., Pan, X.M., Repas, M., Schuchmann, M.N., Schuchmann, H.P., *et al.* (1988). Aspects of the $HO_2\cdot$ elimination reaction from organic peroxyl radicals: some recent examples. *Basic Life Science*, **49**, 55–58.

Das, B.S., Mohanty, S., Mishra, S.K., Patnaik, J.K., Satpathy, S.K., Mohanty, D., *et al.* (1991). Increased cerebrospinal fluid protein and lipid peroxidation products in patients with cerebral malaria. *Transactions of the Royal Society of Tropical Medicine and Hygiene*, **85**, 733–734.

Das, K.C., Lewis, M.Y., and White, C.W. (1995*a*). Activation of NF-kappa B and elevation of MnSOD gene expression by thiol reducing agents in lung adenocarcinoma (A549) cells. *American Journal of Physiology*, **269**, L588–L602.

Das, K.C., Lewis, M.Y., and White, C.W. (1995*b*). Thiol modulation of TNF alpha and IL-1 induced MnSOD gene expression and activation of NF-kappa B. *Molecular and Cellular Biochemistry*, **148**, 45–57.

Daugherty, A., Dunn, J.L., Rateri, D.L., and Heinecke, J.W. (1994). Myeloperoxidase, a catalyst for lipoprotein oxidation, is expressed in human atherosclerotic lesions. *Journal of Clinical Investigation*, **94**, 437–444.

Davidson, V.L. (1989). Steady-state kinetic analysis of the quinoprotein methylamine dehydrogenase from *Paracoccus denitrificans*. *Biochemical Journal*, **261**, 107–111.

Davidson, V.L. (1990). Quinoproteins: a new class of enzymes with potential use as biosensors. *American Biotechnology Laboratory*, **8**, 32–34.

Davidson, V.L., and Jones, L.H. (1991). Inhibition by cyclopropylamine of the quinoprotein methylamine dehydrogenase is mechanism-based and causes covalent cross-linking of alpha and beta subunits. *Biochemistry*, **30**, 1924–1928.

Davidson, V.L., and Jones, L.H. (1992). Cofactor-directed inactivation by nucleophilic amines of the quinoprotein methylamine dehydrogenase from *Paracoccus denitrificans*. *Biochimica et Biophysica Acta*, **1121**, 104–110.

Davidson, V.L., and Jones, L.H. (1995). Reaction mechanism for the inactivation of the quinoprotein methylamine dehydrogenase by phenylhydrazine. *Biochimica et Biophysica Acta*, **1252**, 146–150.

Davidson, V.L., Wu, J., Miller, B., and Jones, L.H. (1992*a*). Factors affecting the stability of methanol dehydrogenase from *Paracoccus denitrificans*. *FEMS Microbiology Letters*, **73**, 53–58.

Davidson, V.L., Kumar, M.A., and Wu, J.Y. (1992*b*). Apparent oxygen-dependent inhibition by superoxide dismutase of the quinoprotein methanol dehydrogenase. *Biochemistry*, **31**, 1504–1508.

Davidson, V.L., Jones, L.H., and Graichen, M.E. (1992*c*). Reactions of benzylamines with methylamine dehydrogenase. Evidence for a carbanionic reaction intermediate and reaction mechanism similar to eukaryotic quinoproteins. *Biochemistry*, **31**, 3385–3390.

Davidson, V.L., Graichen, M.E., and Jones, L.H. (1995). Mechanism of reaction of allylamine with the quinoprotein methylamine dehydrogenase. *Biochemical Journal*, **308**, 487–492.

Davies, J.M., Horwitz, D.A., and Davies, K.J.A (1993). Potential roles of hypochlorous acid and *N*-chloroamines in collagen breakdown by phagocytic cells in synovitis. *Free Radical Biology and Medicine*, **15**, 637–643.

Davies, J.M., Horwitz, D.A., and Davies, K.J.A. (1994). Inhibition of collagenase activity by *N*-chlorotaurine, a product of activated neutrophils. *Arthritis and Rheumatism*, **37**, 424–427.

Davies, J.M., Lowry, C.V., and Davies, K.J. (1995). Transient adaptation to oxidative stress in yeast. *Archives of Biochemistry and Biophysics*, **317**, 1–6.

Davies, K.J., Quintanilha, A.T., Brooks, G.A., and Packer, L. (1982). Free radicals and tissue damage produced by exercise. *Biochemical and Biophysical Research Communications*, **107**, 1198–1205.

Davies, K.J.A. (1985). Free radicals and protein degradation in human red blood cells. *Progress in Clinical Biology Research*, **195**, 15–27.

Davies, K.J.A. (1986). Intracellular proteolytic systems may function as secondary antioxidant defenses: an hypothesis. *Journal of Free Radical Biology and Medicine*, **2**, 155–173.

Davies, K.J.A. (1987). Protein damage and degradation by oxygen radicals. I. General aspects. *Journal of Biological Chemistry*, **262**, 9895–9901.

Davies, K.J.A (1988). A secondary antioxidant defense role for proteolytic systems. *Basic Life Science*, **49**, 575–585.

Davies, K.J.A. (1990). Protein oxidation and proteolytic degradation. General aspects and relationship to cataract formation. *Advances in Experimental Medicine and Biology*, **264**, 503–511.

Davies, K.J.A. (1993). Protein modification by oxidants and the role of proteolytic enzymes. *Biochemical Society Transactions*, **21**, 346–353.

Davies, K.J.A., and Delsignore, M.E. (1987). Protein damage and degradation by oxygen radicals. III. Modification of secondary and tertiary structure. *Journal of Biological Chemistry*, **262**, 9908–9913.

Davies, K.J.A., and Doroshow, J.H. (1986). Redox cycling of anthracyclines by cardiac mitochondria. I. Anthracycline radical formation by NADH dehydrogenase. *Journal of Biological Chemistry*, **261**, 3060–3067.

Davies, K.J.A., and Goldberg, A.L. (1987a). Oxygen radicals stimulate intracellular proteolysis and lipid peroxidation by independent mechanisms in erythrocytes. *Journal of Biological Chemistry*, **262**, 8220–8226.

Davies, K.J.A., and Goldberg, A.L. (1987b). Proteins damaged by oxygen radicals are rapidly degraded in extracts of red blood cells. *Journal of Biological Chemistry*, **262**, 8227–8234.

Davies, K.J.A, and Lin, S.W. (1988a). Degradation of oxidatively denatured proteins in *Escherichia coli*. *Free Radical Biology and Medicine*, **5**, 215–223.

Davies, K.J.A, and Lin, S.W. (1988b). Oxidatively denatured proteins are degraded by an ATP-independent proteolytic pathway in *Escherichia coli*. *Free Radical Biology and Medicine*, **5**, 225–236.

Davies, K.J.A., Sevanian, A., Muakkassah, K.S., and Hochstein, P. (1986). Uric acid-iron ion complexes. A new aspect of the antioxidant functions of uric acid. *Biochemical Journal*, **235**, 747–754.

Davies, K.J.A., Lin, S.W., and Pacifici, R.E. (1987a). Protein damage and degradation by oxygen radicals. IV. Degradation of denatured protein. *Journal of Biological Chemistry*, **262**, 9914–9920.

Davies, K.J.A., Delsignore, M.E., and Lin, S.W. (1987b). Protein damage and degradation by oxygen radicals. II. Modification of amino acids. *Journal of Biological Chemistry*, **262**, 9902–9907.

Davies, M.J. (1987). Applications of electron spin resonance spectroscopy to the identification of radicals produced during lipid peroxidation. *Chemistry and Physics of Lipids*, **44**, 149–173.

Davies, M.J. (1988). Detection of peroxyl and alkoxyl radicals produced by reaction of hydroperoxides with heme-proteins by electron spin resonance spectroscopy. *Biochimica et Biophysica Acta*, **964**, 28–35.

Davies, M.J. (1989a). Direct detection of radical production in the ischaemic and reperfused myocardium: current status. *Free Radical Research Communications*, 7, 275–284.

Davies, M.J. (1989b). Direct detection of peroxyl radicals formed in the reactions of metmyoglobin and methaemoglobin with *t*-butyl hydroperoxide. *Free Radical Research Communications*, 7, 27–32.

Davies, M.J. (1989c). Detection of peroxyl and alkoxyl radicals produced by reaction of hydroperoxides with rat liver microsomal fractions. *Biochemical Journal*, **257**, 603–606.

Davies, M.J. (1990a). Detection of myoglobin-derived radicals on reaction of metmyoglobin with hydrogen peroxide and other peroxidic compounds. *Free Radical Research Communications*, **10**, 361–370.

Davies, M.J. (1990b). Electron spin resonance studies on the degradation of hydroperoxides by rat liver cytosol. *Free Radical Research Communications*, **9**, 251–258.

Davies, M.J. (1991). Identification of a globin free radical in equine myoglobin treated with peroxides. *Biochimica et Biophysica Acta*, **1077**, 86–90.

Davies, M.J. (1993). Detection and identification of macromolecule-derived radicals by EPR spin trapping. *Research on Chemical Intermediates*, **19**, 669–679.

Davies, M.J. (1996). Protein and peptide alkoxyl radicals can give rise to C-terminal decarboxylation and backbone cleavage. *Archives of Biochemistry and Biophysics*, **336**, 163–172.

Davies, M.J., and Gilbert, B.C. (1991). Free radical reactions. fragmentation and rearrangements in aqueous solution. *Advances in Detailed Reaction Mechanisms*, **1**, 35–81.

Davies, M.J., and Puppo, A. (1993). Identification of the site of the globin-derived radical in leghaemoglobins. *Biochimica et Biophysica Acta*, **1202**, 182–188.

Davies, M.J., and Slater, T.F. (1986a). Studies on the photolytic breakdown of hydroperoxides and peroxidized fatty acids by using electron spin resonance spectroscopy. Spin trapping of alkoxyl and peroxyl radicals in organic solvents. *Biochemical Journal*, **240**, 789–795.

Davies, M.J., and Slater, T.F. (1986b). Electron spin resonance spin trapping studies on the photolytic generation of halocarbon radicals. *Chemico-Biological Interactions*, **58**, 137–147.

Davies, M.J., and Slater, T.F. (1987). Studies on the metal-ion and lipoxygenase-catalysed breakdown of hydroperoxides using electron-spin-resonance spectroscopy. *Biochemical Journal*, **245**, 167–173.

Davies, M.J., and Slater, T.F. (1988). The use of electron-spin-resonance techniques to detect free-radical formation and tissue damage. *Proceedings of the Nutrition Society*, **47**, 397–405.

Davies, M.J., and Rice-Evans, C.A. (1993). Detection of radicals in oxidised lipoproteins. *Biochemical Society Transactions*, **21**, 87S.

Davies, M.J., Gilbert, B.C., and Norman, R.O.C. (1983). Electron spin resonance studies. Part 64. The hydroxyl radical-induced decarboxylation of methionine and some related compounds. *Journal of the Chemical Society, Perkin Transactions*, **2**, 731–738.

Davies, M.J., Gilbert, B.C., McCleland, C.W., Thomas, C.B., and Young, J. (1984a). E.s.r. evidence for the multiplicity of side-chain oxidation pathways in the acid-catalysed decomposition of substituted hydroxycyclohexadienyl radicals. *Journal of the Chemical Society, Chemical Communications*, 966–967.

Davies, M.J., Gilbert, B.C., and Norman, R.O.C. (1984b). Electron spin resonance studies. Part 67. Oxidation of aliphatic sulphides and sulphoxides by the sulphate radical anion ($SO_4 \cdot^-$) and of aliphatic radicals by the peroxydisulphate anion ($S_2O_8^{2-}$). *Journal of the Chemical Society, Perkin Transactions*, 2 503–509.

Davies, M.J., Gilbert, B.C., Thomas, C.B., and Young, J. (1985). Electron spin resonance studies. Part 69. Oxidation of some aliphatic carboxylic acids, carboxylate anions, and related compounds by the sulphate radical anion, ($SO_4 \cdot^-$). *Journal of the Chemical Society, Perkin Transactions*, 2 1199–1204.

Davies, M.J., Donkor, R., Dunster, C.A., Gee, C.A., Jonas, S., and Willson, R.L. (1987a). Desferrioxamine (Desferal) and superoxide free radicals. Formation of an enzyme-damaging nitroxide. *Biochemical Journal*, **246**, 725–729.

Davies, M.J., Forni, L.G., and Shuter, S.L. (1987b). Electron spin resonance and pulse radiolysis studies on the spin trapping of sulphur-centered radicals. *Chemico-Biological Interactions*, **61**, 177–188.

Davies, M.J., Forni, L.G., and Willson, R.L. (1988). Vitamin E analogue Trolox C. E.s.r. and pulse-radiolysis studies of free-radical reactions. *Biochemical Journal*, **255**, 513–522.

Davies, M.J., Gilbert, B.C., and Haywood, R.M. (1991). Radical-induced damage to proteins: e.s.r. spin-trapping studies. *Free Radical Research Communications*, **15**, 111–127.

Davies, M.J., Gilbert, B.C., and Haywood, R.M. (1993). Radical-induced damage to bovine serum albumin: role of the cysteine residue. *Free Radical Research Communications*, **18**, 353–367.

Davies, M.J., Fu, S., and Dean, R.T. (1995). Protein hydroperoxides can give rise to reactive free radicals. *Biochemical Journal*, **305**, 643–649.

Davies, M.J., and Puppo, A. (1992). Direct detection of a globin-derived radical in leghaemoglobin treated with peroxides. *Biochemical Journal*, **281**, 197–201.

Davies, M.J., and Timmins, G.S. (1996). EPR spectroscopy of biologically relevant free radicals in cellular, *ex vivo*, and *in vivo* systems. In *Biomedical Applications of Spectroscopy*, (ed. R.J.H. Clark and R.E. Hester), pp. 217–266. John Wiley and Sons, Chichester.

Davis, D.A., Branca, A.A., Pallenberg, A.J., Marschner, T.M., Patt, L.M., Chatlynne, L.G., *et al.* (1995). Inhibition of the human immunodeficiency virus-1 protease and human immunodeficiency virus-1 replication by bathocuproine disulfonic acid Cu^{1+}. *Archives of Biochemistry and Biophysics*, **322**, 127–134.

Davis, D.A., Dorsey, K., Wingfield, P.T., Stahl, S.J., Kaufman, J., Fales, H.M., *et al.* (1996). Regulation of HIV-1 protease activity through cysteine modification. *Biochemistry*, **35**, 2482–2488.

Davis, J.C., and Averill, B.A. (1982). Evidence for a spin-coupled binuclear iron unit at the active site of the purple acid phosphatase from beef spleen. *Proceedings of the National Academy of Science of the United States of America*, **79**, 4623–4627.

Davis, M.D., and Kaufman, S. (1991). Studies on the partially uncoupled oxidation of tetrahydropterins by phenylalanine hydroxylase. *Neurochemistry Research*, **16**, 813–819.

Davis, M.D., Parniak, M.A., Kaufman, S., and Kempner, E. (1996). Structure-function relationships of phenylalanine hydroxylase revealed by radiation target analysis. *Archives of Biochemistry and Biophysics*, **325**, 235–241.

Davison, P.F. (1987). A versatile procedure for the radioiodination of proteins and labeling reagents. *Biochimica et Biophysica Acta*, **926**, 195–202.

Davy, S.L., Osborne, M.J., Breton, J., Moore, G.R., Thomson, A.J., Bertini, I., *et al.* (1995). Determination of the [Fe4S4]Cys4 cluster geometry of *Desulfovibrio africanus* ferredoxin I by ^{1}H NMR spectroscopy. *FEBS Letters*, **363**, 199–204.

Day, N.S., Ge, T., Codina, J., Birnbaumer, L., Vanhoutte, P.M., and Boulanger, C.M. (1995). Gi proteins and the response to 5-hydroxytryptamine in porcine cultured endothelial cells with impaired release of EDRF. *British Journal of Pharmacology*, **115**, 822–827.

de Bono, D.P., Yang, W.D., Davies, M.J., Collis, C.S., and Rice-Evans, C.A. (1994). Effects of *N*-methyl hexanoylhydroxamic acid (NMHH) and myoglobin on endothelial damage by hydrogen peroxide. *Cardiovascular Research*, **28**, 1641–1646.

De Meyer, G.R., Bult, H., and Herman, A.G. (1991). Early atherosclerosis is accompanied by a decreased rather than an increased accumulation of fatty acid hydroxyderivatives. *Biochemical Pharmacology*, **42**, 279–283.

De Sanctis, G., Falcioni, G., Giardina, B., Ascoli, F., and Brunori, M. (1986). Minimyoglobin: preparation and reaction with oxygen and carbon monoxide. *Journal of Molecular Biology*, **188**, 73–76.

de Silva, D., Miller, D.M., Reif, D.W., and Aust, S.D. (1992). *In vitro* loading of apoferritin. *Archives of Biochemistry and Biophysics*, **293**, 409–415.

de Silva, D., and Aust, S.D. (1992). Stoichiometry of Fe(II) oxidation during ceruloplasmin-catalyzed loading of ferritin. *Archives of Biochemistry and Biophysics*, **298**, 259–264.

Dean, R.T. (1975*a*). Lysosomal enzymes as agents of turnover of soluble cytoplasmic proteins. *European Journal of Biochemistry*, **58**, 9–14.

Dean, R.T. (1975*b*). Concerning a possible mechanism for selective capture of cytoplasmic proteins by lysosomes. *Biochemical and Biophysical Research Communications*, **67**, 604–609.

Dean, R.T. (1975*c*). Direct evidence of importance of lysosomes in degradation of intracellular proteins. *Nature*, **257**, 414–416.

Dean, R.T. (1976). The roles of cathepsins B1 and D in the digestion of cytoplasmic protiens *in vitro* by lysosomal extracts. *Biochemical and Biophysical Research Communications*, **68**, 518–523.

Dean, R.T. (1978). Selectivity in endocytosis of serum and cytosol proteins by macrophages in culture. *Biochemical and Biophysical Research Communications*, **85**, 815–819.

Dean, R.T. (1979). Macrophage protein turnover. Evidence for lysosomal participation in basal proteolysis. *Biochemical Journal*, **180**, 339–345.

Dean, R.T. (1980*a*). Lysosomes and protein degradation. *Ciba Foundation Symposia*, **75**, 139–149.

Dean, R.T. (1980*b*). Protein degradation in cell cultures: general considerations on mechanisms and regulation. *Federation Proceedings*, **39**, 15–19.

Dean, R.T. (1987*a*). A mechanism for accelerated degradation of intracellular proteins after limited damage by free radicals. *FEBS Letters*, **220**, 278–282.

Dean, R.T. (1987*b*). Free radicals, membrane damage and cell-mediated cytolysis. *British Journal of Cancer (Supplement)*, **8**, 39–45.

Dean, R.T., and Barrett, A.J. (1976). Lysosomes. *Essays in Biochemistry*, **12**, 1–40.

Dean, R.T., and Cheeseman, K.H. (1987). Vitamin E protects proteins against free radical damage in lipid environments. *Biochemical and Biophysical Research Communications*, **148**, 1277–1282.

Dean, R.T., and Nicholson, P. (1994). The action of nine chelators on iron-dependent radical damage. *Free Radical Research*, **20**, 83–101.

Dean, R.T., and Pollak, J.K. (1985). Endogenous free radical generation may influence proteolysis in mitochondria. *Biochemical and Biophysical Research Communications*, **126**, 1082–1089.

Dean, R.T., and Riley, P.A. (1978). The degradation of normal and analogue-containing proteins in MRC-5 fibroblasts. *Biochimica et Biophysica Acta*, **539**, 230–237.

Dean, R.T., and Schnebli, H.P. (1989). Control of exogenous proteinases and their inhibitors at the macrophage cell surface. *Biochimica et Biophysica Acta*, **992**, 174–180.

Dean, R., and Simpson, J. (1991). Free radical damage to proteins and its role in the immune response. *Molecular Aspects of Medicine*, **12**, 121–128.

Dean, R.T., Roberts, C.R., and Forni, L.G. (1984a). Oxygen-centred free radicals can efficiently degrade the polypeptide of proteoglycans in whole cartilage. *Bioscience Reports*, **4**, 1017–1026.

Dean, R.T., Jessup, W., and Roberts, C.R. (1984b). Effects of exogenous amines on mammalian cells, with particular reference to membrane flow. *Biochemical Journal*, **217**, 27–40.

Dean, R.T., Roberts, C.R., and Jessup, W. (1985). Fragmentation of extracellular and intracellular polypeptides by free radicals. *Progress in Clinical and Biological Research*, **180**, 341–350.

Dean, R.T., Thomas, S.M., Vince, G., and Wolff, S.P. (1986a). Oxidation induced proteolysis and its possible restriction by some secondary protein modifications. *Biomedica et Biochimica Acta*, **45**, 1563–1573.

Dean, R.T., Thomas, S.M., and Garner, A. (1986b). Free-radical-mediated fragmentation of monoamine oxidase in the mitochondrial membrane. Roles for lipid radicals. *Biochemical Journal*, **240**, 489–494.

Dean, R.T., Wolff, S.P., and McElligott, M.A. (1989a). Histidine and proline are important sites of free radical damage to proteins. *Free Radical Research Communications*, **7**, 97–103.

Dean, R.T., Nick, H.P., and Schnebli, H.P. (1989b). Free radicals inactivate human neutrophil elastase and its inhibitors with comparable efficiency. *Biochemical and Biophysical Research Communications*, **159**, 821–827.

Dean, R.T., Hunt, J.V., Grant, A.J., Yamamoto, Y., and Niki, E. (1991). Free radical damage to proteins: the influence of the relative localization of radical generation, antioxidants, and target proteins. *Free Radical Biology and Medicine*, **11**, 161–168.

Dean, R.T., Gebicki, J., Gieseg, S., Grant, A.J., and Simpson, J.A. (1992). Hypothesis: a damaging role in aging for reactive protein oxidation products? *Mutation Research*, **275**, 387–393.

Dean, R.T., Gieseg, S., and Davies, M.J. (1993). Reactive species and their accumulation on radical-damaged proteins. *Trends in Biochemical Science*, **18**, 437–441.

Dean, R.T., Armstrong, S.G., Fu, S., and Jessup, W. (1994). Oxidised proteins and their enzymatic proteolysis in eucaryotic cells: a critical appraisal. In *Free Radicals in the Environment, Medicine and Toxicology*, (ed. H. Nohl, H. Esterbauer, and C. Rice-Evans), pp. 47–79. Richelieu Press, London.

Dean, R.T., Fu, S., Gieseg, G., and Armstrong, S.G. (1996). Protein hydroperoxides, protein hydroxides, and protein-bound DOPA. In *Free Radicals: A Practical Approach*, (ed. N.A. Punchard and F.J. Kelly), pp. 171–183. IRL Press, Oxford.

Dee, G., Rice, E.C., Obeyesekera, S., Meraji, S., Jacobs, M., and Bruckdorfer, K.R. (1991). The modulation of ferryl myoglobin formation and its oxidative effects on low density lipoproteins by nitric oxide. *FEBS Letters*, **294**, 38–42.

Deegan, P.C., Mulloy, E., and McNicholas, W.T. (1995). Topical oropharyngeal anesthesia in patients with obstructive sleep apnea. *American Journal of Respiratory and Cellular Molecular Biology Critical Care Medicine*, **151**, 1108–1112.

DeFelippis, M.R., Faraggi, M., and Klapper, M.H. (1990). Evidence for through-bond long-range electron transfer in peptides. *Journal of the American Chemical Society*, **112**, 5640–5642.

DeGray, J.A., Lassmann, G., Curtis, J.F., Kennedy, T.A., Marnett, L.J., Eling, T.E., et al. (1992). Spectral analysis of the protein-derived tyrosyl radicals from prostaglandin H synthase. *Journal of Biological Chemistry*, **267**, 23583–23588.

Dekker, R.H., Duine, J.A., Frank, J., Verwiel, P.E., and Westerling, J. (1982). Covalent addition of H_2O, enzyme substrates and activators to pyrrolo-quinoline quinone, the coenzyme of quinoproteins. *European Journal of Biochemistry*, **125**, 69–73.

Del, C.J., Bartels, E., and Sobrino, J.A. (1972). Microelectrophoretic application of cholinergic compounds, protein oxidizing agents, and mercurials to the chemically excitable membrane of the electroplax. *Proceedings of the National Academy of Science of the United States of America*, **69**, 2081–2085.

Del Corso, A., Cappiello, M., and Mura, U. (1994). Thiol dependent oxidation of enzymes: the last chance against oxidative stress. *International Journal of Biochemistry*, **26**, 745–750.

Delbarre, B., Delbarre, G., Rochat, C., and Calinon, F. (1995). Effect of piribedil, a D-2 dopaminergic agonist, on dopamine, amino acids, and free radicals in gerbil brain after cerebral ischemia. *Molecular and Chemical Neuropathology*, **26**, 43–52.

Della, R.F., Granata, A., Broccio, M., Zirilli, A., and Broccio, G. (1995). Hemoglobin oxidative stress in cancer. *Anticancer Research*, **15**, 2089–2095.

DeMaster, E.G., Quast, B.J., Redfern, B., and Nagasawa, H.T. (1995). Reaction of nitric oxide with the free sulfydryl group of human serum albumin yields a sulfenic acid and nitrous oxide. *Biochemistry*, **34**, 11494–11499.

Denicola, A., Freeman, B.A., Trujillo, M., and Radi, R. (1996). Peroxynitrate reaction with carbon dioxide/bicarbonate: kinetics and influence on peroxynitrite-mediated oxidations. *Archives of Biochemistry and Biophysics*, **333**, 49–58.

Dennery, P.A., McDonagh, A.F., Spitz, D.R., Rodgers, P.A., and Stevenson, D.K. (1995). Hyperbilirubinemia results in reduced oxidative injury in neonatal Gunn rats exposed to hyperoxia. *Free Radical Biology and Medicine*, **19**, 395–404.

Deno, N.C. (1972). Free-radical chlorinations via nitrogen cation radicals. In *Methods in Free-Radical Chemistry*, (ed. E.S. Huyser), pp. 135–154. Marcel Dekher, New York.

DePillis, G.D., and Ortiz de Montellano, P.R. (1989). Substrate oxidation by the heme edge of fungal peroxidases. Reaction of *Coprinus macrorhizus* peroxidase with hydrazines and sodium azide. *Biochemistry*, **28**, 7947–7952.

Desai, I.D., and Tappel, A.L. (1963). Damage to proteins by peroxidized lipids. *Journal of Lipid Research*, **4**, 204–207.

Desai, I.D., Fletcher, B.L., and Tappel, A.L. (1975). Fluorescent pigments from uterus of vitamin E-deficient rats. *Lipids*, **10**, 307–309.

Desautels, M., and Goldberg, A.L. (1982). Liver mitochondria contain an ATP-dependent, vanadate-sensitive pathway for the degradation of proteins. *Proceedings of the National Academy of Science of the United States of America*, **79**, 1869–1873.

Deshpande, V.V., and Joshi, J.G. (1985). Vit C-Fe(III) induced loss of the covalently bound phosphate and enzyme activity of phosphoglucomutase. *Journal of Biological Chemistry*, **260**, 757–764.

Desos, P., Lepagnol, J.M., Morain, P., Lestage, P., and Cordi, A.A. (1996). Structure-activity relationships in a series of 2(1H)-quinolones bearing different acidic function in the 3-position: 6,7-dichloro-2(1H)-oxoquinoline-3-phosphonic acid, a new potent and selective AMPA/kainate antagonist with neuroprotective properties. *Journal of Medicinal Chemistry*, **39**, 197–206.

Dessauer, F. (1930). The question of the fundamental biological reaction of radiation. *Radiology*, **24**, 1–14.

Di Cola, D., Battista, P., Santarone, S., and Sacchetta, P. (1989). Fragmentation of human hemoglobin by oxidative stress produced by phenylhydrazine. *Free Radical Research Communications*, **6**, 379–386.

Di Simplicio, P., Cheeseman, K.H., and Slater, T.F. (1991). The reactivity of the SH group of bovine serum albumin with free radicals. *Free Radical Research Communications*, **14**, 253–262.

Di Simplicio, P., Lupis, E., and Rossi, R. (1996). Different mechanisms of formation of glutathione-protein mixed disulfides of diamide and *tert*-butyl hydroperoxide in rat blood. *Biochimica et Biophysica Acta*, **1289**, 252–260.

Dias, V.C., Fung, E., Snyder, F.F., Carter, R.J., and Parsons, H.G. (1990). Effects of medium-chain triglyceride feeding on energy balance in adult humans. *Metabolism*, **39**, 887–891.

Dice, J.F. (1987). Molecular determinants of protein half-lives in eukaryotic cells [published erratum appears in *FASEB Journal* (1988), **7**, 2262]. *FASEB Journal*, **1**, 349–357.

Dickson, R.C., and Tappel, A.L. (1969a). Effects of selenocystine and seleno-methionine on activation of sulfydryl enzymes. *Archives of Biochemistry and Biophysics*, **131**, 100–110.

Dickson, R.C., and Tappel, A.L. (1969b). Reduction of selenocystine by cysteine or glutathione. *Archives of Biochemistry and Biophysics*, **130**, 547–550.

Dijkstra, M., Frank, J., Jongejan, J.A., and Duine, J.A. (1984). Inactivation of quinoprotein alcohol dehydrogenases with cyclopropane-derived suicide substrates. *European Journal of Biochemistry*, **140**, 369–373.

Dillard, C.J., and Tappel, A.L. (1971). Fluorescent products of lipid peroxidation of mitochondria and microsomes. *Lipids*, **6**, 715–721.

Dillard, C.J., and Tappel, A.L. (1976). Do carbonylamine browning reactions occur *in vivo*? *Journal of Agricultural and Food Chemistry*, **24**, 74–77.

Dillard, C.J., and Tappel, A.L. (1979). Volatile hydrocarbon and carbonyl products of lipid peroxidation: a comparison of pentane, ethane, hexanal, and acetone as *in vivo* indices. *Lipids*, **14**, 989–995.

Dillard, C.J., and Tappel, A.L. (1984a). Lipid peroxidation and copper toxicity in rats. *Drug and Chemical Toxicology*, **7**, 477–487.

Dillard, C.J., and Tappel, A.L. (1984b). Fluorescent damage products of lipid peroxidation. *Methods in Enzymology*, **105**, 337–341.

Dillard, C.J., and Tappel, A.L. (1986). Mercury, silver, and gold inhibition of selenium-accelerated cysteine oxidation. *Journal of Inorganic Biochemistry*, **28**, 13–20.

Dillard, C.J., and Tappel, A.L. (1989). Lipid peroxidation products in biological tissues. *Free Radical Biology and Medicine*, **7**, 193–196.

Dillard, C.J., Reddy, K., Fletcher, B., Lumen, B.d., Langberg, S., Tappel, A.L., *et al.* (1972). Increased lysosomal enzymes in lungs of ozone-exposed rats. *Archives of Environmental Health*, **25**, 426–431.

Dillard, C.J., Dumelin, E.E., and Tappel, A.L. (1977). Effect of dietary vitamin E on expiration of pentane and ethane by the rat. *Lipids*, **12**, 109–114.

Dillard, C.J., Litov, R.E., Savin, W.M., Dumelin, E.E., and Tappel, A.L. (1978a). Effects of exercise, vitamin E, and ozone on pulmonary function and lipid peroxidation. *Journal of Applied Physiology*, **45**, 927–932.

Dillard, C.J., Litov, R.E., and Tappel, A.L. (1978b). Effects of dietary vitamin E, selenium, and polyunsaturated fats on *in vivo* lipid peroxidation in the rat as measured by pentane production. *Lipids*, **13**, 396–402.

Dillard, C.J., Sagai, M., and Tappel, A.L. (1980). Respiratory pentane: a measure of *in vivo* lipid peroxidation applied to rats fed diets varying in polyunsaturated fats, vitamin E, and selenium and exposed to nitrogen dioxide. *Toxicology Letters*, **6**, 251–256.

Dillard, C.J., Kunert, K.J., and Tappel, A.L. (1982a). Effects of vitamin E, ascorbic acid and mannitol on alloxan-induced lipid peroxidation in rats. *Archives of Biochemistry and Biophysics*, **216**, 204–212.

Dillard, C.J., Kunert, K.J., and Tappel, A.L. (1982b). Lipid peroxidation during chronic inflammation induced in rats by Freund's adjuvant: effect of vitamin E as measured by expired pentane. *Research Communications in Chemical Pathology and Pharmacology*, **37**, 143–146.

Dillard, C.J., Gavino, V.C., and Tappel, A.L. (1983). Relative antioxidant effectiveness of alpha-tocopherol and gamma-tocopherol in iron-loaded rats. *Journal of Nutrition*, **113**, 2266–2273.

Dillard, C.J., Downey, J.E., and Tappel, A.L. (1984). Effect of antioxidants on lipid peroxidation in iron-loaded rats. *Lipids*, **19**, 127–133.

Dillard, C.J., Hu, M.L., and Tappel, A.L. (1987). Effect of aurothioglucose on glutathione and glutathione-metabolizing and related enzymes in rat liver and kidney. *Chemico-Biological Interactions*, **64**, 103–114.

Dillard, C.J., Hu, M.L., and Tappel, A.L. (1991). Vitamin E, diethylmaleate and bromotrichloromethane interactions in oxidative damage *in vivo*. *Free Radical Biology and Medicine*, **10**, 51–60.

Dixon, J.S., and Jen, P.Y. (1995). Development of nerves containing nitric oxide synthase in the human male urogenital organs. *British Journal of Urology*, **76**, 719–725.

Dixon, M., and Meldrum, N.U. (1929). A crystalline tripeptide from living cells. *Nature*, **124**, 512.

Dizdaroglu, M. (1984). The use of capillary gas chromatography-mass spectrometry for identification of radiation-induced DNA base damage and DNA base-amino acid cross-links. *Journal of Chromatography*, **295**, 103–121.

Dizdaroglu, M. (1991). Chemical determination of free radical-induced damage to DNA. *Free Radical Biology and Medicine*, **10**, 225–242.

Dizdaroglu, M. (1992). Oxidative damage to DNA in mammalian chromatin. *Mutation Research*, **275**, 331–342.

Dizdaroglu, M., and Gajewski, E. (1989). Structure and mechanism of hydroxyl radical-induced formation of a DNA-protein cross-link involving thymine and lysine in nucleohistone. *Cancer Research*, **49**, 3463–3467.

Dizdaroglu, M., and Gajewski, E. (1990). Selected-ion mass spectrometry: assays of oxidative DNA damage. *Methods in Enzymology*, **186**, 530–544.

Dizdaroglu, M., and Krutzsch, H.C. (1983). Comparison of reversed-phase and weak anion-exchange high-performance liquid chromatographic methods for peptide separations. *Journal of Chromatography*, **264**, 223–229.

Dizdaroglu, M., and Simic, M.G. (1980). Radiation induced conversion of phenylalanine to tyrosines. *Radiation Research*, **83**, 437.

Dizdaroglu, M., and Simic, M.G. (1983). Isolation and characterization of radiation-induced aliphatic peptide dimers. *International Journal of Radiation Biology and Related Studies in Physics, Chemistry and Medicine*, **44**, 231–239.

Dizdaroglu, M., and Simic, M.G. (1985). Radiation-induced crosslinks between thymine and phenylalanine. *International Journal of Radiation Biology and Related Studies in Physics, Chemistry and Medicine*, **47**, 63–69.

Dizdaroglu, M., Gajewski, E., Simic, M.G., and Krutzsch, H.C. (1983). Identification of some OH radical-induced products of lysozyme. *International Journal of Radiation Biology and Related Studies in Physics, Chemistry and Medicine*, **43**, 185–193.

Dizdaroglu, M., Gajewski, E., and Simic, M.G. (1984). Enzymatic digestibility of peptides cross-linked by ionizing radiation. *International Journal of Radiation Biology and Related Studies in Physics, Chemistry and Medicine*, **45**, 283–295.

Dizdaroglu, M., Gajewski, E., Reddy, P., and Margolis, S.A. (1989). Structure of a hydroxyl radical induced DNA-protein cross-link involving thymine and tyrosine in nucleohistone. *Biochemistry*, **28**, 3625–3628.

Do, N.A. (1976). [Nitrotyrosyl]cytochrome *c*. Studies of the effect of iron binding, protein denaturants and oxidation-reduction potentials. *Biochemical Journal*, **155**, 589–597.

Dodd, N.J.F., Swallow, A.J., and Ley, F.J. (1985). Use of ESR to Identify Irradiated Food. *Radiation Physics and Chemistry*, **26**, 451–453.

Dodds, A.W., Ren, X.D., Willis, A.C., and Law, S.K. (1996). The reaction mechanism of the internal thioester in the human complement component C4. *Nature*, **379**, 177–179.

Doerge, D.R., and Divi, R.L. (1995). Porphyrin pi-cation and protein radicals in peroxidase catalysis and inhibition by anti-thyroid chemicals. *Xenobiotica*, **25**, 761–767.

Doerge, D.R., Cooray, N.M., and Brewster, M.E. (1991). Peroxidase-catalyzed S-oxygenation: mechanism of oxygen transfer for lactoperoxidase. *Biochemistry*, **30**, 8960–8964.

Dogan, I., Steenken, S., Schulte-Frohlinde, D., and Icli, S. (1990). Electron spin resonance and pulse radiolysis studies on the reaction of OH and SO_4^- with five-membered heterocyclic compounds in aqueous solution. *Journal of Physical Chemistry*, **94**, 1887–1894.

Dogterom, P., Mulder, G.J., and Nagelkerke, J.F. (1989). Lipid peroxidation-dependent and -independent protein thiol modifications in isolated rat hepatocytes: differential effects of vitamin E and disulfiram. *Chemico-Biological Interactions*, **71**, 291–306.

Dokter, P., Frank, J., and Duine, J.A. (1986). Purification and characterization of quinoprotein glucose dehydrogenase from *Acinetobacter calcoaceticus L.M.D. 79.41*. *Biochemical Journal*, **239**, 163–167.

Dokter, P., van Wielink, J.E., van Kleet, M.A., and Duine, J.A. (1988). Cytochrome *b*-562 from *Acinetobacter calcoaceticus L.M.D. 79.41*. Its characteristics and role as electron acceptor for quinoprotein glucose dehydrogenase. *Biochemical Journal*, **254**, 131–138.

Dolla, A., Blanchard, L., Guerlesquin, F., and Bruschi, M. (1994). The protein moiety modulates the redox potential in cytochromes *c*. *Biochimie*, **76**, 471–479.

Dolovich, J., Sagona, M., Pearson, F., Buccholz, D., Hiner, E., and Marshall, C. (1987). Sensitization of repeat plasmapheresis donors to ethylene oxide gas. *Transfusion*, **27**, 90–93.

Domigan, N.M., Charlton, T.S., Duncan, M.W., Winterbourn, C.C., and Kettle, A.J. (1995). Chlorination of tyrosyl residues in peptides by myeloperoxidase and human neutrophils. *Journal of Biological Chemistry*, **270**, 16542–16548.

Donatus, I.A., Sardjoko, and Vermeulen, N.P. (1990). Cytotoxic and cytoprotective activities of curcumin. Effects on paracetamol-induced cytotoxicity, lipid peroxidation and glutathione depletion in rat hepatocytes. *Biochemical Pharmacology*, **39**, 1869–1875.

Dong, A.C., Huang, P., and Caughey, W.S. (1992). Redox-dependent changes in beta-extended chain and turn structures of cytochrome *c* in water solution determined by second derivative amide I infrared spectra. *Biochemistry*, **31**, 182–189.

Donnelly, T.J., Pelling, J.C., Anderson, C.L., and Dalbey, D. (1987). Benzoyl peroxide activation of protein kinase C activity in epidermal cell membranes. *Carcinogenesis*, **8**, 1871–1874.

Dooley, D.M., and Brown, D.E. (1995). Resonance Raman spectroscopy of quinoproteins. *Methods in Enzymology*, **258**, 132–140.

Dooley, D.M., McGuirl, M.A., Brown, D.E., Turowski, P.N., McIntire, W.S., and Knowles, P.F. (1991). A Cu(I)-semiquinone state in substrate-reduced amine oxidases. *Nature*, **349**, 262–264.

Dooley, M.M., and Pryor, W.A. (1982). Free radical pathology: inactivation of human alpha-1-proteinase inhibitor by products from the reaction of nitrogen dioxide with hydrogen peroxide and the etiology of emphysema. *Biochemical and Biophysical Research Communications*, **106**, 981–987.

Dorman, C.J. (1995). 1995 Flemming Lecture. DNA topology and the global control of bacterial gene expression: implications for the regulation of virulence gene expression. *Microbiology*, **141**, 1271–1280.

Doroshow, J.H., and Davies, K.J. (1986). Redox cycling of anthracyclines by cardiac mitochondria. II. Formation of superoxide anion, hydrogen peroxide, and hydroxyl radical. *Journal of Biological Chemistry*, **261**, 3068–3074.

Doskeland, A.P., Martinez, A., Knappskog, P.M., and Flatmark, T. (1996). Phosphorylation of recombinant human phenylalanine hydroxylase: effect on catalytic activity, substrate activation and protection against non-specific cleavage of the fusion protein by restriction protease. *Biochemical Journal*, **313**, 409–414.

Douillet, C., Chancerelle, Y., Cruz, C., Maroncles, C., Kergonou, J.F., Renaud, S., *et al.* (1993). High dosage vitamin E effect on oxidative status and serum lipids distribution in streptozotocin-induced diabetic rats. *Biochemistry and Medical Metabolic Biology*, **50**, 265–276.

Downey, J.E., Irving, D.H., and Tappel, A.L. (1978). Effects of dietary antioxidants on *in vivo* lipid peroxidation in the rat as measured by pentane production. *Lipids*, **13**, 403–407.

Downey, J.M., Miura, T., Eddy, L.J., Chambers, D.E., Mellert, T., Hearse, D.J., *et al.* (1987). Xanthine oxidase is not a source of free radicals in the ischemic rabbit heart. *Journal of Molecular and Cellular Cardiology*, **19**, 1053–1060.

Dowton, M., and Austin, A.D. (1995). Increased genetic diversity in mitochondrial genes is correlated with the evolution of parasitism in the Hymenoptera. *Journal of Molecular Evolution*, **41**, 958–965.

Drake, I.M., Davies, M.J., Mapstone, N.P., Dixon, M.F., Schorah, C.J., White, K.L., *et al.* (1996). Ascorbic acid may protect against human gastric cancer by scavenging mucosal oxygen radicals. *Carcinogenesis*, **17**, 559–562.

Drake, M.D., Giffee, J.W., Johnson, D.W., and Koenig, V.L. (1957). Chemical effects of ionising radiation on proteins. I. Effect of gamma-radiation on amino acid content of insulin. *Journal of the American Chemical Society*, **79**, 1395–1401.

Draper, H.H., Agarwal, S., Nelson, D.E., Wee, J.J., Ghoshal, A.K., and Farber, E. (1995). Effects of peroxidative stress and age on the concentration of a deoxy-guanosine-malondialdehyde adduct in rat DNA. *Lipids*, **30**, 959–961.

Dreher, D., Vargas, J.R., Hochstrasser, D.F., and Junod, A.F. (1995). Effects of oxidative stress and Ca^{2+} agonists on molecular chaperones in human umbilical vein endothelial cells. *Electrophoresis*, **16**, 1205–1214.

Drepper, F., Hippler, M., Nitschke, W., and Haehnel, W. (1996). Binding dynamics and electron transfer between plastocyanin and photosystem I. *Biochemistry*, **35**, 1282–1295.

Dreval', A.V., Anykina, N.V., Tishin, D.P., Vysotskii, V.G., Iatsyshina, T.A., Gorodetskii, V.K., *et al.* (1994). Effect of soybean protein isolate on energy substrate oxidation in patients with insulin-dependent diabetes mellitus. *Problems Endokrinology Moskow*, **40**, 21–25.

Droge, W., Schulze, O.K., Mihm, S., Galter, D., Schenk, H., Eck, H.P., *et al.* (1994). Functions of glutathione and glutathione disulfide in immunology and immunopathology. *FASEB Journal*, **8**, 1131–1138.

Dubbelman, T.M., de Goeij, A.F., and van Steveninck, J. (1978). Photodynamic effects of protoporphyrin on human erythrocytes. Nature of the cross-linking of membrane proteins. *Biochimica et Biophysica Acta*, **511**, 141–151.

Dubbelman, T.M., Haasnoot, C., and van Steveninck, J. (1980). Temperature dependence of photodynamic red cell membrane damage. *Biochimica et Biophysica Acta*, **601**, 220–227.

Dubey, A., Forster, M.J., and Sohal, R.S. (1995). Effect of the spin-trapping compound N-tert-butyl-alpha-phenylnitrone on protein oxidation and life span. *Archives of Biochemistry and Biophysics*, **324**, 249–254.

Duda, W. (1981). Effect of γ-irradiation on the α and β chains on bovine hemoglobin and globin. *Radiation Research*, **86**, 123–132.

Dudman, N.P., Wilcken, D.E., and Stocker, R. (1993). Circulating lipid hydroper-oxide levels in human hyperhomocysteinemia. Relevance to development of arteriosclerosis. *Arteriosclerosis and Thrombosis*, **13**, 512–516.

Duh, J.L., Zhu, H., Shertzer, H.G., Nebert, D.W., and Puga, A. (1995). The Y-box motif mediates redox-dependent transcriptional activation in mouse cells. *Journal of Biological Chemistry*, **270**, 30499–30507.

Duine, J.A. (1989). PQQ and quinoprotein research—the first decade. *Biofactors*, **2**, 87–94.

Dumelin, E.E., and Tappel, A.L. (1977). Hydrocarbon gases produced during *in vitro* peroxidation of polyunsaturated fatty acids and decomposition of preformed hydroperoxides. *Lipids*, **12**, 894–900.

Dumelin, E.E., Dillard, C.J., and Tappel, A.L. (1978a). Breath ethane and pentane. *Environmental Research*, **15**, 38–43.

Dumelin, E.E., Dillard, C.J., and Tappel, A.L. (1978b). Effect of vitamin E and ozone on pentane and ethane expired by rats. *Archives of Environmental Health*, **33**, 129–135.

Dunn, J.A., McCance, D.R., Thorpe, S.R., Lyons, T.J., and Baynes, J.W. (1991). Age-dependent accumulation of N-epsilon-(carboxymethyl)lysine and N-epsilon-(carboxymethyl)hydroxylysine in human skin collagen. *Biochemistry*, **30**, 1205–1210.

Duran, L., and Tappel, A.L. (1958). Production of carbonyl compounds and sulfur compounds on irradiation of amino acids. *Radiation Research*, **9**, 498–501.

Durante, W., Kroll, M.H., Orloff, G.J., Cunningham, J.M., Scott, B.T., Vanhoutte, P.M., *et al.* (1996). Regulation of interleukin-1-beta-stimulated inducible nitric oxide synthase expression in cultured vascular smooth muscle cells by hemostatic proteins. *Biochemical Pharmacology*, **51**, 847–853.

Dutton, J., Copeland, L.G., Playfer, J.R., and Roberts, N.B. (1993). Measuring L-dopa in plasma and urine to monitor therapy of elderly patients with Parkinson disease treated with L-dopa and a dopa decarboxylase inhibitor. *Clinical Chemistry*, **39**, 629–634.

Dwyer, S.C., Legendre, L., Low, P.S., and Leto, T.L. (1996). Plant and human neutrophil oxidative burst complexes contain immunologically related proteins. *Biochimica et Biophysica Acta*, **1289**, 231–237.

Dykens, J.A. (1994). Isolated cerebral and cerebellar mitochondria produce free radicals when exposed to elevated CA^{2+} and Na^+: implications for neurodegeneration. *Journal of Neurochemistry*, **63**, 584–591.

Dyrks, T., Dyrks, E., Masters, C.L., and Beyreuther, K. (1993). Amyloidogenicity of rodent and human beta A4 sequences. *FEBS Letters*, **324**, 231–236.

Eager, J.E. (1966). Alanine-3-sulphinic acid in partial hydrolysates of oxidized proteins. *Biochemical Journal*, **100**, 37–38.

Easton, C.J. (1991). α-Carbon-centred radicals from amino acids and their derivatives. In *Advances in Detailed Reaction Mechanisms*, (ed. J.M. Coxon), pp. 83–126. JAI Press, Greenwich, Connecticut.

Easton, C.J. (1997). Free radical reactions in the synthesis of α-amino acids and derivatives. *Chemical Reviews*, **97**, 53–82.

Easton, C.J., and Hay, M.P. (1985). Regioselectivity in formations of amidocarboxy-substituted free radicals. *Journal of the Chemical Society, Chemical Communications*, 425–427.

Easton, C.J., and Hay, M.P. (1986). Preferential reactivity of glycine residues in free radical reactions of amino acid derivatives. *Journal of the Chemical Society, Chemical Communications*, 55–57.

Easton, C.J., Hay, M.P., and Love, S.G. (1988). Regioselective formation of amidocarboxy-substituted free radicals. *Journal of the Chemical Society, Perkin Transactions 1*, 265–268.

Eberhart, M.K. (1974). Radiation induced homolytic aromatic substitution. II. Hydroxylation and phenylation of benzene. *Journal of Physical Chemistry*, **78**, 1795–1797.

Ebert, M., Keene, J.P., Swallow, A.J., and Baxendale, J.H. (1965) *Pulse Radiolysis* Academic Press, New York.

Edelbacher, S. (1924). Oxidative and reductive cleavage of proteins. *Zeitschrift für Physiologische Chemie*, **134**, 129–139.

Edwards, G.W., and Minthorn, M.J. (1968). Preparation and properties of the optical antipodes of beta-methoxyvaline and beta-hydroxyvaline. *Canadian Journal of Biochemistry*, **46**, 1227–1230.

Ehrenberger, K., Felix, D., and Svozil, K. (1995). Origin of auditory fractal random signals in guinea pigs. *Neuroreport*, **6**, 2117–2120.

Eiserich, J.P., Vossen, V., O'Neill, C.A., Halliwell, B., Cross, C.E., and van, d.V.A. (1994). Molecular mechanisms of damage by excess nitrogen oxides: nitration of tyrosine by gas-phase cigarette smoke. *FEBS Letters*, **353**, 53–56.

Eiserich, J.P., van der Vliet, A., Handelman, G.J., Halliwell, B., and Cross, C.E. (1995a). Dietary antioxidants and cigarette smoke-induced biomolecular damage:

a complex interaction. *American Journal of Clinical Nutrition*, **62 (Supplement 6)**, 1490S-1500S.

Eiserich, J.P., Butler, J., van er Vliet, A., Cross, C.E., and Halliwell, B. (1995*b*). Nitric oxide rapidly scavenges tyrosine and tryptophan radicals. *Biochemical Journal*, **310**, 745–749.

Eiserich, J.P., Cross, C.E., Jones, A.D., Halliwell, B., and van der Vliet, A. (1996). Formation of nitrating and chlorinating species by reaction of nitrite with hypochlorous acid. *Journal of Biological Chemistry*, **271**,19199–19208.

Ekberg, M., Sahlin, M., Eriksson, M., Sjoberg, B.-M. (1996). Two conserved tyrosine residues in protein R1 participate in an intermolecular electron transfer in ribonucleotide reductase. *Journal of Biological Chemistry*, **271**, 20655–20659.

Ekert, B., Giocanti, N., and Sabattier, R. (1986). Study of several factors in RNA-protein cross-link formation induced by ionizing radiations within 70S ribosomes of *E. coli* MRE 600. *International Journal of Radiation Biology and Related Studies in Physics, Chemistry and Medicine*, **50**, 507–525.

El, T.M., Pokorny, J., and Janicek, G. (1971). Reaction of oxidized lipids with proteins. 6. Binding of peroxide fractions of oxidized lipids. *Nahrung*, **15**, 663–670.

Elad, D., and Sperling, J. (1969). Photochemical modification of glycine dipeptides. *Journal of the Chemical Society (C)* 1579–1585.

Elgren, T.E., Lynch, J.B., Juarez, G.C., Munck, E., Sjoberg, B.M., and Que, L.J. (1991). Electron transfer associated with oxygen activation in the B2 protein of ribonucleotide reductase from *Escherichia coli*. *Journal of Biological Chemistry*, **266**, 19265–19268.

Elliot, A.J., McEachern, R.J., and Armstrong, D.A. (1981). Oxidation of amino-containing disulphides by $Br_2 \cdot^-$ and HO$\cdot$. A pulse radiolysis study. *Journal of Physical Chemistry*, **85**, 68–75.

Elliot, A.J., Simsons, A.S., and Sopchyshyn, F.C. (1984). Radiolysis of solutions containing organo-disulphides. *Radiation Physics and Chemistry*, **23**, 377–384.

Elmoselhi, A.B., Butcher, A., Samson, S.E., and Grover, A.K. (1994). Free radicals uncouple the sodium pump in pig coronary artery. *American Journal of Physiology*, **266**, C720–C728.

Engels, F., Willems, H., and Nijkamp, F.P. (1986). Cyclooxygenase-catalyzed formation of 9-hydroxylinoleic acid by guinea pig alveolar macrophages under non-stimulated conditions. *FEBS Letters*, **209**, 249–253.

Engfeldt, O. (1922). The action of Dakin hypochlorite solution on certain organic substanes. *Zeitschrift für Physiologische Chemie*, **121**, 18–61.

Englisch, S., Englisch, U., von, d.H.F., and Cramer, F. (1986). The proofreading of hydroxy analogues of leucine and isoleucine by leucyl-tRNA synthetases from *E. coli* and yeast. *Nucleic Acids Research*, **14**, 7529–7539.

Englisch, P.S., von, d.H.F., and Cramer, F. (1990). Fidelity in the aminoacylation of tRNA(Val) with hydroxy analogues of valine, leucine, and isoleucine by valyl-tRNA synthetases from *Saccharomyces cerevisiae* and *Escherichia coli*. *Biochemistry*, **29**, 7953–7958.

Enochs, W.S., Sarna, T., Zecca, L., Riley, P.A., and Swartz, H.M. (1994). The roles of neuromelanin, binding of metal ions, and oxidative cytotoxicity in the pathogenesis of Parkinson's disease: a hypothesis. *Journal of Neural Transmission Parkinson's Disease and Dementia Section*, **7**, 83–100.

Epshtein, Y.A., and Zabozlaeva, E.A. (1955). The digestion by pepsin of serum albumin which has been irradiated with gamma-rays. *Biokhimiya*, **20**, 701–704.

Erben-Russ, M., Michel, C., Bors, W., and Saran, M. (1987). Absolute rate constants of alkoxyl radical reactions in aqueous solution. *Journal of Physical Chemistry*, **91**, 2362–2365.

Erickson, M.C., and Hultin, H.O. (1992). Influence of histidine on lipid peroxidation in sarcoplasmic reticulum. *Archives of Biochemistry and Biophysics*, **292**, 427–432.

Ericsson, M., Tarnvik, A., Kuoppa, K., Sandstrom, G., and Sjostedt, A. (1994). Increased synthesis of DnaK, GroEL, and GroES homologs by *Francisella tularensis* LVS in response to heat and hydrogen peroxide. *Infection and Immunity*, **62**, 178–183.

Eriquez, L.A., and Pisano, M.A. (1979). Isolation and nature of intracellular alpha-aminoadipic acid-containing peptides from *Paecilomyces persicinus P-10*. *Antimicrobial Agents and Chemotherapeutics*, **16**, 392–397.

Erlenmeyer, H., Brintzinger, H., Sigel, H., and Curtius, H.C. (1965). Structure specific oxidative working of peptide-metal complexes. *Experientia*, **21**, 371–372.

Ermacora, M.R., Delfino, J.M., Cuenoud, B., Schepartz, A., and Fox, R.O. (1992). Conformation-dependent cleavage of staphylococcal nuclease with a disulfide-linked iron chelate. *Proceedings of the National Academy of Science of the United States of America*, **89**, 6383–6387.

Erman, J.E., and Yonetani, T. (1975). A kinetic study of the endogenous reduction of the oxidized sites in the primary cytochrome *c* peroxidase-hydrogen peroxide compound. *Biochimica et Biophysica Acta*, **393**, 350–357.

Erman, J.E., Vitello, L.B., Mauro, J.M., and Kraut, J. (1989). Detection of an oxyferryl porphyrin pi-cation-radical intermediate in the reaction between hydrogen peroxide and a mutant yeast cytochrome *c* peroxidase. Evidence for tryptophan-191 involvement in the radical site of compound I. *Biochemistry*, **28**, 7992–7995.

Ermler, U., Siddiqui, R.A., Cramm, R., and Friedrich, B. (1995). Crystal structure of the flavohemoglobin from *Alcaligenes eutrophus* at 1.75 Å resolution. *EMBO Journal*, **14**, 6067–6077.

Erve, J.C., Barofsky, E., Barofsky, D.F., Deinzer, M.L., and Reed, D.J. (1995). Alkylation of *Escherichia coli* thioredoxin by S-(2-chloroethyl)glutathione and identification of the adduct on the active site cysteine-32 by mass spectrometry. *Chemical Research Toxicology*, **8**, 934–941.

Esclade, L., Guillochon, D., and Thomas, D. (1986). Aromatic hydroxylations in peroxidations by haemoglobin systems. *Xenobiotica*, **16**, 615–624.

Eshhar, N., Striem, S., Kohen, R., Tirosh, O., and Biegon, A. (1995). Neuroprotective and antioxidant activities of HU-211, a novel NMDA receptor antagonist. *European Journal of Pharmacology*, **283**, 19–29.

Esposito, F., Agosti, V., Morrone, G., Morra, F., Cuomo, C., Russo, T., *et al*. (1994). Inhibition of the differentiation of human myeloid cell lines by redox changes induced through glutathione depletion. *Biochemical Journal*, **301**, 649–653.

Estell, D.A., Graycar, T.P., and Wells, J.A. (1985). Engineering an enzyme by site-directed mutagenesis to be resistant to chemical oxidation. *Journal of Biological Chemistry*, **260**, 6518–6521.

Esterbauer, H., Gebicki, J., Puhl, H., and Jurgens, G. (1992). The role of lipid peroxidation and antioxidants in oxidative modification of LDL. *Free Radical Biology and Medicine*, **13**, 341–390.

Ettner, N., Metzger, J.W., Lederer, T., Hulmes, J.D., Kisker, C., Hinrichs, W., *et al*. (1995). Proximity mapping of the Tet repressor-tetracycline-Fe^{2+} complex by hydrogen peroxide mediated protein cleavage. *Biochemistry*, **34**, 22–31.

Evans, M.J. (1984). Oxidant gases. *Environmental Health Perspectives*, **55**, 85–95.

Evans, R.F., Ghiron, C.A., Volkert, W.A., and Kuntz, R.R. (1976). Flash photolysis of N-acetyl-L-tryptophanamide; acid-base equilibrium of the radical transients. *Chemical Physics Letters*, **42**, 43–45.

Everett, S.A., and Wardman, P. (1995). Perthiols as antioxidants: radical-scavenging and prooxidative mechanisms. *Methods in Enzymology*, **251**, 55–69.

Everett, S.A., Folkes, L.K., Wardman, P., and Asmus, K.D. (1994). Free-radical repair by a novel perthiol: reversible hydrogen transfer and perthiyl radical formation. *Free Radical Research*, **20**, 387–400.

Everett, S.A., Dennis, M.F., Patel, K.B., Stratford, M.R.L., and Wardman, P. (1996). Oxidative denitrification of N^w-hydroxy-L-arginine by the superoxide radical anion. *Biochemical Journal*, **317**, 17–21.

Fadel, M.M., Foley, P.L., Kassell, N.F., and Lee, K.S. (1995). Histidine attenuates cerebral vasospasm in a rabbit model of subarachnoid hemorrhage. *Surgical Neurology*, **43**, 52–57.

Fagan, J.M., and Goldberg, A.L. (1985). The rate of protein degradation in isolated skeletal muscle does not correlate with reduction-oxidation status. *Biochemical Journal*, **227**, 689–694.

Fagan, J.M., and Waxman, L. (1992). The ATP-independent pathway in red blood cells that degrades oxidant-damaged hemoglobin. *Journal of Biological Chemistry*, **267**, 23015–23022.

Fagan, J.M., Waxman, L., and Goldberg, A.L. (1986). Red blood cells contain a pathway for the degradation of oxidant-damaged hemoglobin that does not require ATP or ubiquitin. *Journal of Biological Chemistry*, **261**, 5705–5713.

Falck, B., Hillarp, N.A., Thieme, G., and Torp, A. (1982). Fluorescence of catechol amines and related compounds condensed with formaldehyde. *Brain Research Bulletin*, **9**, 11–15.

Fan, B.R., Bruni, R., Taeusch, H.W., Findlay, R., and Waring, A.J. (1991). Antibodies against synthetic amphipathic helical sequences of surfactant protein SP-B detect a conformational change in the native protein. *FEBS Letters*, **282**, 220–224.

Fantone, J., Jester, S., and Loomis, T. (1989). Metmyoglobin promotes arachidonic acid peroxidation at acid pH. *Journal of Biological Chemistry*, **264**, 9408–9411.

Faraggi, M., and Klapper, M.H. (1988). Intramolecular long-range electron transfer in the α-hemoglobin subunit. *Journal of the American Chemical Society*, **110**, 5753–5756.

Faraggi, M., Redpath, J.L., and Tal, Y. (1975). Pulse radiolysis studies of electron transfer reaction in molecules of biological interest. I. The reduction of a disulfide bridge by peptide radicals. *Radiation Research*, **64**, 452–466.

Faraggi, M., Klapper, M.H., and Dorfman, L.M. (1978). Fast reaction kinetics of one-electron transfer in proteins. The histidyl radical. Mode of electron migration. *Journal of Physical Chemistry*, **82**, 508–512.

Faraggi, M., Steiner, J.P., and Klapper, M.H. (1985). Intramolecular electron and proton transfer in proteins: CO_2-reduction of riboflavin binding protein and ribonuclease A. *Biochemistry*, **24**, 3273–3279.

Faraggi, M., DeFelippis, M.R., and Klapper, M.H. (1989). Long-range electron transfer between tyrosine and tryptophan in peptides. *Journal of the American Chemical Society*, **111**, 5141–5145.

Farber, J.M., and Levine, R.L. (1986). Sequence of a peptide susceptible to mixed-function oxidation. Probable cation binding site in glutamine synthetase. *Journal of Biological Chemistry*, **261**, 4574–4578.

Fares, F.A., Gruener, N., Carmeli, E., and Reznick, A.Z. (1996). Growth hormone (GH) retardation of muscle damage due to immobilization in old rats. Possible intervention with a new long-acting recombinant GH. *Annals of the New York Academy of Science*, **786**, 430–443.

Farkas, J., and Menzel, E.J. (1995). Proteins lose their nitric oxide stabilizing function after advanced glycosylation. *Biochimica et Biophysica Acta*, **1245**, 305–310.

Farmer, K.J., and Sohal, R.S. (1987). Effects of ambient temperature on free radical generation, antioxidant defenses and life span in the adult housefly, *Musca domestica*. *Experimental Gerontology*, **22**, 59–65.

Farmer, K.J., and Sohal, R.S. (1989). Relationship between superoxide anion radical generation and aging in the housefly, *Musca domestica*. *Free Radical Biology and Medicine*, **7**, 23–29.

Faulstich, H., and Trischmann, H. (1970). Peptide syntheses, XLVI. Synthesis of peptides of gamma-hydroxyleucine. *Justus Liebigs Annalen Chemie*, **741**, 55–63.

Favaudon, V. (1989). Hydroxyl radical-induced crosslinking between double-stranded poly(dA-dT) and tripeptides containing an aromatic residue. *Free Radical Research*, **6**, 157–159.

Favaudon, V., Tourbez, H., Houee, L.C., and Lhoste, J.M. (1990). CO_2·-radical induced cleavage of disulfide bonds in proteins. A gamma-ray and pulse radiolysis mechanistic investigation. *Biochemistry*, **29**, 10978–10989.

Fay, K.C., Brennan, S.O., Costello, J.M., Potter, H.C., Williamson, D.A., Trent, R.J., et al. (1993). Haemoglobin Manukau beta 67[E11] Val⟶Gly: transfusion-dependent haemolytic anaemia ameliorated by coexisting alpha thalassaemia. *British Journal of Haematology*, **85**, 352–355.

Fee, J.A., Findling, K.L., Yoshida, T., Hille, R., Tarr, G.E., Hearshen, D.O., et al. (1984). Purification and characterization of the Rieske iron-sulfur protein from *Thermus thermophilus*. Evidence for a [2Fe-2S] cluster having non-cysteine ligands. *Journal of Biological Chemistry*, **259**, 124–133.

Fehsel, K., Kroncke, K.D., Meyer, K.L., Huber, H., Wahn, V., and Kolb, B.V. (1995). Nitric oxide induces apoptosis in mouse thymocytes. *Journal of Immunology*, **155**, 2858–2865.

Feng, Y., Roder, H., Englander, S.W., Wand, A.J., and Di, S.D. (1989). Proton resonance assignments of horse ferricytochrome c. *Biochemistry*, **28**, 195–203.

Feng, L., Xia, Y., Seiffert, D., and Wilson, C.B. (1995). Oxidative stress-inducible protein tyrosine phosphatase in glomerulonephritis. *Kidney International*, **48**, 1920–1928.

Fenton, H.J.H. (1894). Oxidation of tartaric acid in the presence of iron. *Journal of the Chemical Society*, **65**, 899–910.

Fenton, H.J.H., and Jackson, H. (1899). The oxidation of polyhydric alcohols in the presence of iron. *Journal of the Chemical Society*, **75**, 1–11.

Fenwick, C.W., and English, A.M. (1996). Trapping and LC-MS identification of protein radicals formed in the horse heart metmyoglobin-H_2O_2 reaction. *Journal of the American Chemical Society*, **118**, 12236–12237.

Fernandes, G., Chandrasekar, B., Troyer, D.A., Venkatraman, J.T., and Good, R.A. (1995). Dietary lipids and calorie restriction affect mammary tumor incidence and gene expression in mouse mammary tumor virus/v-Ha-ras transgenic mice. *Proceedings of the National Academy of Science of the United States of America*, **92**, 6494–6498.

Fernau, A., and Pauli, W. (1915). Action of penetration radium rays upon inorganic and bio-colloids. *Biochemical Zeitschrift*, **70**, 426–441.

Fernau, A., and Pauli, W. (1922). The effect of penetrating radium rays on inorganic colloids and biocolloids. II. *Kolloid Zeitschrift*, **30**, 6–13.

Ferrer, I., and Silva, E. (1981). Isolation and photo-oxidation of lysozyme fragments. *Radiation and Environmental Biophysics*, **20**, 67–77.

Finch, J.W., Crouch, R.K., Knapp, D.R., and Schey, K.L. (1993). Mass spectrometric identification of modifications to human serum albumin treated with hydrogen peroxide. *Archives of Biochemistry and Biophysics*, **305**, 595–599.

Finley, J.C., Erickson, J.T., and Katz, D.M. (1995). Galanin expression in carotid body afferent neurons. *Neuroscience*, **68**, 937–942.

Finzel, B.C., Poulos, T.L., and Kraut, J. (1984). Crystal structure of yeast cytochrome c peroxidase refined at 1.7-Å resolution. *Journal of Biological Chemistry*, **259**, 13027–13036.

Fiorino, A., Frigo, G., and Cucchetti, E. (1989). Liquid chromatographic analysis of amino and imino acids in protein hydrolysates by post-column derivatization with o-phthalaldehyde and 3-mercaptopropionic acid. *Journal of Chromatography*, **476**, 83–92.

Fishel, L.A., Villafranca, J.E., Mauro, J.M., and Kraut, J. (1987). Yeast cytochrome c peroxidase: mutagenesis and expression in Escherichia coli show tryptophan-51 is not the radical site in compound I. *Biochemistry*, **26**, 351–360.

Fishel, L.A., Farnum, M.F., Mauro, J.M., Miller, M.A., Kraut, J., Liu, Y.J., *et al.* (1991). Compound I radical in site-directed mutants of cytochrome c peroxidase as probed by electron paramagnetic resonance and electron-nuclear double resonance. *Biochemistry*, **30**, 1986–1996.

Fisher, M.T., and Stadtman, E.R. (1992). Oxidative modification of *Escherichia coli* glutamine synthetase. Decreases in the thermodynamic stability of protein structure and specific changes in the active site conformation. *Journal of Biological Chemistry*, **267**, 1872–1880.

Flanagan, J.M., Kataoka, M., Fujisawa, T., and Engelman, D.M. (1993). Mutations can cause large changes in the conformation of a denatured protein. *Biochemistry*, **32**, 10359–10370.

Flescher, E., Ledbetter, J.A., Schieven, G.L., Vela, R.N., Fossum, D., Dang, H., *et al.* (1994). Longitudinal exposure of human T lymphocytes to weak oxidative stress suppresses transmembrane and nuclear signal transduction. *Journal of Immunology*, **153**, 4880–4889.

Fletcher, B.L., and Tappel, A.L. (1971). Fluorescent modification of serum albumin by lipid peroxidation. *Lipids*, **6**, 172–175.

Fletcher, B.L., and Tappel, A.L. (1973). Protective effects of dietary α-tocopherol in rats exposed to toxic levels of ozone and nitrogen dioxide. *Environmental Research*, **6**, 165–175.

Fletcher, B.L., Dillard, C.J., and Tappel, A.L. (1973). Measurement of fluorescent lipid peroxidation products in biological systems and tissues. *Analytical Biochemistry*, **52**, 1–9.

Fletcher, E.J., Nutt, S.L., Hoo, K.H., Elliott, C.E., Korczak, B., McWhinnie, E.A., *et al.* (1995). Cloning, expression and pharmacological characterization of a human glutamate receptor: hGluR4. *Receptor Channels*, **3**, 21–31.

Fletcher, G.L., and Okada, S. (1961). Radiation induced formation of DOPA from tyrosine and tyrosine-containing peptdies in aqueous solution. *Radiation Research*, **15**, 349–354.

Fliss, H. (1988). Oxidation of proteins in rat heart and lungs by polymorphonuclear leukocyte oxidants. *Molecular and Cellular Biochemistry*, **84**, 177–188.

Fliss, H., and Menard, M. (1994). Rapid neutrophil accumulation and protein oxidation in irradiated rat lungs. *Journal of Applied Physiology*, **77**, 2727–2733.

Florence, T.M. (1985). The degradation of cytochrome *c* by hydrogen peroxide. *Journal of Inorganic Biochemistry*, **23**, 131–141.

Florkowski, C.M., Richardson, M.R., Le, G.C., Jennings, P.E., O'Donnell, M.J., Jones, A.F., *et al.* (1988). Effect of gliclazide on thromboxane B2, parameters of haemostasis, fluorescent IgG and lipid peroxides in non-insulin dependent diabetes mellitus. *Diabetes Research*, **9**, 87–90.

Floyd, R.A., and Carney, J.M. (1992). Free radical damage to protein and DNA: mechanisms involved and relevant observations on brain undergoing oxidative stress. *Annals of Neurology*, **32, (Supplement)**, S22–S27.

Floyd, R.A., and Nagy, I. (1984). Formation of long-lived hydroxyl free radical adducts of proline and hydroxyproline in a Fenton reaction. *Biochimica et Biophysica Acta*, **790**, 94–97.

Fluckiger, R., Paz, M.A., and Gallop, P.M. (1995). Redox-cycling detection of dialyzable pyrroloquinoline quinone and quinoproteins. *Methods in Enzymology*, **258**, 140–149.

Fogliatto, G., Musanti, R., Pirillo, A., and Ghiselli, G. (1995). Oxidized lipoproteins induce long-lasting inhibition of nitric oxide synthase from a murine endothelioma cell line (bEnd.4). *Journal of Cardiovascular Risk*, **2**, 123–130.

Folbergrova, J., Kiyota, Y., Pahlmark, K., Memezawa, H., Smith, M.L., and Siesjo, B.K. (1993). Does ischemia with reperfusion lead to oxidative damage to proteins in the brain? *Journal of Cerebal Blood Flow and Metabolism*, **13**, 145–152.

Folbergrova, J., Zhao, Q., Katsura, K., and Siesjo, B.K. (1995). *N-tert*-butyl-alpha-phenylnitrone improves recovery of brain energy state in rats following transient focal ischemia. *Proceedings of the National Academy of Science of the United States of America*, **92**, 5057–5061.

Folkes, L.K., Candeias, L.P., and Wardman, P. (1995). Kinetics and mechanisms of hypochlorous acid reactions. *Archives of Biochemistry and Biophysics*, **323**, 120–126.

Fong, L.G., Parthasarathy, S., Witztum, J.L., and Steinberg, D. (1987). Non-enzymatic oxidative cleavage of peptide bonds in apoprotein B-100. *Journal of Lipid Research*, **28**, 1466–1477.

Fontecave, M., Gerez, C., Atta, M., and Jeunet, A. (1990). High valent iron oxo intermediates might be involved during activation of ribonucleotide reductase: single oxygen atom donors generate the tyrosyl radical. *Biochemical and Biophysical Research Communications*, **168**, 659–664.

Foote, N., Gadsby, P.M., Berry, M.J., Greenwood, C., and Thomson, A.J. (1987). The formation of ferric haem during low-temperature photolysis of horseradish peroxidase Compound I. *Biochemical Journal*, **246**, 659–668.

Forni, L.G., Mora-Arellano, V.O., Packer, J.E., and Willson, R.L. (1986). Nitrogen dioxide and related free radicals: electron-transfer reactions with organic compounds in solutions containing nitrite or nitrate. *Journal of the Chemical Society, Perkin Transactions 2*, 1–6.

Forrester, K., Ambs, S., Lupold, S.E., Kapust, R.B., Spillare, E.A., Weinberg, W.C., *et al.* (1996). Nitric oxide-induced p53 accumulation and regulation of inducible nitric oxide synthase expression by wild-type p53. *Proceedings of the National Academy of Science of the United States of America*, **93**, 2442–2447.

Forsmark, A.P., Dallner, G., and Ernster, L. (1995). Endogenous ubiquinol prevents protein modification accompanying lipid peroxidation in beef heart submitochondrial particles. *Free Radical Biology and Medicine*, **19**, 749–757.

Forster, M.J., Dubey, A., Dawson, K.M., Stutts, W.A., Lal, H., and Sohal, R.S. (1996). Age-related losses of cognitive function and motor skills in mice are associated with oxidative protein damage in the brain. *Proceedings of the National Academy of Science of the United States of America*, **93**, 4765–4769.

Fossa, A., Beyer, A., Pfitzner, E., Wenzel, B., and Kunau, W.H. (1995). Molecular cloning, sequencing and sequence analysis of the fox-2 gene of *Neurospora crassa* encoding the multifunctional beta-oxidation protein. *Molecular and General Genetics*, **247**, 95–104.

Fossey, J., Lefort, D., and Sobra, J. (1995). *Free Radicals in Organic Chemistry*. Wiley, Chichester.

Foster, A., Fitzsimmons, B., Rokach, J., and Letts, G. (1987). Evidence of *in-vivo* omega-oxidation of peptide leukotrienes in the rat: biliary excretion of $20\text{-}CO_2H$ *N*-acetyl LTE4. *Biochemical and Biophysical Research Communications*, **148**, 1237–1245.

Foster, J.W., and Spector, M.P. (1995). How *Salmonella* survive against the odds. *Annual Reviews of Microbiology*, **49**, 145–174.

Foster, T., and West, P.R. (1973). Electron spin resonance studies in aqueous solution: Fragmentation of radical intermediates derived from β-amino alcohols. *Canadian Journal of Chemistry*, **51**, 4009–4017.

Foster, T., and West, P.R. (1974). Photolysis of aqueous solutions of hydrogen peroxide containing β-ammonio alcohols. *Canadian Journal of Chemistry*, **52**, 3589–3598.

Fox, J.B.J., Nicholas, R.A., Ackerman, S.A., and Swift, C.E. (1974). A multiple wavelength analysis of the reaction between hydrogen peroxide and metmyoglobin. *Biochemistry*, **13**, 5178–5186.

Fox, T., Ferreira, R.L., Hill, B.C., and English, A.M. (1993). Quenching of intrinsic fluorescence of yeast cytochrome *c* peroxidase by covalently- and noncovalently-bound quenchers. *Biochemistry*, **32**, 6938–6943.

Fraga, C.G., and Tappel, A.L. (1988). Damage to DNA concurrent with lipid peroxidation in rat liver slices. *Biochemical Journal*, **252**, 893–896.

Fraga, C.G., Leibovitz, B.E., and Tappel, A.L. (1987). Halogenated compounds as inducers of lipid peroxidation in tissue slices. *Free Radical Biology and Medicine*, **3**, 119–123.

Fraga, C.G., Zamora, R., and Tappel, A.L. (1989). Damage to protein synthesis concurrent with lipid peroxidation in rat liver slices: effect of halogenated compounds, peroxides, and vitamin E1. *Archives of Biochemistry and Biophysics*, **270**, 84–91.

Fraga, C.G., Tappel, A.L., Leibovitz, B.E., Kuypers, F., Chiu, D., Iacono, J.M., *et al.* (1990a). Lability of red blood cell membranes to lipid peroxidation: application to humans fed polyunsaturated lipids. *Lipids*, **25**, 111–114.

Fraga, C.G., Shigenaga, M.K., Park, J.W., Degan, P., and Ames, B.N. (1990b). Oxidative damage to DNA during aging: 8–hydroxy-2'-deoxyguanosine in rat organ DNA and urine. *Proceedings of the National Academy of Science of the United States of America*, **87**, 4533–4537.

Fraga, C.G., Motchnik, P.A., Shigenaga, M.K., Helbock, H.J., Jacob, R.A., and Ames, B.N. (1991). Ascorbic acid protects against endogenous oxidative DNA damage in human sperm. *Proceedings of the National Academy of Science of the United States of America*, **88**, 11003–11006.

Frame, M.C., Wilkie, N.M., Darling, A.J., Chudleigh, A., Pintzas, A., Lang, J.C., *et al.* (1991). Regulation of AP-1/DNA complex formation *in vitro*. *Oncogene*, **6**, 205–209.

Frampton, M.W., Morrow, P.E., Cox, C., Gibb, F.R., Speers, D.M., and Utell, M.J. (1991). Effects of nitrogen dioxide exposure on pulmonary function and airway reactivity in normal humans. *American Reviews of Respiratory Disease*, **143**, 522–527.

Francis, G.A., Mendez, A.J., Bierman, E.L., and Heinecke, J.W. (1993). Oxidative tyrosylation of high density lipoprotein by peroxidase enhances cholesterol removal from cultured fibroblasts and macrophage foam cells. *Proceedings of the National Academy of Science of the United States of America*, **90**, 6631–6635.

Francis, G.L., and Ballard, F.J. (1980). Distribution and partial purification of a liver membrane protein capable of inactivating cytosol enzymes. *Biochemical Journal*, **186**, 571–579.

Francis, G.L., McNamara, P.J., Filsell, O.H., and Ballard, F.J. (1988). Plasma half-lives of native and modified insulin-like growth factor-I in lambs. *Journal of Endocrinology*, **117**, 183–189.

Frank, J.J., van Krimpen, S.H., Verwiel, P.E., Jongejan, J.A., Mulder, A.C., and Duine, J.A. (1989). On the mechanism of inhibition of methanol dehydrogenase by cyclopropane-derived inhibitors. *European Journal of Biochemistry*, **184**, 187–195.

Frantzen, F., Heggli, D.E., and Sundrehagen, E. (1995). Radiolabelling of human haemoglobin using the 125I-Bolton-Hunter reagent is superior to oxidative iodination for conservation of the native structure of the labelled protein. *Biotechnology and Applied Biochemistry*, **22**, 161–167.

Frebort, I., Tamaki, H., Ishida, H., Pec, P., Luhova, L., Tsuno, H., et al. (1996). Two distinct quinoprotein amine oxidases are induced by *n*-butylamine in the mycelia of *Aspergillus niger AKU 3302*. Purification, characterization, cDNA cloning and sequencing. *European Journal of Biochemistry*, **237**, 255–265.

Frederikse, P.H., Garland, D., Zigler, J.J., and Piatigorsky, J. (1996). Oxidative stress increases production of beta-amyloid precursor protein and beta-amyloid (Abeta) in mammalian lenses, and Abeta has toxic effects on lens epithelial cells. *Journal of Biological Chemistry*, **271**, 10169–10174.

Freeman, M.L., and Meredith, M.J. (1989). Measurement of protein thiols after heat shock using 3-(-N-maleimido-propionyl) biocytin labeled proteins separated by SDS-PAGE and electroluted onto nitrocellulose: thiol blotting. *Radiation Research*, **117**, 326–333.

Frei, B. (1995). Cardiovascular disease and nutrient antioxidants: role of low-density lipoprotein oxidation. *Critical Reviews of Food Science and Nutrition*, **35**, 83–98.

Frei, B., Stocker, R., and Ames, B.N. (1988). Antioxidant defenses and lipid peroxidation in human blood plasma. *Proceedings of the National Academy of Science of the United States of America*, **85**, 9748–9752.

Frei, B., and Gaziano, J.M. (1993). Content of antioxidants, preformed lipid hydroperoxides, and cholesterol as predictors of the susceptibility of human LDL to metal ion-dependent and -independent oxidation. *Journal of Lipid Research*, **34**, 2135–2145.

Frei, B., Winterhalter, K.H., and Richter, C. (1985). Quantitative and mechanistic aspects of the hydroperoxide-induced release of Ca^{2+} from rat liver mitochondria. *European Journal of Biochemistry*, **149**, 633–639.

Frei, B., Stocker, R., England, L., and Ames, B.N. (1990). Ascorbate: the most effective antioxidant in human blood plasma. *Advances in Experimental Medical Biology*, **264**, 155–163.

Frei, B., Forte, T.M., Ames, B.N., and Cross, C.E. (1991). Gas phase oxidants of cigarette smoke induce lipid peroxidation and changes in lipoprotein properties in human blood plasma. Protective effects of ascorbic acid. *Biochemical Journal*, **277**, 133–138.

French, S.W., Wong, K., Jui, L., Albano, E., Hagbjork, A.L., and Ingelman, S.M. (1993). Effect of ethanol on cytochrome P450 2E1 (CYP2E1), lipid peroxidation, and serum protein adduct formation in relation to liver pathology pathogenesis. *Experimental Molecular Pathology*, **58**, 61–75.

Fricke, H. (1938). The denaturation of proteins by high-frequencey radiations. *Cold Spring Harbor Symposium on Quantitative Biology*, **6**, 164–169.

Fricke, K., Wirthensohn, K., Laxhuber, R., and Sackmann, E. (1986). Flicker spectroscopy of erythrocytes. A sensitive method to study subtle changes of membrane bending stiffness. *European Biophysical Journal*, **14**, 67–81.

Friedman, A.H., and Morgulis, S. (1936). Oxidation of amino acids with sodium hypobromite. *Journal of the American Chemical Society*, **58**, 909–913.

Friguet, B., Stadtman, E.R., and Szweda, L.I. (1994a). Modification of glucose-6-phosphate dehydrogenase by 4-hydroxy-2-nonenal. Formation of cross-linked protein that inhibits the multicatalytic protease. *Journal of Biological Chemistry*, **269**, 21639–21643.

Friguet, B., Szweda, L.I., and Stadtman, E.R. (1994b). Susceptibility of glucose-6-phosphate dehydrogenase modified by 4-hydroxy-2-nonenal and metal-catalyzed oxidation to proteolysis by the multicatalytic protease. *Archives of Biochemistry and Biophysics*, **311**, 168–173.

Frimer, A.A. (1985). *Singlet O_2*. CRC Press: Boca Raton. .

Fu, W.G., Morgan, T.V., Mortenson, L.E., and Johnson, M.K. (1991). Resonance Raman studies of the [4Fe-4S] to [2Fe-2S] cluster conversion in the iron protein of nitrogenase. *FEBS Letters*, **284**, 165–168.

Fu, M.-X., Wells-Knecht, K.J., Blackledge, J.A., Lyons, T.J., Thorpe, S.R., and Baynes, J.W. (1994). Glycation, glycoxidation, and cross-linking of collagen by glucose. Kinetics, mechanisms, and inhibition of late stages of the Maillard reaction. *Diabetes*, **43**, 676–683.

Fu, M.-W., Requena, J.R., Jenkins, A.J., Lyons, T.J., Baynes, J.W., and Thorpe, S.R. (1996). The advanced glycation end product N^ε-(carboxymethyl)lysine, is a product of both lipid peroxidation and glycoxidation reactions. *Journal of Biological Chemistry*, **271**, 9982–9986.

Fu, S., and Dean, R.T. (1997). Structural characterisation of the products of hydroxyl radical damage to leucine and their detection on proteins. *Biochemical Journal*, **324**, 41–48.

Fu, S., Gebicki, S., Jessup, W., Gebicki, J.M., and Dean, R.T. (1995a). Biological fate of amino acid, peptide and protein hydroperoxides. *Biochemical Journal*, **311**, 821–827.

Fu, S., Hick, L.A., Sheil, M.M., and Dean, R.T. (1995b). Structural identification of valine hydroperoxides and hydroxides on radical-damaged amino acid, peptide, and protein molecules. *Free Radical Biology and Medicine*, **19**, 281–292.

Fucci, L., Oliver, C.N., Coon, M.J., and Stadtman, E.R. (1983). Inactivation of key metabolic enzymes by mixed-function oxidation reactions: possible implication in protein turnover and ageing. *Proceedings of the National Academy of Science of the United States of America*, **80**, 1521–1525.

Fujii, N., Otaka, A., Funakoshi, S., Bessho, K., Watanabe, T., Akaji, K., *et al.* (1987). Studies on peptides. CLI. Syntheses of cystine-peptides by oxidation of

S-protected cysteine-peptides with thallium(III) trifluoroacetate. *Chemical and Pharmaceutical Bulletin Tokyo*, **35**, 2339–2347.

Fujimori, E. (1988). Cross-linking of collagen CNBr peptides by ozone or UV light. *FEBS Letters*, **235**, 98–102.

Fujimori, E. (1989). Cross-linking and fluorescence changes of collagen by glycation and oxidation. *Biochimica et Biophysica Acta*, **998**, 105–110.

Fujino, M., Wakimasu, M., Taketomi, S., and Iwatsuka, H. (1977). Insulin-like activities and insulin-potentiating actions of a modified insulin B21-26 fragment: beta-Ala–Arg–Gly–Phe–Phe–Tyr–NH$_2$. *Endocrinology*, **101**, 360–364.

Fujisawa, R., Wada, Y., Nodasaka, Y., and Kuboki, Y. (1996). Acidic amino acid-rich sequences as binding sites of osteonectin to hydroxyapatite crystals. *Biochimica et Biophysica Acta*, **1292**, 53–60.

Fujiwara, T., and Fukumori, Y. (1996). Cytochrome *cb*-type nitric oxide reductase with cytochrome *c* oxidase activity from *Paracoccus denitrificans ATCC 35512*. *Journal of Bacteriology*, **178**, 1866–1871.

Fukuda, F., Kitada, M., Horie, T., and Awazu, S. (1992). Evaluation of adriamycin-induced lipid peroxidation. *Biochemical Pharmacology*, **44**, 755–760.

Fukui, H., Mizuguchi, H., Liu, Y.Q., Wang, N.P., Hayashi, H., Kangawa, K., *et al.* (1995). Purification and characterization of [3H]mepyramine (histamine H1 antagonist)-binding protein from rat liver: a highly homologous protein with cytochrome P450 2D. *Journal of Biochemistry, Tokyo*, **117**, 993–998.

Fukuo, K., Hata, S., Suhara, T., Nakahashi, T., Shinto, Y., Tsujimoto, Y., *et al.* (1996). Nitric oxide induces upregulation of Fas and apoptosis in vascular smooth muscle. *Hypertension*, **27**, 823–826.

Fukushima, T., Tawara, T., Isobe, A., Hojo, N., Shiwaku, K., and Yamane, Y. (1995). Radical formation site of cerebral complex I and Parkinson's disease. *Journal of Neuroscience Research*, **42**, 385–390.

Fukuzawa, K., and Gebicki, J.M. (1983). Oxidation of alpha-tocopherol in micelles and liposomes by the hydroxyl, perhydroxyl, and superoxide free radicals. *Archives of Biochemistry and Biophysics*, **226**, 242–251.

Fukuzawa, K., Kishikawa, K., Tokumura, A., Tsukatani, H., and Shibuya, M. (1985). Fluorescent pigments by covalent binding of lipid peroxidation by-products to protein and amino acids. *Lipids*, **20**, 854–861.

Fukuzawa, K., Tadokoro, T., Kishikawa, K., Mukai, K., and Gebicki, J.M. (1988*a*). Site-specific induction of lipid peroxidation by iron in charged micelles. *Archives of Biochemistry and Biophysics*, **260**, 146–152.

Fukuzawa, K., Kishikawa, K., Tadokoro, T., Tokumura, A., Tsukatani, H., and Gebicki, J.M. (1988*b*). The effects of alpha-tocopherol on site-specific lipid peroxidation induced by iron in charged micelles. *Archives of Biochemistry and Biophysics*, **260**, 153–160.

Fulceri, R., Pompella, A., Benedetti, A., and Comporti, M. (1990). On the role of lipid peroxidation and protein-bound aldehydes in the haloalkane-induced inactivation of microsomal glucose 6 phosphatase. *Research Communications in Chemical Pathology and Pharmacology*, **68**, 73–88.

Fulks, R.M., and Stadtman, E.R. (1985). Regulation of glutamine synthetase, aspartokinase, and total protein turnover in *Klebsiella aerogenes*. *Biochimica et Biophysica Acta*, **843**, 214–229.

Fulop, V., Ridout, C.J., Greenwood, C., and Hajdu, J. (1995). Crystal structure of the di-haem cytochrome *c* peroxidase from *Pseudomonas aeruginosa*. *Structure*, **3**, 1225–1233.

Fushiki, S., Matsumoto, K., and Nagata, A. (1995). Neurite outgrowth of murine cerebellar granule cells can be enhanced by aniracetam with or without alpha-amino-3-hydroxy-5-methyl-4-isoxazole propionic acid (AMPA). *Neuroscience Letters*, **199**, 171–174.

Gabor, F., Pittner, F., and Spiegl, P. (1995). Drug-protein conjugates: preparation of triamcinolone-acetonide containing bovine serum albumin/keyhole limpet hemo-cyanin-conjugates and polyclonal antibodies. *Archives of Pharmacy, Weinheim*, **328**, 775–780.

Gaertner, H.F., Rose, K., Cotton, R., Timms, D., Camble, R., and Offord, R.E. (1992). Construction of protein analogues by site-specific condensation of unprotected fragments. *Bioconjugate Chemistry*, **3**, 262–268.

Gairi, M., Lloyd, W.P., Albericio, F., and Giralt, E. (1995). Convergent solid-phase peptide synthesis. 12. Chromatographic techniques for the purification of pro-tected peptide segments. *International Journal of Peptide and Protein Research*, **46**, 119–133.

Gajewski, E., and Dizdaroglu, M. (1990). Hydroxyl radical induced cross-linking of cytosine and tyrosine in nucleohistone. *Biochemistry*, **29**, 977–980.

Gajewski, E., Dizdaroglu, M., Krutzsch, H.C., and Simic, M.G. (1984). OH radical-induced crosslinks of methionine peptides. *International Journal of Radiation Biology and Related Studies in Physics, Chemistry and Medicine*, **46**, 47–55.

Gajewski, E., Fuciarelli, A.F., and Dizdaroglu, M. (1988). Structure of hydroxyl radical-induced DNA-protein crosslinks in calf thymus nucleohistone *in vitro*. *International Journal of Radiation Biology and Related Studies in Physics, Chem-istry and Medicine*, **54**, 445–459.

Gajewski, E., Rao, G., Nackerdien, Z., and Dizdaroglu, M. (1990). Modification of DNA bases in mammalian chromatin by radiation-generatred free radicals. *Biochemistry*, **29**, 7876–7882.

Galaris, D., Sevanian, A., Cadenas, E., and Hochstein, P. (1990). Ferrylmyoglobin-catalyzed linoleic acid peroxidation. *Archives of Biochemistry and Biophysics*, **281**, 163–169.

Galinanes, M., and Hearse, D.J. (1990). Diltiazem and/or desferrioxamine administered at the time of reperfusion fail to improve post-ischemic recovery in the isolated rat heart after long-term hypothermic storage. *Journal of Molecular and Cellular Cardiology*, **22**, 1211–1220.

Galinanes, M., Ferrari, R., Qiu, Y., Cargnoni, A., Ezrin, A., and Hearse, D.J. (1992a). PEG-SOD and myocardial antioxidant status during ischaemia and reperfusion: dose-response studies in the isolated blood perfused rabbit heart. *Journal of Molecular and Cellular Cardiology*, **24**, 1021–1030.

Galinanes, M., Qiu, Y., Ezrin, A., and Hearse, D.J. (1992b). PEG-SOD and myocardial protection. Studies in the blood- and crystalloid-perfused rabbit and rat hearts. *Circulation*, **86**, 672–682.

Galinanes, M., Lawson, C.S., Ferrari, R., Limb, G.A., Derias, N.W., and Hearse, D.J. (1993). Early and late effects of leukopenic reperfusion on the recovery of cardiac contractile function. Studies in the transplanted and isolated blood-perfused rat heart. *Circulation*, **88**, 673–683.

Galli, M.C., Cabrini, L., Caboni, F., Cipollone, M., and Landi, L. (1994). Peroxida-tion potential of rat thymus during development and involution. *Comparative Bio-chemistry, Physiology, Pharmacology, Toxicology and Endocrinology*, **107**, 435–440.

Galter, D., Mihm, S., and Droge, W. (1994). Distinct effects of glutathione di-sulphide on the nuclear transcription factor kappa B and the activator protein-1. *European Journal of Biochemistry*, **221**, 639–648.

Gamage, P.T., and Matsushita, S. (1973). Interactions of the autoxidised products of linoleic acid with enzyme proteins. *Agricultural and Biological Chemistry*, **37**, 1–8.

Gambacciani, M., Spinetti, A., Orlandi, R., Piaggesi, L., Cappagli, B., Weiss, C., *et al.* (1995). Effects of a new estrogen/progestin combination in the treatment of postmenopausal syndrome. *Maturitas*, **22**, 115–120.

Ganadu, M.L., Bonomi, F., Pagani, S., and Boelens, R. (1992). ^{1}H NMR studies on the oxidized ferredoxin from Clostridium pasteurianum. *Biochemistry International*, **26**, 577–585.

Gane, A.M., Craik, D., Munro, S.L., Howlett, G.J., Clarke, A.E., and Bacic, A. (1995). Structural analysis of the carbohydrate moiety of arabinogalactan-proteins from stigmas and styles of *Nicotiana alata*. *Carbohydrate Research*, **277**, 67–85.

Gantchev, T.G., and van Liev, J.E. (1995). Catalase inactivation following photosensitization with tetrasulfonated metallophthalocyanines. *Photochemistry and Photobiology*, **62**, 123–134.

Garcia, R., Rodriguez, R., Montesino, R., Besada, V., Gonzalez, J., and Cremata, J.A. (1995). Concanavalin A- and wheat germ agglutinin-conjugated lectins as a tool for the identification of multiple N-glycosylation sites in heterologous protein expressed in yeast. *Analytical Biochemistry*, **231**, 342–348.

Garcia-Castineiras, S., Dillon, J., and Spector, A. (1978). Non-tryptophan fluorescence associated with human lens protein: apparent complexity and isolation of bityrosine and anthranlic acid. *Experimental Eye Research*, **26**, 461–476.

Gardner, H.W. (1979). Lipid hydroperoxide reactivity with proteins and amino acids: a review. *Journal of Agricultural and Food Chemistry*, **27**, 220–229.

Garibaldi, S., Aragno, I., Odetti, P., and Marinari, U.M. (1994). Relationships between protein carbonyls, retinol and tocopherols level in human plasma. *Biochemistry and Molecular Biology International*, **34**, 729–736.

Garland, D. (1990). Role of site-specific, metal-catalyzed oxidation in lens aging and cataract: a hypothesis. *Experimental Eye Research*, **50**, 677–682.

Garland, D., Zigler, J.S., and Kinoshita, J. (1986). Structural changes in bovine lens crystallins induced by ascorbate, metal and oxygen. *Archives of Biochemistry and Biophysics*, **251**, 771–776.

Garlick, P.B., Davies, M.J., Hearse, D.J., and Slater, T.F. (1987). Direct detection of free radicals in the reperfused rat heart using electron spin resonance spectroscopy. *Circulation Research*, **61**, 757–760.

Garner, B., Dean, R.T., and Jessup, W. (1994). Human macrophage-mediated oxidation of low-density lipoprotein is delayed and independent of superoxide production. *Biochemical Journal*, **310**, 421–428.

Garner, M.H., and Spector, A. (1980). Selective oxidation of cysteine and methionine in normal and senile cataractous lenses. *Proceedings of the National Academy of Science of the United States of America*, **77**, 1274–1277.

Garrison, W.M. (1968). Radiation chemistry of organo-nitrogen compounds. *Current Topics in Radiation Research*, **4**, 43–94.

Garrison, W.M. (1972). Radiation-induced reactions of amino acids and peptides. *Radiation Research Reviews*, **3**, 305–326.

Garrison, W.M. (1987). Reaction mechanisms in the radiolysis of peptides, polypeptides, and proteins. *Chemical Reviews*, **87**, 381–398.

Garrison, W.M. (1989a). Comparative free radical chemistry in the radiolytic deamination and dephosphorylation of bio-organic molecules. II. Oxygenated solutions. *Free Radical Biology and Medicine*, **7**, 171–175.

Garrison, W.M. (1989b). Comparative free-radical chemistry in the radiolytic deamination and dephosphorylation of bio-organic molecules. I. Oxygen-free solutions. *Free Radical Biology and Medicine*, **6**, 285–288.

Garrison, W.M., Jayko, M.J., and Bennett, W. (1962). Radiation-induced oxidation of protein in aqueous solution. *Radiation Research*, **16**, 483–502.

Garrison, W.M., Jayko, M.E., and Bennett, W. (1964). Radiation-chemistry oxidation of peptides in solid state. *Science*, **146**, 250–252.

Garrison, W.M., Jayko, M.E., Rodgers, M.A.J., Sokol, H.A., and Bennett-Corniea, W. (1968). Ionization and excitation in peptide radiolysis. In *Radiation Chemistry Vol. 1*, (ed. R.F. Gould), pp. 384–396. American Chemical Society, Washington.

Garrison, W.M., Kland-English, M., Sokol, H.A., and Jayko, M.E. (1970). Radiolytic degradation of the peptide main chain in dilute aqueous solution containing oxygen. *Journal of Physical Chemistry*, **74**, 4506–4509.

Garrison, W.M., Sokol, H.A., and Bennett, C.W. (1973). Radiation chemistry of glycylglycine in oxygen-free systems. *Radiation Research*, **53**, 376–384.

Gast, M.J. (1983). Characterization of preprorelaxin by tryptic digestion and inhibition of its conversion to prorelaxin by amino acid analogs. *Journal of Biological Chemistry*, **258**, 9001–9004.

Gatti, R.M., Radi, R., and Augusto, O. (1994). Peroxynitrite-mediated oxidation of albumin to the protein-thiyl free radical. *FEBS Letters*, **348**, 287–290.

Gaudu, P., Niviere, V., Petillot, Y., Kauppi, B., and Fontecave, M. (1996). The irreversible inactivation of ribonucleotide reductase from *Escherichia coli* by superoxide radicals. *FEBS Letters*, **387**, 137–140.

Gavino, V.C., Dillard, C.J., and Tappel, A.L. (1984). Release of ethane and pentane from rat tissue slices: effect of vitamin E, halogenated hydrocarbons, and iron overload. *Archives of Biochemistry and Biophysics*, **233**, 741–747.

Gavino, V.C., Dillard, C.J., and Tappel, A.L. (1985a). Effect of dietary vitamin E and Santoquin on regenerating rat liver. *Life Science*, **36**, 1771–1777.

Gavino, V.C., Dillard, C.J., and Tappel, A.L. (1985b). The effect of iron overload on urinary excretion of immunoreactive prostaglandin E2. *Archives of Biochemistry and Biophysics*, **237**, 322–327.

Gayda, J.P., Benosman, H., Bertrand, P., More, C., and Asso, M. (1988). EPR determination of interaction redox potentials in a multiheme cytochrome: cytochrome c3 from *Desulfovibrio desulfuricans* Norway. *European Journal of Biochemistry*, **177**, 199–206.

Gaziano, J.M., Hatta, A., Flynn, M., Johnson, E.J., Krinsky, N.I., Ridker, P.M., *et al.* (1995). Supplementation with beta-carotene *in vivo* and *in vitro* does not inhibit low density lipoprotein oxidation. *Atherosclerosis*, **112**, 187–195.

Gebicki, S., and Gebicki, J.M. (1993). Formation of peroxides in amino acids and proteins exposed to oxygen free radicals. *Biochemical Journal*, **289**, 743–749.

Gebicki, S., Bartosz, G., and Gebicki, J.M. (1995). The action of iron on amino acid and protein peroxides. *Biochemical Society Transactions*, **23**, 249S.

Gee, D.L., and Tappel, A.L. (1981a). Production of volatile hydrocarbons by isolated hepatocytes: an *in vitro* model for lipid peroxidation studies. *Toxicology and Applied Pharmacology*, **60**, 112–120.

Gee, D.L., and Tappel, A.L. (1981b). The effect of exhaustive exercise on expired pentane as a measure of *in vivo* lipid peroxidation in the rat. *Life Science*, **28**, 2425–2429.

Gee, D.L., Bechtold, M.M., and Tappel, A.L. (1981). Carbon tetrachloride-induced lipid peroxidation: simultaneous *in vivo* measurements of pentane and chloroform exhaled by the rat. *Toxicology Letters*, **8**, 299–306.

Geeraerts, M.D., Ronveaux, D.M., Lemasters, J.J., and Herman, B. (1991). Cytosolic free Ca^{2+} and proteolysis in lethal oxidative injury in endothelial cells. *American Journal of Physiology*, **261**, C889–C896.

Geerlof, A., Dokter, P., van Wielink, J.E., and Duine, J.A. (1989). Haem-containing protein complexes of *Acinetobacter calcoaceticus* as secondary electron acceptors for quinoprotein glucose dehydrogenase. *Antonie Van Leeuwenhoek*, **56**, 81–84.

Geiger, O., and Gorisch, H. (1989). Reversible thermal inactivation of the quinoprotein glucose dehydrogenase from *Acinetobacter calcoaceticus*. Ca^{2+} ions are necessary for re-activation. *Biochemical Journal*, **261**, 415–421.

Gelvan, D., Moreno, V., Gassmann, W., Hegenauer, J., and Saltman, P. (1992). Metal-ion-directed site-specificity of hydroxyl radical detection. *Biochimica et Biophysica Acta*, **1116**, 183–191.

Geng, Y.J., Hellstrand, K., Wennmalm, A., and Hansson, G.K. (1996). Apoptotic death of human leukemic cells induced by vascular cells expressing nitric oxide synthase in response to gamma-interferon and tumor necrosis factor-alpha. *Cancer Research*, **56**, 866–874.

Gentner, W., and Schwerin, K. (1930). The effect of short wave radiations on proteins. II. The relation between the radiation reaction of the protein and the radiation intensity of the UV rays. *Biochemistry Zeitschrift*, **227**, 286–303.

George, P., and Irvine, D.H. (1951). The reaction between metmyoglobin and hydrogen peroxide. *Erythrocyte Permeability*, **52**, 511–517.

George, P., and Irvine, D.H. (1952). The reaction between metmyoglobin and alkyl hydroperoxides. Metmyoglobin and hydroperoxides, *Nature,*, **55**, 230–236.

Germann, T., Guckes, S., Bongartz, M., Dlugonska, H., Schmitt, E., Kolbe, L., *et al.* (1995). Administration of IL-12 during ongoing immune responses fails to permanently suppress and can even enhance the synthesis of antigen-specific IgE. *International Immunology*, **7**, 1649–1657.

Gershon, H., and Gershon, D. (1970). Detection of inactive enzyme molecules in ageing organisms. *Nature*, **227**, 1214–1216.

Ghio, A.J., Kennedy, T.P., Schapira, R.M., Crumbliss, A.L., and Hoidal, J.R. (1990). Hypothesis: is lung disease after silicate inhalation caused by oxidant generation? *Lancet*, **336**, 967–969.

Ghosh, M., Avezoux, A., Anthony, C., Harlos, K., and Blake, C.C. (1994). X-ray structure of PQQ-dependent methanol dehydrogenase. *EXS*, **71**, 251–260.

Gibson, C., Fogg, G., Okada, N., Geist, R.T., Hanski, E., and Caparon, M. (1995). Regulation of host cell recognition in *Streptococcus pyogenes*. *Developmental Biology Stand*, **85**, 137–144.

Gibson, J.F., and Ingram, D.J.E. (1956). Location of free electrons in porphyrin ring complexes. *Nature*, **178**, 871–872.

Gibson, J.F., and Ingram, D.J.E. (1958). Free radical produced in the reaction of metmyoglobin with hydrogen peroxide. *Nature*, **181**, 1398–1399.

Giese, B. (1986). *Radicals in Organic Synthesis: Formation of Carbon–Carbon Bonds.* Pergamon Press, Oxford.

Giese, R.W., and Riordan, J.F. (1975). Nitrotyrosine internal standard for amino acid analysis. *Analytical Biochemistry*, **64**, 588–592.

Gieseg, S.P., Simpson, J.A., Charlton, T.S., Duncan, M.W., and Dean, R.T. (1993). Protein-bound 3,4-dihydroxyphenylalanine is a major reductant formed during hydroxyl radical damage to proteins. *Biochemistry*, **32**, 4780–4786.

Giessauf, A., Steiner, E., and Esterbauer, H. (1995). Early destruction of trypto-phan residues of apolipoprotein B is a vitamin E-independent process during copper-mediated oxidation of LDL. *Biochimica et Biophysica Acta*, **1256**, 221–232.

Giessauf, A., van Wickern, B., Simat, T., Steinhart, H., and Esterbauer, H. (1996). Formation of *N*-formylkynurenine suggests the involvement of apolipoprotein B-100 centered tryptophan radicals in the initiation of LDL lipid peroxidation. *FEBS Letters*, **389**, 136–140.

Gilbert, B.C., Laue, H.A.H., Norman, R.O.C., and Sealy, R.C. (1975). Electron spin resonance studies. Part XVI. Oxidation of thiols and disulphides in aqueous solution: formation of RS·, RSO·, RSO_2·, RSSR·$^-$, and carbon radicals. *Journal of the Chemical Society, Perkin Transactions 2*, 892–900.

Gilbert, B.C., Holmes, R.G.G., Laue, H.A.H., Norman, R.O.C. (1976). Electron spin resonance studies. Part L. reactions of alkoxyl radicals generated from hydroperoxides and titanium(III) ion in aqueous solution. *Journal of the Chemical Society, Perkin Transactions 2*, 1047–1052.

Gilbert, B.C., Holmes, R.G.G., and Norman, R.O.C. (1977). Electron spin reson-ance studies. Part LII. Reactions of secondary alkoxyl radicals. *Journal of Chemical Research (S)*, 1.

Gilbert, B.C., Marshall, P.D.R., and Norman, R.O.C., Pineda, N., Williams, P.S. (1981). Electron spin resonance studies. Part 61. The generation and reactions of the *t*-butoxyl radical in aqueous solution. *Journal of the Chemical Society, Perkin Transactions 2*, 1392–1400.

Gilbert, H.F., Kruzel, M.L., Lyles, M.M., and Harper, J.W. (1991). Expression and purification of recombinant rat protein disulfide isomerase from *Escherichia coli*. *Protein Experimental Purification*, **2**, 194–198.

Ginsburg, A., and Stadtman, E.R. (1970). Multienzyme systems. *Annual Reviews of Biochemistry*, **39**, 429–472.

Ginsburg, I. (1989). Bacteriolysis is inhibited by hydrogen peroxide and by proteases. *Agents Actions*, **28**, 238–242.

Giron-Calle, J., Zwizinski, C.W., and Schmid, H.H.O. (1994). Peroxidative damage to cardiac mitochondria. II Immunological analysis of modified adenine nucleotide translocase. *Archives of Biochemistry and Biophysics*, **315**, 1–7.

Girotti, A.W., Thomas, J.P., and Jordan, J.E. (1986). Xanthine oxidase-catalyzed crosslinking of cell membrane proteins. *Archives of Biochemistry and Biophysics*, **251**, 639–653.

Giulivi, C., and Cadenas, E. (1993). Inhibition of protein radical reactions of ferrylmyoglobin by the water-soluble analog of vitamin E, Trolox C. *Archives of Biochemistry and Biophysics*, **303**, 152–158.

Giulivi, C., and Davies, K.J. (1990). A novel antioxidant role for hemoglobin. The comproportionation of ferrylhemoglobin with oxyhemoglobin. *Journal of Biological Chemistry*, **265**, 19453–19460.

Giulivi, C., and Davies, K.J. (1993). Dityrosine and tyrosine oxidation products are endogenous markers for the selective proteolysis of oxidatively modified red blood cell hemoglobin by (the 19 S) proteasome. *Journal of Biological Chemistry*, **268**, 8752–8759.

Giulivi, C., and Davies, K.J. (1994a). Hydrogen peroxide-mediated ferrylhemo-globin generation *in vitro* and in red blood cells. *Methods in Enzymology*, **231**, 490–496.

Giulivi, C., and Davies, K.J. (1994b). Dityrosine: a marker for oxidatively modified proteins and selective proteolysis. *Methods in Enzymology*, **233**, 363–371.

Giulivi, C., Romero, F.J., and Cadenas, E. (1992). The interaction of Trolox C, a water-soluble vitamin E analog, with ferrylmyoglobin: reduction of the oxoferryl moiety. *Archives of Biochemistry and Biophysics*, **299**, 302–312.

Giulivi, C., Pacifici, R.E., and Davies, K.J. (1994a). Exposure of hydrophobic moieties promotes the selective degradation of hydrogen peroxide-modified hemoglobin by the multicatalytic proteinase complex, proteasome. *Archives of Biochemistry and Biophysics*, **311**, 329–341.

Giulivi, C., Hochstein, P., and Davies, K.J. (1994b). Hydrogen peroxide production by red blood cells. *Free Radical Biology and Medicine*, **16**, 123–129.

Gladstone, I.J., and Levine, R.L. (1994). Oxidation of proteins in neonatal lungs. *Pediatrics*, **93**, 764–768.

Glatz, Z., Janiczek, O., Wimmerova, M., and Novotny, M.V. (1995). Detection of quinoproteins after electrophoresis in the presence of urea or SDS. *Biochemistry and Molecular Biology International*, **35**, 1–10.

Gmeiner, B.M., and Seelos, C. (1995). Modulation of biological tyrosine reactions by tyrosine phosphorylation. *Wien Klinica Wochenschrift*, **107**, 687–689.

Godovac, Z.J., Krause, I., Buchberger, J., Weiss, G., and Klostermeyer, H. (1990). Genetic variants of bovine beta-lactoglobulin. A novel wild-type beta-lacto-globulin W and its primary sequence. *Biological Chemistry, Hoppe-Seyler*, **371**, 255–260.

Goettlich, R.W., Young, J.O., and Tappel, A.L. (1971). Cathepsins D, A and B, and the effect of pH in the pathway of protein hydrolysis. *Biochimica et Biophysica Acta*, **243**, 137–146.

Goldberg, A.L., and Boches, F.S. (1982). Oxidized proteins in erythrocytes are rapidly degraded by the adenosine triphosphate-dependent proteolytic system. *Science*, **215**, 1107–1109.

Goldberg, A.L., and Dice, J.F. (1974). Intracellular protein degradation in mammalian and bacterial cells. *Annual Reviews of Biochemistry*, **43**, 835–869.

Goldberg, A.L., and St John, A.C. (1976). Intracellular protein degradation in mammalian and bacterial cells: Part 2. *Annual Reviews of Biochemistry*, **45**, 747–803.

Goldsmith, P.C., Leslie, T.A., Hayes, N.A., Levell, N.J., Dowd, P.M., and Foreman, J.C. (1996). Inhibitors of nitric oxide synthase in human skin. *Journal of Investigative Dermatology*, **106**, 113–118.

Goldstein, S., and Czapski, G. (1995). Kinetics of nitric oxide autoxidation in aqueous solution in the absence and presence of various reductants. The nature of the oxidizing intermediates. *Journal of the American Chemical Society*, **117**, 12078–12084.

Goldstone, S.D., Fragonas, J.C., Jeitner, T.M., and Hunt, N.H. (1995). Transcription factors as targets for oxidative signalling during lymphocyte activation. *Biochimica et Biophysica Acta*, **1263**, 114–122.

Gong, H.S., and Ohad, I. (1991). The PQ/PQH2 ratio and occupancy of photosystem II-QB site by plastoquinone control the degradation of D1 protein during photoinhibition *in vivo*. *Journal of Biological Chemistry*, **266**, 21293–21299.

Good, P.F., Werner, P., Hsu, A., Olanow, C.W., and Perl, D.P. (1996). Evidence of neuronal oxidative damage in Alzheimer's disease. *American Journal of Pathology*, **149**, 21–28.

Goodin, D.B., Mauk, A.G., and Smith, M. (1986). Studies of the radical species in compound ES of cytochrome *c* peroxidase altered by site-directed mutagenesis. *Proceedings of the National Academy of Science of the United States of America*, **83**, 1295–1299.

Goodman, Y., and Mattson, M.P. (1996). Ceramide protects hippocampal neurons against excitotoxic and oxidative insults, and amyloid beta-peptide toxicity. *Journal of Neurochemistry*, **66**, 869–872.

Goodwin, J.L., Uemura, E., and Cunnick, J.E. (1995). Microglial release of nitric oxide by the synergistic action of beta-amyloid and IFN-gamma. *Brain Research*, **692**, 207–214.

Gopalakrishna, R., Chen, Z.H., and Gundimeda, U. (1992). Irreversible oxidative inactivation of protein kinase C by photosensitive inhibitor calphostin C. *FEBS Letters*, **314**, 149–154.

Gopaul, N.K., Anggard, E.E., Mallet, A.I., Betteridge, D.J., Wolff, S.P., and Nourooz, Z.J. (1995). Plasma 8-epi-PGF2 alpha levels are elevated in individuals with non-insulin dependent diabetes mellitus. *FEBS Letters*, **368**, 225–229.

Gordon, S., Hart, E.J., Matheson, M.S., Rabani, J., and Thomas, J.K. (1963). Reaction rate constants of the hydrated electron. *Journal of the American Chemical Society*, **85**, 1375–1377.

Gordon, S., Schmidt., K.H., and Hart, E.J. (1977). A pulse radiolysis study of aqueous benzene solutions. *Journal of Physical Chemistry*, **81**, 104–109.

Gordy, W., and Shields, H. (1958). Electron-spin resonance studies of radiation damage to proteins. *Radiation Research*, **9**, 611–625.

Gordy, W., and Miyagawa, I. (1960). Electron spin resonance studies of mechanisms for chemical protection from ionizing radiation. *Radiation Research*, **12**, 211–229.

Gordy, W., Ard, W.B., and Shields, H. (1955a). Microwave spectroscopy of biological susbtances. I Paramagnetic resonance in X-irradiated amino acids and proteins. *Proceedings of the National Academy of Science of the United States of America*, **41**, 983–996.

Gordy, W., Ard, W.B., and Shields, H. (1955b). Microwave spectroscopy of biological substances. II. Paramagnetic resonance in X-irradiated carboxylic and hydroxy acids. *Proceedings of the National Academy of Science of the United States of America*, **41**, 996–1004.

Gorisch, H., and Rupp, M. (1989). Quinoprotein ethanol dehydrogenase from *Pseudomonas*. *Antonie Van Leeuwenhoek*, **56**, 35–45.

Gorman, A.A., Lovering, G., and Rodgers, M.A.J. (1979). The entropy-controlled reactivity of singlet oxygen towards furans and indoles in toluene. Variable temperature study by pulse radiolysis. *Journal of the American Chemical Society*, **101**, 3050–3055.

Gottschall, W.C.J., and Tolbert, B.M. (1968). The radiation chemistry of anhydrous solid state glycine, alanine, and glycine salts. In *Radiation Chemistry Vol. 1*, (ed. R.F. Gould), pp. 374–383. American Chemical Society, Washington.

Gould, A.R., and Eaton, B.T. (1990). The amino acid sequence of the outer coat protein VP2 of neutralizing monoclonal antibody-resistant, virulent and attenuated bluetongue viruses. *Virus Research*, **17**, 161–172.

Gow, A.J., Duran, D., Malcolm, S., and Ischiropoulos, H. (1996a). Effects of peroxynitrite-induced protein modifications on tyrosine phosphorylation and degradation. *FEBS Letters*, **385**, 63–66.

Gow, A., Duran, D., Thom, S.R., and Ischiropoulos, H. (1996b). Carbon dioxide enhancement of peroxynitrite-mediated protein tyrosine nitration. *Archives of Biochemistry and Biophysics*, **333**, 42–48.

Graceffa, P. (1983). Spin labeling of protein sulfydryl groups by spin trapping a sulfur radical: application to bovine serum albumin and myosin. *Archives of Biochemistry and Biophysics*, **225**, 802–808.

Graceffa, P. (1988). Spin trapping the cysteine thiyl radical with phenyl-*N-t*-butylnitrone. *Biochimica et Biophysica Acta*, **954**, 227–230.

Grady, J.K., Chasteen, N.D., and Harris, D.C. (1988). Radicals from 'Good's' buffers. *Analytical Biochemistry*, **173**, 111–115.

Grady, J.K., Chen, Y., Chasteen, N.D., and Harris, D.C. (1989). Hydroxyl radical production during oxidative deposition of iron in ferritin. *Journal of Biological Chemistry*, **264**, 20224–20229.

Graham, A., Hogg, N., Kalyanaraman, B., O'Leary, V., Darley, U.V., and Moncada, S. (1993). Peroxynitrite modification of low-density lipoprotein leads to recognition by the macrophage scavenger receptor. *FEBS Letters*, **330**, 181–185.

Grant, A.J., Jessup, W., and Dean, R.T. (1992). Accelerated endocytosis and incomplete catabolism of radical-damaged protein. *Biochimica et Biophysica Acta*, **1134**, 203–209.

Grant, A.J., Jessup, W., and Dean, R.T. (1993a). Enhanced enzymatic degradation of radical damaged mitochondrial membrane components. *Free Radical Research Communications*, **19**, 125–134.

Grant, A.J., Jessup, W., and Dean, R.T. (1993b). Inefficient degradation of oxidized regions of protein molecules. *Free Radical Research Communications*, **18**, 259–267.

Grattagliano, I., Vendemiale, G., Didonna, D., Errico, F., Bolognino, A., Pistone, A., *et al.* (1995). Oxidative modification of proteins in chronic alcoholics. *Bollettino Societa Italiana Biologia Sperimentale*, **71**, 189–195.

Gray, H.B., and Winkler, J.R. (1996). Electron transfer in proteins. *Annual Reviews of Biochemistry*, **65**, 537–561.

Green, E.S., Evans, H., Rice, E.P., Davies, M.J., Salah, N., and Rice, E.C. (1993a). The efficacy of monohydroxamates as free radical scavenging agents compared with di- and trihydroxamates. *Biochemical Pharmacology*, **45**, 357–366.

Green, E.S., Cooper, C.E., Davies, M.J., and Rice, E.C. (1993b). Antioxidant drugs and the inhibition of low-density lipoprotein oxidation. *Biochemical Society Transactions*, **21**, 362–366.

Green, M. (1982). Incorporation of amino acid analogs interferes with the processing of the asparagine-linked oligosaccharide of the MOPC-46B kappa light chain. *Journal of Biological Chemistry*, **257**, 9039–9042.

Greenaway, F.T., O'Gara, C.Y., Marchena, J.M., Poku, J.W., Urtiaga, J.G., and Zou, Y. (1991). EPR studies of spin-labeled bovine plasma amine oxidase: the nature of the substrate-binding site. *Archives of Biochemistry and Biophysics*, **285**, 291–296.

Greenberg, B.M., Gaba, V., Mattoo, A.K., and Edelman, M. (1987). Identification of a primary *in vivo* degradation product of the rapidly-turning-over 32 kD protein of photosystem II. *EMBO Journal*, **6**, 2865–2869.

Greenberg, B.M., Gaba, V., Canaani, O., Malkin, S., Mattoo, A.K., and Edelman, M. (1989). Separate photosensitizers mediate degradation of the 32-kDa photosystem II reaction center protein in the visible and UV spectral regions. *Proceedings of the National Academy of Science of the United States of America*, **86**, 6617–6620.

Greenberg, J.T., Chou, J.H., Monach, P.A., and Demple, B. (1991). Activation of oxidative stress genes by mutations at the soxQ/cfxB/marA locus of *Escherichia coli*. *Journal of Bacteriology*, **173**, 4433–4439.

Greene, D.A., Sima, A.A., Stevens, M.J., Feldman, E.L., and Lattimer, S.A. (1992). Complications: neuropathy, pathogenetic considerations. *Diabetes Care*, **15**, 1902–1925.

Greenley, T.L., and Davies, M.J. (1992). Detection of radicals produced by reaction of hydroperoxides with rat liver microsomal fractions. *Biochimica et Biophysica Acta*, **1116**, 192–203.

Greenley, T.L., and Davies, M.J. (1993). Radical production from peroxide and peracid tumour promoters: EPR spin trapping studies. *Biochimica et Biophysica Acta*, **1157**, 23–31.

Greenley, T.L., and Davies, M.J. (1994). Direct detection of radical generation in rat liver nuclei on treatment with tumour-promoting hydroperoxides and related compounds. *Biochimica et Biophysica Acta*, **1226**, 56–64.

Greenwell, M.V., Nettleton, G.S., and Feldhoff, R.C. (1983). An investigation of aldehyde fuchsin staining of unoxidized insulin. *Histochemistry*, **77**, 473–483.

Greiner, D.P., Hughes, K.A., Meares, C.F. (1996). Radiolytic protein surface mapping. *Biochemical and Biophysical Research Communications*, **225**, 1006–1008.

Grierson, L., Hildenbrand, K., and Bothe, E. (1992). Intramolecular transformation reaction of the glutathione thiyl radical into a non-sulphur-centred radical: a pulse-radiolysis and EPR study. *International Journal of Radiation Biology and Related Studies in Physics, Chemistry and Medicine*, **62**, 265–277.

Griffiths, H.R., Lunec, J., Gee, C.A., and Willson, R.L. (1988). Oxygen radical-induced alterations in polyclonal IgG. *FEBS Letters*, **230**, 155–158.

Griscavage, J.M., Wilk, S., and Ignarro, L.J. (1996). Inhibitors of the protease some pathway interfere with induction of nitric oxide synthase in macrophages by blocking activation of transcription factor NF-kappa B. *Proceedings of the National Academy of Science of the United States of America*, **93**, 3308–3312.

Grisham, M.B., Jefferson, M.M., Melton, D.F., and Thomas, E.L. (1984). Chlorination of endogenous amines by isolated neutrophils. Ammonia-dependent bactericidal, cytotoxic, and cytolytic activities of the chloramines. *Journal of Biological Chemistry*, **259**, 10404–10413.

Groen, B., Frank, J.J., and Duine, J.A. (1984). Quinoprotein alcohol dehydrogenase from ethanol-grown *Pseudomonas aeruginosa*. *Biochemical Journal*, **223**, 921–924.

Groen, B.W., and Duine, J.A. (1990). Quinoprotein alcohol dehydrogenase from *Pseudomonas aeruginosa* and quinohemoprotein alcohol dehydrogenase from *Pseudomonas testosteroni*. *Methods in Enzymology*, **188**, 33–39.

Groen, B.W., van, d.M.R., and Duine, J.A. (1988). Evidence for PQQ as cofactor in 3,4-dihydroxyphenylalanine (dopa) decarboxylase of pig kidney. *FEBS Letters*, **237**, 98–102.

Groenen, P.J., Seccia, M., Smulders, R.H., Gravela, E., Cheeseman, K.H., Bloemendal, H., *et al.* (1993). Exposure of beta H-crystallin to hydroxyl radicals enhances the transglutaminase-susceptibility of its existing amine-donor and amine-acceptor sites. *Biochemical Journal*, **295**, 399–404.

Gros, D., and Challice, C.E. (1975). The coating of mouse myocardial cells. A cytochemical electron microscopical study. *Journal of Histochemistry and Cytochemistry*, **23**, 727–744.

Gruber, H.A., and Mellon, E.F. (1975). Oxidation products of amino acids and collagens. *Analytical Biochemistry*, **66**, 78–86.

Gruger, E.J., and Tappel, A.L. (1969). Isolation of lipid hydroperoxides by preparative thin-layer chromatography of autoxidized esters of polyunsaturated fatty acids. *Journal of Chromatography*, **40**, 177–181.

Gruger, E.J., and Tappel, A.L. (1970*a*). Reactions of biological antioxidants. II. Fe(3)-catalyzed reactions of methyl linoleate hydroperoxides with derivatives of coenzymes Q and vitamin E. *Lipids*, **5**, 332–336.

Gruger, E.J., and Tappel, A.L. (1970*b*). Reactions of biological antioxidants. I. Fe(3)-catalyzed reactions of lipid hydroperoxides with alpha-tocopherol. *Lipids*, **5**, 326–331.

Gruger, E.J., and Tappel, A.L. (1971). Reactions of biological antioxidants. 3. Composition of biological membranes. *Lipids*, **6**, 147–148.

Grune, T., Reinheckel, T., Joshi, M., and Davies, K.J. (1995). Proteolysis in cultured liver epithelial cells during oxidative stress. Role of the multi-catalytic proteinase complex, proteasome. *Journal of Biological Chemistry*, **270**, 2344–2351.

Grune, T., Reinheckel, T., and Davies, K.J. (1996). Degradation of oxidized proteins in K562 human hematopoietic cells by proteasome. *Journal of Biological Chemistry*, **271**, 15504–15509.

Grzelinska, E., Bartkowiak, A., Bartosz, G., and Leyko, W. (1982). Effect of ·OH scavengers on radiation damage to the erythrocyte membrane. *International Journal of Radiation Biology and Related Studies in Physics, Chemistry and Medicine*, **41**, 473–481.

Guarneri, C., Lugaresi, A., Flamigni, F., Muscari, C., and Caldarera, C.M. (1982). Effect of oxygen radicals and hyperoxia on rate heart ornithine decarboxylase activity. *Biochimica et Biophysica Acta*, **718**, 157–164.

Guelinckx, P.J., Faulkner, J.A., and Essig, D.A. (1988). Neurovascular-anastomosed muscle grafts in rabbits: functional deficits result from tendon repair. *Muscle and Nerve*, **11**, 745–751.

Guengerich, F.P. (1986). Covalent binding to apoprotein is a major fate of heme in a variety of reactions in which cytochrome P-450 is destroyed. *Biochemical and Biophysical Research Communications*, **138**, 193–198.

Guex, N., Henry, H., Flach, J., Richter, H., and Widmer, F. (1995). Glyoxysomal malate dehydrogenase and malate synthase from soybean cotyledons (Glycine max L.): enzyme association, antibody production and cDNA cloning. *Planta*, **197**, 369–375.

Guiles, R.D., Basus, V.J., Sarma, S., Malpure, S., Fox, K.M., Kuntz, I.D., *et al.* (1993). Novel heteronuclear methods of assignment transfer from a diamagnetic to a paramagnetic protein: application to rat cytochrome *b*5. *Biochemistry*, **32**, 8329–8340.

Gunther, M.R., Kelman, D.J., Corbett, J.T., and Mason, R.P. (1995). Self-peroxidation of metmyoglobin results in formation of an oxygen-reactive tryptophan-centered radical. *Journal of Biological Chemistry*, **270**, 16075–16081.

Gupta, S., Rogers, L.K., and Smith, C.V. (1994). Biliary excretion of lysosomal enzymes, iron, and oxidized protein in Fischer-344 and Sprague-Dawley rats and the effects of diquat and acetaminophen. *Toxicology and Applied Pharmacology*, **125**, 42–50.

Guptasarma, P., Balasubramanian, D., Matsugo, S., and Saito, I. (1992). Hydroxyl radical mediated damage to proteins, with special reference to the crystallins [published erratum appears in *Biochemistry* (1992), **46**, 11664]. *Biochemistry*, **31**, 4296–4303.

Guss, J.M., Harrowell, P.R., Murata, M., Norris, V.A., and Freeman, H.C. (1986). Crystal structure analyses of reduced (CuI) poplar plastocyanin at six pH values. *Journal of Molecular Biology*, **192**, 361–387.

Gut, J., Kawato, S., Cherry, R.J., Winterhalter, K.H., and Richter, C. (1985). Lipid peroxidation decreases the rotational mobility of cytochrome P-450 in rat liver microsomes. *Biochimica et Biophysica Acta*, **817**, 217–228.

Gutierrez, S.J., Zentella, d.P.M., and Pina, E. (1993). Acute ethanol intake produces lipid peroxidation in rat red blood cells membranes. *Biochemistry and Molecular Biology International*, **29**, 263–270.

Gutteridge, J.M. (1985). Age pigments and free radicals: fluorescent lipid complexes formed by iron- and copper-containing proteins. *Biochimica et Biophysica Acta*, **834**, 144–148.

Gutteridge, J.M. (1986). Iron promoters of the Fenton reaction and lipid peroxidation can be released from haemoglobin by peroxides. *FEBS Letters*, **201**, 291–295.

Gutteridge, J.M. (1992). Ferrous ions detected in cerebrospinal fluid by using bleomycin and DNA damage. *Clinical Science*, **82**, 315–320.

Gutteridge, J.M., and Smith, A. (1988). Antioxidant protection by haemopexin of haem-stimulated lipid peroxidation. *Biochemical Journal*, **256**, 861–865.

Gutteridge, J.M., Quinlan, G.J., Mumby, S., Heath, A., and Evans, T.W. (1994). Primary plasma antioxidants in adult respiratory distress syndrome patients: changes in iron-oxidizing, iron-binding, and free radical-scavenging proteins. *Journal of Laboratory and Clinical Medicine*, **124**, 263–273.

Gutteridge, J.M.C. (1986). TBA-reactivities following iron-dependent free radical damage to amino acids and carbohydrates. *FEBS Letters*, **128**, 343–346.

Haber, F., and Weiss, J. (1932). Uber die Katalyse des Hydroperoxydes. *Naturwissenschaften*, **20**, 948–950.

Haber, F., and Weiss, J. (1934). The catalytic decomposition of hydrogen peroxide by iron salts. *Proceedings of the National Academy of Science of the Unites Stated of America Royal Society (London) A*, **147**, 332–352.

Haberland, A., Rootwelt, T., Saugstad, O.D., and Schimke, I. (1994). Modulation of the xanthine oxidase/xanthine dehydrogenase ratio by reaction of malondialdehyde with NH_2-groups. *European Journal of Clinical Chemistry and Clinical Biochemistry*, **32**, 267–272.

Haberland, M.E., Olch, C.L., and Folgelman, A.M. (1984). Role of lysines in mediating interaction of modified low density lipoproteins with the scavenger receptor of human monocyte macrophages. *Journal of Biological Chemistry*, **259**, 11305–11311.

Hackman, R.H. (1953). Chemistry of the insect cuticle. 3. Hardening and darkening of the cuticle. *Biochemical Journal*, **54**, 371–377.

Hackman, R.H., and Todd, A.R. (1953). Some observations on the reaction of catechol derivativs with amines and amino acids in the presence of oxidizing agents. *Biochemical Journal*, **55**, 631–637.

Haddad, I.Y., Ischiropoulos, H., Holm, B.A., Beckman, J.S., Baker, J.R., and Matalon, S. (1993). Mechanisms of peroxynitrite-induced injury to pulmonary surfactants. *American Journal of Physiology*, **265**, L555–L564.

Haddad, I.Y., Pataki, G., Hu, P., Galliani, C., Beckman, J.S., and Matalon, S. (1994*a*). Quantitation of nitrotyrosine levels in lung sections of patients and animals with acute lung injury. *Journal of Clinical Investigation*, **94**, 2407–2413.

Haddad, I.Y., Crow, J.P., Hu, P., Ye, Y., Beckman, J., and Matalon, S. (1994*b*). Concurrent generation of nitric oxide and superoxide damages surfactant protein A. *American Journal of Physiology*, **267**, L242–L249.

Haddock, P.S., Woodward, B., and Hearse, D.J. (1995*a*). Cardiac Na^+/K^+ ATPase activity and its relation to myocardial glutathione status: studies in the rat. *Journal of Molecular and Cellular Cardiology*, **27**, 1185–1194.

Haddock, P.S., Shattock, M.J., and Hearse, D.J. (1995*b*). Modulation of cardiac $Na^{(+)}$-K^+ pump current: role of protein and nonprotein sulfydryl redox status. *American Journal of Physiology*, **269**, H297–307.

Haest, C.W., Heller, K., Schwister, K., Kunze, I., Dressler, V., and Deuticke, B. (1983). Concomitant changes of membrane leak permeability and phospholipid dynamics in erythrocytes subjected to chemical and physical membrane perturbation. *Biomedica et Biochimica Acta*, **42**, S127–129.

Hafi, A., Cluet, J.L., Pages, N., Fournier, G., Alcindor, R., and Boudene, C. (1991). Comparison of production of volatile hydrocarbons by phenylhydrazine-induced peroxidation in rats chronically treated with lead. *Research Communications in Chemical Pathology and Pharmacology*, **71**, 105–114.

Hagen, W.R., Wassink, H., Eady, R.R., Smith, B.E., and Haaker, H. (1987). Quantitative EPR of an S = 7/2 system in thionine-oxidized MoFe proteins of nitrogenase. A redefinition of the P-cluster concept. *European Journal of Biochemistry*, **169**, 457–465.

Hainaut, P., and Milner, J. (1993). Redox modulation of p53 conformation and sequence-specific DNA binding *in vitro*. *Cancer Research*, **53**, 4469–4473.

Hainaut, P., Butcher, S., and Milner, J. (1995a). Temperature sensitivity for conformation is an intrinsic property of wild-type p53. *British Journal of Cancer*, **71**, 227–231.

Hainaut, P., Rolley, N., Davies, M., and Milner, J. (1995b). Modulation by copper of p53 conformation and sequence-specific DNA binding: role for Cu(II)/Cu(I) redox mechanism. *Oncogene*, **10**, 27–32.

Haklar, G., Ersahin, C., Moini, H., Sungun, M., Dogan, N., Bilsel, S., *et al.* (1995a). Protective effects of cilazapril against free radical injury in myocardial ischaemia-reperfusion. *Pharmacology Research*, **31**, 33–36.

Haklar, G., Yegenaga, I., and Yalcin, A.S. (1995b). Evaluation of oxidant stress in chronic hemodialysis patients: use of different parameters. *Clinica Chimica Acta*, **234**, 109–114.

Hall, N.C., Carney, J.M., Cheng, M.S., and Butterfield, D.A. (1995a). Ischemia/reperfusion-induced changes in membrane proteins and lipids of gerbil cortical synaptosomes. *Neuroscience*, **64**, 81–89.

Hall, N.C., Carney, J.M., Cheng, M., and Butterfield, D.A. (1995b). Prevention of ischemia/reperfusion-induced alterations in synaptosomal membrane-associated proteins and lipids by N-tert-butyl-alpha-phenylnitrone and difluoromethylornithine. *Neuroscience*, **69**, 591–600.

Haller, I., Hoehn, B., and Henning, U. (1975). Apparent high degree of asymmetry of protein arrangement in the *Escherichia coli* outer cell envelope membrane. *Biochemistry*, **14**, 478–484.

Halliwell, B., and Dizdaroglu, M. (1992). The measurement of oxidative damage to DNA by HPLC and GC/MS techniques. *Free Radical Research Communications*, **16**, 75–87.

Halliwell, B., and Gutteridge, J.M.C. (1989). *Free Radicals in Biology and Medicine*. Clarendon Press, Oxford.

Halliwell, B., Hu, M.L., Louie, S., Duvall, T.R., Tarkington, B.K., Motchnik, P., *et al.* (1992). Interaction of nitrogen dioxide with human plasma. Antioxidant depletion and oxidative damage. *FEBS Letters*, **313**, 62–66.

Hamazume, Y., Mega, T., and Ikenaka, T. (1987). Positions of disulfide bonds in riboflavin-binding protein of hen egg white. *Journal of Biochemistry, Tokyo*, **101**, 217–223.

Hamilton, T.A., Major, J.A., and Chisolm, G.M. (1995). The effects of oxidized low density lipoproteins on inducible mouse macrophage gene expression are gene and stimulus dependent. *Journal of Clinical Investigation*, **95**, 2020–2027.

Hanan, T., and Shaklai, N. (1995). The role of H_2O_2-generated myoglobin radical in crosslinking of myosin. *Free Radical Research*, **22**, 215–227.

Hanawa, T., Yamamoto, T., and Kamiya, S. (1995). Listeria monocytogenes can grow in macrophages without the aid of proteins induced by environmental stresses. *Infection and Immunity*, **63**, 4595–4599.

Handovsky, H. (1928). The oxidation-catalytic action of iron. *Zeitschrift für Physiologische Chemie*, **176**, 79–88.

Hanes, D.M., and Tappel, A.L. (1971). Lysosomal hemochromes and digestion of cytochrome c by the lysosomal protease system. *Biochimica et Biophysica Acta*, **245**, 42–53.

Hansberg, W. (1996). A hyperoxidant state at the start of each developmental stage during *Neurospora crassa* conidiation. *Ciencia e Cultura, Journal of the Brazilian Association for the Advancement of Science*, **48**, 68–74.

Hansberg, W., and Aguirre, J. (1990). Hyperoxidant states cause microbial cell differentiation by cell isolation from dioxygen. *Journal of Theoretical Biology*, **142**, 201–221.

Hansberg, W., De Groot, H., and Sies, H. (1993). Reactive oxygen species associated with cell differentiation in *Neurospora crassa*. *Free Radical Biology and Medicine*, **14**, 287–293.

Hansson, M., Asea, A., Ersson, U., Hermodsson, S., and Hellstrand, K. (1996). Induction of apoptosis in NK cells by monocyte-derived reactive oxygen metabolites. *Journal of Immunology*, **156**, 42–47.

Harada, K., and Yamazaki, I. (1987). Electron spin resonance spectra of free radicals formed in the reaction of metmyoglobins with ethylhydroperoxide. *Journal of Biochemistry, Tokyo*, **101**, 283–286.

Haramaki, N., Marcocci, L., D'Anna, R., Yan, L.J., Kobuchi, H., and Packer, L. (1995). Bio-Catalyzer alpharho No. 11 (Bio-Normalizer) supplementation: effect on oxidative stress to isolated rat hearts. *Biochemistry and Molecular Biology International*, **36**, 1263–1268.

Hardwick, J.S., and Sefton, B.M. (1995). Activation of the Lck tyrosine protein kinase by hydrogen peroxide requires the phosphorylation of Tyr-394. *Proceedings of the National Academy of Science of the United States of America*, **92**, 4527–4531.

Harel, S., and Kanner, J. (1988). The generation of ferryl or hydroxyl radicals during interaction of haemproteins with hydrogen peroxide. *Free Radical Research Communications*, **5**, 21–33.

Harel, S., Salan, M.A., and Kanner, J. (1988). Iron release from metmyoglobin, methaemoglobin and cytochrome c by a system generating hydrogen peroxide. *Free Radical Research Communications*, **5**, 11–19.

Harlow, G.R., and Halpert, J.R. (1996). Mutagenesis study of Asp-290 in cytochrome P450 2B11 using a fusion protein with rat NADPH-cytochrome P450 reductase. *Archives of Biochemistry and Biophysics*, **326**, 85–92.

Harris, D.T. (1926). Observations on the velocity of the photooxidation of proteins and amino acids. *Biochemical Journal*, **20**, 524–532.

Harris, R.Z., Wariishi, H., Gold, M.H., and Ortiz de Montellano, P.R. (1991). The catalytic site of manganese peroxidase. Regiospecific addition of sodium azide and alkylhydrazines to the heme group. *Journal of Biological Chemistry*, **266**, 8751–8758.

Harris, E.D. (1992). The pyrroloquinoline quinone (PQQ) coenzymes: a case of mistaken identity. *Nutrition Reviews*, **50**, 263–267.

Harris, M.E., Carney, J.M., Cole, P.S., Hensley, K., Howard, B.J., Martin, L., et al. (1995a). Beta-amyloid peptide-derived, oxygen-dependent free radicals inhibit glutamate uptake in cultured astrocytes: implications for Alzheimer's disease. Neuroreport, 6, 1875–1879.

Harris, M.E., Hensley, K., Butterfield, D.A., Leedle, R.A., and Carney, J.M. (1995b). Direct evidence of oxidative injury produced by the Alzheimer's beta-amyloid peptide (1–40) in cultured hippocampal neurons. Experimental Neurology, 131, 193–202.

Harris, T.K., and Davidson, V.L. (1993a). Binding and electron transfer reactions between methanol dehydrogenase and its physiologic electron acceptor cytochrome c-551i: a kinetic and thermodynamic analysis. Biochemistry, 32, 14145–14150.

Harris, T.K., and Davidson, V.L. (1993b). A new kinetic model for the steady-state reactions of the quinoprotein methanol dehydrogenase from Paracoccus denitrificans. Biochemistry, 32, 4362–4368.

Harris, T.K., Davidson, V.L., Chen, L., Mathews, F.S., and Xia, Z.X. (1994). Ionic strength dependence of the reaction between methanol dehydrogenase and cytochrome c-551i: evidence of conformationally coupled electron transfer. Biochemistry, 33, 12600–12608.

Harrison, J.E., and Schultz, J. (1976). Studies on the chlorinating activity of myeloperoxidase. Journal of Biological Chemistry, 251, 1371–1374.

Hart, B.A., Eneman, J.D., Gong, Q., and Durieux, L.C. (1995). Increased oxidant resistance of alveolar epithelial type II cells. Isolated from rats following repeated exposure to cadmium aerosols. Toxicology Letters, 81, 131–139.

Hart, E.J., and Anbar, M. (1970). The Hydrated Electron. Wiley-Interscience, New York.

Hart, E.J., and Fielden, E.M., and Anbar, M. (1967). Reactions of carbonylic compounds with hydrated electrons. Journal of Physical Chemistry, 71, 3993–3998.

Hartel, B., Ludwig, P., Schewe, T., and Rapoport, S.M. (1982). Self-inactivation by 13-hydroperoxylinoleic acid and lipohydroperoxidase activity of the reticulocyte lipoxygenase. European Journal of Biochemistry, 126, 353–357.

Hartley, A., Davies, M.J., and Rice, E.C. (1989). Desferrioxamine and membrane oxidation: radical scavenger or iron chelator? Biochemical Society Transactions, 17, 1002–1003.

Hartman, P.S., Eisenstark, A., and Pauw, P.G. (1979). Inactivation of phage T7 by near-ultraviolet radiation plus hydrogen peroxide: DNA-protein crosslinks prevent DNA injection. Proceedings of the National Academy of Science of the United States of America, 76, 3228–3232.

Hartmann, C., and Dooley, D.M. (1995). Detection of reaction intermediates in topa quinone enzymes. Methods in Enzymology, 258, 69–90.

Hashimoto, K., Ivanov, V.V., Inomata, K., Kawai, T., Mizunuma, K., Klimatskaia, L.G., et al. (1995). Biological monitoring of exposure to alkylating xenobiotics by determining them using a new analytical approach in complexes with hemoglobin, plasma proteins and mercapturic acids in urine. II. Acrylamide. Voprosy Medicinska Khimii, 41, 22–25.

Hashimoto, S., Seki, H., Masuda, T., Imamura, M., and Kondo, M. (1981). Dimer formation in radiation-irradiated aqueous solution of lysozyme studied by light-scattering-intensity measurement. International Journal of Radiation Biology and Related Studies in Physics, Chemistry and Medicine, 40, 31–46.

Hasinoff, B.B., and Pecht, I. (1983). Pulse radiolysis kinetics of the reaction of hydrated electrons with ferric-, ferrous-, protoporphyrin IX- and apo-myoglobin. *Biochimica et Biophysica Acta*, **743**, 310–315.

Hatakeyama, T., Yamasaki, N., and Funatsu, G. (1986). Identification of the tryptophan residue located at the low-affinity saccharide binding site of ricin D. *Journal of Biochemistry Tokyo*, **100**, 781–788.

Hatori, M., Sparkman, J., Teixeira, C.C., Grynpas, M., Nervina, J., Olivieri, N., et al. (1995). Effects of deforoximine on chondrocyte alkaline phosphatase activity: proxidant role of deforoximine in thalassemia. *Calcification Tissue International*, **57**, 229–236.

Hatta, A., and Frei, B. (1995). Oxidative modification and antioxidant protection of human low density lipoprotein at high and low oxygen partial pressures. *Journal of Lipid Research*, **36**, 2383–2393.

Haurowitz, F., and Tumer, A. (1949). The proteolytic cleavage of irradiated proteins. *Enzymologia*, **13**, 229–231.

Hawkes, W.C., Lyons, D.E., and Tappel, A.L. (1982). Identification of a selenocysteine-specific aminoacyl transfer RNA from rat liver. *Biochimica et Biophysica Acta*, **699**, 183–191.

Hawkes, W.C., Wilhelmsen, E.C., and Tappel, A.L. (1985). Abundance and tissue distribution of selenocysteine-containing proteins in the rat. *Journal of Inorganic Biochemistry*, **23**, 77–92.

Hawkins, C.L., and Davies, M.J. (1995). Detection of intermediates formed on reaction of hyaluronic acid and related materials with the hydroxyl radical. *Biochemical Society Transactions*, **23**, 248S.

Hawkins, C.L., and Davies, M.J. (1997). Oxidative damage to collagen and related substrates by metal ion/hydrogen peroxide systems: random attack or site-specific damage? *Biochimica et Biophysica Acta*, **1360**, 84–96.

Hayashi, T., Ueno, Y., and Okamoto, T. (1993). Oxidoreductive regulation of nuclear factor kappa B. Involvement of a cellular reducing catalyst thioredoxin. *Journal of Biological Chemistry*, **268**, 11380–11388.

Hayon, E., and Allen, A.O. (1961). Evidence for two kinds of H atoms in the radiation chemistry of water. *Journal of Physical Chemistry*, **65**, 2181–2185.

Hayon, E., and Simic, M. (1971). Pulse radiolysis study of cyclic peptides in aqueous solution. Absorption spectrum of the peptide radical –NHCHCO–. *Journal of the American Chemical Society*, **93**, 6781–6786.

Hazell, L.J., and Stocker, R. (1993). Oxidation of low-density lipoprotein with hypochlorite causes transformation of the lipoprotein into a high-uptake form for macrophages. *Biochemical Journal*, **290**, 165–172.

Hazell, L.J., van, d.B.J., and Stocker, R. (1994). Oxidation of low-density lipoprotein by hypochlorite causes aggregation that is mediated by modification of lysine residues rather than lipid oxidation. *Biochemical Journal*, **302**, 421–428.

Hazell, L.J., Arnold, L., Flowers, D., Waeg, G., Malle, E., and Stocker, R. (1996). Presence of hypochlorite-modified proteins in human atherosclerotic lesions. *Journal of Clinical Investigation*, **97**, 1535–1544.

Hazen, S.L., Hsu, F.F., and Heinecke, J.W. (1996). *p*-Hydroxyphenylacetaldehyde is the major product of L-tyrosine oxidation by activated human phagocytes. A chloride-dependent mechanism for the conversion of free amino acids into reactive aldehydes by myeloperoxidase. *Journal of Biological Chemistry*, **271**, 1861–1867.

Hazlewood, C., and Davies, M.J. (1995*a*). Damage to DNA and RNA by tumour promoter-derived alkoxyl radicals: an EPR spin trapping study. *Biochemical Society Transactions*, **23**, 259S

Hazlewood, C., and Davies, M.J. (1995*b*). EPR spin-trapping studies of the reaction of radicals derived from hydroperoxide tumour-promoters with nucleic acids and their components. *J. Chem. Soc. Perkin Transactions 2*, 895–901.

Häusler, J., Jahn, R., and Schmidt, U. (1978). Radikalisch und photochemisch initiiert Oxidation von Aminosäurederivaten. *Chemistry Berichte*, **111**, 361–366.

He, P., and Yasumoto, K. (1992). Effect of ingestion of excess methionine diet on aging of erythrocytes in mice. *Journal of Nutritional Science and Vitaminology Tokyo*, **38**, 57–68.

Hearse, D.J. (1991*a*). Stunning: a radical re-view. *Cardiovascular Drugs and Therapies*, **5**, 853–876.

Hearse, D.J. (1991*b*). Reperfusion-induced injury: a possible role for oxidant stress and its manipulation. *Cardiovascular Drugs and Therapies*, **2**, 225–235.

Hearse, D.J. (1995). Activation of ATP-sensitive potassium channels: a novel pharmacological approach to myocardial protection? *Cardiovascular Research*, **30**, 1–17.

Hearse, D.J., and Tosaki, A. (1987*a*). Reperfusion-induced arrhythmias and free radicals: studies in the rat heart with DMPO. *Journal of Cardiovascular Pharmacology*, **9**, 641–650.

Hearse, D.J., and Tosaki, A. (1987*b*). Free radicals and reperfusion-induced arrhythmias: protection by spin trap agent PBN in the rat heart. *Circulation Research*, **60**, 375–383.

Hearse, D.J., and Tosaki, A. (1988). Free radicals and calcium: simultaneous interacting triggers as determinants of vulnerability to reperfusion-induced arrhythmias in the rat heart. *Journal of Molecular and Cellular Cardiology*, **20**, 213–223.

Hearse, D.J., Manning, A.S., Downey, J.M., and Yellon, D.M. (1986). Xanthine oxidase: a critical mediator of myocardial injury during ischemia and reperfusion? *Acta Physiologica Scandinavia (Supplement)*, **548**, 65–78.

Hearse, D.J., Kusama, Y., and Bernier, M. (1989). Rapid electrophysiological changes leading to arrhythmias in the aerobic rat heart. Photosensitization studies with rose bengal-derived reactive oxygen intermediates. *Circulation Research*, **65**, 146–153.

Hebbel, R.P., Shalev, O., Foker, W., and Rank, B.H. (1986). Inhibition of erythrocyte Ca^{2+}-ATPase by activated oxygen through thiol- and lipid-dependent mechanisms. *Biochimica et Biophysica Acta*, **862**, 8–16.

Hebbel, R.P., Leung, A., and Mohandas, N. (1990). Oxidation-induced changes in microrheologic properties of the red blood cell membrane. *Blood*, **76**, 1015–1020.

Heilig, K., Willand, J., Gast, M.J., and Hortin, G. (1984). Variable denaturation of ovalbumin by incorporation of amino acid analogs. *Biochemical and Biophysical Research Communications*, **118**, 481–487.

Heim, R., Prasher, D.C., and Tsien, R.Y. (1994). Wavelength mutations and posttranslational autoxidation of green fluorescent protein. *Proceedings of the National Academy of Science of the United States of America*, **91**, 12501–12504.

Heinecke, J.W. (1987). Free radical modification of low-density lipoprotein: mechanisms and biological consequences. *Free Radical Biology and Medicine*, **3**, 65–73.

Heinecke, J.W., and Shapiro, B.M. (1989). Respiratory burst oxidase of fertilization. *Proceedings of the National Academy of Science of the United States of America*, **86**, 1259–1263.

Heinecke, J.W., and Shapiro, B.M. (1990). Superoxide peroxidase activity of ovoperoxidase, the cross-linking enzyme of fertilization. *Journal of Biological Chemistry*, **265**, 9241–9246.

Heinecke, J.W., and Shapiro, B.M. (1992). The respiratory burst oxidase of fertilization. A physiological target for regulation by protein kinase C. *Journal of Biological Chemistry*, **267**, 7959–7962.

Heinecke, J.W., Rosen, H., and Chait, A. (1984). Iron and copper promote modification of low density lipoprotein by human arterial smooth muscle cells in culture. *Journal of Clinical Investigation*, **74**, 1890–1894.

Heinecke, J.W., Rosen, H., Suzuki, L.A., and Chait, A. (1987). The role of sulfur-containing amino acids in superoxide production and modification of low density lipoprotein by arterial smooth muscle cells. *Journal of Biological Chemistry*, **262**, 10098–10103.

Heinecke, J.W., Suits, A.G., Aviram, M., and Chait, A. (1991). Phagocytosis of lipase-aggregated low density lipoprotein promotes macrophage foam cell formation. Sequential morphological and biochemical events. *Arteriosclerosis and Thrombosis*, **11**, 1643–1651.

Heinecke, J.W., Li, W., Francis, G.A., and Goldstein, J.A. (1993a). Tyrosyl radical generated by myeloperoxidase catalyzes the oxidative cross-linking of proteins. *Journal of Clinical Investigation*, **91**, 2866–2872.

Heinecke, J.W., Kawamura, M., Suzuki, L., and Chait, A. (1993b). Oxidation of low density lipoprotein by thiols: superoxide-dependent and -independent mechanisms. *Journal of Lipid Research*, **34**, 2051–2061.

Heinecke, J.W., Li, W., Daehnke, H.D., and Goldstein, J.A. (1993c). Dityrosine, a specific marker of oxidation, is synthesized by the myeloperoxidase-hydrogen peroxide system of human neutrophils and macrophages. *Journal of Biological Chemistry*, **268**, 4069–4077.

Heinecke, J.W., Li, W., Mueller, D.M., Bohrer, A., and Turk, J. (1994). Cholesterol chlorohydrin synthesis by the myeloperoxidase-hydrogen peroxide-chloride system: potential markers for lipoproteins oxidatively damaged by phagocytes. *Biochemistry*, **33**, 10127–10136.

Held, K.D., Sylvester, F.C., Hopcia, K.L., and Biaglow, J.E. (1996). Role of Fenton chemistry in thiol-induced toxicity and apoptosis. *Radiation Research*, **145**, 542–553.

Hendil, K.B. (1980). Intracellular degradation of hemoglobin transferred into fibroblasts by fusion with red blood cells. *Journal of Cellular Physiology*, **105**, 449–460.

Hendriks, W.H., Moughan, P.J., Tarttelin, M.F., and Woolhouse, A.D. (1995). Felinine: a urinary amino acid of Felidae. *Comparative Biochemistry and Physiology B Biochemistry and Molecular Biology*, **112**, 581–588.

Hendrix, L.R., Mallavia, L.P., and Samuel, J.E. (1993). Cloning and sequencing of *Coxiella burnetii* outer membrane protein gene com1. *Infection and Immunity*, **61**, 470–477.

Hennet, T., Peterhans, E., and Stocker, R. (1992). Alterations in antioxidant defences in lung and liver of mice infected with influenza A virus. *Journal of General Virology*, **73**, 39–46.

Henricks, P.A., Engels, F., van, d.V.H., and Nijkamp, F.P. (1991). 9- and 13-hydroxy-linoleic acid possess chemotactic activity for bovine and human polymorphonuclear leukocytes. *Prostaglandins*, **41**, 21–27.

Henriksen, T. (1967). Effect of oxygen on radiation-induced free radicals in proteins. *Radiation Research*, **32**, 892–904.

Henriksen, T., Sanner, T., and Pihl, A. (1963). Secondary processes in proteins irradiated in the dry state. *International Journal of Radiation Biology and Related Studies in Physics, Chemistry and Medicine*, **3**, 351–359.

Henry, R.R., Thorburn, A.W., Beerdsen, P., and Gumbiner, B. (1991). Dose-response characteristics of impaired glucose oxidation in non-insulin-dependent diabetes mellitus. *American Journal of Physiology*, **261**, E132–E140.

Hensley, K., Postlewaite, J., Dobbs, P., and Butterfield, D.A. (1993). Alteration of the erythrocyte membrane via enzymatic degradation of ankyrin (band 2.1): subcellular surgery characterized by EPR spectroscopy. *Biochimica et Biophysica Acta*, **1145**, 205–211.

Hensley, K., Carney, J., Hall, N., Shaw, W., and Butterfield, D.A. (1994a). Electron paramagnetic resonance investigations of free radical-induced alterations in neocortical synaptosomal membrane protein infrastructure. *Free Radical Biology and Medicine*, **17**, 321–331.

Hensley, K., Carney, J.M., Mattson, M.P., Aksenova, M., Harris, M., Wu, J.F., et al. (1994b). A model for beta-amyloid aggregation and neurotoxicity based on free radical generation by the peptide: relevance to Alzheimer disease. *Proceedings of the National Academy of Science of the United States of America*, **91**, 3270–3274.

Hensley, K., Hall, N., Subramaniam, R., Cole, P., Harris, M., Aksenov, M., et al. (1995a). Brain regional correspondence between Alzheimer's disease histopathology and biomarkers of protein oxidation. *Journal of Neurochemistry*, **65**, 2146–2156.

Hensley, K., Howard, B.J., Carney, J.M., and Butterfield, D.A. (1995b). Membrane protein alterations in rodent erythrocytes and synaptosomes due to aging and hyperoxia. *Biochimica et Biophysica Acta*, **1270**, 203–206.

Hensley, K., Aksenova, M., Carney, J.M., Harris, M., and Butterfield, D.A. (1995c). Amyloid beta-peptide spin trapping. I: Peptide enzyme toxicity is related to free radical spin trap reactivity. *Neuroreport*, **6**, 489–492.

Hensley, K., Butterfield, D.A., Mattson, M., Aksenova, M., Harris, M., Wu, J.F., et al. (1995d). A model for beta-amyloid aggregation and neurotoxicity based on the free radical generating capacity of the peptide: implications of 'molecular shrapnel' for Alzheimer's disease. *Proceedings of the America West Pharmacological Society*, **38**, 113–120.

Hensley, K., Aksenova, M., Carney, J.M., Harris, M., and Butterfield, D.A. (1995). Amyloid beta-peptide spin trapping. II: Evidence for decomposition of the PBN spin adduct. *Neuroreport*, **6**, 493–496.

Herbers, K., Monke, G., Badur, R., and Sonnewald, U. (1995). A simplified procedure for the subtractive cDNA cloning of photoassimilate-responding genes: isolation of cDNAs encoding a new class of pathogenesis-related proteins. *Plant Molecular Biology*, **29**, 1027–1038.

Herrada, G., Puppo, A., Moreau, S., Day, D.A., and Rigaud, J. (1993). How is leghemoglobin involved in peribacteroid membrane degradation during nodule senescence? *FEBS Letters*, **326**, 33–38.

Herschberger, L.A., and Tappel, A.L. (1982). Effect of vitamin E on pentane exhaled by rats treated with methyl ethyl ketone peroxide. *Lipids*, **17**, 686–691.

Heym, C., Braun, B., Shuyi, Y., Klimaschewski, L., and Colombo, B.M. (1995). Immunohistochemical correlation of human adrenal nerve fibres and thoracic dorsal root neurons with special reference to substance P. *Histochemistry and Cellular Biology*, **104**, 233–243.

Hicks, M., Delbridge, L., Yue, D.K., and Reeve, T.S. (1988). Catalysis of lipid peroxidation by glucose and glycosylated collagen. *Biochemical and Biophysical Research Communications*, **151**, 649–655.

Hidalgo, F.J., Zamora, R., and Tappel, A.L. (1990a). Damage to red blood cells by halocompounds. *Toxicology Letters*, **52**, 191–199.

Hidalgo, F.J., Zamora, R., and Tappel, A.L. (1990b). Oxidant-induced haemoprotein degradation in rat tissue slices: effect of bromotrichloromethane, antioxidants and chelators. *Biochimica et Biophysica Acta*, **1037**, 313–320.

Higa, T., and Desiderio, D.M. (1988). Chemical degradation of 3H-labeled substance P in tris buffer solution. *Analytical Biochemistry*, **173**, 463–468.

Hildebrandt, P., Matysik, J., Schrader, B., Scharf, B., and Engelhard, M. (1994). Raman spectroscopic study of the blue copper protein halocyanin from *Natronobacterium pharaonis*. *Biochemistry*, **33**, 11426–11431.

Hilgemann, D.W., and Collins, A. (1992). Mechanism of cardiac $Na^{(+)}$-Ca^{2+} exchange current stimulation by MgATP: possible involvement of aminophospholipid translocase. *Journal of Physiology (London)*, **454**, 59–82.

Hill, E., Maclouf, J., Murphy, R.C., and Henson, P.M. (1992). Reversible membrane association of neutrophil 5-lipoxygenase is accompanied by retention of activity and a change in substrate specificity. *Journal of Biological Chemistry*, **267**, 22048–22053.

Hill, K.E., and Burk, R.F. (1984). Influence of vitamin E and selenium on glutathione-dependent protection against microsomal lipid peroxidation. *Biochemical Pharmacology*, **33**, 1065–1068.

Hillar, A., Nicholls, P., Switala, J., and Loewen, P.C. (1994). NADPH binding and control of catalase compound II formation: comparison of bovine, yeast, and *Escherichia coli* enzymes. *Biochemical Journal*, **300**, 531–539.

Hiller, K.-O., Masloch, B., Göbl, M., and Asmus, K.-D. (1981). Mechanism of the OH· radical induced oxidation of methionine in aqueous solution. *Journal of the American Chemical Society*, **103**, 2734–2743.

Hilton, J.C., and Rajagopalan, K.V. (1996). Identification of the molybdenum cofactor of dimethyl sulfoxide reductase from *Rhodobacter sphaeroides f.* sp. denitrificans as bis(molybdopterin guanine dinucleotide)molybdenum. *Archives of Biochemistry and Biophysics*, **325**, 139–143.

Hipkiss, A.R., Carmichael, P.L., and Zimmermann, B. (1991). Metabolism of crystallin fragments in cell-free extracts of bovine lens: effects of ageing and oxygen free-radicals. *Acta Biologica Hungarica*, **42**, 243–263.

Hiramoto, K., Aso, O.R., Ni, I.H., Hikage, S., Kato, T., and Kikugawa, K. (1996). DNA strand break by 2,5-dimethyl-4-hydroxy-3(2H)-furanone, a fragrant compound in various foodstuffs. *Mutation Research*, **359**, 17–24.

Hjelm, H. (1975). Isolation of IgG3 from normal human sera and from a patient with multiple myeloma by using protein A-sepharose 4B. *Scandanavian Journal of Immunology*, **4**, 633–640.

Ho, P.S., Hoffman, B.M., Kang, C.H., and Margoliash, E. (1983). Control of the transfer of oxidizing equivalents between heme iron and free radical site in yeast cytochrome *c* peroxidase. *Journal of Biological Chemistry*, **258**, 4356–4363.

Ho, P.S., Hoffman, B.M., Solomon, N., Kang, C.H., and Margoliash, E. (1984). Kinetics and energetics of intramolecular electron transfer in yeast cytochrome *c* peroxidase. *Biochemistry*, **23**, 4122–4128.

Ho, Y.S., Wang, Y.J., and Lin, J.K. (1996). Induction of p53 and p21/WAF1/CIP1 expression by nitric oxide and their association with apoptosis in human cancer cells. *Molecular Carcinogenesis*, **16**, 20–31.

Hochstein, P., and Jain, S.K. (1981). Association of lipid peroxidation and polymerization of membrane proteins with erythrocyte aging. *Proceedings of the National Academy of Science of the United States of America*, **40**, 183–188.

Hoe, S.T., Bisby, R.H., Cundall, R.B., and Anderson, R.F. (1981). Free radical reactions with proteins and enzymes. The inactivation of bovine carbonic anhydrase B. *Biochimica et Biophysica Acta*, **662**, 55–64.

Hoey, B.M., and Butler, J. (1984). The repair of oxidized amino acids by anti-oxidants. *Biochimica et Biophysica Acta*, **791**, 212–218.

Hoff, H.F., O'Neil, J., Chisolm, G.D., Cole, T.B., Quehenberger, O., Esterbauer, H., *et al.* (1989). Modification of low density lipoprotein with 4-hydroxynonenal induces uptake by macrophages. *Arteriosclerosis*, **9**, 538–549.

Hoffman, B.M., Roberts, J.E., Brown, T.G., Kang, C.H., and Margoliash, E. (1979). Electron-nuclear double resonance of the hydrogen peroxide compound of cytochrome *c* peroxidase: identification of the free radical site with a methionyl cluster. *Proceedings of the National Academy of Science of the United States of America*, **76**, 6132–6136.

Hoffman, B.M., Roberts, J.E., Kang, C.H., and Margoliash, E. (1981). Electron paramagnetic and electron nuclear double resonance of the hydrogen peroxide compound of cytochrome *c* peroxidase. *Journal of Biological Chemistry*, **256**, 6556–6564.

Hofmann, A., Tai, M., Wong, W., and Glabe, C.G. (1995). A sparse matrix screen to establish initial conditions for protein renaturation. *Analytical Biochemistry*, **230**, 8–15.

Hoganson, C.W., and Babcock, G.T. (1992). Protein-tyrosyl radical interactions in photosystem II studied by electron spin resonance and electron nuclear double resonance spectroscopy: comparison with ribonucleotide reductase and *in vitro* tyrosine. *Biochemistry*, **31**, 11874–11880.

Holian, J., and Garrison, W.M. (1968). On the radiation-induced reduction of amide and peptide functions in aquoorganic systems. *Journal of Physical Chemistry*, **72**, 4721–4723.

Holian, J., and Garrison, W.M. (1969). Reconstitution mechanisms in the radiolysis of aqueous biochemical systems: inhibitive effects of thiols. *Nature*, **221**, 175.

Holmberg, S.R., Cumming, D.V., Kusama, Y., Hearse, D.J., Poole, W.P., Shattock, M.J., *et al.* (1991). Reactive oxygen species modify the structure and function of the cardiac sarcoplasmic reticulum calcium-release channel. *Cardioscience*, **2**, 19–25.

Holroyd, R., Glass, J., and Riesz, P. (1970). Radicals formed in proteins by reaction with hydrogen atoms. *Radiation Research*, **44**, 59–67.

Holt, D.B., Eberhart, R.C., and Prager, M.D. (1994). Endothelial cell binding to Dacron modified with polyethylene oxide and peptide. *Asaio Journal*, **40**, M858–M863.

Holzer, P., Jocic, M., and Peskar, B.A. (1995). Mediation by prostaglandins of the nitric oxide-induced neurogenic vasodilatation in rat skin. *British Journal of Pharmacology*, **116**, 2365–2370.

Hommel, R., and Kleber, H.P. (1990). Selective and rapid solubilization of the microbial membrane enzyme aldehyde dehydrogenase. *Journal of Basic Microbiology*, **30**, 297–300.

Hommes, R.W., van Hell, B., Postma, P.W., Neijssel, O.M., and Tempest, D.W. (1985). The functional significance of glucose dehydrogenase in *Klebsiella aerogenes*. *Archives of Microbiology*, **143**, 163–168.

Hong, S.-J., and Piette, L.H. (1989). Electron spin resonance studies of spin-trapped free radicals produced by reaction of metmyoglobins with hydrogen peroxide. *Korean Biochemical Journal*, **22**, 196–201.

Honjoh, K., Yoshimoto, M., Joh, T., Kajiwara, T., Miyamoto, T., and Hatano, S. (1995). Isolation and characterization of hardening-induced proteins in *Chlorella vulgaris C-27*: identification of late embryogenesis abundant proteins. *Plant Cell Physiology*, **36**, 1421–1430.

Hood, D.B., Gettins, P., and Johnson, D.A. (1993). Nitrogen dioxide reactivity with proteins: effects on activity and immunoreactivity with alpha-1-proteinase inhibitor and implications for NO_2-mediated peptide degradation. *Archives of Biochemistry and Biophysics*, **304**, 17–26.

Hopkins, F.G. (1925). Glutathione. Its influence in the oxidation of fats and proteins. *Biochemical Journal*, **19**, 787–819.

Hopkins, F.G., and Elliott, K.A.C. (1931). The relation of glutathione to cell respiration with special reference to hepatic tissue. *Proceedings of the Royal Society (London) B*, **109**, 58–88.

Hori, H., and Yonetani, T. (1985). Powder and single-crystal electron paramagnetic resonance studies of yeast cytochrome *c* peroxidase and its peroxide compound, Compound ES. *Journal of Biological Chemistry*, **260**, 349–355.

Hori, K., Anderson, J.M., Ward, W.W., and Cormier, M.J. (1975). *Renilla luciferin* as the substrate for calcium induced photoprotein bioluminescence. Assignment of *luciferin* tautomers in aequorin and mnemiopsin. *Biochemistry*, **14**, 2371–2376.

Horner, L. (1961). Autoxidation of enols and phenols in the presence of metals. In *Autoxidation and Antioxidants Vol. 1*, (ed. W.O. Lundberg), pp. 171–232. Interscience, New York.

Horstmann, H.J., Rohen, J.W., and Sames, K. (1983). Age-related changes in the composition of proteins in the trabecular meshwork of the human eye. *Mechanisms of Ageing Development*, **21**, 121–136.

Hortin, G., and Boime, I. (1980). Inhibition of preprotein processing in ascites tumor lysates by incorporation of a leucine analog. *Proceedings of the National Academy of Science of the United States of America*, **77**, 1356–1360.

Houee, L.C., Gardes, A.M., Benzineb, K., Ferradini, C., and Hickel, B. (1989). Intramolecular electron transfer in proteins. Radiolysis study of the reductive activation of daunorubicin complexed in egg white apo-riboflavin binding protein. *Biochemistry*, **28**, 9848–9854.

Houseman, A.L., Doan, P.E., Goodin, D.B., and Hoffman, B.M. (1993). Comprehensive explanation of the anomalous EPR spectra of wild-type and mutant cytochrome *c* peroxidase compound ES. *Biochemistry*, **32**, 4430–4443.

Howard, J.A. (1972). Absolute rate constants for reactions of oxyl radicals. *Advances in Free Radical Chemistry*, **4**, 49–173.

Hoyer, D., Cho, H., and Schultz, P.G. (1990). A new strategy for selective protein cleavage. *Journal of the American Chemical Society*, **112**, 3249–3250.

Hsu, K.S., Huang, C.C., and Gean, P.W. (1995). Muscarinic depression of excitatory synaptic transmission mediated by the presynaptic M3 receptors in the rat neostriatum. *Neuroscience Letters*, **197**, 141–144.

Hsuan, J.J. (1987). The cross-linking of tyrosine residues in apo-ovotransferrin by treatment with periodate anions. *Biochemical Journal*, **247**, 467–473.

Hu, J., Speisky, H., and Cotgreave, I.A. (1995). The inhibitory effects of boldine, glaucine, and probucol on TPA-induced down regulation of gap junction function. Relationships to intracellular peroxides, protein kinase C translocation, and connexin 43 phosphorylation. *Biochemical Pharmacology*, **50**, 1635–1643.

Hu, J., Castets, F., Guevara, J.L., and Van, E.L. (1996). S100 beta stimulates inducible nitric oxide synthase activity and mRNA levels in rat cortical astrocytes. *Journal of Biological Chemistry*, **271**, 2543–2547.

Hu, M.L., and Tappel, A.L. (1992a). Potentiation of oxidative damage to proteins by ultraviolet-A and protection by antioxidants. *Photochemistry and Photobiology*, **56**, 357–363.

Hu, M.L., and Tappel, A.L. (1992b). Glutathione and antioxidants protect microsomes against lipid peroxidation and enzyme inactivation. *Lipids*, **27**, 42–45.

Hu, M.L., Dillard, C.J., and Tappel, A.L. (1988a). *In vivo* effects of aurothioglucose and sodium thioglucose on rat tissue sulfydryl levels and plasma sulfydryl reactivity. *Agents and Actions*, **25**, 132–138.

Hu, M.L., Viljoen, A.J., and Tappel, A.L. (1988b). Interactions of gold with cytosolic selenium-containing proteins in rat kidney and liver. *Journal of Inorganic Biochemistry*, **32**, 281–290.

Hu, M.L., Frankel, E.N., Leibovitz, B.E., and Tappel, A.L. (1989). Effect of dietary lipids and vitamin E on *in vitro* lipid peroxidation in rat liver and kidney homogenates. *Journal of Nutrition*, **119**, 1574–1582.

Hu, M.L., Frankel, E.N., and Tappel, A.L. (1990). Effect of dietary menhaden oil and vitamin E on *in vivo* lipid peroxidation induced by iron. *Lipids*, **25**, 194–198.

Hu, M.L., Louie, S., Cross, C.E., Motchnik, P., and Halliwell, B. (1993). Antioxidant protection against hypochlorous acid in human plasma [see comments]. *Journal of Laboratory and Clinical Medicine*, **121**, 257–262.

Huang, R.P., and Adamson, E.D. (1995). A biological role for Egr-1 in cell survival following ultra-violet irradiation. *Oncogene*, **10**, 467–475.

Huggins, T.G., Staton, M.W., Dyer, D.G., Detorie, N.J., Walla, M.D., Baynes, J.W., et al. (1992). *o*-Tyrosine and dityrosine concentrations in oxidized proteins and lens proteins with age. *Annals of the New York Academy of Science*, **663**, 436–437.

Huggins, T.G., Wells, K.M., Detorie, N.A., Baynes, J.W., and Thorpe, S.R. (1993). Formation of *o*-tyrosine and dityrosine in proteins during radiolytic and metal-catalyzed oxidation. *Journal of Biological Chemistry*, **268**, 12341–12347.

Hui, K.S., Lo, E.S., and Hui, M.P. (1994). An endogenous aminoenkephalinase inhibitor: purification and characterization of Arg0–Met5–enkephalin from bovine striatum. *Journal of Neurochemistry*, **63**, 1748–1756.

Huie, R.E. (1994). The reaction kinetics of $NO_2(\cdot)$. *Toxicology*, **89**, 193–216.

Hulsmann, A.R., Raatgeep, H.R., den Hollander, J.C., Bakker, W.H., Saxena, P.R., and de Jongste, J.C. (1996). Permeability of human isolated airways increases after hydrogen peroxide and poly-L-arginine. *American Journal of Respiratory and Cellular Molecular Biology Critical Care Medicine*, **153**, 841–846.

Hume, R., Burchell, A., Allan, B.B., Wolf, C.R., Kelly, R.W., Hallas, A., et al. (1996). The ontogeny of key endoplasmic reticulum proteins in human embryonic and fetal red blood cells. *Blood*, **87**, 762–770.

Hunt, J.V., and Dean, R.T. (1989). Free radical-mediated degradation of proteins: the protective and deleterious effects of membranes. *Biochemical and Biophysical Research Communications*, **162**, 1076–1084.

Hunt, N.H., and Stocker, R. (1990). Oxidative stress and the redox status of malaria-infected erythrocytes. *Blood Cells*, **16**, 499–526.

Hunt, J.V., and Wolff, S.P. (1990). Is glucose the sole source of tissue browning in diabetes mellitus? *FEBS Letters*, **269**, 258–260.

Hunt, J.V., and Wolff, S.P. (1991a). Oxidative glycation and free radical production: a causal mechanism of diabetic complications. *Free Radical Research Communications*, **1**, 115–123.

Hunt, J.V., and Wolff, S.P. (1991*b*). The role of histidine residues in the non-enzymic covalent attachment of glucose and ascorbic acid to protein. *Free Radical Research Communications*, **14**, 279–287.

Hunt, J.V., Dean, R.T., and Wolff, S.P. (1988*a*). Hydroxyl radical production and autoxidative glycosylation. Glucose autoxidation as the cause of protein damage in the experimental glycation model of diabetes mellitus and ageing. *Biochemical Journal*, **256**, 205–212.

Hunt, J.V., Simpson, J.A., and Dean, R.T. (1988*b*). Hydroperoxide-mediated fragmentation of proteins. *Biochemical Journal*, **250**, 87–93.

Hunt, J.V., Smith, C.C., and Wolff, S.P. (1990). Autoxidative glycosylation and possible involvement of peroxides and free radicals in LDL modification by glucose. *Diabetes*, **39**, 1420–1424.

Hunt, J.V., Jiang, Z.Y., and Wolff, S.P. (1992*a*). Formation of hydrogen peroxide by lens proteins: protein-derived hydrogen peroxide as a potential mechanism of oxidative insult to the lens. *Free Radical Biology and Medicine*, **13**, 319–323.

Hunt, J.V., Bottoms, M.A., and Mitchinson, M.J. (1992*b*). Ascorbic acid oxidation: a potential cause of the elevated severity of atherosclerosis in diabetes mellitus? *FEBS Letters*, **311**, 161–164.

Hunt, J.T., Lee, V.G., Liu, E.C., Moreland, S., McMullen, D., Webb, M.L., *et al.* (1993*a*). Control of peptide disulfide regioisomer formation by mixed cysteine-penicillamine bridges. Application to endothelin-1. *International Journal of Peptide and Protein Research*, **42**, 249–258.

Hunt, J.V., Bottoms, M.A., and Mitchinson, M.J. (1993*b*). Oxidative alterations in the experimental glycation model of diabetes mellitus are due to protein-glucose adduct oxidation. Some fundamental differences in proposed mechanisms of glucose oxidation and oxidant production. *Biochemical Journal*, **291**, 529–535.

Hunt, J.V., Bailey, J.R., Schultz, D.L., McKay, A.G., and Mitchinson, M.J. (1994). Apolipoprotein oxidation in the absence of lipid peroxidation enhances LDL uptake by macrophages. *FEBS Letters*, **349**, 375–379.

Hunter, E.P.L., Desrosiers, M.F., and Simic, M.G. (1989). The effect of oxygen, antioxidants and superoxide radical on tyrosine phenoxyl radical dimerisation. *Free Radical Biology and Medicine*, **6**, 581–585.

Hunter, G.C., Dubick, M.A., Keen, C.L., and Eskelson, C.D. (1991). Effects of hypertension on aortic antioxidant status in human aneurysmal and occlusive disease. *Proceedings of the Society for Experimental Biology and Medicine*, **196**, 273–279.

Hunter, M.J., and Komives, E.A. (1995). Deprotection of S-acetamidomethyl cysteine-containing peptides by silver trifluoromethanesulfonate avoids the oxidation of methionines. *Analytical Biochemistry*, **228**, 173–177.

Husain, M., Davidson, V.L., Gray, K.A., and Knaff, D.B. (1987). Redox properties of the quinoprotein methylamine dehydrogenase from paracoccus denitrificans. *Biochemistry*, **26**, 4139–4143.

Husain, S., and Hadi, S.M. (1995). Strand scission in DNA induced by L-DOPA in the presence of Cu(II). *FEBS Letters*, **364**, 75–78.

Hussey, R.G., and Thompson, W.R. (1923*a*). The effect of radioactive radiations and X-rays on enzymes. I. The effect of radiation from radium emanation on solutions of trypsin. *Journal of General Physiology*, **5**, 647–659.

Hussey, R.G., and Thompson, W.R. (1923*b*). The effect of radioactive emanations and X-rays on enzymes. II. The effect of radiations from radium emanations on pepsin in solution. *Journal of General Physiology*, **6**, 1–5.

Huttenhofer, A., and Noller, H.F. (1992). Hydroxyl radical cleavage of tRNA in the ribosomal P site. *Proceedings of the National Academy of Science of the United States of America*, **89**, 7851–7855.

Hutton, J.J., Witkop, B., Kurtz, J., Berger, A., and Udenfriend, S. (1968). Synthetic polypeptides as substrates and inhibitors of collagen proline hydroxylase. *Archives of Biochemistry and Biophysics*, **125**, 779–785.

Huynh, B.H., Moura, J.J., Moura, I., Kent, T.A., LeGall, J., Xavier, A.V., et al. (1980). Evidence for a three-iron center in a ferredoxin from *Desulfovibrio gigas*. Mossbauer and EPR studies. *Journal of Biological Chemistry*, **255**, 3242–3244.

Huyser, E.S. (1970). *Free Radical Chain Reactions*. Wiley-Interscience, New York.

Hyun, Y.L., and Davidson, V.L. (1995a). Unusually large isotope effect for the reaction of aromatic amine dehydrogenase. A common feature of quinoproteins? *Biochimica et Biophysica Acta*, **1251**, 198–200.

Hyun, Y.L., and Davidson, V.L. (1995b). Mechanistic studies of aromatic amine dehydrogenase, a tryptophan tryptophylquinone enzyme. *Biochemistry*, **34**, 816–823.

Ichikawa, H., Ronowicz, K., Hicks, M., and Gebicki, J.M. (1987). Lipid peroxidation is not the cause of lysis of human erythrocytes exposed to inorganic or methylmercury. *Archives of Biochemistry and Biophysics*, **259**, 46–51.

Ignarro, L.J., Wood, K.S., Ballot, B., and Wolin, M.S. (1984). Guanylate cyclase from bovine lung. Evidence that enzyme activation by phenylhydrazine is mediated by iron-phenyl hemoprotein complexes. *Journal of Biological Chemistry*, **259**, 5923–5931.

Iheanacho, E.N., Stocker, R., and Hunt, N.H. (1993). Redox metabolism of vitamin C in blood of normal and malaria-infected mice. *Biochimica et Biophysica Acta*, **1182**, 15–21.

Iijima, M., Mihara, K., Kondo, T., Tsuji, T., Ishioka, C., and Namba, M. (1996). Mutation in p53 and de-regulation of p53-related gene expression in three human cell lines immortalized with 4-nitroquinoline 1–oxide or 60Co gamma rays. *International Journal of Cancer*, **66**, 698–702.

Ijioma, S.C., Challiss, R.A., and Boyle, J.P. (1995). Comparative effects of activation of soluble and particulate guanylyl cyclase on cyclic GMP elevation and relaxation of bovine tracheal smooth muscle. *British Journal of Pharmacology*, **115**, 723–732.

Ilan, Y., Rabani, J., and Henglein, A. (1976). Pulse radiolytic investigations of peroxy radicals produced from 2-propanol and methanol. *Journal of Physical Chemistry*, **80**, 1558–1565.

Imai, S., Hukuda, S., and Maeda, T. (1995). Dually innervating nociceptive networks in the rat lumbar posterior longitudinal ligaments. *Spine*, **20**, 2086–2092.

Inanami, O., Kuwabara, M., Hayashi, M., Yoshii, G., Syuto, B., and Sato, F. (1986). Reaction of the hydrated electron with histone H1 and related compounds studied by e.s.r. and spin-trapping. *International Journal of Radiation Biology and Related Studies in Physics, Chemistry and Medicine*, **49**, 47–56.

Inanami, O., Kuwabara, M., and Sato, F. (1988). ESR and spin-trapping study of free radicals in gamma-irradiated solid lysozyme. *Free Radical Research Communications*, **5**, 43–49.

Inglis, A.S., Rivett, D.E., and McMahon, D.T. (1979). The identification of tryptophan residues in proteins as oxidised derivatives during amino acid sequence determinations. *FEBS Letters*, **104**, 115–118.

Ingold, K.U., Bowry, V.W., Stocker, R., and Walling, C. (1993). Autoxidation of lipids and antioxidation by alpha-tocopherol and ubiquinol in homogeneous solution and in aqueous dispersions of lipids: unrecognized consequences of lipid particle size as exemplified by oxidation of human low density lipoprotein. *Proceedings of the National Academy of Science of the United States of America*, **90**, 45–49.

Innes, J.B., and Brudvig, G.W. (1989). Location and magnetic relaxation properties of the stable tyrosine radical in photosystem II. *Biochemistry*, **28**, 1116–1125.

Ischiropoulos, H., and al-Mehdi, A.B. (1995). Peroxynitrite-mediated oxidative protein modifications. *FEBS Letters*, **364**, 279–282.

Ischiropoulos, H., Zhu, L., Chen, J., Tsai, M., Martin, J.C., Smith, C.D., *et al.* (1992). Peroxynitrite-mediated tyrosine nitration catalyzed by superoxide dismutase. *Archives of Biochemistry and Biophysics*, **298**, 431–437.

Ischiropoulos, H., Duran, D., and Horwitz, J. (1995*a*). Peroxynitrite-mediated inhibition of DOPA synthesis in PC12 cells. *Journal of Neurochemistry*, **65**, 2366–2372.

Ischiropoulos, H., al-Mehdi, A., and Fisher, A.B. (1995*b*). Reactive species in ischemic rat lung injury: contribution of peroxynitrite. *American Journal of Physiology*, **269**, L158–164.

Ischiropoulos, H., Beers, M.F., Ohnishi, S.T., Fisher, D., Garner, S.E., and Thom, S.R. (1996). Nitric oxide production and perivascular nitration in brain after carbon monoxide poisoning in the rat [see comments]. *Journal of Clinical Investigation*, **97**, 2260–2267.

Ishida, H., Tamai, S., Yajima, H., Inoue, K., Ohgushi, H., and Dohi, Y. (1996). Histologic and biochemical analysis of osteogenic capacity of vascularized periosteum. *Plastic and Reconstructive Surgery*, **97**, 512–518.

Ishii, T., Aoki, N., Noda, A., Adachi, T., Nakamura, R., and Matsuda, T. (1995). Carboxy-terminal cytoplasmic domain of mouse butyrophilin specifically associates with a 150–kDa protein of mammary epithelial cells and milk fat globule membrane. *Biochimica et Biophysica Acta*, **1245**, 285–292.

Isied, S.S., Ogawa, M.Y., and Wishart, J.F. (1992). Peptide-mediated intramolecular electron transfer: long-range distance dependence. *Chemical Reviews*, **92**, 381–394.

Israel, N., Gougerot, P.M., Aillet, F., and Virelizier, J.L. (1992). Redox status of cells influences constitutive or induced NF-kappa B translocation and HIV long terminal repeat activity in human T and monocytic cell lines. *Journal of Immunology*, **149**, 3386–3393.

Iszard, M.B., Liu, J., and Klaassen, C.D. (1995). Effect of several metallothionein inducers on oxidative stress defense mechanisms in rats. *Toxicology*, **104**, 25–33.

Itakura, K., Uchida, K., and Kawakishi, S. (1994). Selective formation of oxindole- and formylkynurenine-type products from tryptophan and its peptides treated with a superoxide-generating system in the presence of iron(III)-EDTA: a possible involvement with iron-oxygen complex. *Chemical Research in Toxicology*, **7**, 185–190.

Ito, K., and Kawanishi, S. (1991). Site-specific fragmentation and modification of albumin by sulfite in the presence of metal ions or peroxidase/H_2O_2: role of sulfate radical. *Biochemical and Biophysical Research Communications*, **176**, 1306–1312.

Ito, N., Phillips, S.E., Stevens, C., Ogel, Z.B., McPherson, M.J., Keen, J.N., *et al.* (1991). Novel thioether bond revealed by a 1.7 Å crystal structure of galactose oxidase. *Nature*, **350**, 87–90.

Ito, S., Kato, T., Shinpo, K., and Fujita, K. (1984). Oxidation of tyrosine residues by tyrosinase—formation of protein-bound 3,4-dihydroxyphenylalanine and 5-S-cysteinyl-3,4-dihydroxyphenylalanine. *Biochemical Journal*, **222**, 407–411.

Ito, S., Kato, T., and Fujita, K. (1988). Covalent binding of catechols to protein through the suphydyrl group. *Biochemical Pharmacology*, **37**, 1707–1710.

Itoh, F., Minamide, Y., Horie, T., and Awazu, S. (1990). Fluorescent proteins formed in peroxidized microsomes of rat liver. *Pharmacology and Toxicology*, **67**, 178–181.

Ivancich, A., Jouve, H.M., and Gaillard. J. (1996). EPR evidence for a tyrosyl radical intermediate in bovine liver catalase. *Journal of the American Chemical Society*, **118**, 12852–12853.

Ivanov, V.N., Deng, G., Podack, E.R., and Malek, T.R. (1995). Pleiotropic effects of Bcl-2 on transcription factors in T cells: potential role of NF-kappa B p50–p50 for the anti-apoptotic function of Bcl-2. *International Immunology*, **7**, 1709–1720.

Iwamura, H., Moore, A.R., and Willoughby, D.A. (1993). Interaction between neutrophil-derived elastase and reactive oxygen species in cartilage degradation. *Biochimica et Biophysica Acta*, **1156**, 295–301.

Jabbar, S.A., Hoffbrand, A.V., and Wickremasinghe, R.G. (1994). Redox reagents and staurosporine inhibit stimulation of the transcription regulator NF-kappa B following tumour necrosis factor treatment of chronic B-leukaemia cells. *Leukocyte Research*, **18**, 523–530.

Jabbar, S.A., Hoffbrand, A.V., and Wickremasinghe, R.G. (1995). Defects in signal transduction pathways in chronic B lymphocytic leukemia cells. *Leukocyte Lymphoma*, **18**, 163–170.

Jacks, T.J., Hensarling, T.P., Muller, L.L., St, A.A., and Neucere, N.J. (1982). Peroxide-induced conformational transitions of peanut storage protein (arachin). *International Journal of Peptide and Protein Research*, **20**, 149–153.

Jacob, D.F., Pinkner, J., Xu, Z., Striker, R., Padmanhaban, A., and Hultgren, S.J. (1994). PapD chaperone function in pilus biogenesis depends on oxidant and chaperone-like activities of DsbA. *Proceedings of the National Academy of Science of the United States of America*, **91**, 11552–11556.

Jacobs, A.A., Paul, B.B., Strauss, R.R., and Sbarra, A.J. (1970). The Role of the Phagocyte in Host-Parasite Interactions. XXIII. Relation of Bactericidal Activity to Peroxidase-Associated Decarboxylation and Deamination. *Biochemical and Biophysical Research Communications*, **39**, 284–289.

Jaeger, J., Sorensen, K., and Wolff, S.P. (1994). Peroxide accumulation in detergents. *Journal of Biochemical and Biophysical Methods*, **29**, 77–81.

Jamieson, D.J., Rivers, S.L., and Stephen, D.W. (1994). Analysis of *Saccharomyces cerevisiae* proteins induced by peroxide and superoxide stress. *Microbiology*, **140**, 3277–3283.

Janata, E., and Schuler, R.H. (1982). Rate constant for scavenging e^-_{aq} in N_2O-saturated solutions. *Journal of Physical Chemistry*, **86**, 2078–2084.

Janero, D.R., and Yarwood, C. (1995). Oxidative modulation and inactivation of rabbit cardiac adenylate deaminase. *Biochemical Journal*, **306**, 421–427.

Janes, S.M., and Klinman, J.P. (1995). Isolation of 2,4,5-trihydroxyphenylalanine quinone (topa quinone) from copper amine oxidases. *Methods in Enzymology*, **258**, 20–34.

Janes, S.M., Palcic, M.M., Scaman, C.H., Smith, A.J., Brown, D.E., Dooley, D.M., *et al.* (1992). Identification of topaquinone and its consensus sequence in copper amine oxidases. *Biochemistry*, **31**, 12147–12154.

Janoff, A., Carp, H., Lee, D.K., and Drew, R.T. (1979). Cigarette smoke inhalation decreases alpha 1–antitrypsin activity in rat lung. *Science*, **206**, 1313–1314.

Janzen, E.G. (1971). Spin Trapping. *Accounts of Chemical Research*, **4**, 31–40.

*Janzen, E.G., and Haire, D.L. (1990). Two Decades of Spin Trapping. *Advances in Free Radical Chemistry*, **1**, 253–295.

Jasin, H.E. (1987). Cross-linking of immune complexes by human mononuclear phagocytes. *Inflammation*, **11**, 117–129.

Jayko, M.E., and Garrison, W.M. (1956). Indirect action of radiation on the $-NH-CH^2-$ linkage in diethylamina (a mechanism for radiation induced decomposition of the peptide chain). *Journal of Chemical Physics*, **25**, 1084.

Jayko, M.E., and Garrison, W.M. (1958). Formation of $>C=O$ bonds in the radiation-induced oxidation of protein in aqueous systems. *Nature*, **181**, 413–414.

Jayko, M.E., Tung, T.L., Welch, G.P., and Garrison, W.M. (1976). Methodology in the radiolysis of biochemical compounds with cyclotron beams at low flux densities. *Biochemical and Biophysical Research Communications*, **68**, 307–312.

Jayson, G.G., Scholes, G., and Weiss, J. (1954). Formation of formylkynurenine by the action of X-rays on trytophan in aqueous solution. *Biochemical Journal*, **57**, 386–390.

Jayson, G.G., Stirling, D.A., and Swallow, A.J. (1971). Pulse- and X-radiolysis of 2-mercaptoethanol in aqueous solution. *International Journal of Radiation Biology and Related Studies in Physics, Chemistry and Medicine*, **19**, 143–156.

Jeding, I., Evans, P.J., Akanmu, D., Dexter, D., Spencer, J.D., Aruoma, O.I., et al. (1995). Characterization of the potential antioxidant and pro-oxidant actions of some neuroleptic drugs. *Biochemical Pharmacology*, **49**, 359–365.

Jeng, M.F., and Dyson, H.J. (1996). Direct measurement of the aspartic acid 26 pK_a for reduced *Escherichia coli* thioredoxin by 13C NMR. *Biochemistry*, **35**, 1–6.

Jeng, D.K., and Woodworth, A.G. (1990). Chlorine dioxide gas sterilization of oxygenators in an industrial scale sterilizer: a successful model. *Artifical Organs*, **14**, 361–368.

Jeong, K.S., Lee, I.J., Roberts, B.J., Soh, Y., Yoo, J.K., Lee, J.W., et al. (1996). Transcriptional inhibition of cytochrome P4502E1 by a synthetic compound, YH439. *Archives of Biochemistry and Biophysics*, **326**, 137–144.

Jeppesen, P., and Morten, H. (1985). Effects of sulphydryl reagents on the structure of dehistonized metaphase chromosomes. *Journal of Cell Science*, **73**, 245–260.

Jessup, W., Jurgens, G., Lang, J., Esterbauer, H., and Dean, R.T. (1986). Interaction of 4-hydroxynonenal-modified low-density lipoproteins with the fibroblast apolipoprotein B/E receptor. *Biochemical Journal*, **234**, 245–248.

Jessup, W., and Dean, R.T. (1993). Autoinhibition of murine macrophage-mediated oxidation of low-density lipoprotein by nitric oxide synthesis. *Atherosclerosis*, **101**, 145–155.

Jessup, W. (1993). Cellular modification of low-density lipoproteins. *Biochemical Society Transactions*, **21**, 321–325.

Jessup, W., Bedwell, S., Kwok, K., and Dean, R.T. (1988). Oxidative modification of low-density lipoprotein: initiation by free radicals and protection by antioxidants. *Agents and Actions (Supplement)*, **26**, 241–246.

Jessup, W., Dean, R.T., de, W.C., Rankin, S.M., and Leake, D.S. (1990a). The role of oxidative modification and antioxidants in LDL metabolism and atherosclerosis. *Advances in Experimental Medicine and Biology*, **264**, 139–142.

Jessup, W., Rankin, S.M., De Whalley, C.V., Hoult, J.R., Scott, J., and Leake, D.S. (1990b). Alpha-tocopherol consumption during low-density-lipoprotein oxidation. *Biochemical Journal*, **265**, 399–405.

Jessup, W., Mohr, D., Gieseg, S.P., Dean, R.T., and Stocker, R. (1992a). The participation of nitric oxide in cell free- and its restriction of macrophage-mediated oxidation of low-density lipoprotein. *Biochimica et Biophysica Acta*, **1180**, 73–82.

Jessup, W., Mander, E.L., and Dean, R.T. (1992*b*). The intracellular storage and turnover of apolipoprotein B of oxidized LDL in macrophages. *Biochimica et Biophysica Acta*, **1126**, 167–177.

Jessup, W., Simpson, J.A., and Dean, R.T. (1993). Does superoxide radical have a role in macrophage-mediated oxidative modification of LDL? *Atherosclerosis*, **99**, 107–120.

Jessup, W., Dean, R.T., and Gebicki, J.M. (1994). Iodometric determination of hydroperoxides in lipids and proteins. *Methods in Enzymology*, **233**, 289–303.

Jiang, Z.Y., Woollard, A.C., and Wolff, S.P. (1990). Hydrogen peroxide production during experimental protein glycation. *FEBS Letters*, **268**, 69–71.

Jiang, Z.Y., Woollard, A.C., and Wolff, S.P. (1991). Lipid hydroperoxide measurement by oxidation of Fe^{2+} in the presence of xylenol orange. Comparison with the TBA assay and an iodometric method. *Lipids*, **26**, 853–856.

Jiang, Z.Y., Zhou, Q.L., Eaton, J.W., Koppenol, W.H., Hunt, J.V., and Wolff, S.P. (1991). Spirohydantoin inhibitors of aldose reductase inhibit iron- and copper-catalysed ascorbate oxidation *in vitro*. *Biochemical Pharmacology*, **42**, 1273–1278.

Jiang, Z.Y., Hunt, J.V., and Wolff, S.P. (1992). Ferrous ion oxidation in the presence of xylenol orange for detection of lipid hydroperoxide in low density lipoprotein. *Analytical Biochemistry*, **202**, 384–389.

Jin, F., Leitich, J., and von Sonntag, C. (1993). The superoxide radical reacts with tyrosine-derived phenoxyl radicals by addition rather than by electron transfer. *Journal of the Chemical Society, Perkin Transactions*, **2**, 1583–1588.

Johansson, S., Kjellen, L., Hook, M., and Timpl, R. (1981). Substrate adhesion of rat hepatocytes: a comparison of laminin and fibronectin as attachment proteins. *Journal of Cell Biology*, **90**, 260–264.

Johnson, E.A., Levine, R.L., and Lin, E.C. (1985). Inactivation of glycerol dehydrogenase of *Klebsiella pneumoniae* and the role of divalent cations. *Journal of Bacteriology*, **164**, 479–483.

Johnson, G.R.A., Scholes, G., and Weiss, J. (1951). Formation of alpha-keto acids from alpha-amino acids by the action of free radicals in aqueous solution. *Science*, **114**, 412–412.

Johnson, M.K., Thomson, A.J., Robinson, A.E., Rao, K.K., and Hall, D.O. (1981). Low-temperature magnetic circular dichroism spectra and magnetisation curves of 4Fe clusters in iron-sulphur proteins from *Chromatium* and *Clostridium pasteurianum*. *Biochimica et Biophysica Acta*, **667**, 433–451.

Johnson, R.A., and Greene, F.D. (1975). Chlorination with *N*-chloro amides. I. Inter- and intramolecular chlorination. *Journal of Organic Chemistry*, **40**, 2186–2192.

Johnson, R.M., Ravindranath, Y., el Alfy, M., and Goyette, G. (1994). Oxidant damage to erythrocyte membrane in glucose-6-phosphate dehydrogenase deficiency: correlation with *in vivo* reduced glutathione concentration and membrane protein oxidation. *Blood*, **83**, 1117–1123.

Johnson, S.A., Bisby, R.H., Tavender, S.M., and Parker, A.W. (1996). The free radical site in pea seedling copper amine oxidase probed by resonance Raman spectroscopy and generated by photolysis of caged substrate. *FEBS Letters*, **380**, 183–187.

Johnston, H.M., and Morris, B.J. (1994). NMDA and nitric oxide increase microtubule-associated protein 2 gene expression in hippocampal granule cells. *Journal of Neurochemistry*, **63**, 379–382.

Jonak, J., Petersen, T.E., Meloun, B., and Rychlik, I. (1984). Histidine residues in elongation factor EF-tu from *Escherichia coli* protected by aminoacyl-tRNA against photo-oxidation. *European Journal of Biochemistry*, **144**, 295–303.

Jones, A.F., and Lunec, J. (1987). Protein fluorescence and its relationship to free radical activity. *British Journal of Cancer (Supplement)*, **8**, 60–65.

Jones, A.F., Winkles, J.W., Thornalley, P.J., Lunec, J., Jennings, P.E., and Barnett, A.H. (1987). Inhibitory effect of superoxide dismutase on fructosamine assay. *Clinical Chemistry*, **33**, 147–149.

Jones, A.F., Jennings, P.E., Wakefield, A., Winkles, J.W., Lunec, J., and Barnett, A.H. (1988). The fluorescence of serum proteins in diabetic patients with and without retinopathy. *Diabetes Medica*, **5**, 547–551.

Jones, R.H., and Hothersall, J.S. (1993). The effect of diabetes and dietary ascorbate supplementation on the oxidative modification of rat lens beta L-crystallin. *Biochemical and Medical Metabolism and Biology*, **50**, 197–209.

Josimovic, L.J., Jankovic, I., AND Jovanovic, S.V. (1993). Radiation induced decomposition of tryptophan in the presence of oxygen. *Radiation Physics and Chemistry*, **41**, 835–841.

Jourlin, C., Simon, G., Pommier, J., Chippaux, M., and Mejean, V. (1996). The periplasmic TorT protein is required for trimethylamine N-oxide reductase gene induction in *Escherichia coli*. *Journal of Bacteriology*, **178**, 1219–1223.

Jovanovic, S.V., and Simic, M.G. (1985). Repair of tryptophan radicals by antioxidants. *Journal of Free Radical Biology and Medicine*, **1**, 125–129.

Jovanovic, S.L., AND Steenken, S. (1992). Substituent effects on the spectral, acid-base, and redox properties of indolyl radicals: a pulse radiolysis study. *Journal of Physical Chemistry*, **96**, 6674–6679.

Jovanovic, S.V., Steenken, S., AND Simic, M.G. (1991). Kinetics and energetics of one-electron-transfer reactions involving tryptophan neutral and cation radicals. *Journal of Physical Chemistry*, **95**, 684–687.

Junek, H., Kirk, K.L., and Cohen, L.A. (1969). The oxidative cleavage of tyrosyl–peptide bonds during iodination. *Biochemistry*, **8**, 1844–1848.

Jung, C., Hui, B.H.G., Davydov, D., Gill, E., and Heremans, K. (1995). Compressibility of the heme pocket of substrate analogue complexes of cytochrome P-450cam–CO. The effect of hydrostatic pressure on the Soret band. *European Journal of Biochemistry*, **233**, 600–606.

Jurgens, G., Hoff, H.F., Chisolm, G.d., and Esterbauer, H. (1987). Modification of human serum low density lipoprotein by oxidation—characterization and pathophysiological implications. *Chemistry and Physics of Lipids*, **45**, 315–336.

Jzn, J.F., Duine, J.A., and Balny, C. (1991). Preliminary studies on quinoprotein glucose dehydrogenase under extreme conditions of temperature and pressure. *Biochimie*, **73**, 611–613.

Kadoya, K., Azuma, M., David, L.L., and Shearer, T.R. (1993). Role of calpain in hydrogen peroxide induced cataract. *Current Eye Research*, **12**, 341–346.

Kagan, H.M. (1994). Lysyl oxidase: mechanism, regulation and relationship to liver fibrosis. *Pathology Research Practice*, **190**, 910–919.

Kagan, H.M., Reddy, V.B., Narasimhan, N., and Csiszar, K. (1995). Catalytic properties and structural components of lysyl oxidase. *Ciba Foundation Symposia*, **192**, 100–115.

Kahane, I., Shifter, A., and Rachmilewitz, E.A. (1978). Cross-linking of red blood cell membrane proteins induced by oxidative stress in beta thalassemia. *FEBS Letters*, **85**, 267–270.

Kako, A., Kato, M., Matsuoka, T., Mustapha, A. (1988). Depression of membrane-bound Na^+-K^+-ATPase activity induced by free radicals and by ischemia of kidney. *American Journal of Physiology*, **254**, C330–C337.

Kako, K.J. (1987). Free radical effects on membrane protein in myocardial ischemia/reperfusion injury. *Journal of Molecular and Cellular Cardiology*, **19**, 209–211.

Kalant, N., and McCormick, S. (1992). Inhibition by serum components of oxidation and collagen-binding of low-density lipoprotein. *Biochimica et Biophysica Acta*, **1128**, 211–219.

Kalhan, S.C. (1993). Rates of urea synthesis in the human newborn: effect of maternal diabetes and small size for gestational age. *Pediatric Research*, **34**, 801–804.

Kaluza, J., and Szydlowska, H. (1972). A comparative histochemical study on the functional groups in proteins and some oxidizing-reducing enzymes in reactive glia and glial tumours. I. Glial tumours. *Neuropathology (Poland)*, **10**, 249–254.

Kalyanaraman, B., Darley-Usmar, V., Struck, A., Hogg, N., and Parthasarathy, S. (1995). Role of apolipoprotein B-derived radical and α-tocopheroxyl radical in peroxidase-dependent oxidation of low density lipoprotein. *Journal of Lipid Research*, **36**, 1037–1045.

Kamal, A., and Garrison, W.M. (1965). Radiolytic degradation of aqueous cytosine: enhancement by a second organic solute. *Nature*, **206**, 1315–1317.

Kamat, J.P., and Devasagayam, T.P. (1995). Tocotrienols from palm oil as potent inhibitors of lipid peroxidation and protein oxidation in rat brain mitochondria. *Neuroscience Letters*, **195**, 179–182.

Kamei, A. (1993). Glutathione levels of the human crystalline lens in aging and its antioxidant effect against the oxidation of lens proteins. *Biological Pharmacology Bulletin*, **16**, 870–875.

Kaminsky, S.M., and Richards, F.M. (1992). Differences in hydrogen exchange behavior between the oxidized and reduced forms of *Escherichia coli* thioredoxin. *Protein Science*, **1**, 10–21.

Kanazawa, K., and Ashida, H. (1991). Target enzymes on hepatic dysfunction caused by dietary products of lipid peroxidation. *Archives of Biochemistry and Biophysics*, **288**, 71–78.

Kandzia, J., Scholz, W., Anderson, M.J., and Muller, R.W. (1985). Magnetic albumin/protein A immunomicrospheres. II. Specificity, reproducibility, and resolution of the magnetic cell separation technique. *Diagnostic Immunology*, **3**, 83–88.

Kaneko, I., Yamada, N., Sakuraba, Y., Kamenosono, M., and Tutumi, S. (1995). Suppression of mitochondrial succinate dehydrogenase, a primary target of beta-amyloid, and its derivative racemized at Ser residue. *Journal of Neurochemistry*, **65**, 2585–2593.

Kaneko, M., Masuda, H., Suzuki, H., Matsumoto, Y., Kobayashi, A., and Yamazaki, N. (1993). Modification of contractile proteins by oxygen free radicals in rat heart. *Molecular and Cellular Biochemistry*, **125**, 163–169.

Kang, J.O., Chan, P.O., and Kesner, L. (1985). Peroxidation of lysozyme treated with Cu(II) and hydrogen peroxide. *Inorganica Chimica Acta*, **107**, 253–258.

Kanner, J., and Harel, S. (1985a). Initiation of membranal lipid peroxidation by activated metmyoglobin and methemoglobin. *Archives of Biochemistry and Biophysics*, **237**, 314–321.

Kanner, J., and Harel, S. (1985b). Lipid peroxidation and oxidation of several compounds by H_2O_2 activated metmyoglobin. *Lipids*, **20**, 625–628.

Kappus, H. (1987). Oxidative stress in chemical toxicity. *Archives of Toxicology*, **60**, 144–149.

Kaput, J., Goltz, S., and Blobel, G. (1982). Nucleotide sequence of the yeast nuclear gene for cytochrome *c* peroxidase precursor. Functional implications of the pre sequence for protein transport into mitochondria. *Journal of Biological Chemistry*, **257**, 15054–15058.

Karam, L.R., Dizdaroglu, M., and Simic, M.G. (1984). OH radical-induced products of tyrosine peptides. *International Journal of Radiation Biology and Related Studies in Physics, Chemistry and Medicine*, **46**, 715–724.

Karapetian, A.V., Kamalian, M.G., and Nalbandyan, R.M. (1986). A copper-containing protein that inhibits nitrite reductase from *Pseudomonas aeruginosa*. *FEBS Letters*, **203**, 131–134.

Karel, M., Schaich, K., and Roy, R.B. (1975). Interaction of peroxidizing methyl linoleate with some proteins and amino acids. *Journal of Agricultural and Food Chemistry*, **23**, 159–163.

Karlstrom, A.R., and Levine, R.L. (1991). Copper inhibits the protease from human immunodeficiency virus 1 by both cysteine-dependent and cysteine-independent mechanisms. *Proceedings of the National Academy of Science of the United States of America*, **88**, 5552–5556.

Karlstrom, A.R., Shames, B.D., and Levine, R.L. (1993). Reactivity of cysteine residues in the protease from human immunodeficiency virus: identification of a surface-exposed region which affects enzyme function. *Archives of Biochemistry and Biophysics*, **304**, 163–169.

Karpel, R., Marx, G., and Chevion, M. (1991). Free radical-induced fibrinogen coagulation: modulation of neofibe formation by concentration, pH and temperature. *Israeli Journal of Medical Science*, **27**, 61–66.

Karthein, R., Dietz, R., Nastainczyk, W., and Ruf, H.H. (1988). Higher oxidation states of prostaglandin H synthase. EPR study of a transient tyrosyl radical in the enzyme during the peroxidase reaction. *European Journal of Biochemistry*, **171**, 313–320.

Kato, T., Hinoo, H., Terui, Y., Kikuchi, J., and Shoji, J. (1988). The structures of katanosins A and B [published erratum appears in *Journal of Antibiotics, Tokyo* (1989), **42**, C-2]. *Journal of Antibiotics, Tokyo*, **41**, 719–725.

Kato, Y., Uchida, K., and Kawakishi, S. (1992). Oxidatie fragmentation of collagen and prolyl peptide by $Cu(II)/H_2O_2$. *Journal of Biological Chemistry*, **267**, 23646–23651.

Katrantzis, M., Baker, M.S., Handley, C.J., and Lowther, D.A. (1991). The oxidant hypochlorite (OCl^-), a product of the myeloperoxidase system, degrades articular cartilage proteoglycan aggregate. *Free Radical Biology and Medicine*, **10**, 101–109.

Kaur, H., and Halliwell, B. (1994). Evidence for nitric oxide-mediated oxidative damage in chronic inflammation. Nitrotyrosine in serum and synovial fluid from rheumatoid patients. *FEBS Letters*, **350**, 9–12.

Kautiainen, A. (1992). Determination of hemoglobin adducts from aldehydes formed during lipid peroxidation *in vitro*. *Chemico-Biological Interactions*, **83**, 55–63.

Kawahara, H., Nakamura, M., Ishizaki, N., Yamada, T., Kawamoto, T., Hikari, S., *et al.* (1979). Solubility of metallic mercury into the solutions containing various amino acids (trans. author). *Shika Rikogaku Zasshi*, **20**, 137–141.

Kawamura, M., Heinecke, J.W., and Chait, A. (1994). Pathophysiological concentrations of glucose promote oxidative modification of low density lipoprotein by a superoxide-dependent pathway. *Journal of Clinical Investigation*, **94**, 771–778.

Kawasaki, I., and Wakakura, M. (1995). Possible role of the AMPA/KA receptors in cultured Muller cells]. *Nippon Ganka Gakkai Zasshi*, **99**, 1214–1221.

Kay, M.M., Lake, D., and Cover, C. (1995). Band 3 and its peptides during aging, radiation exposure, and Alzheimer's disease: alterations and self-recognition. *Advances in Experimental Medical Biology*, **383**, 167–193.

Kaye, N.M., and Weitzman, P.D. (1976). Rose Bengal immobilized on Sepharose-a new tool for protein photo-oxidation. *FEBS Letters*, **62**, 334–337.

Kaytka, V.V., and Donchenko, H.V. (1995). Antioxidant properties of products of the interaction of amino acids with carbohydrates under conditions of the Maillard reaction. *Ukrainskii Biokhimichiskii Zhurnal*, **67**, 71–75.

Keaney, J.J., Gaziano, J.M., Xu, A., Frei, B., Curran, C.J., Shwaery, G.T., *et al.* (1994). Low-dose alpha-tocopherol improves and high-dose alpha-tocopherol worsens endothelial vasodilator function in cholesterol-fed rabbits. *Journal of Clinical Investigation*, **93**, 844–851.

Keaney, J.J., Xu, A., Cunningham, D., Jackson, T., Frei, B., and Vita, J.A. (1995). Dietary probucol preserves endothelial function in cholesterol-fed rabbits by limiting vascular oxidative stress and superoxide generation. *Journal of Clinical Investigation*, **95**, 2520–2529.

Keck, R.G. (1996). The use of *t*-butyl hydroperoxide as a probe for methionine oxidation in proteins. *Analytical Biochemistry*, **236**, 56–62.

Kelder, P.P., Fischer, M.J., de Mol, N.J., and Janssen, L.H. (1991*a*). Oxidation of chlorpromazine by methemoglobin in the presence of hydrogen peroxide. Formation of chlorpromazine radical cation and its covalent binding to met-hemoglobin. *Archives of Biochemistry and Biophysics*, **284**, 313–319.

Kelder, P.P., de Mol, N.J., and Janssen, L.H. (1991*b*). Mechanistic aspects of the oxidation of phenothiazine derivatives by methemoglobin in the presence of hydrogen peroxide. *Biochemical Pharmacology*, **42**, 1551–1559.

Kelder, P.P., de Mol, N.J., Fischer, M.J., and Janssen, L.H. (1994). Kinetic evaluation of the oxidation of phenothiazine derivatives by methemoglobin and horseradish peroxidase in the presence of hydrogen peroxide. Implications for the reaction mechanisms. *Biochimica et Biophysica Acta*, **1205**, 230–238.

Keller, R.J., Halmes, N.C., Hinson, J.A., and Pumford, N.R. (1993). Immuno-chemical detection of oxidized proteins. *Chemical Research in Toxicology*, **6**, 430–433.

Kelly, F.J., and Birch, S. (1993). Ozone exposure inhibits cardiac protein synthesis in the mouse. *Free Radical Biology and Medicine*, **14**, 443–446.

Kelman, D.J., and Mason, R.P. (1992). The myoglobin-derived radical formed on reaction of metmyoglobin with hydrogen peroxide is not a tyrosine peroxyl radical. *Free Radical Research Communications*, **16**, 27–33.

Kelman, D.J., and Mason, R.P. (1993). Characterization of the rat hemoglobin thiyl free radical formed upon reaction with phenylhydrazine. *Archives of Biochemistry and Biophysics*, **306**, 439–442.

Kelman, D.J., DeGray, J.A., and Mason, R.P. (1994). Reaction of myoglobin with hydrogen peroxide forms a peroxyl radical which oxidizes substrates. *Journal of Biological Chemistry*, **269**, 7458–7463.

Kempner, E.S., Miller, J.H., and McCreery, M.J. (1986). Radiation target analysis of glycoproteins. *Analytical Biochemistry*, **156**, 140–146.

Kenar, J.A., Havrilla, C.M., Porter, N.A., Guyton, J.R., Brown, S.A., Klemp, K.F., *et al.* (1996). Identification and quantification of the regioisomeric cholesteryl linoleate hydroperoxides in oxidised human low denisty lipoprotein and high density lipoprotein. *Chemical Research in Toxicology*, **9**, 737–744.

Kensler, T., Guyton, K., Egner, P., McCarthy, T., Lesko, S., and Akman, S. (1995). Role of reactive intermediates in tumor promotion and progression. *Progress in Clinical Biology Research*, **391**, 103–116.

Kepp, R.K., and Michel, K.F. (1953). Action of X-rays on aqueous protein solutions. *Strahlentherapie*, **92**, 416–422.

Keren, N., Gong, H., and Ohad, I. (1995). Oscillations of reaction center II-D1 protein degradation *in vivo* induced by repetitive light flashes. Correlation between the level of RCII-QB- and protein degradation in low light. *Journal of Biological Chemistry*, **270**, 806–814.

Kessler, M., Arai, A., Quan, A., and Lynch, G. (1996). Effect of cyclothiazide on binding properties of AMPA-type glutamate receptors: lack of competition between cyclothiazide and GYKI 52466. *Molecular Pharmacology*, **49**, 123–131.

Kettle, A.J. (1996). Neutrophils convert tyrosyl residues in albumin to chlorotyrosine. *FEBS Letters*, **379**, 103–106.

Khazipov, R., Congar, P., and Ben, A.Y. (1995). Hippocampal CA1 lacunosummoleculare interneurons: comparison of effects of anoxia on excitatory and inhibitory postsynaptic currents. *Journal of Neurophysiology*, **74**, 2138–2149.

Khoroshilova, E.V., Repeyev, Y.A., and Nikogosyan, D.N. (1990). UV photolysis of aromatic amino acids and related dipeptides and tripeptides. *Journal of Photochemistry and Photobiology B: Biology*, **7**, 159–172.

Khramtsov, V.V., Yelinova, V.I., Weiner, L.M., Berezina, T.A., Martin, V.V., and Volodarsky, L.B. (1989). Quantitative determination of SH groups in low- and high-molecular-weight compounds by an electron spin resonance method. *Analytical Biochemistry*, **182**, 58–63.

Kikugawa, K., Kato, T., and Okamoto, Y. (1994). Damage of amino acids and proteins induced by nitrogen dioxide, a free radical toxin, in air. *Free Radical Biology and Medicine*, **16**, 373–382.

Kim, H.J., Mee, L.K., Adelstein, S.J., Taub, I.A., Carr, S.A., and Reinhold, V.N. (1984a). Binding site specificity of gamma-radiation-induced crosslinking between phenylalanine and a phenylalanine-containing tetrapeptide. *Radiation Research*, **100**, 30–40.

Kim, H.J., Mee, L.K., Adelstein, S.J., and Taub, I.A. (1984b). Binding-site specificity of the radiolytically induced crosslinking of phenylalanine to glucagon. *Radiation Research*, **98**, 26–36.

Kim, H.S., Oh, S.H., Kim, D.I., Kim, I.C., Cho, K.H., and Park, Y.B. (1995). Chemical synthesis of 15-ketosterols and their inhibitions of cholesteryl ester transfer protein. *Bioorganic Medicine and Chemistry*, **3**, 367–374.

Kim, K., Rhee, S.G., and Stadtman, E.R. (1985). Nonenzymatic cleavage of proteins by reactive oxygen species generated by dithiothreitol and iron. *Journal of Biological Chemistry*, **260**, 15394–15397.

Kim, K., Kim, I.H., Lee, K.Y., Rhee, S.G., and Stadtman, E.R. (1988). The isolation and purification of a specific 'protector' protein which inhibits enzyme inactivation by a thiol/Fe(III)/O_2 mixed-function oxidation system. *Journal of Biological Chemistry*, **263**, 4704–4711.

Kim, M.J., Dawes, J., and Jessup, W. (1994). Transendothelial transport of modified low-density lipoproteins. *Atherosclerosis*, **108**, 5–17.

Kim, M.-S., and Akera, T. (1987). O_2 free radicals: cause of ischemia-reperfusion injury to cardiac Na^+-K^+-ATPase. *American Journal of Physiology*, **252**, H252–H257.

Kim, S.W., Luykx, D.M., de Vries, S., and Duine, J.A. (1996). A second molybdoprotein aldehyde dehydrogenase from *Amycolatopsis methanolica NCIB 11946*. *Archives of Biochemistry and Biophysics*, **325**, 1–7.

Kim, Y.M., Bergonia, H.A., Muller, C., Pitt, B.R., Watkins, W.D., and Lancaster, J.J. (1995). Nitric oxide and intracellular heme. *Advances in Pharmacology*, **34**, 277–291.

Kimura, K., and Sugano, S. (1992). Inactivation of *Bacillus subtilis* glutamine synthetase by metal-catalyzed oxidation. *Journal of Biochemistry, Tokyo*, **112**, 828–833.

King, D.S., and Reichard, P. (1995). Mass spectrometric determination of the radical scission site in the anaerobic ribonucleotide reductase of *Escherichia coli*. *Biochemical and Biophysical Research Communications*, **206**, 731–735.

King, F.J., Anderson, M.L., and Steinberg, M.L. (1962). Reaction of cod acto-myosine with linoleic and linolenic acids. *Journal of Food Science*, **27**, 363–366.

King, N.K., and Winfield, M.E. (1963). The mechanism of metmyoglobin oxidation. *Journal of Biological Chemistry*, **238**, 1520–1528.

King, N.K., Looney, F.D., and Winfield, M.E. (1967). Amino acid free radicals in oxidised metmyoglobin. *Biochimica et Biophysica Acta*, **133**, 65–82.

Kinoshita, T., Iinuma, F., Atsumi, K., and Tsuji, A. (1977). A fluorometric assay of proteins on Kieselguhr plates using sodium hypochlorite and thiamine. *Analytical Biochemistry*, **77**, 471–477.

Kirilovsky, D.L., Boussac, A.G., van Mieghem, F., Ducruet, J.M., Setif, P.R., Yu, J.J., *et al.* (1992). Oxygen-evolving photosystem II preparation from wild type and photosystem II mutants of *Synechocystis* sp. PCC 6803. *Biochemistry*, **31**, 2099–2107.

Kirkland, J.B. (1991). Lipid peroxidation, protein thiol oxidation and DNA damage in hydrogen peroxide-induced injury to endothelial cells: role of activation of poly(ADP-ribose)polymerase. *Biochimica et Biophysica Acta*, **1092**, 319–325.

Kirkpatrick, D.L., Sa'da, I.A., Chernoff, W., and Kuperus, M. (1994). Disulfide cytotoxicity under hypoxia. *Oncology Research*, **6**, 545–552.

Kiso, Y. (1995). Design and synthesis of HIV protease inhibitors containing allo-phenylnorstatine as a transition-state mimic. *Advances in Experimental Medical Biology*, **362**, 413–423.

Kitazawa, M., and Iwasaki, K. (1996). Suppression of iron catalyzed free radical generation by iron tyrosinate protein models. *Biochemical and Biophysical Research Communications*, **220**, 36–41.

Kittridge, K.J., and Willson, R.L. (1984). Uric acid substantially enhances the free radical-induced inactivation of alcohol dehydrogenase. *FEBS Letters*, **170**, 162–164.

Klapper, M.H., and Faraggi, M. (1979). Application of pulse radiolysis to protein chemistry. *Quarterly Review of Biophysics*, **12**, 465–519.

Klebanoff, S.J., Kinsella, M.G., and Wight, T.N. (1993). Degradation of endothelial cell matrix heparan sulfate proteoglycan by elastase and the myeloperoxidase-H_2O_2-chloride system. *American Journal of Pathology*, **143**, 907–917.

Kleinveld, H.A., Swaak, A.J., Hack, C.E., and Koster, J.F. (1989). Interactions between oxygen free radicals and proteins. Implications for rheumatoid arthritis. An overview. *Scandanavian Journal of Rheumatology*, **18**, 341–352.

Klinman, J.P., Dooley, D.M., Duine, J.A., Knowles, P.F., Mondovi, B., and Villafranca, J.J. (1991). Status of the cofactor identity in copper oxidative enzymes. *FEBS Letters*, **282**, 1–4.

Klug-Roth, D., and Rabani, J. (1976). Pulse radiolytic studies on the reactions of aqueous superoxide radicals with copper(II) complexes. *Journal of Physical Chemistry*, **80**, 588–591.

Knappe, J., Neugebauer, F.A., Blaschkowski, H.P., and Ganzler, M. (1984). Post-translational activation introduces a free radical into pyruvate formate-lyase. *Proceedings of the National Academy of Science of the United States of America*, **81**, 1332–1335.

Knappe, J., Elbert, S., Frey, M., and Wagner, A.F. (1993). Pyruvate formate-lyase mechanism involving the protein-based glycyl radical. *Biochemical Society Transactions*, **21**, 731–734.

Knecht, K.J., Feather, M.S., and Baynes, J.W. (1992). Detection of 3-deoxyfructose and 3-deoxyglucosone in human urine and plasma: evidence for intermediate stages of the Maillard reaction *in vivo*. *Archives of Biochemistry and Biophysics*, **294**, 130–137.

Kneepkens, C.M., Lepage, G., and Roy, C.C. (1994). The potential of the hydro-carbon breath test as a measure of lipid peroxidation [published erratum appears in *Free Radical Biology and Medicine* (1994), **17**, 609]. *Free Radical Biology and Medicine*, **17**, 127–160.

Knight, K.L., and Mudd, J.B. (1984). The reaction of ozone with glyceralde-hyde-3-phosphate dehydrogenase. *Archives of Biochemistry and Biophysics*, **229**, 259–269.

Knight, K.R., MacPhadyen, K., Lepore, D.A., Kuwata, N., Eadie, P.A., and O'Brien, B.M. (1991). Enhancement of ischaemic rabbit skin flap survival with the antioxidant and free-radical scavenger *N*-acetylcysteine. *Clinical Science*, **81**, 31–36.

Knott, T.J., Pease, R.J., Powell, L.M., Wallis, S.C., Rall, S.C.J., Innerarity, T.L., *et al.* (1986). Complete protein sequence and identification of structural domains of human apolipoprotein B. *Nature*, **323**, 734–742.

Knowles, R.G., and Burchell, B. (1977). A simple method for purification of epoxide hydratase from rat liver. *Biochemical Journal*, **163**, 381–383.

Koc, O.N., Allay, J.A., Lee, K., Davis, B.M., Reese, J.S., and Gerson, S.L. (1996). Transfer of drug resistance genes into hematopoietic progenitors to improve chemotherapy tolerance. *Seminars in Oncology*, **23**, 46–65.

Kochi, J.K. (1973). Oxidation-reduction reactions of free radicals and metal complexes. In *Free Radicals*, (ed. J.K. Kochi), pp. 591–683. John Wiley and Sons, New York.

Kohar, I., Baca, M., Suarna, C., Stocker, R., and Southwell, K.P. (1995). Is alpha-tocopherol a reservoir for alpha-tocopheryl hydroquinone? *Free Radical Biology and Medicine*, **19**, 197–207.

Kohen, R., and Chevion, M. (1988). Cytoplasmic membrane is the target organelle for transition metal mediated damage induced by paraquat in *Escherichia coli*. *Biochemistry*, **27**, 2597–2603.

Kohno, T., Yamada, Y., Hata, T., Mori, H., Yamamura, M., Tomonaga, M., *et al.* (1996). Relation of oxidative stress and glutathione synthesis to CD95(Fas/APO-1)-mediated apoptosis of adult T cell leukemia cells. *Journal of Immunology*, **156**, 4722–4728.

Konat, G.W. (1985). Effect of reactive oxygen species on myelin membrane proteins. *Journal of Neurochemistry*, **45**, 1113–1118.

Konen, D.A., Silbert, L.S., and Pfeffer, P.E. (1975). α Anions. VII. Direct oxidation of enolate anions to 2-hydroperoxy- and 2-hydroxycarboxylic acids and esters. *Journal of Organic Chemistry*, **40**, 3253–3258.

Kong, S.B., Cutnell, J.D., and La Mar, G.N. (1983). Proton nuclear magnetic resonance study of the dynamic stability of the heme pocket of soybean leghemoglobin A. Exchange rates for the labile proton of the proximal histidyl imidazole. *Journal of Biological Chemistry*, **258**, 3843–3849.

Konig, S., Ugi, I., and Schramm, H.J. (1995). Facile syntheses of C2-symmetrical HIV-1 protease inhibitors. *Archives of Pharmacology (Weinheim)*, **328**, 699–704.

Kontush, A., Kohlschutter, A., and Beisiegel, U. (1995). Physical properties of oxidized lipoproteins. *Biochemistry and Molecular Biology International*, **37**, 707–716.

Kooy, N.W., Royall, J.A., Ye, Y.Z., Kelly, D.R., and Beckman, J.S. (1995). Evidence for in vivo peroxynitrite production in human acute lung injury. *American Journal of Respiratory and Cellular Molecular Biology Critical Care Medicine*, **151**, 1250–1254.

Kopoldova, J. (1968). Effect of γ-irradiation on aqueous solutions of the cyclic dodecapeptide polymyxin B. In *Radiation Chemistry Vol. 1*, (ed. R.F. Gould), pp. 472–479. American Chemical Society, Washington.

Kopoldova, J., and Hrneir, S. (1977). Gamma-radiolysis of aqueous solution of histidine. *Zeitschrift für Naturforschung. C: Bioscience*, **32c**, 482–487.

Kopoldova, J., Liebster, J., and Babicky, A. (1963a). The mechanism of the radiation chemical degradation of amino acids—III. Radiolysis of norvaline in aqueous oxygenated and oxygen-free solutions. *International Journal of Applied Radiation and Isotopes*, **14**, 455–460.

Kopoldova, J., Liebster, J., and Babicky, A. (1963b). The mechanism of the radiation chemical degradation of amino acids—IV. Radiolysis of valine in aqueous oxygenated and oxygen-free solutions. *International Journal of Applied Radiation and Isotopes*, **14**, 489–492.

Kopoldova, J., Liebster, J., and Babicky, A. (1963c). The mechanism of the radiation chemical degradation of amino acids—V. Radiolysis of norleucine, leucine and isoleucine in aqueous solution. *International Journal of Applied Radiation and Isotopes*, **14**, 493–498.

Kopoldova, J., Liebster, J., and Gross, E. (1967). Radiation chemical reactions in aqueous solutions of methionine and its peptides. *Radiation Research*, **30**, 261–274.

Koppenol, W.H. (1994). Thermodynamic considerations on the formation of reactive species from hypochlorite, superoxide and nitrogen monoxide. Could nitrosyl chloride be produced by neutrophils and macrophages? *FEBS Letters*, **347**, 5–8.

Kopriva, S., and Bauwe, H. (1995). H-protein of glycine decarboxylase is encoded by multigene families in *Flaveria pringlei* and *F. cronquistii* (*Asteraceae*). *Molecular and General Genetics*, **249**, 111–116.

Korchagin, V.P., Bratkovskaia, L.B., Shvedova, A.A., Arkhipenko, I., and Kagan, V.E. (1980). Oligomerization of integral membrane proteins under lipid peroxidation. *Biokhimiia*, **45**, 1767–1772.

Kornhauser, A. (1976). UV induced DNA-protein cross-links *in vitro* and *in vivo*. *Photochemistry and Photobiology*, **23**, 457–460.

Kortt, A.A., and Liu, T.Y. (1973). On the mechanism of action of streptococcal proteinase. 3. The effect of pH, organic solvents, and deuterium oxide on the proteinase-catalyzed hydrolysis of *N*-acylamino acid esters. *Biochemistry*, **12**, 338–345.

Kostner, G.M., Oettl, K., Jauhiainen, M., Ehnholm, C., Esterbauer, H., and Dieplinger, H. (1995). Human plasma phospholipid transfer protein accelerates exchange/transfer of alpha-tocopherol between lipoproteins and cells. *Biochemical Journal*, **305**, 659–667.

Kowanko, I.C., Bates, E.J., and Ferrante, A. (1989). Mechanisms of human neutrophil-mediated cartilage damage *in vitro*: the role of lysosomal enzymes, hydrogen peroxide and hypochlorous acid. *Immunology and Cellular Biology*, **67**, 321–329.

Kowluru, A., Seavey, S.E., Rhodes, C.J., and Metz, S.A. (1996). A novel regulatory mechanism for trimeric GTP-binding proteins in the membrane and secretory granule fractions of human and rodent beta cells. *Biochemical Journal*, **313**, 97–107.

Kramer, J.H., Arroyo, C.M., Dickens, B.F., and Weglicki, W.B. (1987). Spin-trapping evidence that graded myocardial ischemia alters post-ischemic superoxide production. *Free Radical Biology and Medicine*, **3**, 153–159.

Krause, G.S., DeGracia, D.J., Skjaerlund, J.M., and O'Neil, B.J. (1992). Assessment of free radical-induced damage in brain proteins after ischemia and reperfusion. *Resuscitation*, **23**, 59–69.

Krems, B., Charizanis, C., and Entian, K.D. (1996). The response regulator-like protein Pos9/Skn7 of *Saccharomyces cerevisiae* is involved in oxidative stress resistance. *Current Genetics*, **29**, 327–334.

Kretsinger, R.H. (1968). A crystallographic study of iodinated sperm whale metmyoglobin. *Journal of Molecular Biology*, **31**, 315–318.

Krijnse, L.J., Parton, R.G., Fuller, S.D., Griffiths, G., and Dotti, C.G. (1995). The organization of the endoplasmic reticulum and the intermediate compartment in cultured rat hippocampal neurons. *Molecular Biology of the Cell*, **6**, 1315–1332.

Krishna, C.M., Kondo, T., and Riesz, P. (1988). Sonochemistry of nucleic acid constituents in aqueous solution: a spin-trapping study. *Basic Life Science*, **49**, 433–436.

Krishnamoorthi, R., Markley, J.L., Cusanovich, M.A., Przysiecki, C.T., and Meyer, T.E. (1986). Hydrogen-1 nuclear magnetic resonance investigation of high-potential iron-sulfur proteins from *Ectothiorhodospira halophila* and *Ectothiorhodospira vacuolata*: a comparative study of hyperfine-shifted resonances. *Biochemistry*, **25**, 60–67.

Kritharides, L., Jessup, W., Gifford, J., and Dean, R.T. (1993). A method for defining the stages of low-density lipoprotein oxidation by the separation of cholesterol- and cholesteryl ester-oxidation products using HPLC. *Analytical Biochemistry*, **213**, 79–89.

Kritharides, L., Jessup, W., and Dean, R.T. (1995*a*). Macrophages require both iron and copper to oxidize low-density lipoprotein in Hanks' balanced salt solution. *Archives of Biochemistry and Biophysics*, **323**, 127–136.

Kritharides, L., Jessup, W., and Dean, R.T. (1995*b*). EDTA differentially and incompletely inhibits components of prolonged cell-mediated oxidation of low-density lipoprotein. *Free Radical Research*, **22**, 399–417.

Kritharides, L., Jessup, W., Mander, E.L., and Dean, R.T. (1995*c*). Apolipoprotein A-I-mediated efflux of sterols from oxidized LDL-loaded macrophages. *Arteriosclerosis Thrombosis and Vascular Biology*, **15**, 276–289.

Kroese, E.D., Bannenberg, G., Dogterom, P., Noach, A.B., Nagelkerke, J.F., and Meerman, J.H. (1990). Lipid peroxidation and protein thiol depletion are not involved in the cytotoxicity of *N*-hydroxy-2-acetylaminofluorene in isolated rat hepatocytes. *Biochemical Pharmacology*, **40**, 1885–1892.

Krsek, S.J., and Webster, R.O. (1993). Ceruloplasmin inhibits carbonyl formation in endogenous cell proteins. *Free Radical Biology and Medicine*, **14**, 115–125.

Ku, H.H., and Sohal, R.S. (1993). Comparison of mitochondrial pro-oxidant generation and anti-oxidant defenses between rat and pigeon: possible basis of variation in longevity and metabolic potential. *Mechanisms of Ageing Development*, **72**, 67–76.

Ku, H.H., Brunk, U.T., and Sohal, R.S. (1993). Relationship between mitochondrial superoxide and hydrogen peroxide production and longevity of mammalian species. *Free Radical Biology and Medicine*, **15**, 621–627.

Kuhn, H., Heydeck, D., and Sprecher, H. (1991). On the mechanistic reasons for the dual positional specificity of the reticulocyte lipoxygenase. *Biochimica et Biophysica Acta*, **1081**, 129–134.

Kuhn, T.S. (1970). *The Structure of Scientific Revolutions*. University of Chicago Press, Chicago.

Kukreja, R.C., Okabe, E., Schrier, G.M., and Hess, M.L. (1988). Oxygen radical-mediated lipid peroxidation and inhibition of Ca^{2+}-ATPase avtivity of cardiac sarcoplasmic reticulum. *Archives of Biochemistry and Biophysics*, **261**, 447–457.

Kulmacz, R.J., Ren, Y., Tsai, A.L., and Palmer, G. (1990). Prostaglandin H synthase: spectroscopic studies of the interaction with hydroperoxides and with indomethacin. *Biochemistry*, **29**, 8760–8771.

Kulmacz, R.J., Palmer, G., and Tsai, A.L. (1993). Substrate-induced free radicals in prostaglandin H synthase. *Journal of Lipid Mediators*, **6**, 145–154.

Kumta, U.S., Shimazu, F., and Tappel, A.L. (1962). Decrease of radiation damage to proteins by sulfydryl protectors. *Radiation Research*, **16**, 679–685.

Kumta, V.S., and Tappel, A.L. (1961). Radiation damage to proteins. *Nature*, **191**, 1304–1305.

Kunert, K.J., and Tappel, A.L. (1983). The effect of vitamin C on *in vivo* lipid peroxidation in guinea pigs as measured by pentane and ethane production. *Lipids*, **18**, 271–274.

Kupke, T., Kempter, C., Jung, G., and Gotz, F. (1995). Oxidative decarboxylation of peptides catalyzed by flavoprotein EpiD. Determination of substrate specificity using peptide libraries and neutral loss mass spectrometry. *Journal of Biological Chemistry*, **270**, 11282–11289.

Kurosaki, F. (1996). Transacylase-like structure and its role in substrate channeling of 6-hydroxymellein synthase, a multifunctional polyketide biosynthetic enzyme in carrot cell extracts. *FEBS Letters*, **379**, 97–102.

Kurtel, H., Granger, D.N., Tso, P., and Grisham, M.B. (1992). Vulnerability of intestinal interstitial fluid to oxidant stress. *American Journal of Physiology*, **263**, G573–578.

Kusama, Y., Bernier, M., and Hearse, D.J. (1989). Singlet oxygen-induced arrhythmias. Dose- and light-response studies for photoactivation of Rose Bengal in the rat heart. *Circulation*, **80**, 1432–1448.

Kusama, Y., Bernier, M., and Hearse, D.J. (1990). Photoactivation of porphyrins: studies of reactive oxygen intermediates and arrhythmogenesis in the aerobic rat heart. *Cardiovascular Research*, **24**, 676–682.

Kusama, Y., Hearse, D.J., and Avkiran, M. (1992). Diabetes and susceptibility to reperfusion-induced ventricular arrhythmias. *Journal of Molecular and Cellular Cardiology*, **24**, 411–421.

Kusunose, M., Matsumoto, J., Ichihara, K., Kusunose, E., and Nozaka, J. (1967). Requirement of three proteins for hydrocarbon oxidation. *Journal of Biochemistry, Tokyo*, **61**, 665–667.

Kutty, R.K., Kutty, G., Wiggert, B., Chader, G.J., Darrow, R.M., and Organisciak, D.T. (1995). Induction of heme oxygenase 1 in the retina by intense visible light: suppression by the antioxidant dimethylthiourea. *Proceedings of the National Academy of Science of the United States of America*, **92**, 1177–1181.

Kuypers, F.A., Scott, M.D., Schott, M.A., Lubin, B., and Chiu, D.T. (1990). Use of ektacytometry to determine red cell susceptibility to oxidative stress. *Journal of Laboratory and Clinical Medicine*, **116**, 535–545.

Kwon, N.S., Chan, P.C., and Kesner, L. (1990). Inactivation of alpha 1-proteinase inhibitor by Cu(II) and hydrogen peroxide. *Agents and Actions*, **29**, 388–393.

L'vov, K.M. (1965). Studies on the recombination of free radicals in irradiated proteins. *Biofizika*, **10**, 212–216.

L'vov, K.M., and Bekmurzaev, B.M. (1990). Accumulation of UV-induced radicals in proteins with various degree of aggregation]. Biofizika, **35**, 421–424.

L'vov, K.M., and Iskakov, A.A. (1993a). Study of free radical reactions in proteins by a recombination-kinetic method. *Biofizika*, **38**, 411–416.

L'vov, K.M., and Iskakov, A.A. (1993b). Mechanisms of death of free radical states in proteins. *Biofizika*, **38**, 7–11.

L'vov, K.M., Ovcharenko, V.P., and L'vova, O.F. (1978). Effect of luminescence quenchers on the maximum concentration of radicals in proteins following UV-irradiation (77 K). *Biofizika*, **23**, 970–973.

Laboissiere, M.C., Chivers, P.T., and Raines, R.T. (1995). Production of rat protein disulfide isomerase in *Saccharomyces cerevisiae*. *Protein Expression and Purification*, **6**, 700–706.

Lacampagne, A., Duittoz, A., Bolanos, P., Peineau, N., and Argibay, J.A. (1995). Effect of sulfydryl oxidation on ionic and gating currents associated with L-type calcium channels in isolated guinea-pig ventricular myocytes. *Cardiovascular Research*, **30**, 799–806.

Ladenheim, H.S., Mistchenko, A.S., and Drut, R. (1995). Expression of early and late adenoviral proteins in fatal adenovirus bronchopneumonia. *Pediatric Pathology and Laboratory Medicine*, **15**, 291–298.

Laerum, O.D., Sletvold, O., Bjerknes, R., Eriksen, J.A., Johansen, J.H., Schanche, J.S., et al. (1988). The dimer of hemoregulatory peptide (HP5B) stimulates mouse and human myelopoiesis *in vitro*. *Experimental Hematology*, **16**, 274–280.

Laffranchi, R., Gogvadze, V., Richter, C., and Spinas, G.A. (1995). Nitric oxide (nitrogen monoxide, NO) stimulates insulin secretion by inducing calcium release from mitochondria. *Biochemical and Biophysical Research Communications*, **217**, 584–591.

Laguzza, B.C., Nichols, C.L., Briggs, S.L., Cullinan, G.J., Johnson, D.A., Starling, J.J., et al. (1989). New antitumor monoclonal antibody-vinca conjugates LY203725 and related compounds: design, preparation, and representative *in vivo* activity. *Journal of Medicinal Chemistry*, **32**, 548–555.

Lambeir, A.M., Markey, C.M., Dunford, H.B., and Marnett, L.J. (1985). Spectral properties of the higher oxidation states of prostaglandin H synthase. *Journal of Biological Chemistry*, **260**, 14894–14896.

Lamboy, J.S., Staples, R.C., and Hoch, H.C. (1995). Superoxide dismutase: a differentiation protein expressed in *Uromyces* germlings during early appressorium development. *Experimental Mycology*, **19**, 284–296.

Land, E.J., and Ebert, M. (1967). Pulse radiolysis of aqueous phenol. Water elimination from dihydroxycyclohexadienyl radicals to form phenoxyl. *Transactions of the Faraday Society*, **63**, 1181–1190.

Land, E.J., and Prutz, W.A. (1977). Fast one-electron oxidation of tryptophan by azide radicals. *International Journal of Radiation Biology and Related Studies in Physics, Chemistry and Medicine*, **32**, 203–207.

Land, E.J., and Prutz, W.A. (1979). Reaction of azide radicals with amino acids and proteins. *International Journal of Radiation Biology and Related Studies in Physics, Chemistry and Medicine*, **36**, 75–83.

Lander, H.M., Ogiste, J.S., Teng, K.K., and Novogrodsky, A. (1995). p21ras as a common signaling target of reactive free radicals and cellular redox stress. *Journal of Biological Chemistry*, **270**, 21195–21198.

Landry, L.G., Chapple, C.C., and Last, R.L. (1995). Arabidopsis mutants lacking phenolic sunscreens exhibit enhanced ultraviolet-B injury and oxidative damage. *Plant Physiology*, **109**, 1159–1166.

Lane, R.W., Ibers, J.A., Frankel, R.B., and Holm, R.H. (1975). Synthetic analogs of active sites of iron-sulfur proteins: bis (o-xylyldithiolato) ferrate (III) monoanion, a structurally unconstrained model for the rubredoxin Fe-S4 unit. *Proceedings of the National Academy of Science of the United States of America*, **72**, 2868–2872.

Lapolla, A., Fedele, D., Seraglia, R., Catinella, S., Baldo, L., Aronica, R., *et al.* (1995). A new effective method for the evaluation of glycated intact plasma proteins in diabetic subjects. *Diabetologia*, **38**, 1076–1081.

Lariviere, F., Kupranycz, D.B., Chiasson, J.L., and Hoffer, L.J. (1992). Plasma leucine kinetics and urinary nitrogen excretion in intensively treated diabetes mellitus. *American Journal of Physiology*, **263**, E173–179.

Larson, D.E., Rising, R., Ferraro, R.T., and Ravussin, E. (1995). Spontaneous overfeeding with a 'cafeteria diet' in men: effects on 24-hour energy expenditure and substrate oxidation. *International Journal of Obesity and Related Metabolic Disorders*, **19**, 331–337.

Larsson, A., and Sjoberg, B.M. (1986). Identification of the stable free radical tyrosine residue in ribonucleotide reductase. *EMBO Journal*, **5**, 2037–2040.

Lass, A., Belkner, J., Esterbauer, H., and Kuhn, H. (1996). Lipoxygenase treatment renders low-density lipoprotein susceptible to Cu^{2+}-catalysed oxidation. *Biochemical Journal*, **314**, 577–585.

Lassmann, G., and Potsch, S. (1995). Structure of transient radicals from cytostatic-active p-alkoxyphenols by continuous-flow EPR. *Free Radical Biology and Medicine*, **19**, 533–539.

Lassmann, G., Odenwaller, R., Curtis, J.F., DeGray, J.A., Mason, R.P., Marnett, L.J., *et al.* (1991). Electron spin resonance investigation of tyrosyl radicals of prostaglandin H synthase. Relation to enzyme catalysis [published erratum appears in *Journal of Biological Chemistry* (1992), **267**, 6449]. *Journal of Biological Chemistry*, **266**, 20045–20055.

Lassmann, G., Thelander, L., and Graslund, A. (1992). EPR stopped-flow studies of the reaction of the tyrosyl radical of protein R2 from ribonucleotide reductase with hydroxyurea. *Biochemical and Biophysical Research Communications*, **188**, 879–887.

Lassmann, G., Curtis, J., Liermann, B., Mason, R.P., and Eling, T.E. (1993). ESR studies on reactivity of protein-derived tyrosyl radicals formed by prostaglandin H synthase and ribonucleotide reductase. *Archives of Biochemistry and Biophysics*, **300**, 132–136.

Latarjet, R., and Loiseleur, J. (1942). Modalités de la Fixation de L'Oxygène en Radiobiologie. *Societe de Biologie Comptes Rendue*, **136**, 60–63.

Latour, B., and Woolgar, S. (1979). *Laboratory Life: the Social Construction of Scientific Facts*. Sage, Beverly Hills.

Lau, R.C., and Rinehart, K.L. (1994). Berninamycins B, C, and D, minor metabolites from *Streptomyces bernensis* [published erratum appears in *Journal Antibiotics, Tokyo* (1995), **48**, C-1]. *Journal of Antibiotics, Tokyo*, **47**, 1466–1472.

Laudenbach, D.E., Herbert, S.K., McDowell, C., Fork, D.C., Grossman, A.R., and
Straus, N.A. (1990). Cytochrome *c*-553 is not required for photosynthetic activity
in the cyanobacterium *Synechococcus*. *Plant Cell*, **2**, 913–924.

Lauffer, R.B., Antanaitis, B.C., Aisen, P., and Que, L.J. (1983). ^{1}H NMR studies
of porcine uteroferrin. Magnetic interactions and active site structure. *Journal of
Biological Chemistry*, **258**, 14212–14218.

Laverty, G., and Wideman, R.J. (1985). Avian renal responses to oxidized and
nonoxidized bPTH(1-34). *General and Comprehensive Endocrinology*, **59**, 391–398.

Lavrovsky, Y., Schwartzman, M.L., and Abraham, N.G. (1993). Novel regulatory
sites of the human heme oxygenase-1 promoter region. *Biochemical and Biophysical Research Communications*, **196**, 336–341.

Lawson, C.S., Coltart, D.J., and Hearse, D.J. (1993). The antiarrhythmic action of
ischaemic preconditioning in rat hearts does not involve functional Gi proteins
[see comments]. *Cardiovascular Research*, **27**, 681–687.

Le Guen, C.A., Jones, A.F., Barnett, A.H., and Lunec, J. (1992). Role of reactive
oxygen species in the generation of fluorescence by glycation. *Annals of Clinical
Biochemistry*, **29**, 184–189.

Le Prince, G., Delaere, P., Fages, C., Lefrancois, T., Touret, M., Salanon, M., *et al.*
(1995). Glutamine synthetase (GS) expression is reduced in senile dementia of the
Alzheimer type. *Neurochemistry Research*, **20**, 859–862.

Leader, D.P. (1980). Phosphorylated and other modified forms of eukaryotic ribosomal protein S3 analysed by two-dimensional gel electrophoresis. *Biochemical
Journal*, **189**, 241–245.

Leader, D.P., and Mosson, G.J. (1980). The anomalous migration during two-
dimensional gel electrophoresis of eukaryotic ribosomal proteins with oxidised
thiol groups. *Biochimica et Biophysica Acta*, **622**, 360–364.

Leaver, H.A., Yap, P.L., Rogers, P., Wright, I., Smith, G., Williams, P.E., *et al.* (1995).
Peroxides in human leucocytes in acute septic shock: a preliminary study of acute
phase changes and mortality. *European Journal of Clinical Investigation*, **25**, 777–783.

Leboeuf, R.C., Tolson, D., and Heinecke, J.W. (1995). Dissociation between tissue
iron concentrations and transferrin saturation among inbred mouse strains.
Journal of Laboratory and Clinical Medicine, **126**, 128–136.

Lecomte, E., Artur, Y., Chancerelle, Y., Herbeth, B., Galteau, M.M., Jeandel, C., *et
al.* (1993). Malondialdehyde adducts to, and fragmentation of, apolipoprotein B
from human plasma. *Clinica Chimica Acta*, **218**, 39–46.

Ledwozyw, A. (1995). The influence of proline analogs on bleomycin-induced lung
injury in rats. *Acta Physiologica Hungarica*, **83**, 195–202.

Lee, J., Trad, C.H., and Butterfield, D.A. (1993). Electron paramagnetic resonance
studies of the effects of methoxyacetic acid, a teratologic toxin, on human
erythrocyte membranes. *Toxicology*, **83**, 131–148.

Lee, J.J., and Berns, D.S. (1968). Protein aggregation. The effect of deuterium oxide
on large protein aggregates of C-phycocyanin. *Biochemical Journal*, **110**, 465–470.

Lee, M.H., and Park, J.W. (1995). Lipid peroxidation products mediate damage of
superoxide dismutase. *Biochemistry and Molecular Biology International*, **35**,
1093–1102.

Lee, Y., and Shacter, E. (1995). Role of carbohydrates in oxidative modification of
fibrinogen and other plasma proteins. *Archives of Biochemistry and Biophysics*,
321, 175–181.

Lee, Y.S., Park, S.C., Goldberg, A.L., and Chung, C.H. (1988). Protease So from *Escherichia coli* preferentially degrades oxidatively damaged glutamine synthetase. *Journal of Biological Chemistry*, **263**, 6643–6646.

Legler, G., Muller, P.C., Mentges, H.M., Pflieger, G., and Julich, E. (1985). On the chemical basis of the Lowry protein determination. *Analytical Biochemistry*, **150**, 278–287.

Lehr, H.A., Frei, B., Olofsson, A.M., Carew, T.E., and Arfors, K.E. (1995). Protection from oxidized LDL-induced leukocyte adhesion to microvascular and macrovascular endothelium *in vivo* by vitamin C but not by vitamin E. *Circulation*, **91**, 1525–1532.

Lehrer, S.S., and Fasman, G.D. (1967). Ultraviolet irradiation effects in poly-L-tyrosine and model compounds. Identification of bityrosine as a photoproduct. *Biochemistry*, **6**, 757–767.

Leibowitz, A.I., Vladutiu, A.O., and Nolan, J.P. (1979). Immunoradiometric assay of endotoxin in serum. *Clinical Chemistry*, **25**, 68–70.

Leibovitz, B., Hu, M.L., and Tappel, A.L. (1990). Dietary supplements of vitamin E, beta-carotene, coenzyme Q10 and selenium protect tissues against lipid peroxidation in rat tissue slices. *Journal of Nutrition*, **120**, 97–104.

Leibovitz, B.E., Hu, M.L., and Tappel, A.L. (1990). Lipid peroxidation in rat tissue slices: effect of dietary vitamin E, corn oil-lard and menhaden oil. *Lipids*, **25**, 125–129.

Lenssen, W., and Wiegand, G. (1942) Treating textiles with peroxide-containing liquors, *German Patent*, **728**, 171.

Lenz, A.G., Costabel, U., Shaltiel, S., and Levine, R.L. (1989). Determination of carbonyl groups in oxidatively modified proteins by reduction with tritiated sodium borohydride. *Analytical Biochemistry*, **177**, 419–425.

Lepoittevin, J.P., and Karlberg, A.T. (1994). Interactions of allergenic hydroperoxides with proteins: a radical mechanism? *Chemical Research in Toxicology*, **7**, 130–133.

Lertsiri, S., Fujimoto, K., and Miyazawa, T. (1995). Pyrone hydroperoxide formation during the Maillard reaction and its implication in biological systems. *Biochimica et Biophysica Acta*, **1245**, 278–284.

Levine, R.L. (1977). Fluorescence-quenching studies of the binding of bilirubin to albumin. *Clinical Chemistry*, **23**, 2292–2301.

Levine, R.L. (1983*a*). Oxidative modification of glutamine synthetase. II. Characterization of the ascorbate model system. *Journal of Biological Chemistry*, **258**, 11828–11833.

Levine, R.L. (1983*b*). Oxidative modification of glutamine synthetase. I. Inactivation is due to loss of one histidine residue. *Journal of Biological Chemistry*, **258**, 11823–11827.

Levine, R.L. (1984). Mixed-function oxidation of histidine residues. *Methods in Enzymology*, **107**, 370–376.

Levine, R.L. (1985). Covalent modification of proteins by mixed function oxidation. *Current Topics in Cell Regulation*, **27**, 305–316.

Levine, R.L. (1989). Proteolysis induced by metal-catalyzed oxidation. *Revisiones Sobre Biologia Cellular*, **21**, 347–360.

Levine, R.L. (1993). Ischemia: from acidosis to oxidation. *FASEB Journal*, **7**, 1242–1246.

Levine, R.L., and Federici, M.M. (1982). Quantitation of aromatic residues in proteins: model compounds for second-derivative spectroscopy. *Biochemistry*, **21**, 2600–2606.

Levine, R.L., and Lehrman, S.R. (1984). Identification of amino acid phenyl-thiohydantoins by multicomponent analysis of ultraviolet spectra. *Journal of Chromatography*, **288**, 111–116.

Levine, R.L., and Rivett, A.J. (1988). Oxidative modification of glutamine synthetase: covalent and conformational changes which control susceptibility to proteolysis. *Basic Life Science*, **49**, 541–544.

Levine, R.L., Oliver, C.N., Fulks, R.M., and Stadtman, E.R. (1981). Turnover of bacterial glutamine synthetase: oxidative inactivation precedes proteolysis. *Proceedings of the National Academy of Science of the United States of America*, **78**, 2120–2124.

Levine, R.L., Garland, D., Oliver, C.N., Amici, A., Climent, I., Lenz, A.G., et al. (1990). Determination of carbonyl content in oxidatively modified proteins. *Methods in Enzymology*, **186**, 464–478.

Levine, R.L., Williams, J.A., Stadtman, E.R., and Shacter, E. (1994). Carbonyl assays for determination of oxidatively modified proteins. *Methods in Enzymology*, **233**, 346–357.

Levitzki, A., and Anbar, M. (1967). Modification of the radiolytic oxidation of ribonuclease induced by bound copper. *Journal of the American Chemical Society*, **89**, 4185–4189.

Levitzki, A., and Berger, A. (1971). Specific oxidation of copper binding sites in copper(II)-oligopeptide complexes. *Biochemistry*, **10**, 64–66.

Levitzki, A., Anbar, M., and Berger, A. (1967). Specific oxidation of peptides via their copper complexes. *Biochemistry*, **6**, 3757–3765.

Levitzki, A., Pecht, I., and Berger, A. (1972). The copper-poly-L-histidine complexes. II. Physicochemical properties. *Journal of the American Chemical Society*, **94**, 6844–6848.

Lewisch, S.A., and Levine, R.L. (1995). Determination of 2-oxohistidine by amino acid analysis. *Analytical Biochemistry*, **231**, 440–446.

Li, D., Cottrell, C.E., and Cowan, J.A. (1995). ^{15}N resonance assignments of oxidized and reduced *Chromatium vinosum* high-potential iron protein. *Journal of Protein Chemistry*, **14**, 115–126.

Li, S., Schoneich, C., and Borchardt, R.T. (1995a). Chemical pathways of peptide degradation. VIII. Oxidation of methionine in small model peptides by prooxidant/transition metal ion systems: influence of selective scavengers for reactive oxygen intermediates. *Pharmacuetical Research*, **12**, 348–355.

Li, S., Schoneich, C., Wilson, G.S., and Borchardt, R.T. (1993). Chemical pathways of peptide degradation. V. Ascorbic acid promotes rather than inhibits the oxidation of methionine to methionine sulfoxide in small model peptides. *Pharmaceutical Research*, **10**, 1572–1579.

Li, S., Nguyen, T.H., Schoneich, C., and Borchardt, R.T. (1995b). Aggregation and precipitation of human relaxin induced by metal-catalyzed oxidation. *Biochemistry*, **34**, 5762–5772.

Li, W., Zhao, Y., and Chou, I.N. (1993). Alterations in cytoskeletal protein sulfydryls and cellular glutathione in cultured cells exposed to cadmium and nickel ions. *Toxicology*, **77**, 65–79.

Li, W.C., Wang, G.M., Wang, R.R., and Spector, A. (1994). The redox active components H_2O_2 and N-acetyl-L-cysteine regulate expression of c-jun and c-fos in lens systems. *Experimental Eye Research*, **59**, 179–190.

Liang, J.N., and Rossi, M.T. (1990). *In vitro* non-enzymatic glycation and formation of browning products in the bovine lens alpha-crystallin. *Experimental Eye Research*, **50**, 367–371.

Liao, F., Andalibi, A., deBeer, F.C., Fogelman, A.M., and Lusis, A.J. (1993). Genetic control of inflammatory gene induction and NF-kappa B-like transcription factor activation in response to an atherogenic diet in mice. *Journal of Clinical Investigation*, **91**, 2572–2579.

Liao, J.C., Roider, J., and Jay, D.G. (1994). Chromophore-assisted laser inactivation of proteins is mediated by the photogeneration of free radicals. *Proceedings of the National Academy of Science of the United States of America*, **91**, 2659–2663.

Liao, L., Aw, T.Y., Kvietys, P.R., and Granger, D.N. (1995). Oxidized LDL-induced microvascular dysfunction. Dependence on oxidation procedure. *Arteriosclerosis Thrombosis and Vascular Biology*, **15**, 2305–2311.

Licht, S., Gerfen, G.J., and Stubbe, J. (1996). Thiyl radicals in ribonucleotide reductases. *Science*, **271**, 477–481.

Lii, C.K., Chai, Y.C., Zhao, W., Thomas, J.A., and Hendrich, S. (1994). S-thiolation and irreversible oxidation of sulfydryls on carbonic anhydrase III during oxidative stress: a method for studying protein modification in intact cells and tissues. *Archives of Biochemistry and Biophysics*, **308**, 231–239.

Lima, C.D., Wang, J.C., and Mondragon, A. (1993). Crystallization of a 67 kDa fragment of *Escherichia coli* DNA topoisomerase I. *Journal of Molecular Biology*, **232**, 1213–1216.

Lin, G., McKay, G., Hubbard, J.W., and Midha, K.K. (1994). Decomposition of clozapine N-oxide in the qualitative and quantitative analysis of clozapine and its metabolites. *Journal of Pharmaceutical Science*, **83**, 1412–1417.

Lindstedt, K.A., Kokkonen, J.O., and Kovanen, P.T. (1993). Inhibition of copper-mediated oxidation of LDL by rat serosal mast cells. A novel cellular protective mechanism involving proteolysis of the substrate under oxidative stress. *Arteriosclerosis and Thrombosis*, **13**, 23–32.

Lindvall, S., and Rydell, G. (1994). Influence of various compounds on the degradation of hyaluronic acid by a myeloperoxidase system. *Chemico-Biological Interactions*, **90**, 1–12.

Linetsky, M., and Ortwerth, B.J. (1996). Quantitation of the reactive oxygen species generated by the UVA irradiation of ascorbic acid-glycated lens proteins. *Photochemistry and Photobiology*, **63**, 649–655.

Ling, J., Sahlin, M., Sjoberg, B.M., Loehr, T.M., and Sanders, L.J. (1994). Dioxygen is the source of the mu-oxo bridge in iron ribonucleotide reductase. *Journal of Biological Chemistry*, **269**, 5595–5601.

Lion, Y., Denis, G., Mossoba, M.M., and Riesz, P. (1983). E.s.r. of spin-trapped radicals in gamma-irradiated polycrystalline DL-alanine. A quantitative determination of radical yield. *International Journal of Radiation Biology and Related Studies in Physics, Chemistry and Medicine*, **43**, 71–83.

Lion, Y.F., Kuwabara, M., and Riesz, P. (1980). UV photolysis of aqueous solutions of aliphatic peptides. An ESR and spin-trapping study. *Journal of Physical Chemistry*, **84**, 3378–3384.

Lipman, R.M., Tripathi, B.J., and Tripathi, R.C. (1988). Cataracts induced by microwave and ionizing radiation. *Surgical Ophthalmology*, **33**, 200–210.

Lipton, B.A., Parthasarathy, S., Ord, V.A., Clinton, S.K., Libby, P., and Rosenfeld, M.E. (1995). Components of the protein fraction of oxidized low density lipoprotein stimulate interleukin-1 alpha production by rabbit arterial macrophage-derived foam cells. *Journal of Lipid Research*, **36**, 2232–2242.

Lipton, S.H., Bodwell, C.E., and Coleman, A.J. (1977). Amino acid analyzer studies of the products of peroxide oxidation of cystine, lanthionine, and homocystine. *Journal of Agricultural and Food Chemistry*, **25**, 624–628.

Lissi, E.A., and Clavero, N. (1990). Inactivation of lysozyme by alkylperoxyl radicals. *Free Radical Research Communications*, **10**, 177–184.

Lissi, E.A., Salim, H.M., Faure, M., and Videla, L.A. (1991). 2,2'-Azo-bis-amidinopropane as a radical source for lipid peroxidation and enzyme inactivation studies. *Xenobiotica*, **21**, 995–1001.

Litov, R.E., Irving, D.H., Downey, J.E., and Tappel, A.L. (1978). Lipid peroxidation: a mechanism involved in acute ethanol toxicity as demonstrated by *in vivo* pentane production in the rat. *Lipids*, **13**, 305–307.

Litov, R.E., Gee, D.L., Downey, J.E., and Tappel, A.L. (1981a). The role of peroxidation during chronic and acute exposure to ethanol as determined by pentane expiration in the rat. *Lipids*, **16**, 52–63.

Litov, R.E., Matthews, L.C., and Tappel, A.L. (1981b). Vitamin E protection against *in vivo* lipid peroxidation initiated in rats by methyl ethyl ketone peroxide as monitored by pentane. *Toxicology and Applied Pharmacology*, **59**, 96–106.

Little, C., and O'Brien, P.J. (1967). Products of oxidation of a protein thiol group after reaction with various oxidizing agents. *Archives of Biochemistry and Biophysics*, **122**, 406–410.

Little, C., and O'Brien, P.J. (1968). The effectiveness of a lipid peroxide in oxidizing protein and non-protein thiols. *Biochemical Journal*, **106**, 419–423.

Liu, B., Hackshaw, K.V., and Whisler, R.L. (1996). Calcium signals and protein tyrosine kinases are required for the induction of c-jun in Jurkat cells stimulated by the T cell-receptor complex and oxidative signals. *Journal of Interferon and Cytokine Research*, **16**, 77–90.

Liu, H., Lightfoot, R., and Stevens, J.L. (1996). Activation of heat shock factor by alkylating agents is triggered by glutathione depletion and oxidation of protein thiols. *Journal of Biological Chemistry*, **271**, 4805–4812.

Liu, L., and Wells, P.G. (1994). *In vivo* phenytoin-initiated oxidative damage to proteins and lipids in murine maternal hepatic and embryonic tissue organelles: potential molecular targets of chemical teratogenesis. *Toxicology and Applied Pharmacology*, **125**, 247–255.

Liu, L., and Wells, P.G. (1995). Potential molecular targets mediating chemical teratogenesis: *in vitro* peroxidase-catalyzed phenytoin metabolism and oxidative damage to proteins and lipids in murine maternal hepatic microsomes and embryonic 9000 g supernatant. *Toxicology and Applied Pharmacology*, **134**, 71–80.

Liu, R.Q., Geren, L., Anderson, P., Fairris, J.L., Peffer, N., McKee, A., *et al.* (1995). Design of ruthenium-cytochrome *c* derivatives to measure electron transfer to cytochrome *c* peroxidase. *Biochimie*, **77**, 549–561.

Liu, X.D., and Thiele, D.J. (1996). Oxidative stress induced heat shock factor phosphorylation and HSF-dependent activation of yeast metallothionein gene transcription. *Genes and Development*, **10**, 592–603.

Liu, Y., Rosenthal, R.E., Starke, R.P., and Fiskum, G. (1993). Inhibition of postcardiac arrest brain protein oxidation by acetyl-L-carnitine. *Free Radical Biology and Medicine*, **15**, 667–670.

Livesey, G., and Elia, M. (1988). Estimation of energy expenditure, net carbohydrate utilization, and net fat oxidation and synthesis by indirect calorimetry: evaluation of errors with special reference to the detailed composition of fuels [published erratum appears in *American Journal of Clinical Nutrition* (1989), **50**, 1475]. *American Journal of Clinical Nutrition*, **47**, 608–628.

Livingstone, R., and Zeldes, H. (1966). Paramagnetic resonance study of liquids during photolysis. III. Aqueous solutions of alcohols with hydrogen peroxide. *Journal of the American Chemical Society*, **88**, 4333–4336.

Lizard, G., Deckert, V., Dubrez, L., Moisant, M., Gambert, P., and Lagrost, L. (1996). Induction of apoptosis in endothelial cells treated with cholesterol oxides. *American Journal of Pathology*, **148**, 1625–1638.

Lloyd, J.B., and Mason, R.W. (1996). Biology of the lysosome. *Subcellular Biochemistry*, Vol. 27 (ed. J.B. Lloyd and R.W. Mason), pp. 409. Plenum: New York.

Lode, H.N., Bruchelt, G., Rieth, A.G., and Niethammer, D. (1990). Release of iron from ferritin by 6-hydroxydopamine under aerobic and anaerobic conditions. *Free Radical Research Communications*, **11**, 153–158.

Loiseleur, J., Latarjet, R., and Crovisier, C. (1942). Formation of hydroperoxides in aqueous solutions of organic substances under the action of X-rays. *Compte Rendu Academy Science (Paris)*, **136**, 57–60.

Lou, M.F., Xu, G.T., and Cui, X.L. (1995). Further studies on the dynamic changes of glutathione and protein-thiol mixed disulfides in H_2O_2 induced cataract in rat lenses: distributions and effect of aging. *Current Eye Research*, **14**, 951–958.

Lougheed, M., Zhang, H.F., and Steinbrecher, U.P. (1991). Oxidized low density lipoprotein is resistant to cathepsins and accumulates within macrophages. *Journal of Biological Chemistry*, **266**, 14519–14525.

Loughran, M.G., Hall, J.M., Turner, A.P., and Davidson, V.L. (1995). Amperometric detection of histamine at a quinoprotein dehydrogenase enzyme electrode. *Biosensors and Bioelectronics*, **10**, 569–576.

Louie, S., Arata, M.A., Offerdahl, S.D., and Halliwell, B. (1993). Effect of tracheal insufflation of deferoxamine on acute ozone toxicity in rats. *Journal of Laboratory and Clinical Medicine*, **121**, 502–509.

Lovering, K.E., and Dean, R.T. (1991). Restriction of the participation of copper in radical-generating systems by zinc. *Free Radical Research Communications*, **14**, 217–225.

Lubec, B., Golej, J., Marx, M., Weninger, M., and Hoeger, H. (1995). L-arginine reduces kidney lipid peroxidation, glycoxidation and collagen accumulation in the aging NMRI mouse. *Renal Physiology and Biochemistry*, **18**, 97–102.

Lucesoli, F., and Fraga, C.G. (1995). Oxidative damage to lipids and DNA concurrent with decrease of antioxidants in rat testes after acute iron intoxication. *Archives of Biochemistry and Biophysics*, **316**, 567–571.

Lundqvist, H., Follin, P., Khalfan, L., and Dahlgren, C. (1996). Phorbol myristate acetate-induced NADPH oxidase activity in human neutrophils: only half the story has been told. *Journal of Leukocyte Biology*, **59**, 270–279.

Lung, C.C., Pinnas, J.L., Yahya, M.D., Meinke, G.C., and Mooradian, A.D. (1993). Malondialdehyde modified proteins and their antibodies in the plasma of control and streptozotocin induced diabetic rats [published erratum appears in *Life Science* (1993), **52**, 1327]. *Life Science*, **52**, 329–337.

Luttinger, A. (1995). The twisted 'life' of DNA in the cell: bacterial topoisomerases. *Molecular Microbiology*, **15**, 601–606.

Lymar, S.V., Jiang, Q., and Hurst, J.K. (1996). Mechanism of carbon dioxide-catalyzed oxidation of tyrosine by peroxynitrite. *Biochemistry*, **35**, 7855–7861.

Lynch, S.M., and Frei, B. (1993). Mechanisms of copper- and iron-dependent oxidative modification of human low density lipoprotein. *Journal of Lipid Research*, **34**, 1745–1753.

Lynch, S.M., and Frei, B. (1995). Reduction of copper, but not iron, by human low density lipoprotein (LDL). Implications for metal ion-dependent oxidative modification of LDL. *Journal of Biological Chemistry*, **270**, 5158–5163.

Lynn, K.R., and Purdie, J.W. (1976). Some pulse radiolysis studies of tyrosine and its glycyl peptides. *International Journal of Radiation and Physical Chemistry*, **8**, 685–689.

Lyons, T.J., Bailie, K.E., Dyer, D.G., Dunn, J.A., and Baynes, J.W. (1991). Decrease in skin collagen glycation with improved glycemic control in patients with insulin-dependent diabetes mellitus. *Journal of Clinical Investigation*, **87**, 1910–1915.

Lyras, L., Evans, P.J., Shaw, P.J., Ince, P.G., and Halliwell, B. (1996). Oxidative damage and motor neurone disease. Difficulties in the measurement of protein carbonyls in human brain tissue. *Free Radical Research*, **24**, 397–406.

Maccarrone, M., Veldink, G.A., and Vliegenthart, J.F. (1991). An investigation on the quinoprotein nature of some fungal and plant oxidoreductases. *Journal of Biological Chemistry*, **266**, 21014–21017.

Mackiewicz, P., and Furstoss, R. (1978). Radicaux amidyl: structure et reactivite. *Tetrahedron*, **34**, 3241–3260.

MacLean, S.J., and Huber, R.E. (1971). The effects of DL-*p*-fluorophenylalanine and L-3-nitrotyrosine on the growth and biochemistry of the Taper liver tumor. *Cancer Research*, **31**, 1669–1672.

Madabushi, H.T., De Mulder, C.L., and Tappel, A.L. (1996). Vitamin E protects chick tissues against *ex vivo* oxidation of heme protein. *Lipids*, **31**, 43–46.

Maeba, R., Shimasaki, H., and Ueta, N. (1994). Conformational changes in oxidized LDL recognized by mouse peritoneal macrophages. *Biochimica et Biophysica Acta*, **1215**, 79–86.

Magdalou, J., Kiffel, L., Balland, M., Thirion, C., Le Meste, M., and Siest, G. (1982). Conformational study of purified epoxide hydrolase from rat liver. *Chemico-Biological Interactions*, **39**, 245–256.

Maggi, E., Bellazzi, R., Gazo, A., Seccia, M., and Bellomo, G. (1994). Autoantibodies against oxidatively-modified LDL in uremic patients undergoing dialysis. *Kidney International*,, **46**, 869–876.

Magliozzo, R.S., McIntosh, B.A., and Sweeney, W.V. (1982). Origin of the pH dependence of the midpoint reduction potential in *Clostridium pasteurianum* ferredoxin: oxidation state-dependent hydrogen ion association. *Journal of Biological Chemistry*, **257**, 3506–3509.

Magner, E., and McLendon, G. (1989). Photochemical generation and reactions of heme cation radicals in heme proteins. *Biochemical and Biophysical Research Communications*, **159**, 472–476.

Maguire, J.J., Kellogg, E.D., and Packer, L. (1982). Protection against free radical formation by protein bound iron. *Toxicology Letters*, **14**, 27–34.

Mahadevan, S., Dillard, C.J., and Tappel, A.L. (1969). A modified colorimetric micro method for long-chain fatty acids and its application for assay of lipolytic enzymes. *Analytical Biochemistry*, **27**, 387–396.

Mahmoodi, H., Hadley, M., Chang, Y.X., and Draper, H.H. (1995). Increased formation and degradation of malondialdehyde-modified proteins under conditions of peroxidative stress. *Lipids*, **30**, 963–966.

Mahon, T.M., Brennan, P., and O'Neill, L.A. (1993). Evidence for a redox-sensitive protein tyrosine kinase in nuclear factor kappa B activation and interleukin 2 production in EL4.NOB1 cells. *Biochemical Society Transactions*, **21**, 389S.

Maiorino, M., Chu, F.F., Ursini, F., Davies, K.J., Doroshow, J.H., and Esworthy, R.S. (1991). Phospholipid hydroperoxide glutathione peroxidase is the 18-kDa selenoprotein expressed in human tumor cell lines. *Journal of Biological Chemistry*, **266**, 7728–7732.

Makada, H.A., and Garrison, W.M. (1972). Radiolytic oxidation of peptide derivatives of glycine in aqueous solution. *Radiation Research*, **50**, 48–55.

Makino, K. (1979). Studies on spin-trapped radicals in γ-irradiated aqueous solutions of DL-methionine by high performance liquid chromatography and ESR spectroscopy. *Journal of Physical Chemistry*, **83**, 2520–2523.

Makino, K. (1980a). Studies on spin-trapped radicals in γ-irradiated aqueous solutions of L-isoleucine and L-leucine by high-performance liquid chromatography and ESR spectroscopy. *Journal of Physical Chemistry*, **84**, 1968–1974.

Makino, K. (1980b). Studies on spin-trapped radicals in γ-irradiated aqueous L-valine solutions by high-performance liquid chromatogrpahy and ESR spectroscopy. *Journal of Physical Chemistry*, **84**, 1016–1019.

Makino, K., and Riesz, P. (1982). E.S.R. of spin-trapped radicals in gamma-irradiated polycrystalline amino acids. Chromatographic separation of radicals. *International Journal of Radiation Biology and Related Studies in Physics, Chemistry and Medicine*, **41**, 615–624.

Makino, S., and Nakashima, H. (1982). Behavior of fragmented band 3 from chymotrypsin-treated bovine erythrocyte membrane in nonionic detergent solution. *Journal of Biochemistry, Tokyo*, **92**, 1069–1077.

Malencik, D.A., and Anderson, S.R. (1996). Dityrosine formation in calmodulin: cross-linking and polymerization catalyzed by *Arthromyces peroxidase*. *Biochemistry*, **35**, 4375–4386.

Malle, E., Hazell, L., Stocker, R., Sattler, W., Esterbauer, H., and Waeg, G. (1995). Immunologic detection and measurement of hypochlorite-modified LDL with specific monoclonal antibodies. *Arteriosclerosis Thrombosis and Vascular Biology*, **15**, 982–989.

Mallery, S.R., Bailer, R.T., Hohl, C.M., Ng, B.C., Ness, G.M., Livingston, B.E., *et al.* (1995). Cultured AIDS-related Kaposi's sarcoma (AIDS-KS) cells demonstrate impaired bioenergetic adaptation to oxidant challenge: implication for oxidant stress in AIDS-KS pathogenesis. *Journal of Cellular Biochemistry*, **59**, 317–328.

Malone, J.I., Lowitt, S., and Cook, W.R. (1990). Nonosmotic diabetic cataracts. *Pediatric Research*, **27**, 293–296.

Malshet, V.G., Tappel, A.L., and Burns, V.M. (1974). Fluorescent products of lipid peroxidation. II. Methods for analysis and characterization. *Lipids*, **9**, 328–332.

Mandai, M., Mittag, T.W., Kogishi, J., Iwaki, M., Hangai, M., and Yoshimura, N. (1996). Role of nitric oxide synthase isozymes in endotoxin-induced uveitis. *Investigative Ophthalmology and Vision Science*, **37**, 826–832.

Mander, E.L., Dean, R.T., Stanley, K.K., and Jessup, W. (1994). Apolipoprotein B of oxidized LDL accumulates in the lysosomes of macrophages. *Biochimica et Biophysica Acta*, **1212**, 80–92.

Manelli, A.M., and Puttfarcken, P.S. (1995). Beta-amyloid-induced toxicity in rat hippocampal cells: *in vitro* evidence for the involvement of free radicals. *Brain Research Bulletin*, **38**, 569–576.

Mann, G.J., Graslund, A., Ochiai, E., Ingemarson, R., and Thelander, L. (1991). Purification and characterization of recombinant mouse and herpes simplex virus ribonucleotide reductase R2 subunit. *Biochemistry*, **30**, 1939–1947.

Manneberg, M., Lahm, H.W., and Fountoulakis, M. (1995). Quantification of cysteine residues following oxidation to cysteic acid in the presence of sodium azide. *Analytical Biochemistry*, **231**, 349–353.

Manning, M.C., Patel, K., and Borchardt, R.T. (1989). Stability of protein pharmaceuticals. *Pharmaceutical Research*, **6**, 903–918.

Mansoor, M.A., Svardal, A.M., and Ueland, P.M. (1992a). Determination of the *in vivo* redox status of cysteine, cysteinylglycine, homocysteine, and glutathione in human plasma. *Analytical Biochemistry*, **200**, 218–229.

Mansoor, M.A., Svardal, A.M., Schneede, J., and Ueland, P.M. (1992b). Dynamic relation between reduced, oxidized, and protein-bound homocysteine and other thiol components in plasma during methionine loading in healthy men. *Clinical Chemistry* , **38**, 1316–1321.

Mao, S.S., Yu, G.X., Chalfoun, D., and Stubbe, J. (1992a). Characterization of C439SR1, a mutant of *Escherichia coli* ribonucleotide diphosphate reductase: evidence that C439 is a residue essential for nucleotide reduction and C439SR1 is a protein possessing novel thioredoxin-like activity. *Biochemistry*, **31**, 9752–9759.

Mao, S.S., Holler, T.P., Bollinger, J.J., Yu, G.X., Johnston, M.I., and Stubbe, J. (1992b). Interaction of C225SR1 mutant subunit of ribonucleotide reductase with R2 and nucleoside diphosphates: tales of a suicidal enzyme. *Biochemistry*, **31**, 9744–9751.

Maples, K.R., Jordan, S.J., and Mason, R.P. (1988a). *In vivo* rat hemoglobin thiyl free radical formation following phenylhydrazine administration. *Molecular Pharmacology*, **33**, 344–350.

Maples, K.R., Jordan, S.J., and Mason, R.P. (1988b). *In vivo* rat hemoglobin thiyl free radical formation following administration of phenylhydrazine and hydrazine-based drugs. *Drug Metabolism and Disposition*, **16**, 799–803.

Maples, K.R., Eyer, P., and Mason, R.P. (1990a). Aniline-, phenylhydroxylamine-, nitrosobenzene-, and nitrobenzene-induced hemoglobin thiyl free radical formation *in vivo* and *in vitro*. *Molecular Pharmacology*, **37**, 311–318.

Maples, K.R., Kennedy, C.H., Jordan, S.J., and Mason, R.P. (1990b). *In vivo* thiyl free radical formation from hemoglobin following administration of hydroperoxides. *Archives of Biochemistry and Biophysics*, **277**, 402–409.

Marcillat, O., Zhang, Y., Lin, S.W., and Davies, K.J. (1988). Mitochondria contain a proteolytic system which can recognize and degrade oxidatively-denatured proteins. *Biochemical Journal*, **254**, 677–683.

Marcillat, O., Zhang, Y., and Davies, K.J. (1989). Oxidative and non-oxidative mechanisms in the inactivation of cardiac mitochondrial electron transport chain components by doxorubicin. *Biochemical Journal*, **259**, 181–189.

Marcolongo, R., Calabria, A.A., Lalumera, M., Gerli, R., Alessandrini, C., and Cavallo, G. (1988). The 'switch-off' mechanism of spontaneous resolution of acute gout attack. *Journal of Rheumatology*, **15**, 101–109.

Marcus, R.A. (1956). On the theory of oxidation-reduction reactions involving electron transfer. I. *Journal of Chemical Physics*, **24**, 966–978.

Marcus, R.A., and Sutin, N. (1985). Electron transfers in chemistry and biology. *Biochimica et Biophysica Acta*, **811**, 265–322.

Maret, W. (1994). Oxidative metal release from metallothionein via zinc-thiol/ disulfide interchange. *Proceedings of the National Academy of Science of the United States of America*, **91**, 237–241.

Margolis, S.A., Coxon, B., Gajewski, E., and Dizdaroglu, M. (1988). Structure of a hydroxyl radical induced cross-link of thymine and tyrosine. *Biochemistry*, **27**, 6353–6359.

Maria, C.S., Revilla, E., Ayala, A., de la Cruz, C.P., and Machado, A. (1995). Changes in the histidine residues of Cu/Zn superoxide dismutase during aging. *FEBS Letters*, **374**, 85–88.

Mark, R.J., Hensley, K., Butterfield, D.A., and Mattson, M.P. (1995). Amyloid beta-peptide impairs ion-motive ATPase activities: evidence for a role in loss of neuronal Ca^{2+} homeostasis and cell death. *Journal of Neuroscience*, **15**, 6239–6249.

Markley, J.L., Ulrich, E.L., Berg, S.P., and Krogmann, D.W. (1975). Nuclear magnetic resonance studies of the copper binding sites of blue copper proteins: oxidized, reduced, and apoplastocyanin. *Biochemistry*, **14**, 4428–4433.

Marquez, L.A., and Dunford, H.B. (1994). Chlorination of taurine by myeloperoxidase. Kinetic evidence for an enzyme-bound intermediate. *Journal of Biological Chemistry*, **269**, 7950–7956.

Marquez, L.A., and Dunford, H.B. (1995). Kinetics of oxidation of tyrosine and dityrosine by myeloperoxidase compounds I and II. Implications for lipoprotein peroxidation studies. *Journal of Biological Chemistry*, **270**, 30434–30440.

Marsh, E.N. (1995a). A radical approach to enzyme catalysis. *Bioessays*, **17**, 431–441.

Marsh, E.N. (1995b). Tritium isotope effects in adenosylcobalamin-dependent glutamate mutase: implications for the mechanism. *Biochemistry*, **34**, 7542–7547.

Martin, D., Tayyeb, M.I., and Swartzwelder, H.S. (1995). Ethanol inhibition of AMPA and kainate receptor-mediated depolarizations of hippocampal area CA1. *Alcohol Clinical Experimental Research*, **19**, 1312–1316.

Marui, N., Offermann, M.K., Swerlick, R., Kunsch, C., Rosen, C.A., Ahmad, M., *et al.* (1993). Vascular cell adhesion molecule-1 (VCAM-1) gene transcription and expression are regulated through an antioxidant-sensitive mechanism in human vascular endothelial cells. *Journal of Clinical Investigation*, **92**, 1866–1874.

Maruthamuthu, P., and Neta, P. (1977). Reactions of phosphate radicals with organic compounds. *Journal of Physical Chemistry*, **81**, 1622–1625.

Maruthamuthu, P., and Neta, P. (1978). Phosphate radicals. Spectra, acid-base equilibria, and reactions with inorganic compounds. *Journal of Physical Chemistry*, **82**, 710–713.

Marx, G. (1991). Immunological monitoring of Fenton fragmentation of fibrinogen. *Free Radical Research Communications*, **2**, 517–520.

Marx, G., and Chevion, M. (1985). Fibrinogen coagulation without thrombin: reaction with vitamin C and copper(II). *Thrombosis Research*, **40**, 11–18.

Marx, G., and Chevion, M. (1986). Site-specific modification of albumin by free radicals. Reaction with copper(II) and ascorbate. *Biochemical Journal*, **236**, 397–400.

Marzabadi, M.R., Sohal, R.S., and Brunk, U.T. (1988). Effect of ferric iron and desferrioxamine on lipofuscin accumulation in cultured rat heart myocytes. *Mechanisms of Ageing Development*, **46**, 145–157.

Marzabadi, M.R., Sohal, R.S., and Brunk, U.T. (1990). Effect of alpha-tocopherol and some metal chelators on lipofuscin accumulation in cultured neonatal rat cardiac myocytes. *Analytical Cell Pathology*, **2**, 333–346.

Marzabadi, M.R., Sohal, R.S., and Brunk, U.T. (1991). Mechanisms of lipofuscinogenesis: effect of the inhibition of lysosomal proteinases and lipases under varying concentrations of ambient oxygen in cultured rat neonatal myocardial cells. *Apmis*, **99**, 416–426.

Maskos, Z., Rush, J.D., Koppenol, W.H. (1992). The hydroxylation of phenylalanine and tyrosine: a comparison with salicylate and tryptophan. *Archives of Biochemistry and Biophysics*, **262**, 521–529.

Mason, R.P. (1982). Free-radical intermediates in the metabolism of toxic chemicals. In *Free Radicals in Biology*, (ed. W.A. Pryor), pp. 161–222. Academic Press, New York.

Mason, V.C., Rudemo, M., and Bech, A.S. (1980). Hydrolysate preparation for amino acid determinations in feed constituents. 6. The influence of phenol and formic acid on the recovery of amino acids from oxidized feed proteins. *Z Tierphysiol Tierernahr Futtermittelkd*, **43**, 35–48.

Masuda, Y., and Murano, T. (1979). Effect of linoleic acid hydroperoxide on liver microsomal enzymes *in vitro*. *Japanese Journal of Pharmacology*, **29**, 179–186.

Masuda, Y., Park, S.M., Ohta, A., and Takagi, M. (1995). Cloning and characterization of the POX2 gene in *Candida maltosa*. *Gene*, **167**, 157–161.

Matheson, N.R., and Travis, J. (1985). Differential effects of oxidizing agents on human plasma alpha 1-proteinase inhibitor and human neutrophil myeloperoxidase. *Biochemistry*, **24**, 1941–1945.

Mathews, F.S. (1995). X-ray studies of quinoproteins. *Methods in Enzymology*, **258**, 191–216.

Matsuda, T., Nakashima, I., Kato, Y., and Nakamura, R. (1987). Antibody response to haptenic sugar antigen: immunodominancy of protein-bound lactose formed by amino-carbonyl reaction. *Molecular Immunology*, **24**, 421–425.

Matsueda, R., Maruyama, H., Kitazawa, E., Takagi, H., and Mukaiyama, T. (1975). Letter: Solid phase peptide synthesis by oxidation-reduction condensation. *Journal of the American Chemical Society*, **97**, 2573–2575.

Matsugo, S., Yan, L.J., Han, D., and Packer, L. (1995). Induction of protein oxidation in human low density lipoprotein by the photosensitive organic hydroperoxide, N,N'-bis(2-hydroxyperoxy-2-methoxyethyl)-1,4,5,8-naphthalene-tetra-carb oxylic-diimide. *Biochemical and Biophysical Research Communications*, **206**, 138–145.

Matsui, M.S., Mintz, E., and DeLeo, V.A. (1995). Effect of benzoyl peroxide on protein kinase C in cultured human epidermal keratinocytes. *Skin Pharmacology*, **8**, 130–138.

Matsumoto, T., Takahashi, K., Nagafuji, T., Kubo, S., and Kumazawa, J. (1995). Effect of inhibitors of protein kinase C on enhanced superoxide production of human leucocytes by ofloxacin and fleroxacin. *Drugs*, **2**, 286–288.

Matsushima, A., Yamazaki, S., Shibata, K., and Inada, Y. (1972). The reactivity of amino groups in proteins and peptides to *tert*-butyl hypochlorite. *Biochimica et Biophysica Acta*, **271**, 243–251.

Matsushima, A., Yamazaki, S., and Inada, Y. (1974). Reactivity of peptide imino groups in proteins with *tert*-butyl hypochlorite in relation to secondary structure. *Journal of Biochemistry, Tokyo*, **75**, 875–879.

Matsushita, K., Shinagawa, E., Adachi, O., and Ameyama, M. (1989). Reactivity with ubiquinone of quinoprotein D-glucose dehydrogenase from *Gluconobacter suboxydans*. *Journal of Biochemistry, Tokyo*, **105**, 633–637.

Matsuzaki, R., Fukui, T., Sato, H., Ozaki, Y., and Tanizawa, K. (1994). Generation of the topa quinone cofactor in bacterial monoamine oxidase by cupric ion-dependent autooxidation of a specific tyrosyl residue. *FEBS Letters*, **351**, 360–364.

Matsuzaki, R., Suzuki, S., Yamaguchi, K., Fukui, T., and Tanizawa, K. (1995). Spectroscopic studies on the mechanism of the topa quinone generation in bacterial monoamine oxidase. *Biochemistry*, **34**, 4524–4530.

Matthews, J.R., Wakasugi, N., Virelizier, J.L., Yodoi, J., and Hay, R.T. (1992). Thioredoxin regulates the DNA binding activity of NF-kappa B by reduction of a disulphide bond involving cysteine 62. *Nucleic Acids Research*, **20**, 3821–3830.

Matthews, J.R., Kaszubska, W., Turcatti, G., Wells, T.N., and Hay, R.T. (1993). Role of cysteine 62 in DNA recognition by the P50 subunit of NF-kappa B. *Nucleic Acids Research*, **21**, 1727–1734.

Matthews, W., Driscoll, J., Tanaka, K., Ichihara, A., and Goldberg, A.L. (1989). Involvement of the proteasome in various degradative processes in mammalian cells [published erratum appears in *Proceedings of the National Academy of Science of the United States of America* (1989), **86**, 5350]. *Proceedings of the National Academy of Science of the United States of America*, **86**, 2597–2601.

Mattson, M.P. (1994). Calcium and neuronal injury in Alzheimer's disease. Contributions of beta-amyloid precursor protein mismetabolism, free radicals, and metabolic compromise. *Annals of the New York Academy of Science*, **747**, 50–76.

Mattson, M.P. (1995). Degenerative and protective signaling mechanisms in the neurofibrillary pathology of AD. *Neurobiology and Aging*, **16**, 447–457.

Mattson, M.P., Carney, J.W., and Butterfield, D.A. (1995). A tombstone in Alzheimer's? *Nature*, **373**, 481.

Matuk, Y., Lou, P., and Parker, J.A. (1977). Biosynthesis of proteins by the retina. Inactivation by near-ultraviolet light and the effects of tryptophan, epinephrine, and catalase. *Investigations in Ophthalmology and Vision Science*, **16**, 1104–1109.

Maubert, A., Jalonstre, L., Lemau, P., and Guilbert, C. (1924). Action of X-rays on the catalase of the liver. *Comptes Rendu*, **178**, 889–891.

Maupin, F.J., and Ferry, J.G. (1996). Characterization of the cdhD and cdhE genes encoding subunits of the corrinoid/iron-sulfur enzyme of the CO dehydrogenase complex from *Methanosarcina thermophila*. *Journal of Bacteriology*, **178**, 340–346.

Maxwell, C.R., Peterson, D.D., and Shrpless, N.E. (1954). The effect of ionizing radiation on amino acids. I. The effect of X-rays on aqueous solution. *Radiation Research*, **1**, 530–545.

Maxwell, C.R., Peterson, D.C., and White, C. (1955). Effect of ionising radiation on amino acids. III. Effect of electron irradiation on aqueous solutions of glycine. *Radiation Research*, **2**, 431–438.

Maxwell, M.P., Hearse, D.J., and Yellon, D.M. (1989). Inability of desferrioxamine to limit tissue injury in the ischaemic and reperfused rabbit heart. *Journal of Cardiovascular Pharmacology*, **13**, 608–615.

Mazumder, S., Nath, I., and Dhar, M.M. (1993). Immunomodulation of human T cell responses with receptor selective enkephalins. *Immunology Letters*, **35**, 33–38.

McAndrew, S.J., Chen, N.Y., Kelder, B., Cioffi, J.A., and Kopchick, J.J. (1991). Effects of a leucine analog on growth hormone processing and secretion by cultured cells. *Journal of Biological Chemistry*, **266**, 15016–15020.

McArdle, F.J., and Desrosier, N.W. (1955). Influences of ionising radiation on the protein components of selected foods. *Food Technology*, **9**, 527–532.

McArthur, K.M., and Davies, M.J. (1993). Detection and reactions of the globin radical in haemoglobin. *Biochimica et Biophysica Acta*, **1202**, 173–181.

McBrien, K.D., Berry, R.L., Lowe, S.E., Neddermann, K.M., Bursuker, I., Huang, S., et al. (1995). Rakicidins, new cytotoxic lipopeptides from *Micromonospora* sp. fermentation, isolation and characterization. *Journal of Antibiotics, Tokyo*, **48**, 1446–1452.

McCance, D.R., Dyer, D.G., Dunn, J.A., Bailie, K.E., Thorpe, S.R., Baynes, J.W., et al. (1993). Maillard reaction products and their relation to complications in insulin-dependent diabetes mellitus. *Journal of Clinical Investigation*, **91**, 2470–2478.

McClarty, G.A., Chan, A.K., Engstrom, Y., Wright, J.A., and Thelander, L. (1987). Elevated expression of M1 and M2 components and drug-induced posttranscriptional modulation of ribonucleotide reductase in a hydroxyurea-resistant mouse cell line. *Biochemistry*, **26**, 8004–8011.

McClarty, G.A., Chan, A.K., Choy, B.K., Thelander, L., and Wright, J.A. (1988). Molecular mechanisms responsible for the drug-induced posttranscriptional modulation of ribonucleotide reductase levels in a hydroxyurea-resistant mouse L cell line. *Biochemistry*, **27**, 7524–7531.

McDonald, M.R. (1954). The effects of X-rays on dilute solutions of crystalline trypsin by X-radiation: continued inactivation after termination of irradiation. *British Journal of Radiology*, **27**, 62–63.

McGowan, J.I., and Josephy, P.D. (1990). Hydroperoxidase I catalyzes peroxidative activation of 3,3'-dichlorobenzidine to a mutagen in *Salmonella typhimurium*. *Archives of Biochemistry and Biophysics*, **282**, 352–357.

McGowan, S.E., and Murray, J.J. (1987). Direct effects of neutrophil oxidants on elastase-induced extracellular matrix proteolysis. *American Review of Respiratory Diseases*, **135**, 1286–1293.

McGuirl, M.A., McCahon, C.D., McKeown, K.A., and Dooley, D.M. (1994). Purification and characterization of pea seedling amine oxidase for crystallization studies. *Plant Physiology*, **106**, 1205–1211.

McIntire, W.S. (1994). Quinoproteins. *FASEB Journal*, **8**, 513–521.

McIntire, W.S., Bates, J.L., Brown, D.E., and Dooley, D.M. (1991). Resonance Raman spectroscopy of methylamine dehydrogenase from bacterium W3A1. *Biochemistry*, **30**, 125–133.

McKenna, S.M., and Davies, K.J. (1988a). Bacterial killing by phagocytes: potential role(s) of hypochlorous acid and hydrogen peroxide in protein turnover, DNA synthesis, and RNA synthesis. *Basic Life Science*, **49**, 829–832.

McKenna, S.M., and Davies, K.J. (1988b). The inhibition of bacterial growth by hypochlorous acid. Possible role in the bactericidal activity of phagocytes. *Biochemical Journal*, **254**, 685–692.

McLane, K.E., Wu, X.D., Diethelm, B., and Conti, T.B. (1991). Structural determinants of alpha-bungarotoxin binding to the sequence segment 181-200 of the muscle nicotinic acetylcholine receptor alpha subunit: effects of cysteine/cystine modification and species-specific amino acid substitutions. *Biochemistry*, **30**, 4925–4934.

McNamara, M., and Augusteyn, R.C. (1984). The effects of hydrogen peroxide on lens proteins: a possible model for nuclear cataract. *Experimental Eye Research*, **38**, 45–56.

Mecham, R.P., Broekelmann, T., Davis, E.C., Gibson, M.A., and Brown, A.P. (1995). Elastic fibre assembly: macromolecular interactions. *Ciba Foundation Symposium*, **192**, 172–181.

Medvedev, A., Kirkel, A., Kamyshanskaya, N., and Gorkin, V. (1993). Lipid peroxidation affects catalytic properties of rat liver mitochondrial monoamine oxidases and their sensitivity to proteolysis. *International Journal of Biochemistry*, **25**, 1791–1799.

Mee, L.K., and Adelstein, S.J. (1981). Predominance of core histones in formation of DNA-protein crosslinks in gamma-irradiated chromatin. *Proceedings of the National Academy of Science of the United States of America*, **78**, 2194–2198.

Mee, L.K., and Adelstein, S.J. (1987). Radiation damage to histone H2A by the primary aqueous radicals. *Radiation Research*, **110**, 155–160.

Mee, L.K., and Stein, G. (1956). The reduction of cytochrome c by free radicals in irradiated solutions. *Biochemical Journal*, **62**, 377–380.

Mehlhorn, R.J., and Gomez, J. (1993). Hydroxyl and alkoxyl radical production by oxidation products of metmyoglobin. *Free Radical Research Communications*, **18**, 29–41.

Mehlhorn, R.J., and Swanson, C.E. (1992). Nitroxide-stimulated H_2O_2 decomposition by peroxidases and pseudoperoxidases. *Free Radical Research Communications*, **17**, 157–175.

Mehta, R.A., Fawcett, T.W., Porath, D., and Mattoo, A.K. (1992). Oxidative stress causes rapid membrane translocation and *in vivo* degradation of ribulose-1, 5-bisphosphate carboxylase/oxygenase. *Journal of Biological Chemistry*, **267**, 2810–2816.

Mehvar, R., Jamali, F., Watson, M.W., and Skelton, D. (1986). Direct injection high-performance liquid chromatography of tetrabenazine and its metabolite in plasma of humans and rats. *Journal of Pharmacological Science*, **75**, 1006–1009.

Mekhfi, H., Veksler, V., Mateo, P., Maupoil, V., Rochette, L., and Ventura, C.R. (1996). Creatine kinase is the main target of reactive oxygen species in cardiac myofibrils. *Circulation Research*, **78**, 1016–1027.

Mellors, A., and Tappel, A.L. (1966). The inhibition of mitochondrial peroxidation by ubiquinone and ubiquinol. *Journal of Biological Chemistry*, **241**, 4353–4356.

Melo, T.B. (1973). Radiation damage to proteins—an e.s.r. study of a single crystal of glycyl-glycine at low temperatures. *International Journal of Radiation Biology and Related Studies in Physics, Chemistry and Medicine*, **23**, 247–261.

Menendez, M.C., Domenech, P., Prieto, J., and Garcia, M.J. (1995). Cloning and expression of the *Mycobacterium fortuitum* superoxide dismutase gene. *FEMS Microbiology Letters*, **134**, 273–278.

Menon, S.D., Qin, S., Guy, G.R., and Tan, Y.H. (1993). Differential induction of nuclear NF-kappa B by protein phosphatase inhibitors in primary and transformed human cells. Requirement for both oxidation and phosphorylation in nuclear translocation. *Journal of Biological Chemistry*, **268**, 26805–26812.

Messmer, U.K., and Brune, B. (1996). Nitric oxide (NO) in apoptotic versus necrotic RAW 264.7 macrophage cell death: the role of NO-donor exposure, NAD^+ content, and p53 accumulation. *Archives of Biochemistry and Biophysics*, **327**, 1–10.

Messmer, U.K., Ankarcrona, M., Nicotera, P., and Brune, B. (1994). p53 expression in nitric oxide-induced apoptosis. *FEBS Letters*, **355**, 23–26.

Messmer, U.K., Lapetina, E.G., and Brune, B. (1995). Nitric oxide-induced apoptosis in RAW 264.7 macrophages is antagonized by protein kinase C- and protein kinase A-activating compounds. *Molecular Pharmacology*, **47**, 757–765.

Messmer, U.K., Reimer, D.M., Reed, J.C., and Brune, B. (1996). Nitric oxide induced poly(ADP-ribose) polymerase cleavage in RAW 264.7 macrophage apoptosis is blocked by Bcl-2. *FEBS Letters*, **384**, 162–166.

Meucci, E., Mordente, E., and Martorana, G.E. (1991). Metal-catalysed oxidation of human serum albumin: conformational and functional changes. *Journal of Biological Chemistry*, **266**, 4692–4699.

Meybeck, A., and Meybeck, J. (1967). Photo-oxidation of the peptide group. II. Solid state peptides and polyaminoacids. *Photochemistry and Photobiology*, **6**, 365–378.

Meyer, B.U., Schneider, W., and Elstner, E.F. (1992). Peroxide-dependent amino acid oxidation and chemiluminescence catalysed by magnesium-pyridoxal phosphate-glutamate complex. *Biochemical Pharmacology*, **44**, 505–508.

Meyer, M., Pahl, H.L., and Baeuerle, P.A. (1994). Regulation of the transcription factors NF-kappa B and AP-1 by redox changes. *Chemico-Biological Interactions*, **91**, 91–100.

Michaud, S.I., Daniel, R., Chopard, C., Mansuy, D., Cucurou, C., Ullrich, V., *et al.* (1990). Soybean lipoxygenases-1, -2a, -2b and -2c do not contain PQQ. *Biochemical and Biophysical Research Communications*, **172**, 1122–1128.

Michejda, C.J., Campbell, D.H., Sieh, D.H., and Koepke, S.R. (1978). The chemistry of some nitrogen-centered radicals. In *Organic Free Radicals*, (ed. W.A. Pryor), pp. 292–308. American Chemical Society, Washington.

Mickel, H.S., Oliver, C.N., and Starke, R.P. (1990). Protein oxidation and myelinolysis occur in brain following rapid correction of hyponatremia. *Biochemical and Biophysical Research Communications*, **172**, 92–97.

Middendorff, R., Davidoff, M.S., Mayer, B., and Holstein, A.F. (1995). Neuroendocrine characteristics of human Leydig cell tumours. *Andrologia*, **27**, 351–355.

Mieden, O.J., and von Sonntag, C. (1989). Peptide free-radicals: The reactions of OH radicals with glycine anhydride and its methyl derivatives sarconine and alanine anhydride. A pulse radiolysis and product study. *Zeitschrift feur Naturforschung*, **44b**, 959–974.

Mieden, O.J., Schuchmann, M.N., and von Sonntag, C. (1993). Peptide peroxyl radicals: Base-induced $O_2^{\cdot-}$ elimination versus bimolecular decay. A pulse radiolysis and product study. *Journal of Physical Chemistry*, **97**, 3783–3790.

Miglietta, A., Bonelli, G., and Gabriel, L. (1984). Effect of lipid peroxidation on microtubular protein. *Research Communications in Chemical Pathology and Pharmacology*, **44**, 331–334.

Miki, H., Harada, K., and Yamazaki, I. (1988). Light- or oxidant-induced generation of free radicals in hemoproteins. *Radiation Physics and Chemistry*, **32**, 375–378.

Miki, M., Tamai, H., Mino, M., Yamamoto, Y., and Niki, E. (1987). Free-radical chain oxidation of rat red blood cells by molecular oxygen and its inhibition by alpha-tocopherol. *Archives of Biochemistry and Biophysics*, **258**, 373–380.

Miklavc, A. (1996). Temperature-nearly-independent binding constant in several biochemical systems. The underlying entropy-driven binding mechanism and its practical significance. *Biochemical Pharmacology*, **51**, 723–729.

Milagres, L.G., Lemos, A.P., Meles, C.E., Silva, E.L., Ferreira, L.H., Souza, J.A., *et al.* (1995). Antibody response after immunization of Brazilian children with serogroup C meningococcal polysaccharide noncovalently complexed with outer membrane proteins. *Brazilian Journal of Medical and Biological Research*, **28**, 981–989.

Miller, B.T. (1996). Acylation of peptide hydroxyl groups with the Bolton-Hunter reagent. *Biochemical and Biophysical Research Communications*, **218**, 377–382.

Miller, M.A., Vitello, L., and Erman, J.E. (1995). Regulation of interprotein electron transfer by Trp 191 of cytochrome *c* peroxidase. *Biochemistry*, **34**, 12048–12058.

Miller, M.J., Thompson, J.H., Zhang, X.J., Sadowska, K.H., Kakkis, J.L., Munshi, U.K., *et al.* (1995). Role of inducible nitric oxide synthase expression and peroxynitrite formation in guinea pig ileitis. *Gastroenterology*, **109**, 1475–1483.

Miller, N.J., Rice-Evans,C., and Davies, M.J. (1993a). A new method for measuring antioxidant activity. *Biochemical Society Transactions*, **21**, 95S.

Miller, N.J., Rice-Evans, C., Davies, M.J., Gopinathan, V., and Milner, A. (1993b). A novel method for measuring antioxidant capacity and its application to monitoring the antioxidant status in premature neonates. *Clinical Science*, **84**, 407–412.

Miller, R.W., Smith, B.E., and Eady, R.R. (1993). Energy transduction by nitrogenase: binding of MgADP to the MoFe protein is dependent on the oxidation state of the iron-sulphur 'P' clusters. *Biochemical Journal*, **291**, 709–711.

Miller, Y.I., Felikman, Y., and Shaklai, N. (1996). Hemoglobin induced apolipoprotein B crosslinking in low-density lipoprotein peroxidation. *Archives of Biochemistry and Biophysics*, **326**, 252–260.

Miller, V.P., Goodin, D.B., Friedman, A.E., Hartmann, C., and Ortiz, d.M.P. (1995). Horseradish peroxidase Phe172 ⟶ Tyr mutant. Sequential formation of compound I with a porphyrin radical cation and a protein radical. *Journal of Biological Chemistry*, **270**, 18413–18419.

Milne, D.M., Campbell, L.E., Campbell, D.G., and Meek, D.W. (1995). p53 is phosphorylated *in vitro* and *in vivo* by an ultraviolet radiation-induced protein kinase characteristic of the c-Jun kinase, JNK1. *Journal of Biological Chemistry*, **270**, 5511–5518.

Milne, D.B., and Nielsen, F.H. (1996). Effects of a diet low in copper on copper-status indicators in postmenopausal women. *American Journal of Clinical Nutrition*, **63**, 358–364.

Milne, H.B., and Carpenter, F.H. (1968). Peptide synthesis via oxidation of N-acyl-alpha-amino acid phenylhydrazides. III. Dialanyl-insulin and diphenylalanyl-insulin. *Journal of Organic Chemistry*, **33**, 4476–4479.

Milne, H.B., and Most, C.J. (1968). Peptide synthesis via oxidation of N-acyl-alpha-amino acid phenylhydrazides. II. Benzyloxycarbonyl peptide phenylhydrazides. *Journal of Organic Chemistry*, **33**, 169–175.

Milton, R.C., Mayer, E., Walsh, J.H., Rivier, J.E., Dykert, J., Lee, T.D., *et al.* (1988). Solid phase synthesis and characterization of two canine gut gastrin-releasing peptides. *International Journal of Peptide and Protein Research*, **32**, 141–152.

Minamide, Y., Horie, T., and Awazu, S. (1992). Fluorospectroscopic analysis of the fluorescent substances in peroxidized microsomes of rat liver. *Lipids*, **27**, 354–359.

Minegishi, A., Bergene, R., and Riesz, P. (1980). E.s.r. of spin-trapped radicals in aqueous solutions of deuterated amino acids and alcohols. *International Journal of Radiation Biology and Related Studies in Physics, Chemistry and Medicine*, **38**, 395–415.

Minetti, G., Balduini, C., and Brovelli, A. (1994). Reduction of DABS-L-methionine-DL-sulfoxide by protein methionine sulfoxide reductase from polymorphonuclear leukocytes: stereospecificity towards the L-sulfoxide. *Italian Journal of Biochemistry*, **43**, 273–283.

Miquel, J., Tappel, A.L., Dillard, C.J., Herman, M.M., and Bensch, K.G. (1974). Fluorescent products and lysosomal components in aging *Drosophila melanogaster*. *Journal of Gerontology*, **29**, 622–637.

Mirza, U.A., Chait, B.T., and Lander, H.M. (1995). Monitoring reactions of nitric oxide with peptides and proteins by electrospray ionization-mass spectrometry. *Journal of Biological Chemistry*, **270**, 17185–17188.

Mishra, O.P., Delivoria, P.M., Cahillane, G., and Wagerle, L.C. (1990). Lipid peroxidation as the mechanism of modification of brain 5'-nucleotidase activity *in vitro*. *Neurochemistry Research*, **15**, 237–242.

Misra, M., Olinski, R., Dizdaroglu, M., and Kasprzak, K.S. (1993). Enhancement by L-histidine of nickel(II)-induced DNA-protein cross-linking and oxidative DNA base damage in the rat kidney. *Chemical Research in Toxicology*, **6**, 33–37.

Mistry, R., Snashall, P.D., Totty, N., Guz, A., and Tetley, T.D. (1991). Isolation and characterization of sheep alpha 1-proteinase inhibitor. *Biochemical Journal*, **273**, 685–690.

Mitomo, K., Nakayama, K., Fujimoto, K., Sun, X., Seki, S., and Yamamoto, K. (1994). Two different cellular redox systems regulate the DNA-binding activity of the p50 subunit of NF-kappa B *in vitro*. *Gene*, **145**, 197–203.

Mittal, J.P., and Hayon, E. (1974). Interaction of hydrated electrons with phenylalanine and related compounds. *Journal of Physical Chemistry*, **78**, 1790–1794.

Miura, S., and Ichikawa, Y. (1991). Conformational change of adrenodoxin induced by reduction of iron-sulfur cluster. Proton nuclear magnetic resonance study. *Journal of Biological Chemistry*, **266**, 6252–6258.

Miura, T., Muraoka, S., and Ogiso, T. (1993). Inhibition of hydroxyl radical-induced protein damages by trolox. *Biochemistry and Molecular Biology International*, **31**, 125–133.

Miyamae, T., Yue, J.L., Okumura, Y., Goshima, Y., and Misu, Y. (1995). Loss of tonic neuronal activity to release L-DOPA in the caudal ventrolateral medulla of spontaneously hypertensive rats. *Neuroscience Letters*, **198**, 37–40.

Mizutani, T., Nakahori, Y., and Yamamoto, K. (1994). *p*-Dichlorobenzene-induced hepatotoxicity in mice depleted of glutathione by treatment with buthionine sulfoximine. *Toxicology*, **94**, 57–67.

Mo, J.Q., Hom, D.G., and Andersen, J.K. (1995). Decreases in protective enzymes correlates with increased oxidative damage in the aging mouse brain. *Mechanisms in Ageing Development*, **81**, 73–82.

Moan, J., and Kaalhaus, O. (1974). Ultraviolet- and X-ray-induced radicals in frozen polar solutions of L-tryptophan. *Journal of Chemical Physics*, **61**, 3556–3566.

Moenne, L.P., Nakamura, N., Steinebach, V., Duine, J.A., Mure, M., Klinman, J.P., *et al.* (1995). Characterization of the topa quinone cofactor in amine oxidase from *Escherichia coli* by resonance Raman spectroscopy. *Biochemistry*, **34**, 7020–7026.

Mohr, D., and Stocker, R. (1994). Radical-mediated oxidation of isolated human very-low-density lipoprotein. *Arteriosclerosis and Thrombosis*, **14**, 1186–1192.

Mohr, D., Bowry, V.W., and Stocker, R. (1992). Dietary supplementation with coenzyme Q10 results in increased levels of ubiquinol-10 within circulating lipoproteins and increased resistance of human low-density lipoprotein to the initiation of lipid peroxidation. *Biochimica et Biophysica Acta*, **1126**, 247–254.

Mohsenin, V., and Gee, J.L. (1989). Oxidation of alpha 1-protease inhibitor: role of lipid peroxidation products. *Journal of Applied Physiology*, **66**, 2211–2215.

Molitor, J.A., Ballard, D.W., and Greene, W.C. (1991). Kappa B-specific DNA binding proteins are differentially inhibited by enhancer mutations and biological oxidation. *New Biology*, **3**, 987–996.

Molyneux, M.J., and Davies, M.J. (1995). Direct evidence for hydroxyl radical-induced damage to nucleic acids by chromium(VI)-derived species: implications for chromium carcinogenesis. *Carcinogenesis*, **16**, 875–882.

Monboisse, J.C., Braquet, P., Randoux, A., and Borel, J.P. (1983). Non-enzymatic degradation of acid-soluble calf skin collagen by superoxide ion: protective effect of flavonoides. *Biochemical Pharmacology*, **32**, 53–58.

Moncada, C., Torres, V., Varghese, G., Albano, E., and Israel, Y. (1994). Ethanol-derived immunoreactive species formed by free radical mechanisms. *Molecular Pharmacology*, **46**, 786–791.

Monig, J., Chapman, R., Asmus, K.-D. (1985). Effect of the portonation state of the amino group on the OH radical induced decarboxylation of amino acids in aqueous solution. *Journal of Physical Chemistry*, **89**, 3139–3144.

Montine, T.J., Amarnath, V., Martin, M.E., Strittmatter, W.J., and Graham, D.G. (1996). E-4-hydroxy-2-nonenal is cytotoxic and cross-links cytoskeletal proteins in P19 neuroglial cultures. *American Journal of Pathology*, **148**, 89–93.

Moore, R.B., Hulgan, T.M., Green, J.W., and Jenkins, L.D. (1992). Increased susceptibility of the sickle cell membrane $Ca^{2+} + Mg^{(2+)}$-ATPase to t-butylhydroperoxide: protective effects of ascorbate and desferal. *Blood*, **79**, 1334–1341.

Moore, W.G. (1986). Behavior of chymotrypsinogen during low pH gel electrophoresis is altered by persulfate. *Biochimica et Biophysica Acta*, **870**, 372–374.

Morand, K., Talbo, G., and Mann, M. (1993). Oxidation of peptides during electrospray ionization. *Rapid Communications in Mass Spectrometry*, **7**, 738–743.

Mordente, A., Miggiano, G.A., Martorana, G.E., Meucci, E., Santini, S.A., and Castelli, A. (1987). Alkaline phosphatase inactivation by mixed function oxidation systems. *Archives of Biochemistry and Biophysics*, **258**, 176–185.

Mordente, A., Santini, S.A., Miggiano, A.G., Martorana, G.E., Petiti, T., Minotti, G., *et al.* (1994a). The interaction of short chain coenzyme Q analogs with different redox states of myoglobin. *Journal of Biological Chemistry*, **269**, 27394–27400.

Mordente, A., Martorana, G.E., Miggiano, G.A., Petitti, T., Giardina, B., Littarru, G.P., *et al.* (1994b). Free radical production by activated haem proteins: protective effect of coenzyme Q. *Molecular Aspects of Medicine*, **15 (Supplement)**, S109-S115.

Moreau, S., Puppo, A., and Davies, M.J. (1995a). The reactivity of ascorbate with different redox states of leghaemoglobin. *Phytochemistry*, **39**, 1281–1286.

Moreau, S., Davies, M.J., and Puppo, A. (1995b). Reaction of ferric leghemoglobin with H_2O_2: formation of heme-protein cross-links and dimeric species. *Biochimica et Biophysica Acta*, **1251**, 17–22.

Moreau, S., Davies, M.J., Mathieu, C., Herouart, D., and Puppo, A. (1996). Leghemoglobin-derived radicals. Evidence for multiple protein-derived radicals and the initiation of peribacteroid membrane damage. *Journal of Biological Chemistry*, **271**, 32557–32562.

Morel, M.H., and Autran, J.C. (1990). Separation of durum wheat proteins by ultrathin-layer isoelectric focusing: a new tool for the characterization and quantification of low molecular weight glutenins. *Electrophoresis*, **11**, 392–399.

Moreno, J.J., and Pryor, W.A. (1992). Inactivation of alpha 1-proteinase inhibitor by peroxynitrite. *Chemical Research in Toxicology*, **5**, 425–431.

Morgan, C.A., Pilling, M.J., Tulloch, J.M., Ruiz, R.P., and Bayes, K.D. (1982). Direct determination of the equilibrium constant and thermodynamic parameters for the reaction $C_3H_5 + O_2 = C_3H_5O_2$. *Journal of the Chemical Society, Faraday Transactions. 2*, **78**, 1323–1330.

Morgan, R.W., Christman, M.F., Jacobson, F.S., Storz, G., and Ames, B.N. (1986). Hydrogen peroxide-inducible proteins in *Salmonella typhimurium* overlap with heat shock and other stress proteins. *Proceedings of the National Academy of Science of the United States of America*, **83**, 8059–8063.

Morris, J.W., Mercola, D.A., and Arquilla, E.R. (1970). Preparation and properties of 3-nitrotyrosine insulins. *Biochemistry*, **9**, 3930–3937.

Morrow, J.D., Frei, B., Longmire, A.W., Gaziano, J.M., Lynch, S.M., Shyr, Y., *et al.* (1995). Increase in circulating products of lipid peroxidation (F2-isoprostanes) in smokers. Smoking as a cause of oxidative damage. *New England Journal of Medicine*, **332**, 1198–1203.

Mortimore, G.E., and Ward, W.F. (1976). Behavior of the lysosomal system during organ perfusion. An inquiry into the mechanism of hepatic proteolysis. *Frontiers of Biology*, **45**, 157–184.

Moseley, R., Waddington, R., Evans, P., Halliwell, B., and Embery, G. (1995). The chemical modification of glycosaminoglycan structure by oxygen-derived species *in vitro*. *Biochimica et Biophysica Acta*, **1244**, 245–252.

Moshchinskii, P., and Pych, R. (1976). Obtaining complexes of thiamine with proteins. *Prikl Biokhimia Mikrobiologia*, **12**, 162–170.

Moskovitz, J., Rahman, M.A., Strassman, J., Yancey, S.O., Kushner, S.R., Brot, N., *et al.* (1995). *Escherichia coli* peptide methionine sulfoxide reductase gene: regulation of expression and role in protecting against oxidative damage. *Journal of Bacteriology*, **177**, 502–507.

Moskovitz, J., Jenkins, N.A., Gilbert, D.J., Copeland, N.G., Jursky, F., Weissbach, H., *et al.* (1996). Chromosomal localization of the mammalian peptide-methionine sulfoxide reductase gene and its differential expression in various tissues. *Proceedings of the National Academy of Science of the United States of America*, **93**, 3205–3208.

Moss, J., Stanley, S.J., and Levine, R.L. (1990). Inactivation of bacterial glutamine synthetase by ADP-ribosylation. *Journal of Biological Chemistry*, **265**, 21056–21060.

Motherwell, W.B., and Crich, D. (1992) *Free Radical Chain Reactions in Organic Synthesis*. Academic Press, New York.

Motsenbocker, M.A., and Tappel, A.L. (1982). Selenium and selenoproteins in the rat kidney. *Biochimica et Biophysica Acta*, **709**, 160–165.

Mottley, C., Trice, T.B., and Mason, R.P. (1982). Direct detection of the sulfur trioxide radical anion during the horseradish peroxidase-hydrogen peroxide oxidation of sulfite (aqueous sulfur dioxide). *Molecular Pharmacology*, **22**, 732–737.

Mönig, J., Chapman, R., and Asmus, K.-D. (1985). Effect of the protonation state of the amino group on the ·OH radical induced decarboxylation of amino acids in aqueous solution. *Journal of Physical Chemistry*, **89**, 3139–3144.

Mu, D., and Klinman, J.P. (1995). Cloning of mammalian topa quinone-containing enzymes. *Methods in Enzymology*, **258**, 114–122.

Mu, D., Janes, S.M., Smith, A.J., Brown, D.E., Dooley, D.M., and Klinman, J.P. (1992). Tyrosine codon corresponds to topa quinone at the active site of copper amine oxidases. *Journal of Biological Chemistry*, **267**, 7979–7982.

Mukaiyama, T., Ueki, M., Maruyama, H., and Matsueda, R. (1968). A new method for peptide synthesis by oxidation-reduction condensation. *Journal of the American Chemical Society*, **90**, 4490–4491.

Mukaiyama, T., Matsueda, R., Maruyama, H., and Ueki, M. (1969). The effects of metal components and acids on racemization in the synthesis of peptides by the oxidation-reduction condensation. *Journal of the American Chemical Society*, **91**, 1554–1555.

Mukhopadhyay, C.K., and Chatterjee, I.B. (1994*a*). NADPH-initiated cytochrome P450-mediated free metal ion-independent oxidative damage of microsomal proteins. Exclusive prevention by ascorbic acid. *Journal of Biological Chemistry*, **269**, 13390–13397.

Mukhopadhyay, C.K., and Chatterjee, I.B. (1994*b*). Free metal ion-independent oxidative damage of collagen. Protection by ascorbic acid. *Journal of Biological Chemistry*, **269**, 30200–30205.

Mukhopadhyay, C.K., Ghosh, M.K., and Chatterjee, I.B. (1995). Ascorbic acid prevents lipid peroxidation and oxidative damage of proteins in guinea pig extrahepatic tissue microsomes. *Molecular and Cellular Biochemistry*, **142**, 71–78.

Mukhopadhyay, M., Mukhopadhyay, C.K., and Chatterjee, I.B. (1993). Protective effect of ascorbic acid against lipid peroxidation and oxidative damage in cardiac microsomes. *Molecular and Cellular Biochemistry*, **126**, 69–75.

Mullarkey, C.J., Edelstein, D., and Brownlee, M. (1990). Free radical generation by early glycation products: a mechanism for accelerated atherogenesis in diabetes. *Biochemical and Biophysical Research Communications*, **173**, 932–939.

Mullen, W.H., Churchouse, S.J., and Vadgama, P.M. (1985). Enzyme electrode for glucose based on the quinoprotein glucose dehydrogenase. *Analyst*, **110**, 925–928.

Mulliez, E., Fontecave, M., Gaillard, J., and Reichard, P. (1993). An iron-sulfur center and a free radical in the active anaerobic ribonucleotide reductase of *Escherichia coli*. *Journal of Biological Chemistry*, **268**, 2296–2299.

Multhaup, G., Schlicksupp, A., Hesse, L., Beher, D., Ruppert, T., Masters, C.L., *et al.* (1996). The amyloid precursor protein of Alzheimer's disease in the reduction of copper(II) to copper(I). *Science*, **271**, 1406–1409.

Murakami, K., Jahngen, J.H., Lin, S.W., Davies, K.J., and Taylor, A. (1990). Lens proteasome shows enhanced rates of degradation of hydroxyl radical modified alpha-crystallin. *Free Radical Biology and Medicine*, **8**, 217–222.

Murase, K., Hattori, A., Kohno, M., and Hayashi, K. (1993). Stimulation of nerve growth factor synthesis/secretion in mouse astroglial cells by coenzymes. *Biochemistry and Molecular Biology International*, **30**, 615–621.

Murata, A., Kawasaki, M., Motomatsu, H., and Kato, F. (1986). Virus-inactivating effect of D-isoascorbic acid. *Journal of Nutritional Science and Vitaminology Tokyo*, **32**, 559–567.

Mure, M., and Klinman, J.P. (1995). Model studies of topa quinone: synthesis and characterization of topa quinone derivatives. *Methods in Enzymology*, **258**, 39–52.

Murohara, T., Kugiyama, K., and Yasue, H. (1996). Interactions of nitrovaso-dilators, atrial natriuretic peptide and endothelium-derived nitric oxide. *Journal of Vascular Research*, **33**, 78–85.

Murphy, M.E., and Kehrer, J.P. (1989). Oxidation state of tissue thiol groups and content of protein carbonyl groups in chickens with inherited muscular dystrophy. *Biochemical Journal*, **260**, 359–364.

Murphy, P.G., Myers, D.S., Webster, N.R., Jones, J.G., and Davies, M.J. (1991). Direct detection of free radical generation in an *in vivo* model of acute lung injury. *Free Radical Research Communications*, **15**, 167–176.

Murphy, P.G., Myers, D.S., Davies, M.J., Webster, N.R., and Jones, J.G. (1992). The antioxidant potential of propofol (2,6-diisopropylphenol). *British Journal of Anaesthesia*, **68**, 613–618.

Musci, G., Bonaccorsi, d.P.M., and Calabrese, L. (1995). Modulation of the redox state of the copper sites of human ceruloplasmin by chloride. *Journal of Protein Chemistry*, **14**, 611–619.

Mushegian, A.R., and Koonin, E.V. (1995). A putative FAD-binding domain in a distinct group of oxidases including a protein involved in plant development. *Protein Science*, **4**, 1243–1244.

Mustafa, M.G., and Tierney, D.F. (1978). Biochemical and metabolic changes in the lung with oxygen, ozone, and nitrogen dioxide toxicity. *American Review of Respiratory Disease*, **118**, 1061–1090.

Mutsvangwa, T., Buchanan, S.J., and McBride, B.W. (1996). Interactions between ruminal degradable nitrogen intake and *in vitro* addition of substrates on patterns of amino acid metabolism in isolated ovine hepatocytes. *Journal of Nutrition*, **126**, 209–218.

Nackerdien, Z., Rao, G., Cacciuttolo, M.A., Gajewski, E., and Dizdaroglu, M. (1991). Chemical nature of DNA-protein cross-links produced in mammalian chromatin by hydrogen peroxide in the presence of iron or copper ions. *Biochemistry*, **30**, 4873–4879.

Nadkarni, D.V., and Sayre, L.M. (1995). Structural definition of early lysine and histidine adduction chemistry of 4-hydroxynonenal. *Chemical Research Toxicology*, **8**, 284–291.

Nagaraj, R.H., Portero, O.M., and Monnier, V.M. (1996). Pyrraline ether crosslinks as a basis for protein crosslinking by the advanced Maillard reaction in aging and diabetes. *Archives of Biochemistry and Biophysics*, **325**, 152–158.

Nagasawa, T., and Yamada, H. (1987). Nitrile hydratase is a quinoprotein. A possible new function of pyrroloquinoline quinone: activation of H_2O in an enzymatic hydration reaction. *Biochemical and Biophysical Research Communications*, **147**, 701–709.

Nagata, S., Bakthavatsalam, S., Galkin, A.G., Asada, H., Sakai, S., Esaki, N., *et al.* (1995). Gene cloning, purification, and characterization of thermostable and halophilic leucine dehydrogenase from a halophilic thermophile, *Bacillus licheniformis TSN9*. *Applied Microbiology and Biotechnology*, **44**, 432–438.

Nagelkerke, J.F., Dogterom, P., De Bont, H.J., and Mulder, G.J. (1989). Prolonged high intracellular free calcium concentrations induced by ATP are not immediately cytotoxic in isolated rat hepatocytes. Changes in biochemical parameters implicated in cell toxicity. *Biochemical Journal*, **263**, 347–353.

Nagy, I., and Floyd, R.A. (1984). Hydroxyl free radical reactions with amino acids and proteins studied by electron spin resonance spectroscopy and spin-trapping. *Biochimica et Biophysica Acta*, **790**, 238–250.

Nagy, I.Z. (1995). Semiconduction of proteins as an attribute of the living state: the ideas of Albert Szent-Gyorgyi revisited in light of the recent knowledge regarding oxygen free radicals. *Experimental Gerontology*, **30**, 327–335.

Nair, K.S. (1987). Hyperglucagonemia increases resting metabolic rate in man during insulin deficiency. *Journal of Clinical Endocrinology and Metabolism*, **64**, 896–901.

Naish-Byfield, S., and Dean, R.T. (1989). Antioxidants and the influence of free radical damage to proteins on proteolysis in and around mammalian cells. *Revisiones Sobre Biologia Cellular*, **21**, 361–375.

Naito, A., Akasaka, K., and Hatano, H. (1981). Dimer cation radicals of *N*-acetyl methionine: E.S.R. and ENDOR studies. *Molecular Physics*, **44**, 427–443.

Nakagawa, Y., Moldeus, P., and Cotgreave, I.A. (1992). The S-thiolation of hepatocellular protein thiols during diquat metabolism. *Biochemical Pharmacology*, **43**, 2519–2525.

Nakamura, H., Matsuda, M., Furuke, K., Kitaoka, Y., Iwata, S., Toda, K., *et al.* (1994). Adult T cell leukemia-derived factor/human thioredoxin protects endothelial F-2 cell injury caused by activated neutrophils or hydrogen peroxide [published erratum appears in *Immunological Letters* (1994), **42**, 213]. *Immunological Letters*, **42**, 75–80.

Nakamura, K., and Stadtman, E.R. (1984). Oxidative inactivation of glutamine synthetase subunits. *Proceedings of the National Academy of Science of the United States of America*, **81**, 2011–2015.

Nakamura, K., Oliver, C., and Stadtman, E.R. (1985). Inactivation of glutamine synthetase by a purified rabbit liver microsomal cytochrome P-450 system. *Archives of Biochemistry and Biophysics*, **240**, 319–329.

Nakamura, N., Matsuzaki, R., Choi, Y.H., Tanizawa, K., and Sanders, L.J. (1996). Biosynthesis of topa quinone cofactor in bacterial amine oxidases. Solvent origin of C-2 oxygen determined by Raman spectroscopy. *Journal of Biological Chemistry*, **271**, 4718–4724.

Nakanishi, Y., Isohashi, F., Matsunaga, T., and Sakamoto, Y. (1985). Oxidative inactivation of an extramitochondrial acetyl-CoA hydrolase by autoxidation of L-ascorbic acid. *European Journal of Biochemistry*, **152**, 337–342.

Nakano, K., Chijiiwa, K., Okamoto, S., Yamashita, H., Kuroki, S., and Tanaka, M. (1995). Hepatic cholesterol 7 alpha-hydroxylase activity and serum 7 alpha-hydroxy-cholesterol level during liver regeneration after partial hepatectomy in rats. *European Surgical Research*, **27**, 389–395.

Nakano, M. (1992). Free radicals and their biological significance: present and future. *Human Cell*, **5**, 334–340.

Nakao, H.J., Ito, H., and Kawashima, S. (1992). An oxidative mechanism is involved in high glucose-induced serum protein modification causing inhibition of endothelial cell proliferation. *Atherosclerosis*, **97**, 89–95.

Nakata, T., and Hearse, D.J. (1990). Species differences in vulnerability to injury by oxidant stress: a possible link with calcium handling? *Cardiovascular Research*, **24**, 857–864.

Nakazawa, H., Ichomori, K., Shinozaki, Y., Okino, H., and Hori, S. (1988). Is superoxide demonstration by electron-spin resonance spectroscopy really superoxide? *American Journal of Physiology*, **255**, H213-H215.

Nappi, A.J., and Vass, E. (1994). The effects of glutathione and ascorbic acid on the oxidations of 6-hydroxydopa and 6-hydroxydopamine. *Biochimica et Biophysica Acta*, **1201**, 498–504.

Nappi, A.J., and Vass, E. (1996). Hydrogen peroxide generation associated with the oxidations of the eumelanin precursors 5,6-dihydroxyindole and 5,6-dihydroxyindole-2-carboxylic acid. *Melanoma Research*, **6**, 341–349.

Narita, H., and Morishita, E. (1995). Production and application of monoclonal antibodies specific to pyrroloquinoline quinone. *Journal of Biochemistry, Tokyo*, **117**, 830–835.

Nashed, N.T., Michaud, D.P., Levin, W., and Jerina, D.M. (1986). 7-Dehydrocholesterol 5,6 beta-oxide as a mechanism-based inhibitor of microsomal cholesterol oxide hydrolase. *Journal of Biological Chemistry*, **261**, 2510–2513.

Natake, M., and Ueda, M. (1986). Changes in food proteins reacted with nitrite at gastric pH. *Nutrition and Cancer*, **8**, 41–45.

Nath, J., Ohno, Y., Gallin, J.I., and Wright, D.G. (1992). A novel post-translational incorporation of tyrosine into multiple proteins in activated human neutrophils. Correlation with phagocytosis and activation of the NADPH oxidase-mediated respiratory burst. *Journal of Immunology*, **149**, 3360–3371.

Navab, M., Fogelman, A.M., Berliner, J.A., Territo, M.C., Demer, L.L., Frank, J.S., et al. (1995). Pathogenesis of atherosclerosis. *American Journal of Cardiology*, **76**, 18C-23C.

Navok, T., and Chevion, M. (1984). Transition metals mediate enzymatic inactivation caused by favism-inducing agents. *Biochemical and Biophysical Research Communications*, **122**, 297–303.

Nazir, M., and Shah, F.H. (1990). Stability of fatty acids and leaf protein concentrate of Persian clover (*Trifolium resupinatum*). *Plant Foods and Human Nutrition*, **40**, 283–288.

Neale, R.S. (1971). Nitrogen radicals as synthesis intermediates. *N*-Halamide rearrangements and additions to unsatruated hydrocarbons. *Synthesis*, **1**, 1–15.

Nedved, M.L., and Moe, G.R. (1994). Cooperative, non-specific binding of a zinc finger peptide to DNA. *Nucleic Acids Research*, **22**, 4705–4711.

Needles, H.L. (1977). Peroxydisulfate anion-induced crosslinking of proteins. *Advances in Experimental Medicine and Biology*, **86A**, 549–556.

Negelein, E. (1923). The reactivity of various amino acids to blood charcoals; also to hydrogen peroxide. *Biochemal Zeitschrift*, **142**, 493–505.

Nelsen, S.F. (1973). Nitrogen-Centered Radicals. In *Free Radicals*, (ed. J.K. Kochi), pp. 527–593. Wiley-Interscience.

Nelson, C.E., Sitzman, E.V., Kang, C.H., and Margoliash, E. (1977). Preparation of cytochrome *c* peroxidase from baker's yeast. *Analytical Biochemistry*, **83**, 622–631.

Nelson, K.M., Long, C.L., Bailey, R., Smith, R.J., Laws, H.L., and Blakemore, W.S. (1992). Regulation of glucose kinetics in trauma patients by insulin and glucagon. *Metabolism*, **41**, 68–75.

Nelson, M.J., and Cowling, R.A. (1990). Observation of a peroxyl radical in samples of 'purple' lipoxygenase. *Journal of the American Chemical Society*, **112**, 2820–2821.

Nesbitt, W.E., Beem, J.E., Leung, K.P., Stroup, S., Swift, R., McArthur, W.P., *et al.* (1996). Inhibition of adherence of *Actinomyces naeslundii* (*Actinomyces viscosus*) *T14V-J1* to saliva-treated hydroxyapatite by a monoclonal antibody to type 1 fimbriae. *Oral Microbiology and Immunology*, **11**, 51–58.

Nese, C., Schuchmann, M.N., Steenken, S., and von Sonntag, C. (1995). Oxidation *vs.* fragmentation in radiosensitization. Reactions of α-alkoxyalkyl radicals with 4-nitrobenzonitrile and oxygen. A pulse radiolysis and product analysis study. *Journal of the Chemical Society*, **2**, 1037–1044.

Neta, P., and Fessenden, R.W. (1971*a*). Electron spin resonance study of radicals produced in irradiated aqueous solutions of thiols. *Journal of Physical Chemistry*, **75**, 2277–2283.

Neta, P., and Fessenden, R.W. (1971*b*). Electron spin resonance study of radicals produced in irradiated aqueous solutions of amines and amino acids. *Journal of Physical Chemistry*, **75**, 738–748.

Neta, P., and Huie, R.E. (1985). Free-radical chemistry of sulfite. *Environmental Health Perspectives*, **64**, 209–217.

Neta, P., and Schuler, R.H. (1972). Rate constants for reaction of hydrogen atoms with aromatic and heterocyclic compounds. The electrophilic nature of hydrogen atoms. *Journal of the American Chemical Society*, **95**, 1056–1059.

Neta, P., Simic, M.G., and Hayon, E. (1970). Pulse radiolysis of aliphatic acids in aqueous solution. III. Simple amino acids. *Journal of Physical Chemistry*, **74**, 1214–1220.

Neta, P., Simic, M., and Hayon, E. (1972). On the pK_a of the $^+NH_3 \cdot CHCOOH$ radical. *Journal of Physical Chemistry*, **76**, 3507–3508.

Neta, P., Dizdaroglu, M., and Simic, M.G. (1984). Radiolytic studies of the cumyloxyl radical in aqueous solutions. *Israel Journal of Chemistry*, **24**, 25–28.

Neta, P., Huie, R.E., and Ross, A.B. (1988). Rate Constants for reactions of Inorganic Radicals in Aqueous Solution. *Journal of Physical Chemistry Reference Data*, **17**, 1027–1284.

Neta, P., Huie, R.E., Ross, A.B. (1990). Rate constants for reactions of peroxyl radicals in fluid solutions. *Journal of Physical Chemistry Reference Data*, **19**, 413–513.

Neta, R. (1990). Radioprotection and therapy of radiation injury with cytokines. *Progress in Clinical Biology Research*, **352**, 471–478.

Nettesheim, D.G., Harder, S.R., Feinberg, B.A., and Otvos, J.D. (1992). Sequential resonance assignments of oxidized high-potential iron-sulfur protein from *Chromatium vinosum*. *Biochemistry*, **31**, 1234–1244.

Neurath, A.R., Jiang, S., Strick, N., Lin, K., Li, Y.Y., and Debnath, A.K. (1996). Bovine beta-lactoglobulin modified by 3-hydroxyphthalic anhydride blocks the CD4 cell receptor for HIV. *Nature (Medicine)*, **2**, 230–234.

Neuzil, J., and Stocker, R. (1993). Bilirubin attenuates radical-mediated damage to serum albumin. *FEBS Letters*, **331**, 281–284.

Neuzil, J., and Stocker, R. (1994). Free and albumin-bound bilirubin are efficient co-antioxidants for alpha-tocopherol, inhibiting plasma and low density lipoprotein lipid peroxidation. *Journal of Biological Chemistry*, **269**, 16712–16719.

Neuzil, J., Gebicki, J.M., and Stocker, R. (1993). Radical-induced chain oxidation of proteins and its inhibition by chain-breaking antioxidants. *Biochemical Journal*, **293**, 601–606.

Neuzil, J., Thomas, S.R., and Stocker, R. (1997). Requirement for promotion or inhibition by alpha-tocopherol of radical-induced initiation of plasma lipoprotein lipid peroxidation. *Free Radical Biology and Medicine*, **22**, 57–71.

Newcomer, T.A., Palmer, A.M., Rosenberg, P.A., and Aizenman, E. (1993). Non-enzymatic conversion of 3,4-dihydroxyphenylalanine to 2,4,5-trihydroxyphenyl-alanine and 2,4,5-trihydroxyphenylalanine quinone in physiological solutions. *Journal of Neurochemistry*, **61**, 911–920.

Newcomer, T.A., Rosenberg, P.A., and Aizenman, E. (1995a). TOPA quinone, a kainate-like agonist and excitotoxin is generated by a catecholaminergic cell line. *Journal of Neuroscience*, **15**, 3172–3177.

Newcomer, T.A., Rosenberg, P.A., and Aizenman, E. (1995b). Iron-mediated oxidation of 3,4-dihydroxyphenylalanine to an excitotoxin. *Journal of Neuro-chemistry*, **64**, 1742–1748.

Newman, E.S., Rice, E.C., and Davies, M.J. (1991). Identification of initiating agents in myoglobin-induced lipid peroxidation. *Biochemical and Biophysical Research Communications*, **179**, 1414–1419.

Nichol, K.A., Schulz, M.W., and Bennett, M.R. (1995). Nitric oxide-mediated death of cultured neonatal retinal ganglion cells: neuroprotective properties of glutamate and chondroitin sulfate proteoglycan. *Brain Research*, **697**, 1–16.

Nicholson, A.C., Frieda, S., Pearce, A., and Silverstein, R.L. (1995). Oxidized LDL binds to CD36 on human monocyte-derived macrophages and transfected cell lines. Evidence implicating the lipid moiety of the lipoprotein as the binding site. *Arteriosclerosis Thrombosis and Vascular Biology*, **15**, 269–275.

Nicol, C.J., Harrison, M.L., Laposa, R.R., Gimelshtein, I.L., and Wells, P.G. (1995). A teratologic suppressor role for p53 in benzo[a]pyrene-treated transgenic p53-deficient mice. *Nature (Genetics)*, **10**, 181–187.

Nielsen, H. (1978). Reaction between peroxidized phospholipid and protein: I. Covalent binding of peroxidized cardiolipin to albumin. *Lipids*, **13**, 253–258.

Nielsen, H. (1979). Reaction between peroxidized phospholipid and protein: II. Molecular weight and phosphorus content of albumin after reaction with peroxidized cardiolipin. *Lipids*, **14**, 900–906.

Nielsen, H.K. (1981). Covalent binding of peroxidised phospholipid to protein: III. Reaction of individual phospholipids with different proteins. *Lipids*, **16**, 215–222.

Nielsen, H.K., Loliger, J., and Hurrell, R.F. (1985). Reactions of proteins with oxidizing lipids. 1. Analytical measurements of lipid oxidation and of amino acid losses in a whey protein-methyl linolenate model system. *British Journal of Nutrition*, **53**, 61–73.

Niimura, Y., Poole, L.B., and Massey, V. (1995). *Amphibacillus xylanus* NADH oxidase and *Salmonella typhimurium* alkyl-hydroperoxide reductase flavoprotein components show extremely high scavenging activity for both alkyl hydroperoxide and hydrogen peroxide in the presence of *S. typhimurium* alkyl-hydroperoxide reductase 22-kDa protein component. *Journal of Biological Chemistry*, **270**, 25645–25650.

Nikandrov, V.N., and Kaziuchits, O.A. (1988). Study of the role of tryptophan residues in streptokinase molecules using a chemical modification method. *Biokhimiia*, **53**, 508–515.

Nishiyama, Y., Suwa, H., Okamoto, K., Fukumoto, M., Hiai, H., and Toyokuni, S. (1995). Low incidence of point mutations in H-, K- and N-ras oncogenes and p53 tumor suppressor gene in renal cell carcinoma and peritoneal mesothelioma of Wistar rats induced by ferric nitrilotriacetate. *Journal of Cancer Research*, **86**, 1150–1158.

Noble, L.J., Cortez, S.C., and Ellison, J.A. (1990). Endogenous peroxidatic activity in astrocytes after spinal cord injury. *Journal of Comparative Neurology*, **296**, 674–685.

Nofre, C., Welin, L., Parnet, J., and Cier, A. (1961). Action du radical libre hydroxyle sur les acide amines. *Bulletin Societe Chimique Biologique*, **43**, 1237–1245.

Noguchi, N., and Niki, E. (1994). Apolipoprotein B protein oxidation in low-density lipoproteins. *Methods in Enzymology*, **233**, 490–494.

Noguchi, N., Gotoh, N., and Niki, E. (1994). Effects of ebselen and probucol on oxidative modifications of lipid and protein of low density lipoprotein induced by free radicals. *Biochimica et Biophysica Acta*, **1213**, 176–182.

Nohl, H. (1979). Influence of age on thermotropic kinetics of enzymes involved in mitochondrial energy-metabolism. *Zeitscrift fur Gerontology*, **12**, 9–18.

Nohl, H., and Stolze, K. (1993). Chemiluminescence from activated heme compounds detected in the reaction of various xenobiotics with oxyhemoglobin: comparison with several heme/hydrogen peroxide systems. *Free Radical Biology and Medicine*, **15**, 257–263.

Nomura, K., and Suzuki, N. (1995). Sea urchin ovoperoxidase:solubilization and isolation from the fertilization envelope, some structural and functional properties, and degradation by hatching enzyme. *Archives of Biochemistry and Biophysics*, **319**, 525–534.

Nonhebel, D.C., Tedder, J.M., and Walton, J.C. (1977). *Radicals*. Cambridge University Press, Cambridge.

Nordlund, P., and Eklund, H. (1993). Structure and function of the *Escherichia coli* ribonucleotide reductase protein R2. *Journal of Molecular Biology*, **232**, 123–164.

Nordlund, P., Sjoberg, B.M., and Eklund, H. (1990). Three-dimensional structure of the free radical protein of ribonucleotide reductase. *Nature*, **345**, 593–598.

Nordstrom, G., Saljo, A., and Hasselgren, P.O. (1988). Studies on the possible role of oxygen-derived free radicals for impairment of protein and energy metabolism in liver ischemia. *Circulatory Shock*, **26**, 115–126.

Nosworthy, J., and Allsop, C.B. (1956). Effects of X-rays on dilute aqueous solutions of amino acids. *Journal of Colloid Science*, 11, 565–574.

Nourooz, Z.J., Tajaddini, S.J., and Wolff, S.P. (1994). Measurement of plasma hydroperoxide concentrations by the ferrous oxidation-xylenol orange assay in conjunction with triphenylphosphine. *Analytical Biochemistry*, 220, 403–409.

Nourooz, Z.J., Tajaddini, S.J., McCarthy, S., Betteridge, D.J., and Wolff, S.P. (1995). Elevated levels of authentic plasma hydroperoxides in NIDDM. *Diabetes*, 44, 1054–1058.

Nourooz, Z.J., Tajaddini, S.J., Ling, K.L., and Wolff, S.P. (1996). Low-density lipoprotein is the major carrier of lipid hydroperoxides in plasma. Relevance to determination of total plasma lipid hydroperoxide concentrations. *Biochemical Journal*, 313, 781–786.

Nurnberger. (1937). Ionization theory and radio-biological reactions. *Proceedings of the National Academy of Science of the United States of America*, 23, 189–193.

O'Connell, M.J., and Peters, T.J. (1987). Ferritin and haemosiderin in free radical generation, lipid peroxidation and protein damage. *Chemistry and Physics of Lipids*, 45, 241–249.

O'Connell, M.J., Baum, H., and Peters, T.J. (1986). Haemosiderin-like properties of free-radical-modified ferritin. *Biochemical Journal*, 240, 297–300.

O'Donnell, M.J., and Smith, B.E. (1978). Electron-paramagnetic-resonance studies on the redox properties of the molybdenum-iron protein of nitrogenase between +50 and -450 mV. *Biochemical Journal*, 173, 831–839.

O'Neill, C.A., Halliwell, B., van der Vliet, A., Davis, P.A., Packer, L., Tritschler, H., et al. (1994). Aldehyde-induced protein modifications in human plasma: protection by glutathione and dihydrolipoic acid. *Journal of Laboratory and Clinical Medicine*, 124, 359–370.

O'Neill, P., Schulte-Frohlinde, D., Steenken, S. (1977). Formation of radical cations and zwitterions *versus* methoxylation in the reaction of OH with a series of methoxylated benzenes and benzoic acids. An example of the electrphilic nature of the OH radical. *Journal of the Chemical Society, Faraday Discussions*, 63, 141–148.

O'Neill, P., Fielden, E.M., Finazzi, A.A., and Avigliano, L. (1983). Pulse-radiolysis studies on the interaction of one-electron-reduced species with ascorbate oxidase in aqueous solution. *Biochemical Journal*, 209, 167–174.

Obara, Y. (1995). The oxidative stress in the cataract formation. *Nippon Ganka Gakkai Zasshi*, 99, 1303–1341.

Oberley, T.D., Sempf, J.M., and Oberley, L.W. (1995). Immunohistochemical localization of antioxidant enzymes during hamster kidney development. *Histochemistry Journal*, 27, 575–586.

Oda, T., Wals, P., Osterburg, H.H., Johnson, S.A., Pasinetti, G.M., Morgan, T.E., et al. (1995). Clusterin (apoJ) alters the aggregation of amyloid beta-peptide (A beta 1-42) and forms slowly sedimenting A beta complexes that cause oxidative stress. *Experimental Neurology*, 136, 22–31.

Ogino, T., and Okada, S. (1995). Oxidative damage of bovine serum albumin and other enzyme proteins by iron-chelate complexes. *Biochimica et Biophysica Acta*, 1245, 359–365.

Ogura, Y., Takanashi, T., Ishigooka, H., and Ogino, N. (1991). Quantitative analysis of lens changes after vitrectomy by fluorophotometry. *American Journal of Ophthalmology*, 111, 179–183.

Oh, B.H., Westler, W.M., Darba, P., and Markley, J.L. (1988). Protein carbon-13 spin systems by a single two-dimensional nuclear magnetic resonance experiment. *Science*, 240, 908–911.

Oh, U., Ho, Y.K., and Kim, D. (1995). Modulation of the serotonin-activated K^+ channel by G protein subunits and nucleotides in rat hippocampal neurons. *Journal of Membrane Biology*, **147**, 241–253.

Ohad, I., Kyle, D.J., and Arntzen, C.J. (1984). Membrane protein damage and repair: removal and replacement of inactivated 32-kilodalton polypeptides in chloroplast membranes. *Journal of Cellular Biology*, **99**, 481–485.

Ohki, K., Yoshida, K., Hagiwara, M., Harada, T., Takamura, M., Ohashi, T., *et al.* (1995). Nitric oxide induces c-fos gene expression via cyclic AMP response element binding protein (CREB) phosphorylation in rat retinal pigment epithelium. *Brain Research*, **696**, 140–144.

Ohnishi, K., Niimura, Y., Yokoyama, K., Hidaka, M., Masaki, H., Uchimura, T., *et al.* (1994). Purification and analysis of a flavoprotein functional as NADH oxidase from *Amphibacillus xylanus* overexpressed in *Escherichia coli*. *Journal of Biological Chemistry*, **269**, 31418–31423.

Ohnishi, K., Niimura, Y., Hidaka, M., Masaki, H., Suzuki, H., Uozumi, T., *et al.* (1995). Role of cysteine 337 and cysteine 340 in flavoprotein that functions as NADH oxidase from *Amphibacillus xylanus* studied by site-directed mutagenesis. *Journal of Biological Chemistry*, **270**, 5812–5817.

Ohshima, H., Friesen, M., Brouet, I., and Bartsch, H. (1990). Nitrotyrosine as a new marker for endogenous nitrosation and nitration of proteins. *Food and Chemical Toxicology*, **28**, 647–652.

Ohshima, H., Brouet, I., Friesen, M., and Bartsch, H. (1991). Nitrotyrosine as a new marker for endogenous nitrosation and nitration. *IARC Science Publications*, **1991**, 443–448.

Ohyashiki, T., Ohtsuka, T., and Mohri, T. (1988). Increase of the molecular rigidity of the protein conformation in the intestinal brush-border membranes by lipid peroxidation. *Biochimica et Biophysica Acta*, **939**, 383–392.

Ohyashiki, T., Sakata, N., Kamata, K., and Matsui, K. (1991). A study on peroxidative damage of the porcine intestinal brush-border membranes using a fluorogenic thiol reagent, N-(1-pyrene)maleimide. *Biochimica et Biophysica Acta*, **1067**, 159–165.

Okada, S. (1957). Inactivation of DNAase by X rays. I. Mechanism of inactivation in aqueous solution. *Archives of Biochemistry and Biophysics*, **67**, 95–101.

Okada, S. (1958). Formation of hydroperoxides from certain amino acids and peptides in aqueous solution by irradiation in the presence of oxygen. In *Organic Peroxides in Radiobiology*, (ed. R. Latarjet), pp. 46–58. Pergamon, London.

Okada, S. (1961). Active site of DNAse 1. I. The nature of the active site of DNAse I. *Radiation Research*, **15**, 452–459.

Okada, S., and Gehrmann, G. (1957). Inactivation of DNAse by X rays. IV. Changes in amino acid composition and UV absorption induced by ionizing radiation. *Biochimica et Biophysica Acta*, **25**, 179–182.

Okada, S., Kraunz, R., and Gassner, E. (1960). Radiation induced changes in susceptibility of substrates to enzymatic degradation. *Radiation Research*, **13**, 607–612.

Okamoto, T., Ogiwara, H., Hayashi, T., Mitsui, A., Kawabe, T., and Yodoi, J. (1992). Human thioredoxin/adult T cell leukemia-derived factor activates the enhancer binding protein of human immunodeficiency virus type 1 by thiol redox control mechanism. *International Immunology*, **4**, 811–819.

Okano, K., Kuraishi, Y., and Satoh, M. (1995). Effects of repeated cold stress on aversive responses produced by intrathecal excitatory amino acids in rats. *Biological Pharmacology Bulletin*, **18**, 1602–1604.

Okuno, H., Akahori, A., Sato, H., Xanthoudakis, S., Curran, T., and Iba, H. (1993). Escape from redox regulation enhances the transforming activity of Fos. *Oncogene*, **8**, 695–701.

Olin, K.L., Shigenaga, M.K., Ames, B.N., Golub, M.S., Gershwin, M.E., Hendrickx, A.G., *et al.* (1993). Maternal dietary zinc influences DNA strand break and 8-hydroxy-2'-deoxyguanosine levels in infant rhesus monkey liver. *Proceedings of the National Academy of Science of the United Stated of America*, **203**, 461–466.

Olinski, R., Nackerdien, Z., and Dizdaroglu, M. (1992). DNA-protein cross-linking between thymine and tyrosine in chromatin of gamma-irradiated or H_2O_2-treated cultured human cells. *Archives of Biochemistry and Biophysics*, **297**, 139–143.

Oliver, C.N. (1985). Inactivation of enzymes by activated human neutrophils. *Current Topics in Cell Regulation*, **27**, 335–343.

Oliver, C.N. (1987). Inactivation of enzymes and oxidative modification of proteins by stimulated neutrophils. *Archives of Biochemistry and Biophysics*, **253**, 62–72.

Oliver, C.N. (1988). Oxidative modification of enzymes by stimulated neutrophils. *Basic Life Science*, **49**, 839–844.

Oliver, C.N. (1990). Measurement of oxidized proteins in systems involving activated neutrophils or HL-60 cells. *Methods in Enzymology*, **186**, 575–579.

Oliver, C.N., and Stadtman, E.R. (1983). A proteolytic artifact associated with the lysis of bacteria by egg white lysozyme. *Proceedings of the National Academy of Science of the United States of America*, **80**, 2156–2160.

Oliver, C.N., Ahn, B.W., Moerman, E.J., Goldstein, S., and Stadtman, E.R. (1987). Age-related changes in oxidized proteins. *Journal of Biological Chemistry*, **262**, 5488–5491.

Oliver, C.N., Starke, R.P., Stadtman, E.R., Liu, G.J., Carney, J.M., and Floyd, R.A. (1990). Oxidative damage to brain proteins, loss of glutamine synthetase activity, and production of free radicals during ischemia/reperfusion-induced injury to gerbil brain. *Proceedings of the National Academy of Science of the United States of America*, **87**, 5144–5147.

Omaye, S.T., and Tappel, A.L. (1974). Glutathione peroxidase, glutathione reductase, and thiobarbituric acid-reactive products in muscles of chickens and mice with genetic muscular dystrophy. *Life Science*, **15**, 137–145.

Opanashuk, L.A., and Finkelstein, J.N. (1995). Relationship of lead-induced proteins to stress response proteins in astroglial cells. *Journal of Neuroscience Research*, **42**, 623–632.

Ormo, M., Regnstrom, K., Wang, Z., Que, L.J., Sahlin, M., and Sjoberg, B.M. (1995). Residues important for radical stability in ribonucleotide reductase from *Escherichia coli*. *Journal of Biological Chemistry*, **270**, 6570–6576.

Orr, C.W. (1966). The inhibition of catalase by ascorbic acid. *Biochemical and Biophysical Research Communications*, **23**, 854–860.

Orr, C.W. (1967a). Studies on ascorbic acid. I. Factors influencing the ascorbate-mediated inhibition of catalase. *Biochemistry*, **6**, 2995–3000.

Orr, C.W. (1967b). Studies on ascorbic acid. II. Physical changes in catalase following incubation with ascorbate or ascorbate and copper (II). *Biochemistry*, **6**, 3000–3006.

Orr, W.C., and Sohal, R.S. (1992). The effects of catalase gene overexpression on life span and resistance to oxidative stress in transgenic *Drosophila melanogaster*. *Archives of Biochemistry and Biophysics*, **297**, 35–41.

Orr, W.C., and Sohal, R.S. (1993). Effects of Cu-Zn superoxide dismutase overexpression of life span and resistance to oxidative stress in transgenic *Drosophila melanogaster*. *Archives of Biochemistry and Biophysics*, **301**, 34–40.

Orr, W.C., and Sohal, R.S. (1994). Extension of life-span by overexpression of superoxide dismutase and catalase in *Drosophila melanogaster*. *Science*, **263**, 1128–1130.

Orr, W.C., Arnold, L.A., and Sohal, R.S. (1992). Relationship between catalase activity, life span and some parameters associated with antioxidant defenses in *Drosophila melanogaster*. *Mechanisms of Ageing and Development*, **63**, 287–296.

Ortiz de Montellano, P.R. (1987). Control of the catalytic activity of prosthetic heme by the structure of hemoproteins. *Accounts of Chemical Research*, **20**, 289–294.

Ortiz de Montellano, P.R. (1990). Free radical modification of prosthetic heme groups. *Pharmacology and Theraputics*, **48**, 95–120.

Ortiz de Montellano, P.R. (1992). Catalytic sites of hemoprotein peroxidases. *Annual Reviews on Pharmacology and Toxicology*, **32**, 89–107.

Ortiz de Montellano, P.R. (1995). Arylhydrazines as probes of hemoprotein structure and function. *Biochimie*, **77**, 581–593.

Ortiz de Montellano, P.R., and Catalano, C.E. (1985). Epoxidation of styrene by hemoglobin and myoglobin. Transfer of oxidizing equivalents to the protein surface. *Journal of Biological Chemistry*, **260**, 9265–9271.

Ortwerth, B.J., Linetsky, M., and Olesen, P.R. (1995). Ascorbic acid glycation of lens proteins produces UVA sensitizers similar to those in human lens. *Photochemistry and Photobiology*, **62**, 454–462.

Osswald, W.F., Schutz, W., and Elstner, E.F. (1989). Cysteine and crocin oxidation catalyzed by horseradish peroxidase. *Free Radical Research Communications*, **5**, 259–265.

Ostdal, H., Daneshvar, B., and Skibsted, L.H. (1996). Reduction of ferrylmyoblobin by β-lactoglobulin. *Free Radical Research*, **24**, 429–438.

Ostermeier, M., De Sutter, K., and Georgiou, G. (1996). Eukaryotic protein disulfide isomerase complements *Escherichia coli* dsbA mutants and increases the yield of a heterologous secreted protein with disulfide bonds. *Journal of Biological Chemistry*, **271**, 10616–10622.

Oteiza, P.I., Olin, K.L., Fraga, C.G., and Keen, C.L. (1995). Zinc deficiency causes oxidative damage to proteins, lipids and DNA in rat testes. *Journal of Nutrition*, **125**, 823–829.

Ottnad, E., Parthasarathy, S., Sambrano, G.R., Ramprasad, M.P., Quehenberger, O., Kondratenko, N., *et al.* (1995). A macrophage receptor for oxidized low density lipoprotein distinct from the receptor for acetyl low density lipoprotein: partial purification and role in recognition of oxidatively damaged cells. *Proceedings of the National Academy of Science of the United States of America*, **92**, 1391–1395.

Ottonello, L., Dapino, P., Scirocco, M., Dallegri, F., and Sacchetti, C. (1994). Proteolytic inactivation of alpha-1-antitrypsin by human neutrophils: involvement of multiple and interlinked cell responses to phagocytosable targets. *European Journal of Clinical Investigation*, **24**, 42–49.

Ou, P., and Wolff, S.P. (1993). Aminoguanidine: a drug proposed for prophylaxis in diabetes inhibits catalase and generates hydrogen peroxide *in vitro*. *Biochemical Pharmacology*, **46**, 1139–1144.

Ou, P., and Wolff, S.P. (1994). Erythrocyte catalase inactivation (H_2O_2 production) by ascorbic acid and glucose in the presence of aminotriazole: role of transition metals and relevance to diabetes. *Biochemical Journal*, **303**, 935–939.

Ou, P., Tritschler, H.J., and Wolff, S.P. (1995). Thioctic (lipoic) acid: a therapeutic metal-chelating antioxidant? *Biochemical Pharmacology*, **50**, 123–126.

Ou, X., Thomas, G.R., Chacon, M.R., Tang, L., and Selkirk, M.E. (1995). *Brugia malayi*: differential susceptibility to and metabolism of hydrogen peroxide in adults and microfilariae. *Experimental Parasitology*, **80**, 530–540.

Oury, T.D., Tatro, L., Ghio, A.J., and Piantadosi, C.A. (1995). Nitration of tyrosine by hydrogen peroxide and nitrite. *Free Radical Research*, **23**, 537–547.

Oxlund, H., Barckman, M., Ortoft, G., and Andreassen, T.T. (1995). Reduced concentrations of collagen cross-links are associated with reduced strength of bone. *Bone*, **17 (Supplement)**, 365S–371S.

Paardekooper, M., Van den Broek, P.J., De Bruijne, A.W., Elferink, J.G., Dubbelman, T.M., and Van Steveninck, J. (1992). Photodynamic treatment of yeast cells with the dye toluidine blue: all-or-none loss of plasma membrane barrier properties. *Biochimica et Biophysica Acta*, **1108**, 86–90.

Paardekooper, M., De Bruijne, A.W., Van Steveninck, J., and Van den Broek, P.J. (1993). Inhibition of transport systems in yeast by photodynamic treatment with toluidine blue. *Biochimica et Biophysica Acta*, **1151**, 143–148.

Paardekooper, M., De Bruijne, A.W., Van Steveninck, J., and Van den Broek, P.J. (1995). Intracellular damage in yeast cells caused by photodynamic treatment with toluidine blue. *Photochemistry and Photobiology*, **61**, 84–89.

Pacifici, R.E., and Davies, K.J. (1990). Protein degradation as an index of oxidative stress. *Methods in Enzymology*, **186**, 485–502.

Pacifici, R.E., and Davies, K.J. (1991). Protein, lipid and DNA repair systems in oxidative stress: the free-radical theory of aging revisited. *Gerontology*, **37**, 166–180.

Pacifici, R.E., Lin, S.W., and Davies, K.J. (1988). The measurement of protein degradation in response to oxidative stress. *Basic Life Science*, **49**, 531–535.

Pacifici, R.E., Salo, D.C., and Davies, K.J. (1989). Macroxyproteinase (M.O.P.): a 670 kDa proteinase complex that degrades oxidatively denatured proteins in red blood cells [published erratum appears in *Free Radical Biology and Medicine* (1990), **8**, 211–2]. *Free Radical Biology and Medicine*, **7**, 521–536.

Pacifici, R.E., Kono, Y., and Davies, K.J. (1993). Hydrophobicity as the signal for selective degradation of hydroxyl radical-modified hemoglobin by the multi-catalytic proteinase complex, proteasome. *Journal of Biological Chemistry*, **268**, 15405–15411.

Packer, E.L., and Sternlicht, H. (1975). The use of 13C nuclear magnetic resonance of aromatic amino acid residues to determine the midpoint oxidation-reduction potential of each iron-sulfur cluster of *Clostridium acidi-urici* and *Clostridium pasteurianum* ferredoxins. *Journal of Biological Chemistry*, **250**, 2062–2072.

Packer, J.E., Mahood, J.S., Willson, R.L., and Wolfenden, B.S. (1981). Reactions of the trichloromethylperoxy free radical (Cl3COO) with tryptophan, tryptophanyl-tyrosine and lysozyme. *International Journal of Radiation Biology and Related Studies in Physics, Chemistry and Medicine*, **39**, 135–141.

Packer, L., Valenza, M., Serbinova, E., Starke, R.P., Frost, K., and Kagan, V. (1991). Free radical scavenging is involved in the protective effect of L-propionyl-carnitine against ischemia-reperfusion injury of the heart. *Archives of Biochemistry and Biophysics*, **288**, 533–537.

Padilla, C.A., Martinez, G.E., Lopez, B.J., Holmgren, A., and Barcena, J.A. (1992). Immunolocalization of thioredoxin and glutaredoxin in mammalian hypophysis. *Molecular and Cellular Endocrinology*, **85**, 1–12.

Pahlmark, K., Folbergrova, J., Smith, M.L., and Siesjo, B.K. (1993). Effects of dimethylthiourea on selective neuronal vulnerability in forebrain ischemia in rats. *Stroke*, **24**, 731–736.

Palamanda, J.R., and Kehrer, J.P. (1992). Inhibition of protein carbonyl formation and lipid peroxidation by glutathione in rat liver microsomes. *Archives of Biochemistry and Biophysics*, **293**, 103–109.

Palcic, M.M., and Janes, S.M. (1995). Spectrophotometric detection of topa quinone. *Methods in Enzymology*, **258**, 34–38.

Palcic, M.M., Scaman, C.H., and Alton, G. (1995). Stereochemistry and cofactor identity status of semicarbazide-sensitive amine oxidases. *Progress in Brain Research*, **106**, 41–47.

Palladini, G., Finardi, G., and Bellomo, G. (1996). Disruption of actin microfilament organization by cholesterol oxides in 73/73 endothelial cells. *Experimental Cell Research*, **223**, 72–82.

Pan, X.-M., Schuchmann, M.N., von Sonntag, C. (1993). Oxidation of benzene by the OH radical. A product and pulse radiolysis study in oxygenated aqueous solution. *Journal of the Chemical Society, Perkin Transactions*, **2**, 289–297.

Panasenko, O.M., Evgina, S.A., Aidyraliev, R.K., Sergienko, V.I., and Vladimirov, Y.A. (1994). Peroxidation of human blood lipoproteins induced by exogenous hypochlorite or hypochlorite generated in the system of 'myeloperoxidase + H_2O_2 + Cl^-'. *Free Radical Biology and Medicine*, **16**, 143–148.

Pande, J., Lomakin, A., Fine, B., Ogun, O., Sokolinski, I., and Benedek, G. (1995). Oxidation of gamma II-crystallin solutions yields dimers with a high phase separation temperature. *Proceedings of the National Academy of Science of the United States of America*, **92**, 1067–1071.

Paneque, A., Barcena, J.A., Cordero, N., Revilla, E., and Liobell, A. (1982). Benzyl viologen-mediated *in vivo* and *in vitro* inactivation of glutamine synthetase in *Azotobacter chorococcum*. *Molecular and Cellular Biochemistry*, **49**, 33–41.

Papov, V.V., Diamond, T.V., Biemann, K., and Waite, J.H. (1995). Hydroxy-arginine-containing polyphnolic proteins in the adhesive plaque of the marine mussel *Mytilus edulis*. *Journal of Biological Chemistry*, **270**, 20183–20192.

Parhami, F., Fang, Z.T., Fogelman, A.M., Andalibi, A., Territo, M.C., and Berliner, J.A. (1993). Minimally modified low density lipoprotein-induced inflammatory responses in endothelial cells are mediated by cyclic adenosine monophosphate. *Journal of Clinical Investigation*, **92**, 471–478.

Parinandi, N.L., Weis, B.K., Natarajan, V., and Schmid, H.H. (1990). Peroxidative modification of phospholipids in myocardial membranes. *Archives of Biochemistry and Biophysics*, **280**, 45–52.

Parinandi, N.L., Zwizinski, C.W., and Schmid, H.H. (1991). Free radical-induced alterations of myocardial membrane proteins. *Archives of Biochemistry and Biophysics*, **289**, 118–123.

Park, E.M., Shigenaga, M.K., Degan, P., Korn, T.S., Kitzler, J.W., Wehr, C.M., *et al.* (1992). Assay of excised oxidative DNA lesions: isolation of 8-oxoguanine and its nucleoside derivatives from biological fluids with a monoclonal antibody column. *Proceedings of the National Academy of Science of the United States of America*, **89**, 3375–3379.

Park, J.H., Lee, Y.S., Chung, C.H., and Goldberg, A.L. (1988). Purification and characterization of protease Re, a cytoplasmic endoprotease in *Escherichia coli*. *Journal of Bacteriology*, **170**, 921–926.

Park, J.R., and Tappel, A.L. (1991). Protein damage and lipid peroxidation: effects of diethyl maleate, bromotrichloromethane and vitamin E on ammonia, urea and enzymes involved in ammonia metabolism. *Toxicology Letters*, **58**, 29–36.

Park, J.Y., Shigenaga, M.K., and Ames, B.N. (1996). Induction of cytochrome P4501A1 by 2,3,7,8-tetrachlorodibenzo-*p*-dioxin or indolo(3,2-b)carbazole is associated with oxidative DNA damage. *Proceedings of the National Academy of Science of the United States of America*, **93**, 2322–2327.

Park, Y., and Kehrer, J.P. (1991). Oxidative changes in hypoxic-reoxygenated rabbit heart: a consequence of hypoxia rather than reoxygenation. *Free Radical Research Communications*, **14**, 179–185.

Park, Y., Kanekal, S., and Kehrer, J.P. (1991). Oxidative changes in hypoxic rat heart tissue. *American Journal of Physiology*, **260**, H1395–H1405.

Parker, C.W., Huber, M.M., Hoffman, M.K., and Falkenhein, S.F. (1979). Characterization of the two major species of slow reacting substance from rat basophilic leukemia cells as glutathionyl thioethers of eicosatetraenoic acids oxygenated at the 5 position. Evidence that peroxy groups are present and important for spasmogenic activity. *Prostaglandins*, **18**, 673–686.

Parker, K.C., Shields, M., DiBrino, M., Brooks, A., and Coligan, J.E. (1995). Peptide binding to MHC class I molecules: implications for antigenic peptide prediction. *Immunological Research*, **14**, 34–57.

Pascoe, G.A., and Reed, D.J. (1989). Cell calcium, vitamin E, and the thiol redox system in cytotoxicity. *Free Radical Biology and Medicine*, **6**, 209–224.

Patel, K.B., and Willson, R.L. (1973). Semiquinone free radicals and oxygen. Pulse radiolysis study of one electron transfer equilibria. *Journal of the Chemical Society, Faraday Transactions 1*, **69**, 814–825.

Pattanayak, S., Arora, D.D., Sehgal, C.L., Raghavan, N.G., Topa, P.K., and Subrahmanyam, Y.K. (1970). Comparative studies of smallpox vaccination by the bifurcated needle and rotary lancet techniques. *Bulletin World Health Organisation*, **42**, 305–310.

Patten, R.A., and Gordy, W. (1964). Further studies of radiation effects on proteins and their constituents. *Radiation Research*, **22**, 29–44.

Patton, W., Bacon, V., Duffield, A.M., Halpern, B., Hoyano, Y., Pereira, W., *et al.* (1972). Chlorination Studies. I. The reaction of aqueous hypochlorous acid with cytosine. *Biochemical and Biophysical Research Communications*, **48**, 880–884.

Pau, R.N., and Kelly, C. (1975). The hydroxylation of tyrosine by an enzyme from third-instar larvae of the blowfly *Calliphora erythrocephala*. *Biochemical Journal*, **147**, 565–573.

Paul, H., and Fischer, H. (1969). Elektronenspinresonanz kurzleiger Radikale aus einigen Aminosäuren und Amiden. *Berichte Bunsengelles*, **73**, 972–980.

Paul, H., and Fischer, H. (1971). ESR studies on hydroxyl radical reactions with glycine. *Helvetica Chimica Acta*, **54**, 485–491.

Pavlik, A., and Pilar, J. (1989). Protection of cell proteins against free-radical attack by nootropic drugs: scavenger effect of pyritinol confirmed by electron spin resonance spectroscopy. *Neuropharmacology*, **28**, 557–561.

Paz, M.A., Gallop, P.M., Torrelio, B.M., and Fluckiger, R. (1988). The amplified detection of free and bound methoxatin (PQQ) with nitroblue tetrazolium redox reactions: insights into the PQQ-locus. *Biochemical and Biophysical Research Communications*, **154**, 1330–1337.

Paz, M.A., Fluckiger, R., Torrelio, B.M., and Gallop, P.M. (1989). Methoxatin (PQQ), coenzyme for copper-dependent amine and mixed-function oxidation in mammalian tissues. *Connective Tissue Research*, **20**, 251–257.

Paz, M.A., Fluckiger, R., Boak, A., Kagan, H.M., and Gallop, P.M. (1991). Specific detection of quinoproteins by redox-cycling staining. *Journal of Biological Chemistry*, **266**, 689–692.

Peak, J.G., Peak, M.J., Sikorski, R.S., and Jones, C.A. (1985). Induction of DNA-protein crosslinks in human cells by ultraviolet and visible radiations: action spectrum. *Photochemistry and Photobiology*, **41**, 295–302.

Peak, M.J., Peak, J.G., and Jones, C.A. (1985). Different (direct and indirect) mechanisms for the induction of DNA-protein crosslinks in human cells by far- and near-ultraviolet radiations (290 and 405 nm). *Photochemistry and Photobiology*, **42**, 141–146.

Pecht, I., Levitzki, A., and Anbar, M. (1967). The copper-poly-L-histidine complex. I. The environmental effect of the polyelectrolyte on the oxidase activity of copper ions. *Journal of the American Chemical Society*, **89**, 1587–1591.

Pedersen, A.O., Schonheyder, F., and Brodersen, R. (1977). Photooxidation of human serum albumin and its complex with bilirubin. *European Journal of Biochemistry*, **72**, 213–221.

Pedersen, J.Z., and Finazzi, A.A. (1993). Protein-radical enzymes. *FEBS Letters*, **325**, 53–58.

Pellmar, T.C. (1995). Use of brain slices in the study of free-radical actions. *Journal of Neuroscience Methods*, **59**, 93–98.

Peng, M., Huang, L., Xie, Z.J., Huang, W.H., and Askari, A. (1995). Oxidant-induced activations of nuclear factor-kappa B and activator protein-1 in cardiac myocytes. *Cellular and Molecular Biology Research*, **41**, 189–197.

Penning, L.C., Rasch, M.H., Ben, H.E., Dubbelman, T.M., Havelaar, A.C., Van der Zee, J., *et al.* (1992). A role for the transient increase of cytoplasmic free calcium in cell rescue after photodynamic treatment. *Biochimica et Biophysica Acta*, **1107**, 255–260.

Penning, L.C., Tijssen, K., Boegheim, J.P., van Steveninck, J., and Dubbelman, T.M. (1994). Relationship between photodynamically induced damage to various cellular parameters and loss of clonogenicity in different cell types with hemato-porphyrin derivative as sensitizer. *Biochimica et Biophysica Acta*, **1221**, 250–258.

Pennington, M.W., and Byrnes, M.E. (1995). Evaluation of $TiCl_4$-mediated reduction of methionine sulfoxide in peptides with oxidizable or reducible residues. *Peptide Research*, **8**, 39–43.

Pereira, W.E., Hoyano, Y., Summons, R.E., Bacon, V.A., and Duffield, A.M. (1973). Chlorination Studies. II. The reaction of aqueous hypochlorous acid with α-amino acids and dipeptides. *Biochimica et Biophysica Acta.*, **313**, 170–180.

Perkins, M.J. (1980). Spin Trapping. *Advances in Physical Organic Chemistry*, **17**, 1–64.

Perriello, G., Misericordia, P., Volpi, E., Santucci, A., Santucci, C., Ferrannini, E., *et al.* (1994). Acute antihyperglycemic mechanisms of metformin in NIDDM. Evidence for suppression of lipid oxidation and hepatic glucose production. *Diabetes*, **43**, 920–928.

Pesonen, K. (1991). Variation of hydrophobicity of human urinary epidermal growth factor. *Journal of Chromatography*, **568**, 226–231.

Peter, F.A., and Neta, P. (1972). The effect of ionic dissociation of organic compounds on their rate of reaction with hydrated electrons. *Journal of Physical Chemistry*, **76**, 630–635.

Petersen, R.L., Symons, M.C.R., and Taiwo, F.A. (1989). Application of radiation and electron spin resonance spectroscopy to the study of ferryl myoglobin. *Journal of the Chemical Society, Faraday Transactions*, **1**, 2435–2443.

Peterson, D.B., Holian, J., and Garrison, W.M. (1969). Radiation chemistry of the alpha-amino acids. Gamma radiolysis of solid cysteine. *Journal of Physical Chemistry*, **73**, 1568–1572.

Petersson, L., Graslund, A., Ehrenberg, A., Sjoberg, B.M., and Reichard, P. (1980). The iron center in ribonucleotide reductase from *Escherichia coli*. *Journal of Biological Chemistry*, **255**, 6706–6712.

Petit, E., Chancerelle, Y., Dumont, E., Divoux, D., Kergonou, F., and Nouvelot, A. (1995). Polyclonal antibodies against malondialdehyde-modified proteins: characterization and application in study of *in vitro* lipid peroxidation of cellular membranes. *Biochemistry and Molecular Biology International*, **36**, 355–364.

Phelps, R.A., Neet, K.E., Lynn, L.T., and Putnam, F.W. (1961). The cupric ion catalysis of the cleavage of gamma-globulin and other proteins by hydrogen peroxide. *Journal of Biological Chemistry*, **236**, 96–105.

Pichorner, H., Metodiewa, D., and Winterbourn, C.C. (1995). Generation of superoxide and tyrosine peroxide as a result of tyrosyl radical scavenging by glutathione. *Archives of Biochemistry and Biophysics*, **323**, 429–437.

Pierce, S., and Tappel, A.L. (1978). Glutathione peroxidase activities from rat liver. *Biochimica et Biophysica Acta*, **523**, 27–36.

Pietri, S., Culcasi, M., and Cozzone, P.J. (1989). Real-time continuous-flow spin trapping of hydroxyl free radical in the ischemic and post-ischemic myocardium. *European Journal of Biochemistry*, **186**, 163–173.

Pigeolet, E., and Remacle, J. (1991). Susceptibility of glutathione peroxidase to proteolysis after oxidative alteration by peroxides and hydroxyl radicals. *Free Radical Biology and Medicine*, **11**, 191–195.

Piper, P.W. (1995). The heat shock and ethanol stress responses of yeast exhibit extensive similarity and functional overlap. *FEMS Microbiology Letters*, **134**, 121–127.

Pirnay, F., Lacroix, M., Mosora, F., Luyckx, A., and Lefebvre, P. (1977). Effect of glucose ingestion on energy substrate utilization during prolonged muscular exercise. *European Journal of Applied Physiology*, **36**, 247–254.

Pittman, T., Williams, D., Rathore, M., Knutsen, A.P., and Mueller, K.R. (1994). The role of ethylene oxide allergy in sterile shunt malfunctions. *British Journal of Neurosurgery*, **8**, 41–45.

Platis, I.E., Ermacora, M.R., and Fox, R.O. (1993). Oxidative polypeptide cleavage mediated by EDTA-Fe covalently linked to cysteine residues. *Biochemistry*, **32**, 12761–12767.

Pogozheva, I.D., Fedorovich, I.B., Ostrovskii, M.A., and Emanuel, N.M. (1981). Photodamage of rhodopsin molecule. Oxidation of SH-group. *Biofizika*, **26**, 398–403.

Pokorny, J., and Janicek, G. (1971). Reaction of oxidized lipids with proteins. 5. Reaction with paracasein. *Nahrung*, **15**, 317–318.

Pokorny, J., and Janicek, G. (1975). [Interaction between proteins and oxidized lipids]. *Nahrung*, **19**, 911–920.

Pokorny, J., Phan, T.T., Nguyen, T.L., and Janicek, G. (1973). Reactions of oxidized lipids with proteins. 8. Reactions of alkanals with proteins. *Nahrung*, **17**, 621–627.

Pokorny, J., El, Z.A., Nguyen, T.L., and Janicek, G. (1976a). Nonenzymic browning. XV. Effect of unsaturation on browning reactions of oxidized lipids with protein. *Z Lebensm Unters Forsch*, **161**, 271–272.

Pokorny, J., Kocourek, V., and Zajic, J. (1976b). Reactions of oxidized lipids with protein. XIII. Interactions of polar groups of lipids with nonlipidic substances. *Nahrung*, **20**, 707–714.

Pokorny, J., Kminek, M., Janitz, W., Novotna, E., and Davidek, J. (1985). Reactions of oxidized lipids with protein. Part 13. Autoxidation of hexanal in presence of nonlipidic components. *Nahrung*, **29**, 459–465.

Pokorny, J., Davidek, J., Novotna, E., Valentova, H., Janitz, W., and Kminek, M. (1986). Effect of lipid hydroperoxides on animal proteins under conditions of storage and food preparation. *Nahrung*, **30**, 416–418.

Pokorny, J., Davidek, J., Tran, H.C., Valentova, H., Matejicek, J., and Dlaskova, Z. (1988). Reactions of oxidized lipids with protein. Part 15. Mechanism of lipoprotein formation from interactions of oxidized ethyl linoleate with egg albumin. *Nahrung*, **32**, 343–350.

Poli, G., Gravela, E., Albano, E., and Dianzani, M.U. (1979). Studies on fatty liver with isolated hepatocytes. II. The action of carbon tetrachloride on lipid peroxidation, protein, and triglyceride synthesis and secretion. *Experimental Molecular Pathology*, **30**, 116–127.

Pompella, A., Romani, A., Benedetti, A., and Comporti, M. (1991). Loss of membrane protein thiols and lipid peroxidation in allyl alcohol hepatotoxicity. *Biochemical Pharmacology*, **41**, 1255–1259.

Pompella, A., Cambiaggi, C., Dominici, S., Paolicchi, A., Tongiani, R., and Comporti, M. (1996). Single-cell investigation by laser scanning confocal microscopy of cytochemical alterations resulting from extracellular oxidant challenge. *Histochemistry Cellular Biology*, **105**, 173–178.

Porter, N.A., Weber, B.A., Weenan, H., and Khan, J.A. (1980). Autoxidation of polyunsaturated lipids. Factors controlling the streochemistry of product hydroperoxides. *Journal of the American Chemical Society*, **102**, 5597–5601.

Porter, N.A., Lehman, L.S., Weber, B.A., and Smith, K.J. (1981). Unified mechanism for polyunsaturated fatty acid autoxidation. Competition of peroxy radical hydrogen atom abstraction, β-scission, and cyclization. *Journal of the American Chemical Society*, **103**, 6447–6455.

Posener, M.L., Adams, G.E., and Wardman, P. (1976). Mechanism of tryptophan oxidation by some inorganic radical-anions: A pulse radiolysis study. *Journal of the Chemical Society, Faraday Transactions 1*, **72**, 2231–2239.

Posewitz, M.C., and Wilcox, D.E. (1995). Properties of the Sp1 zinc finger 3 peptide: coordination chemistry, redox reactions, and metal binding competition with metallothionein. *Chemical Research in Toxicology*, **8**, 1020–1028.

Poston, J.M., and Parenteau, G.L. (1992). Biochemical effects of ischemia on isolated, perfused rat heart tissues. *Archives of Biochemistry and Biophysics*, **295**, 35–41.

Prabhakaram, M., and Ortwerth, B.J. (1991). The glycation-associated crosslinking of lens proteins by ascorbic acid is not mediated by oxygen free radicals. *Experimental Eye Research*, **53**, 261–268.

Presnell, B., Conti, A., Erhardt, G., Krause, I., and Godovac, Z.J. (1990). A rapid microbore HPLC method for determination of primary structure of beta-lactoglobulin genetic variants. *Journal of Biochemical and Biophysical Methods*, **20**, 325–333.

Prezioso, J.A., Wang, J., Kim, M., Duty, L., Tweardy, D.J., and Gorelik, E. (1995). Augmentation of TNF cytotoxicity by protein kinase C inhibitors: role of arachidonic acid and manganese superoxide dismutase. *Cytokine*, **7**, 517–525.

Prinsze, C., Dubbelman, T.M., and Van Steveninck, J. (1990). Protein damage, induced by small amounts of photodynamically generated singlet oxygen or hydroxyl radicals. *Biochimica et Biophysica Acta*, **1038**, 152–157.

Prinsze, C., Tijssen, K., Dubbelman, T.M., and Van Steveninck, J. (1991a). Potentiation of hyperthermia-induced haemolysis of human erythrocytes by photodynamic treatment. Evidence for the involvement of the anion transporter in this synergistic interaction. *Biochemical Journal*, **271**, 183–188.

Prinsze, C., Dubbelman, T.M., and Van Steveninck, J. (1991*b*). Potentiation of thermal inactivation of glyceraldehyde-3-phosphate dehydrogenase by photodynamic treatment. A possible model for the synergistic interaction between photodynamic therapy and hyperthermia. *Biochemical Journal*, **276**, 357–362.

Pritchard, K.J., Groszek, L., Smalley, D.M., Sessa, W.C., Wu, M., Villalon, P., *et al.* (1995). Native low-density lipoprotein increases endothelial cell nitric oxide synthase generation of superoxide anion. *Circulation Research*, **77**, 510–518.

Prokopenko, V.M., Arutiunian, A.V., Kuz'minykh, T.U., Govorova, E.E., and Frolova, E.V. (1995). Free radical oxidation in placental tissues in preterm delivery. *Voprosy Medicinska Khimii*, **41**, 53–56.

Proudfoot, A.E., Rose, K., and Wallace, C.J. (1989). Conformation-directed recombination of enzyme-activated peptide fragments: a simple and efficient means to protein engineering. Its use in the creation of cytochrome *c* analogues for structure-function studies. *Journal of Biological Chemistry*, **264**, 8764–8770.

Prutz, W.A. (1986). Nitro-tyrosine as promoter of free radical damage in a DNA model system. *Free Radical Research Communications*, **2**, 77–83.

Prutz, W.A. (1990). Free radical transfer involving sulphur peptide functions. In *Sulfur-Centered Reactive Intermediates in Chemistry and Biology*, (ed. C. Chatgilialoglu and K.D. Asmus), pp. 389–399. Plenum Press, New York.

Prutz, W.A. (1992). Catalytic reduction of Fe(III)-cytochrome-c involving stable radiolysis products derived from disulphides, proteins and thiols. *International Journal of Radiation Biology and Related Studies in Physics, Chemistry and Medicine*, **61**, 593–602.

Prutz, W.A., and Land, E.J. (1979). Charge transfer in peptides. Pulse radiolysis investigation of one-electron reactions in dipeptides of tryptophan and tyrosine. *International Journal of Radiation Biology and Related Studies in Physics, Chemistry and Medicine*, **36**, 513–520.

Prutz, W.A., Butler, J., Land, E.J., and Swallow, A.J. (1980). Direct demonstration of electron transfer between tryptophan and tyrosine in proteins. *Biochemical and Biophysical Research Communications*, **96**, 408–414.

Prutz, W.A., Land, E.J., and Sloper, R.W. (1981). Charge transfer in peptides. Effects of temperature, peptide length and solvent conditions upon intramolecular one-electron reactions involving tryptophan and tyrosine. *Journal of the Chemical Society, Faraday Transactions 1*, **77**, 281–292.

Prutz, W.A., Siebert, F., Butler, J., Land, E.J., Menez, A., and Montenay-Garestier, T. (1982). Charge transfer in peptides. Intramolecular radical transformations involving methionine, tryptophan and tyrosine. *Biochimica et Biophysica Acta*, **705**, 139–149.

Prutz, W.A., Butler, J., and Land, E.J. (1983). Phenol coupling initiated by one-electron oxidation of tyrosine units in peptides and histone. *International Journal of Radiation Biology and Related Studies in Physics, Chemistry and Medicine*, **44**, 183–196.

Prutz, W.A., Butler, J., and Land, E.J. (1985). Methionyl-tyrosyl radical transitions initiated by Br2$^-$. in peptide model systems and ribonuclease A. *International Journal of Radiation Biology and Related Studies on Physics, Chemistry and Medicine*, **47**, 149–156.

Prutz, W.A., Butler, J., Land, E.J., and Swallow, A.J. (1986). Unpaired electron migration between aromatic and sulfur peptide units. *Free Radical Research Communications*, **2**, 69–75.

Prutz, W.A., Butler, J., Land, E.J., and Swallow, A.J. (1989). The role of sulphur peptide functions in free radical transfer: a pulse radiolysis study. *International Journal of Radiation Biology and Related Studies in Physics, Chemistry and Medicine*, **55**, 539–556.

Pryor, W.A. (1966) *Free Radicals*. McGraw-Hill, New York.

Pryor, W.A. (1992). Biological effects of cigarette smoke, wood smoke, and the smoke from plastics: the use of electron spin resonance. *Free Radical Biology and Medicine*, **13**, 659–676.

Pryor, W.A., Lightsey, J.W., and Church, D.F. (1982). Reaction of nitrogen dioxide with alkenes and polyunsaturated fatty acids: addition and hydrogen abstraction mechanisms. *Journal of the American Chemical Society*, **104**, 6685–6692.

Pryor, W.A., Dooley, M.M., and Church, D.F. (1985). Mechanisms of cigarette smoke toxicity: the inactivation of human alpha-1-proteinase inhibitor by nitric oxide/isoprene mixtures in air. *Chemico-Biological Interactions*, **54**, 171–183.

Pryor, W.A., Cueto, R., Jin, X., Koppenol, W.H., Ngu, S.M., Squadrito, G.L., *et al.* (1995). A practical method for preparing peroxynitrite solutions of low ionic strength and free of hydrogen peroxide. *Free Radical Biology and Medicine*, **18**, 75–83.

Puchala, M., and Schuessler, H. (1986). Radiation-induced binding of methanol, ethanol and 1-butanol to haemoglobin. *International Journal of Radiation Biology and Related Studies in Physics, Chemistry and Medicine*, **50**, 535–546.

Puchala, M., and Schuessler, H. (1993). Oxygen effect in the radiolysis of proteins. III. Haemoglobin. *International Journal of Radiation Biology and Related Studies in Physics, Chemistry and Medicine*, **64**, 149–156.

Puchala, M., and Schuessler, H. (1995). Oxygen effect in the radiolysis of proteins. IV. Myoglobin. *International Journal of Peptide and Protein Research*, **46**, 326–332.

Puhl, H., Waeg, G., and Esterbauer, H. (1994). Methods to determine oxidation of low-density lipoproteins. *Methods in Enzymology*, **233**, 425–441.

Pumiglia, K.M., Lau, L.F., Huang, C.K., Burroughs, S., and Feinstein, M.B. (1992). Activation of signal transduction in platelets by the tyrosine phosphatase inhibitor pervanadate (vanadyl hydroperoxide). *Biochemical Journal*, **286**, 441–449.

Punchard, N.A., and Kelly, F.J. (eds.) (1996). *Free Radicals. A Practical Approach*. IRL Press, Oxford.

Puppo, A., and Davies, M.J. (1995). The reactivity of thiol compounds with different redox states of leghaemoglobin: evidence for competing reduction and addition pathways. *Biochimica et Biophysica Acta*, **1246**, 74–81.

Puppo, A., and Halliwell, B. (1988*a*). Formation of hydroxyl radicals in biological systems. Does myoglobin stimulate hydroxyl radical formation from hydrogen peroxide? *Free Radical Research Communications*, **4**, 415–422.

Puppo, A., and Halliwell, B. (1988*b*). Formation of hydroxyl radicals from hydrogen peroxide in the presence of iron. Is haemoglobin a biological Fenton reagent? *Biochemical Journal*, **249**, 185–190.

Puppo, A., Monny, C., and Davies, M.J. (1993). Glutathione-dependent conversion of ferryl leghaemoglobin into the ferric form: a potential protective process in soybean (Glycine max) root nodules. *Biochemical Journal*, **289**, 435–438.

Purdie, J.W. (1967). γ-Radiolysis of cystine in aqueous solution. Dose-rate effects and a proposed mechanism. *Journal of the American Chemical Society*, **89**, 226–230.

Purdie, J.W., and Lynn, K.R. (1973). The influence of gamma-radiation on the structure and biological activity of oxytocin, a cyclic oligopeptide. *International*

Journal of Radiation Biology and Related Studies in Physics, Chemistry and Medicine, **23**, 583–589.

Purdy, R.E., and Tappel, A.L. (1979). Permeation chromatography of fluorescent products from tissues and peroxidized lipids. *Journal of Chromatography*, **170**, 217–220.

Puttfarcken, P.S., Manelli, A.M., Neilly, J., and Frail, D.E. (1996). Inhibition of age-induced beta-amyloid neurotoxicity in rat hippocampal cells. *Experimental Neurology*, **138**, 73–81.

Qin, J., Clore, G.M., and Gronenborn, A.M. (1996). Ionization equilibria for side-chain carboxyl groups in oxidized and reduced human thioredoxin and in the complex with its target peptide from the transcription factor NF kappa B. *Biochemistry*, **35**, 7–13.

Qin, S., Inazu, T., Takata, M., Kurosaki, T., Homma, Y., and Yamamura, H. (1996). Cooperation of tyrosine kinases p72syk and p53/56lyn regulates calcium mobilization in chicken B cell oxidant stress signaling. *European Journal of Biochemistry*, **236**, 443–449.

Qiu, Y., Bernier, M., and Hearse, D.J. (1990). The influence of *N*-acetylcysteine on cardiac function and rhythm disorders during ischemia and reperfusion. *Cardioscience*, **1**, 65–74.

Qiu, Y., Galinanes, M., Ferrari, R., Cargnoni, A., Ezrin, A., and Hearse, D.J. (1992). PEG-SOD improves postischemic functional recovery and antioxidant status in blood-perfused rabbit hearts. *American Journal of Physiology*, **263**, H1243–1249.

Quillet, M.A., Mansat, V., Duchayne, E., Come, M.G., Allouche, M., Bailly, J.D., *et al.* (1996). Daunorubicin-induced internucleosomal DNA fragmentation in acute myeloid cell lines. *Leukemia*, **10**, 417–425.

Quinkal, I., Kyritsis, P., Kohzuma, T., Im, S.C., Sykes, A.G., and Moulis, J.M. (1996). The influence of conserved aromatic residues on the electron transfer reactivity of 2[4Fe-4S] ferredoxins. *Biochimica et Biophysica Acta*, **1295**, 201–208.

Quinlan, G.J., Evans, T.W., and Gutteridge, J.M. (1994). Oxidative damage to plasma proteins in adult respiratory distress syndrome. *Free Radical Research*, **20**, 289–298.

Quintanilha, A.T., and Davies, K.J. (1982). Vitamin E deficiency and photo-sensitization of electron-transport carriers in microsomes. *FEBS Letters*, **139**, 241–244.

Quintanilha, A.T., Packer, L., Davies, J.M., Racanelli, T.L., and Davies, K.J. (1982). Membrane effects of vitamin E deficiency: bioenergetic and surface charge density studies of skeletal muscle and liver mitochondria. *Annals of the New York Academy of Science*, **393**, 32–47.

Rabani, J., Klug-Roth, D., and Henglein, A. (1974). Pulse radiolytic investigations of $OHCH_2O_2$ radicals. *Journal of Physical Chemistry*, **78**, 2089–2093.

Rabgaoui, N., Slaoui, H.A., and Torreilles, J. (1993). Boomerang effect between [Met]-enkephalin derivatives and human polymorphonuclear leukocytes. *Free Radical Biology and Medicine*, **14**, 519–529.

Rabilloud, T., Berthier, R., Vincon, M., Ferbus, D., Goubin, G., and Lawrence, J.J. (1995). Early events in erythroid differentiation: accumulation of the acidic peroxidoxin (PRP/TSA/NKEF-B). *Biochemical Journal*, **312**, 699–705.

Rabinovitch, C.H., Cook, M.J., Breton, J.C., and Rigaud, M. (1992). Purification of lipoxygenase and hydroperoxide dehydrase in flaxseeds: interaction between these enzymatic activities. *Biochemical and Biophysical Research Communications*, **188**, 858–864.

Raffioni, S., Luporini, P., and Bradshaw, R.A. (1989). Purification, characterization, and amino acid sequence of the mating pheromone Er-10 of the ciliate *Euplotes raikovi*. *Biochemistry*, **28**, 5250–5256.

Raghavan, N.V., and Steenken, S. (1980). Electrophilic reaction of the OH radical with phenol. Determination of the distribution of isomeric dihydroxycyclo-hexadienyl radicals. *Journal of the American Chemical Society*, **102**, 3495–3499.

Raghothama, C., and Rao, P. (1994). Increased proteolysis of oxidatively damaged hemoglobin in erythrocyte lysates in diabetes mellitus. *Clinica Chimica Acta*, **225**, 65–70.

Rainwater, R., Parks, D., Anderson, M.E., Tegtmeyer, P., and Mann, K. (1995). Role of cysteine residues in regulation of p53 function. *Molecular and Cellular Biology*, **15**, 3892–3903.

Rajavashisth, T.B., Yamada, H., and Mishra, N.K. (1995). Transcriptional activation of the macrophage-colony stimulating factor gene by minimally modified LDL. Involvement of nuclear factor-kappa B. *Arteriosclerosis Thrombosis and Vascular Biology*, **15**, 1591–1598.

Rajewsky, B. (1929). Reactions of protein following UV and roentgen irradiations. *Strahlentherapie*, **33**, 362–374.

Rajewsky, I.B. (1930). The effect of short wave radiation on proteins. I. *Biochem Zeitschrift*, **227**, 272–285.

Rajguru, S.U., Yeargans, G.S., and Seidler, N.W. (1994). Exercise causes oxidative damage to rat skeletal muscle microsomes while increasing cellular sulfydryls. *Life Science*, **54**, 149–157.

Rall, D.P. (1974). Review of the health effects of sulfur oxides. *Environmental Health Perspectives*, **8**, 97–121.

Ramakrishnan, N., Kalinich, J.F., and McClain, D.E. (1996). Ebselen inhibition of apoptosis by reduction of peroxides. *Biochemical Pharmacology*, **51**, 1443–1451.

Ramos, C.L., Pou, S., and Rosen, G.M. (1995). Effect of anti-inflammatory drugs on myeloperoxidase-dependent hydroxyl radical generation by human neutrophils. *Biochemical Pharmacology*, **49**, 1079–1084.

Ramprasad, M.P., Fischer, W., Witztum, J.L., Sambrano, G.R., Quehenberger, O., and Steinberg, D. (1995). The 94- to 97-kDa mouse macrophage membrane protein that recognizes oxidized low density lipoprotein and phosphatidylserine-rich liposomes is identical to macrosialin, the mouse homologue of human CD68. *Proceedings of the National Academy of Science of the United States of America*, **92**, 9580–9584.

Ramsey, A.J., Daubner, S.C., Ehrlich, J.I., and Fitzpatrick, P.F. (1995). Identification of iron ligands in tyrosine hydroxylase by mutagenesis of conserved histidinyl residues. *Protein Science*, **4**, 2082–2086.

Rana, T.M., and Meares, C.F. (1990). Specific cleavage of a protein by an attached iron chelate. *Journal of the American Chemical Society*, **112**, 2457–2458.

Rana, T.M., and Meares, C.F. (1991a). Transfer of oxygen from an artificial protease to peptide carbon during proteolysis. *Proceedings of the National Academy of Science of the United States of America*, **88**, 10578–10582.

Rana, T.M., and Meares, C.F. (1991b). Iron Chelate Mediated Proteolysis: Protein Structure Dependence. *Journal of the American Chemical Society*, **113**, 1859–1861.

Rao, P.S., and Hayon, E. (1974). Interaction of hydrated electrons with the peptide linkage. *Journal of Physical Chemistry*, **78**, 1193–1196.

Rao, P.S., and Hayon, E. (1975). Reactions of hydroxyl radicals with oligopeptides in aqueous solutions. *Journal of Physical Chemistry*, **79**, 109–115.

Rao, P.S., Simic, M., and Hayon, E. (1975). Pulse radiolysis study of imidazole and histidine in water. *Journal of Physical Chemistry*, **79**, 1260–1263.

Rao, S.I., Wilks, A., and Ortiz, d.M.P. (1993). The roles of His-64, Tyr-103, Tyr-146, and Tyr-151 in the epoxidation of styrene and beta-methylstyrene by recombinant sperm whale myoglobin. *Journal of Biological Chemistry*, **268**, 803–809.

Rao, S.I., Wilks, A., Hamberg, M., and Ortiz, d.M.P. (1994). The lipoxygenase activity of myoglobin. Oxidation of linoleic acid by the ferryl oxygen rather than protein radical. *Journal of Biological Chemistry*, **269**, 7210–7216.

Rao, V.S., Chaves, M.C., and Ribeiro, R.A. (1995). Nitric oxide synthase inhibition and the uterotrophic response to oestrogen in immature rats. *Journal of Reproductive Fertility*, **105**, 303–306.

Raper. (1932). Note on the oxidation of tyrosine, tyramine and phenylalanine with hydrogen peroxide. *Biochemical Journal*, **26**, 2000–2004.

Raschke, P., Massoudy, P., and Becker, B.F. (1995). Taurine protects the heart from neutrophil-induced reperfusion injury. *Free Radical Biology and Medicine*, **19**, 461–471.

Rassat, A., and Rey, P. (1967). Nitroxides. 23. Preparation of amino acid free radicals and their complex salts. *Bulletin Societe Chimique France*, **3**, 815–818.

Rauk, A., Yu, D., and Armstrong, D.A. (1997). Toward site specificity of oxidative damage in proteins: C–H and C–C bond dissociation energies and reduction potentials of the radicals of alanine, serine, and threonine residues—an ab initio study. *Journal of the American Chemical Society*, **119**, 208–217.

Ravi, N., Moura, I., Costa, C., Teixeira, M., LeGall, J., Moura, J.J., *et al.* (1992). Mossbauer characterization of the tetraheme cytochrome *c*3 from *Desulfovibrio baculatus (DSM 1743)*. Spectral deconvolution of the heme components. *European Journal of Biochemistry*, **204**, 779–782.

Ravichandran, V., Seres, T., Moriguchi, T., Thomas, J.A., and Johnston, R.J. (1994). S-thiolation of glyceraldehyde-3-phosphate dehydrogenase induced by the phagocytosis-associated respiratory burst in blood monocytes. *Journal of Biological Chemistry*, **269**, 25010–25015.

Rawlings, J., Stephens, P.J., Nafie, L.A., and Kamen, M.D. (1977). Near-infrared magnetic circular dichroism of cytochrome *c'*. *Biochemistry*, **16**, 1725–1729.

Ray, B.R., Davisson, E.O., and Crespi, H.L. (1954). Experiments on the degradation of lipoproteins from serum. *Journal of Physical Chemistry*, **58**, 841–846.

Reaven, P.D., Herold, D.A., Barnett, J., and Edelman, S. (1995). Effects of Vitamin E on susceptibility of low-density lipoprotein and low-density lipoprotein subfractions to oxidation and on protein glycation in NIDDM. *Diabetes Care*, **18**, 807–816.

Reddy, K., and Tappel, A.L. (1974). Effect of dietary selenium and autoxidized lipids on the glutathione peroxidase system of gastrointestinal tract and other tissues in the rat. *Journal of Nutrition*, **104**, 1069–1078.

Reddy, S., Bichler, J., Wells-Knecht, K.J., Thorpe, S.R., and Baynes, J.W. (1995). N^{ε}-(Carboxymethyl)lysine is a dominant advanced glycation end product (AGE) antigen in tissue proteins. *Biochemistry*, **34**, 10872–10878.

Reddy, V.Y., Desorchers, P.E., Pizzo, S.V., Gonias, S.L., Sahakian, J.A., Levine, R.L., *et al.* (1994). Oxidative dissociation of human alpha 2-macroglobulin tetramers into dysfunctional dimers. *Journal of Biological Chemistry*, **269**, 4683–4691.

Redpath, J.L., and Willson, R.L. (1975). Chain reactions and radiosensitization: model enzyme studies. *International Journal of Radiation Biology and Related Studies in Physics, Chemistry and Medicine*, **27**, 389–398.

Redpath, J.L., Santus, R., Ovadia, J., and Grossweiner, L.I. (1975a). The role of metal ions in the radiosensitivity of metalloproteins. Model experiments with bovine carbonic anhydrase. *International Journal of Radiation Biology and Related Studies in Physics, Chemistry and Medicine*, **28**, 243–253.

Redpath, J.L., Santus, R., Ovadia, J., and Grossweiner, L.I. (1975b). The oxidation of tryptophan by radical anions. *International Journal of Radiation Biology and Related Studies in Physics, Chemistry and Medicine*, **27**, 201–204.

Reeves, J.P., Bailey, C.A., and Hale, C.C. (1986). Redox modification of sodium-calcium exchange activity in cardiac sarcolemmal vesicles. *Journal of Biological Chemistry*, **261**, 4948–4955.

Reif, D.W., Schubert, J., and Aust, S.D. (1988). Iron release from ferritin and lipid peroxidation by radiolytically generated reducing radicals. *Archives of Biochemistry and Biophysics*, **264**, 238–243.

Reinhart, W.H., Sung, L.P., and Chien, S. (1986). Quantitative relationship between Heinz body formation and red blood cell deformability [see comments]. *Blood*, **68**, 1376–1383.

Reinheckel, T., Wiswedel, I., Noack, H., and Augustin, W. (1995). Electrophoretic evidence for the impairment of complexes of the respiratory chain during iron/ascorbate induced peroxidation in isolated rat liver mitochondria. *Biochimica et Biophysica Acta*, **1239**, 45–50.

Reiss, U., and Tappel, A.L. (1973). Decreased activity in protein synthesis systems from liver of vitamin E-deficient rats. *Biochimica et Biophysica Acta*, **312**, 608–615.

Reiss, U., Tappel, A.L., and Chio, K.S. (1972). DNA-malonaldehyde reaction: formation of fluorescent products. *Biochemical and Biophysical Research Communications*, **48**, 921–926.

Reiter, R.J. (1995a). The role of the neurohormone melatonin as a buffer against macromolecular oxidative damage. *Neurochemistry International*, **27**, 453–460.

Reiter, R.J. (1995b). Functional pleiotropy of the neurohormone melatonin: antioxidant protection and neuroendocrine regulation. *Frontiers of Neuroendocrinology*, **16**, 383–415.

Remmer, H., Kessler, W., Einsele, H., Hintze, T., Diaz, d.T.G., Gharaibeh, A.M., et al. (1989). Ethanol promotes oxygen-radical attack on proteins but not on lipids. *Drug Metabolism Reviews*, **20**, 219–232.

Requena, J.R., Vidal, P., and Cabezas, C.J. (1992). Aminoguanidine inhibits the modification of proteins by lipid peroxidation derived aldehydes: a possible antiatherogenic agent. *Diabetes Research*, **20**, 43–49.

Reszka, K.J., Bilski, P., Chignell, C.F., and Dillon, J. (1996). Free Radical Reactions Photosensitized by the Human Lens Component, Kynurenine: An EPR and Spin Trapping Investigation. *Free Radical Biology and Medicine*, **20**, 23–24.

Retsky, K.L., and Frei, B. (1995). Vitamin C prevents metal ion-dependent initiation and propagation of lipid peroxidation in human low-density lipoprotein. *Biochimica et Biophysica Acta*, **1257**, 279–287.

Retsky, K.L., Freeman, M.W., and Frei, B. (1993). Ascorbic acid oxidation product(s) protect human low density lipoprotein against atherogenic modification. Anti- rather than prooxidant activity of vitamin C in the presence of transition metal ions. *Journal of Biological Chemistry*, **268**, 1304–1309.

Reznick, A.Z., Kagan, V.E., Ramsey, R., Tsuchiya, M., Khwaja, S., Serbinova, E.A., et al. (1992a). Antiradical effects in L-propionyl carnitine protection of the heart against ischemia-reperfusion injury: the possible role of iron chelation. *Archives of Biochemistry and Biophysics*, **296**, 394–401.

Reznick, A.Z., Witt, E., Matsumoto, M., and Packer, L. (1992*b*). Vitamin E inhibits protein oxidation in skeletal muscle of resting and exercised rats. *Biochemical and Biophysical Research Communications*, **189**, 801–806.

Reznick, A.Z., Cross, C.E., Hu, M.L., Suzuki, Y.J., Khwaja, S., Safadi, A., et al. (1992*c*). Modification of plasma proteins by cigarette smoke as measured by protein carbonyl formation. *Biochemical Journal*, , **286**, 607–611.

Rhee, S.G., Chock, P.B., and Stadtman, E.R. (1985). Glutamine synthetase from *Escherichia coli*. *Methods in Enzymology*, **113**, 213–241.

Rhee, S.G., Chock, P.B., and Stadtman, E.R. (1989). Regulation of *Escherichia coli* glutamine synthetase. *Advances in Enzymology and Related Areas in Molecular Biology*, **62**, 37–92.

Rhee, S.G., Kim, K., Kim, I.H., and Stadtman, E.R. (1990). Protein that prevents mercaptan-mediated protein oxidation. *Methods in Enzymology*, **186**, 478–485.

Rhee, S.G., Kim, K.H., Chae, H.Z., Yim, M.B., Uchida, K., Netto, L.E., et al. (1994). Antioxidant defense mechanisms: a new thiol-specific antioxidant enzyme. *Annals of the New York Academy of Science*, **738**, 86–92.

Rice, G.E., and Barnea, A. (1983). A possible role for copper-mediated oxidation of thiols in the regulation of the release of luteinizing hormone releasing hormone from isolated hypothalamic granules. *Journal of Neurochemistry*, **41**, 1672–1679.

Rice, R.H., Lee, Y.M., and Brown, W.D. (1983). Interactions of heme proteins with hydrogen peroxide: protein crosslinking and covalent binding of benzo[a]pyrene and 17 beta-estradiol. *Archives of Biochemistry and Biophysics*, **221**, 417–427.

Richards, D.M., Dean, R.T., and Jessup, W. (1988). Membrane proteins are critical targets in free radical mediated cytolysis. *Biochimica et Biophysica Acta*, **946**, 281–288.

Richards, P.G., Coles, B., Heptinstall, J., and Walton, D.J. (1994). Electrochemical modification of lysozyme: anodic reaction of tyrosine residues. *Enzyme Microbology Technology*, **16**, 795–801.

Richards, P.G., Walton, D.J., and Heptinstall, J. (1996). The effects of tyrosine nitration on the structure and function of hen egg-white lysozyme. *Biochemical Journal*, **315**, 473–479.

Richardson, J.S., Zhou, Y., and Kumar, U. (1996). Free radicals in the neurotoxic actions of beta-amyloid. *Annals of the New York Academy of Science*, **777**, 362–367.

Richter, C. (1987). Biophysical consequences of lipid peroxidation in membranes. *Chemistry and Physics of Lipids*, **44**, 175–189.

Richter, C. (1992). Reactive oxygen and DNA damage in mitochondria. *Mutation Research*, **275**, 249–255.

Richter, C. (1995). Oxidative damage to mitochondrial DNA and its relationship to ageing. *International Journal of Biochemistry Cellular Biology*, **27**, 647–653.

Richter, C., and Schlegel, J. (1993). Mitochondrial calcium release induced by prooxidants. *Toxicology Letters*, **67**, 119–127.

Richter, C., Frei, B., and Cerutti, P.A. (1987). Mobilization of mitochondrial Ca^{2+} by hydroperoxy-eicosatetraenoic acid. *Biochemical and Biophysical Research Communications*, **143**, 609–616.

Richter, C., Park, J.W., and Ames, B.N. (1988). Normal oxidative damage to mitochondrial and nuclear DNA is extensive. *Proceedings of the National Academy of Science of the United States of America*, **85**, 6465–6467.

Richter, C., Schlegel, J., and Schweizer, M. (1992). Prooxidant-induced Ca^{2+} release from liver mitochondria. Specific versus nonspecific pathways. *Annals of the New York Academy of Science*, **663**, 262–268.

Richter, C., Gogvadze, V., Schlapbach, R., Schweizer, M., and Schlegel, J. (1994). Nitric oxide kills hepatocytes by mobilizing mitochondrial calcium. *Biochemical and Biophysical Research Communications*, **205**, 1143–1150.

*Richter, C., Gogvadze, V., Laffranchi, R., Schlapbach, R., Schweizer, M., Suter, M., et al. (1995). Oxidants in mitochondria: from physiology to diseases. *Biochimica et Biophysica Acta*, **1271**, 67–74.

Richter, F., and Kuhn, F. (1924). Oxidation of amino acids with hydrogen peroxide and at the anode. *Helvetica Chimica Acta*, **7**, 167–172.

Riedl, A., Anderton, M., Shamsi, Z., Goldfarb, P., and Wiseman, A. (1995). Structural modulation of lipid peroxidation by the proteins within membranes: model protein studies with liposomes. *Biochemical Society Transactions*, **23**, 251S.

Rieser, P. (1956). Radiation induced alteration of fibrinogen clotting rate and clot lability. *Proceedings of the Society for Experimental Biology and Medicine*, **91**, 654–657.

Rieser, P., and Rutman, R.J. (1957). On the nature of the clotting defect in irradiated fibrinogen. *Archives of Biochemistry and Biophysics*, **66**, 247–249.

Riesz, P., and White, F.H. (1968). Tritiated free radical scavengers in the study of the irradiated protein molecule. In *Radiation Chemistry Vol. 1*, (ed. R.F. Gould), pp. 496–520. American Chemical Society, Washington.

Riesz, P., Smitherman, T.C., and Scher, C.D. (1970). Hydrogen transfer from exchangeable to carbon-bound sites in gamma-irradiated proteins and nucleic acids: the mechanism of radical saturation. *International Journal of Radiation Biology and Related Studies in Physics, Chemistry and Medicine*, **17**, 389–393.

Rikans, L.E., and Cai, Y. (1993). Diquat-induced oxidative damage in BCNU-pretreated hepatocytes of mature and old rats. *Toxicology and Applied Pharmacology*, **118**, 263–270.

Riley, M.L., and Harding, J.J. (1993). The reaction of malondialdehyde with lens proteins and the protective effect of aspirin. *Biochimica et Biophysica Acta*, **1158**, 107–112.

Rimoldi, J.M., Wang, Y.X., Nimkar, S.K., Kuttab, S.H., Anderson, A.H., Burch, H., et al. (1995). Probing the mechanism of bioactivation of MPTP type analogs by monoamine oxidase B: structure-activity studies on substituted 4-phenoxy-, 4-phenyl-, and 4-thiophenoxy-1-cyclopropyl-1,2,3,6-tetrahydropyridines. *Chemical Research Toxicology*, **8**, 703–710.

Riordan, J.F., Wacker, W.E., and Vallee, B.L. (1965). *N*-Acetylimidazole: A reagent for determination of 'free' tyrosyl residues of proteins. *Biochemistry*, **4**, 1758–1765.

Riva, E., Manning, A.S., and Hearse, D.J. (1987). Superoxide dismutase and the reduction of reperfusion-induced arrhythmias: *in vivo* dose-response studies in the rat. *Cardiovascular Drugs and Therapies*, **1**, 133–139.

Rivett, A.J., and Levine, R.L. (1987). Enhanced proteolytic susceptibility of oxidized proteins. *Biochemical Society Transactions*, **15**, 816–818.

Rivett, A.J., and Levine, R.L. (1990). Metal-catalyzed oxidation of *Escherichia coli* glutamine synthetase: correlation of structural and functional changes. *Archives of Biochemistry and Biophysics*, **278**, 26–34.

Rivett, A.J., Roseman, J.E., Oliver, C.N., Levine, R.L., and Stadtman, E.R. (1985). Covalent modification of proteins by mixed-function oxidation: recognition by intracellular proteases. *Progress in Clinical Biological Research*, **180**, 317–328.

Roberts, C.R., and Dean, R.T. (1986). Degradation of cartilage by macrophages in culture: evidence for the involvement of an enzyme which is associated with the cell surface. *Connective Tissue Research*, **14**, 199–212.

Roberts, C.R., Roughley, P.J., and Mort, J. (1987). Treatment of cartilage aggregate with hydrogen peroxide. Relationship between observed degradation products and those that occur naturally during aging. *Biochemical Journal*, **247**, 349–357.

Roberts, C.R., Roughley, P.J., and Mort, J.S. (1989). Degradation of human proteoglycan aggregate induced by hydrogen peroxide. Protein fragmentation, amino acid modification and hyaluronic acid cleavage. *Biochemical Journal*, **259**, 805–811.

Robinson, M.G., Weiss, J.J., and Wheeler, C.M. (1966a). Irradiation deoxyribonucleohistone solutions. I. Amino acid destruction. *Biochimica et Biophysica Acta*, **124**, 176–180.

Robinson, M.G., Weiss, J.J., and Wheeler, C.M. (1966b). Irradiation of deoxyribonucleohistone solutions. II. Labilization of the DNA-histone linkage. *Biochimica et Biophysica Acta*, **124**, 181–186.

Rocha, V., Deeley, M., and Crawford, I.P. (1979). Conservation of primary structure of the pyridoxyl peptide of *Escherichia coli* and *Serratia marcescens* tryptophan synthase beta2 protein. *Journal of Bacteriology*, **137**, 700–703.

Rodgers, M.A., and Garrison, W.M. (1968). Excited-molecule reactions in the radiolysis of peptides in concentrated aqueous solution. *Journal of Physical Chemistry*, **72**, 758–759.

Rodgers, M.A., Sokol, H.A., and Garrison, W.M. (1968). The radiation-induced 'hydrolysis' of the peptide bond. *Journal of the American Chemical Society*, **90**, 795–796.

Rodgers, M.A., Sokol, H.A., and Garrison, W.M. (1970). Radiolytic cleavage of the peptide main-chain in concentrated aqueous solution: energy level of excited-molecule intermediates. *Biochemical and Biophysical Research Communications*, **40**, 622–627.

Rodriguez, L.J., Banon, A.M., Martinez, O.F., Tudela, J., Acosta, M., Varon, R., *et al.* (1992). Catalytic oxidation of 2,4,5-trihydroxyphenylalanine by tyrosinase: identification and evolution of intermediates. *Biochimica et Biophysica Acta*, **1160**, 221–228.

Roebke, W., Renz, M., and Henglein, A. (1969). Pulseradiolyse der anionen $S_2O_8^{2-}$ und HSO_5^- in wassriger Losung. *International Journal of Radiation and Physical Chemistry*, **1**, 39–44.

Roginsky, V.A., Mohr, D., and Stocker, R. (1996). Reduction of ubiquinone-1 by ascorbic acid is a catalytic and reversible process controlled by the concentration of molecular oxygen. *Redox Report*, **2**, 55–62.

Roh, J.H., Takenaka, Y., Suzuki, H., Yamamoto, K., and Kumagai, H. (1995). Escherichia coli K-12 copper-containing monoamine oxidase: investigation of the copper binding ligands by site-directed mutagenesis, elemental analysis and topa quinone formation. *Biochemical and Biophysical Research Communications*, **212**, 1107–1114.

Rokutan, K., Thomas, J.A., and Sies, H. (1989). Specific S-thiolation of a 30-kDa cytosolic protein from rat liver under oxidative stress. *European Journal of Biochemistry*, **179**, 233–239.

Rokutan, K., Thomas, J.A., and Johnston, R.B. (1991). Phagocytosis and stimulation of the respiratory burst by phorbol diester initiate S-thiolation of specific proteins in macrophages. *Journal of Immunology*, **147**, 260–264.

Rokutan, K., Johnston, R.J., and Kawai, K. (1994). Oxidative stress induces S-thiolation of specific proteins in cultured gastric mucosal cells. *American Journal of Physiology*, **266**, G247–254.

Roma, P., Bernini, F., Fogliatto, R., Bertulli, S.M., Negri, S., Fumagalli, R., et al. (1992). Defective catabolism of oxidized LDL by J774 murine macrophages. Journal of Lipid Research, 33, 819–829.

Romani, R.J., and Tappel, A.L. (1959). Anaerobic irradiation of alcohol dehydrogenase, aldolase and ribonuclease. Archives of Biochemistry and Biophysics, 79, 323–329.

Romani, R.J., and Tappel, A.L. (1960). Irradiation of egg albumin solutions uner anaerobic conditions. Radiation Research, 12, 526–531.

Romero, F.J., Ordonez, I., Arduini, A., and Cadenas, E. (1992). The reactivity of thiols and disulfides with different redox states of myoglobin. Redox and addition reactions and formation of thiyl radical intermediates. Journal of Biological Chemistry, 267, 1680–1688.

Roseman, J.E., and Levine, R.L. (1987). Purification of a protease from Escherichia coli with specificity for oxidized glutamine synthetase. Journal of Biological Chemistry, 262, 2101–2110.

Rosenberg, P.A., Loring, R., Xie, Y., Zaleskas, V., and Aizenman, E. (1991). 2,4,5-trihydroxyphenylalanine in solution forms a non-N-methyl-D-aspartate glutamatergic agonist and neurotoxin. Proceedings of the National Academy of Science of the United States of America, 88, 4865–4869.

Rosenfeld, M.E., Palinski, W., Yla, H.S., and Carew, T.E. (1990). Macrophages, endothelial cells, and lipoprotein oxidation in the pathogenesis of atherosclerosis. Toxicolology and Pathology, 18, 560–571.

Rosenfeld, M.E., Khoo, J.C., Miller, E., Parthasarathy, S., Palinski, W., and Witztum, J.L. (1991). Macrophage-derived foam cells freshly isolated from rabbit atherosclerotic lesions degrade modified lipoproteins, promote oxidation of low-density lipoproteins, and contain oxidation-specific lipid-protein adducts. Journal of Clinical Investigation, 87, 90–99.

Rosenthal, I., Mossoba, M.M., and Riesz, P. (1981). Dibenzoyl peroxide induced photodecarboxylation of amino acids and peptides. A spin-trapping study. Journal of Physical Chemistry, 85, 2398–2403.

Rosselli, F., Ridet, A., Soussi, T., Duchaud, E., Alapetite, C., and Moustacchi, E. (1995). p53-dependent pathway of radio-induced apoptosis is altered in Fanconi anemia. Oncogene, 10, 9–17.

Rossi, F., De Togni, P., Bellavite, P., Della Bianca, V., and Grzeskowiak, M. (1983). Relationship between the binding of N-formylmethionylleucylphenylalanine and the respiratory response in human neutrophils. Biochimica et Biophysica Acta, 758, 168–175.

Roubal, W.T. (1970). Trapped radicals in dry lipid-protein systems undergoing oxidation. Journal of the American Oil and Chemical Society, 47, 141–144.

Roubal, W.T. (1971). Free radicals, malonaldehyde and protein damage in lipid-protein systems. Lipids, 6, 62–64.

Roubal, W.T., and Tappel, A.L. (1966a). Polymerization of proteins induced by free-radical lipid peroxidation. Archives of Biochemistry and Biophysics, 113, 150–155.

Roubal, W.T., and Tappel, A.L. (1966b). Damage to proteins, enzymes, and amino acids by peroxidizing lipids. Archives of Biochemistry and Biophysics, 113, 5–8.

Rowbottom, J. (1955). The radiolysis of aqueous solutions of tyrosine. Journal of Biological Chemistry, 212, 877–885.

Roy, B., Lepoivre, M., Henry, Y., and Fontecave, M. (1995). Inhibition of ribonucleotide reductase by nitric oxide derived from thionitrites: reversible modifications of both subunits. Biochemistry, 34, 5411–5418.

Royall, J.A., Kooy, N.W., and Beckman, J.S. (1995). Nitric oxide-related oxidants in acute lung injury. *New Horizons*, **3**, 113–122.

Rozell, B., Barcena, J.A., Martinez, G.E., Padilla, C.A., and Holmgren, A. (1993). Immunochemical characterization and tissue distribution of glutaredoxin (thioltransferase) from calf. *European Journal of Cellular Biology*, **62**, 314–323.

Ruch, F.J., Lin, E.C., Kowit, J.D., Tang, C.T., and Goldberg, A.L. (1980). *In vivo* inactivation of glycerol dehydrogenase in *Klebsiella aerogenes*: properties of active and inactivated proteins. *Journal of Bacteriology*, **141**, 1077–1085.

Rudie, N.G., Porter, D.J.T., and Bright, H.J. (1980). Chlorination of an active site tyrosyl residue in D-amino acid oxidase by *N*-chloro-D-leucine. *Journal of Biological Chemistry*, **255**, 498–508.

Rumsby, P.C., Davies, M.J., and Evans, J.G. (1994). Screening for p53 mutations in C3H/He mouse liver tumors derived spontaneously or induced with diethylnitrosamine or phenobarbitone. *Molecular Carcinology*, **9**, 71–75.

Rupp, M., and Gorisch, H. (1988). Purification, crystallisation and characterization of quinoprotein ethanol dehydrogenase from *Pseudomonas aeruginosa*. *Biological Chemistry, Hoppe-Seyler*, **369**, 431–439.

Ruppen, M.E., and Switzer, R.L. (1983). Degradation of *Bacillus subtilis* gluatmine phosphoribosyl-pyrophosphate amidotransferase *in vivo*. *Journal of Biological Chemistry*, **258**, 2843–2851.

Rush, J.D., and Bielski, B.H. (1995). The oxidation of amino acids by ferrate(V). A pre-mix pulse radiolysis study. *Free Radical Research*, **22**, 571–579.

Russell, G.A. (1957). Deuterium-isotope effects in the autoxidation of aralkyl hydrocarbons. Mechanism of the interaction of peroxy radicals. *Journal of the American Chemical Society*, **79**, 3871–3877.

Russo, T., Zambrano, N., Esposito, F., Ammendola, R., Cimino, F., Fiscella, M., *et al.* (1995). A p53-independent pathway for activation of WAF1/CIP1 expression following oxidative stress. *Journal of Biological Chemistry*, **270**, 29386–29391.

Rustgi, S.N., and Riesz, P. (1978*a*). An e.s.r. and spin-trapping study of the reactions of the SO_4^- radical with protein and nucleic acid constituents. *International Journal of Radiation Biology and Related Studies in Physics, Chemistry and Medicine*, **34**, 301–316.

Rustgi, S., and Riesz, P. (1978*b*). E.s.r. and spin-trapping studies of the reactions of hydrated electrons with dipeptides. *International Journal of Radiation Biology and Related Studies in Physics, Chemistry and Medicine*, **34**, 127–148.

Rustgi, S., and Riesz, P. (1978*c*). Hydrated electron-initiated main-chain scission in peptides: an e.s.r. and spin-trapping study. *International Journal of Radiation Biology and Related Studies in Physics, Chemistry and Medicine*, **34**, 449–460.

Rustgi, S., Joshi, A., Moss, H., and Riesz, P. (1977*a*). E.s.r. of spin-trapped radicals in aqueous solutions of amino acids. Reactions of the hydroxyl radical. *International Journal of Radiation Biology and Related Studies in Physics, Chemistry and Medicine*, **31**, 415–440.

Rustgi, S., Joshi, A., Riesz, P., and Friedberg, F. (1977*b*). E.s.r. of spin-trapped radicals in aqueous solutions of amino acids. Reactions of the hydrated electron. *International Journal of Radiation Biology and Related Studies in Physics, Chemistry and Medicine*, **32**, 533–552.

Rydon, H.N., and Smith, P.W.G. (1952). A new method for the detection of peptides and similar compounds on paper chromatograms. *Nature*, **169**, 922–923.

Ryle, M.J., Lanzilotta, W.N., Seefeldt, L.C., Scarrow, R.C., and Jensen, G.M. (1996). Circular dichroism and X-ray spectroscopies of *Azotobacter vinelandii* nitrogenase iron protein. MgATP and MgADP induced protein conformational changes affecting the [4Fe-4S] cluster and characterization of a [2Fe-2S] form. *Journal of Biological Chemistry*, **271**, 1551–1557.

Rzepecki, L.M., and Waite, J.H. (1993). The byssus of the zebra mussel, *Dreissena polymorpha*. I: Morphology and *in situ* protein processing during maturation. *Molecular Marine Biology and Biotechnology*, **2**, 255–266.

Rzepecki, L.M., and Waite, J.H. (1995). Wresting the muscle from mussel beards: research and applications. *Molecular Marine Biology and Biotechnology*, **4**, 313–322.

Sagai, M., and Tappel, A.L. (1979). Lipid peroxidation induced by some halomethanes as measured by *in vivo* pentane production in the rat. *Toxicology and Applied Pharmacology*, **49**, 283–291.

Sagara, Y., Dargusch, R., Klier, F.G., Schubert, D., and Behl, C. (1996). Increased antioxidant enzyme activity in amyloid beta protein-resistant cells. *Journal of Neuroscience*, **16**, 497–505.

Saha, A., Mandal, P.C., and Bhattacharyya, S.N. (1992). Radiation-induced inactivation of dihydroorotate dehydrogenase in dilute aqueous solution. *Radiation Research*, **132**, 7–12.

Sahakian, J.A., Szweda, L.I., Friguet, B., Kitani, K., and Levine, R.L. (1995). Aging of the liver: proteolysis of oxidatively modified glutamine synthetase. *Archives of Biochemistry and Biophysics*, **318**, 411–417.

Sahlin, M., Graslund, A., Ehrenberg, A., and Sjoberg, B.M. (1982). Structure of the tyrosyl radical in bacteriophage T4-induced ribonucleotide reductase. *Journal of Biological Chemistry*, **257**, 366–369.

Sahlin, M., Petersson, L., Graslund, A., Ehrenberg, A., Sjoberg, B.M., and Thelander, L. (1987). Magnetic interaction between the tyrosyl free radical and the antiferromagnetically coupled iron center in ribonucleotide reductase. *Biochemistry*, **26**, 5541–5548.

Sahlin, M., Lassmann, G., Potsch, S., Slaby, A., Sjoberg, B.M., and Graslund, A. (1994). Tryptophan radicals formed by iron/oxygen reaction with *Escherichia coli* ribonucleotide reductase protein R2 mutant Y122F. *Journal of Biological Chemistry*, **269**, 11699–11702.

Sahu, S.C. (1990). Oncogenes, oncogenesis, and oxygen radicals. *Biomedical and Environmental Science*, **3**, 183–201.

Sahu, S.C., and Washington, M.C. (1992). Effect of ascorbic acid and curcumin on quercetin-induced nuclear DNA damage, lipid peroxidation and protein degradation. *Cancer Letters*, **63**, 237–241.

Sakiyama, F., and Natsuki, R. (1976). Identification of tryptophan 62 as an ozonization-sensitive residue in hen egg-white lysozyme. *Journal of Biochemistry Tokyo*, **79**, 225–228.

Saldise, L., Martinez, A., Montuenga, L.M., Treston, A., Springall, D.R., Polak, J.M., *et al.* (1996). Distribution of peptidyl-glycine alpha-amidating mono-oxygenase (PAM) enzymes in normal human lung and in lung epithelial tumors. *Journal of Histochemistry and Cytochemistry*, **44**, 3–12.

Salemme, F.R. (1977). Structure and function of cytochromes c. *Annual Reviews of Biochemistry*, **46**, 299–329.

Salganik, R.I., Shabalina, I.G., Solovyova, N.A., Kolosova, N.G., Solovyov, V.N., and Kolpakov, A.R. (1994). Impairment of respiratory functions in mitochondria of rats with an inherited hyperproduction of free radicals. *Biochemical and Biophysical Research Communications*, **205**, 180–185.

Salman, T.S., Guerin, M.C., and Torreilles, J. (1995). Nitration of tyrosyl-residues from extra- and intracellular proteins in human whole blood. *Free Radical Biology and Medicine*, **19**, 695–698.

Salminen, A., Liu, P.K., and Hsu, C.Y. (1995). Alteration of transcription factor binding activities in the ischemic rat brain. *Biochemical and Biophysical Research Communications*, **212**, 939–944.

Salo, D.C., Lin, S.W., Pacifici, R.E., and Davies, K.J. (1988). Superoxide dismutase is preferentially degraded by a proteolytic system from red blood cells following oxidative modification by hydrogen peroxide. *Free Radical Biology and Medicine*, **5**, 335–339.

Salo, D.C., Pacifici, R.E., Lin, S.W., Giulivi, C., and Davies, K.J. (1990). Superoxide dismutase undergoes proteolysis and fragmentation following oxidative modification and inactivation. *Journal of Biological Chemistry*, **265**, 11919–11927.

Salo, D.C., Donovan, C.M., and Davies, K.J. (1991). HSP70 and other possible heat shock or oxidative stress proteins are induced in skeletal muscle, heart, and liver during exercise. *Free Radical Biology and Medicine*, **11**, 239–246.

Samuni, A., and Czapski, G. (1978). Radiation-induced damage in *Escherichia coli* B: the effect of superoxide radicals and molecular oxygen. *Radiation Research*, **76**, 624–632.

Samuni, A., and Neta, P. (1973). Electron spin resonance study of the reaction of hydroxyl radicals with pyrrole, imidazole, and related compounds. *Journal of Physical Chemistry*, **77**, 1629–1635.

Samuni, A., Chevion, M., Halpern, Y.S., Ilan, Y.A., and Czapski, G. (1978). Radiation-induced damage in T4 bacteriophage: the effect of superoxide radicals and molecular oxygen. *Radiation Research*, **75**, 489–496.

Samuni, A., Chevion, M., and Czapski, G. (1981). Unusual copper-induced sensitization of the biological damage due to superoxide radicals. *Journal of Biological Chemistry*, **256**, 12632–12635.

Samuni, A., Aronovitch, J., Godinger, D., Chevion, M., and Czapski, G. (1983). On the cytotoxicity of vitamin C and metal ions. A site-specific Fenton mechanism. *European Journal of Biochemistry*, **137**, 119–124.

Samuni, A., Chevion, M., and Czapski, G. (1984). Roles of copper and O(2) in the radiation-induced inactivation of T7 bacteriophage. *Radiation Research*, **99**, 562–572.

Sanchez, A., Alvarez, A.M., Benito, M., and Fabregat, I. (1996). Apoptosis induced by transforming growth factor-beta in fetal hepatocyte primary cultures: involvement of reactive oxygen intermediates. *Journal of Biological Chemistry*, **271**, 7416–7422.

Sandhu, I.S., Ware, K., and Grisham, M.B. (1992). Peroxyl radical-mediated hemolysis: role of lipid, protein and sulfydryl oxidation. *Free Radical Research Communications*, **16**, 111–122.

Sano, M., Motchnik, P.A., and Tappel, A.L. (1986). Halogenated hydrocarbon and hydroperoxide-induced peroxidation in rat tissue slices. *Journal of Free Radical Biology and Medicine*, **2**, 41–48.

Santamaria, R., Granato, C.G., and Santamaria, R. (1972). Rheological study of photo-oxidized contractile proteins. *Research Progress in Organic Biological and Medicinal Chemistry*, **1**, 259–269.

Santiago, R.Z., Williams, J.S., Gorenstein, D.G., and Andrisani, O.M. (1993). Bacterial expression and characterization of the CREB bZip module: circular dichroism and 2D ^{1}H-NMR studies. *Protein Science*, **2**, 1461–1471.

Sapezhinskii, I.I., Gudkova, N.A., Dontsova, E.G., Smirnov, L.D., and Kuz'min, V.I. (1980). Effect of different substances on the X-ray chemiluminescence of solutions of serum albumin and glycyltryptophan. *Biofizika*, **25**, 30–35.

Sapezhinskii, I.I., Dontsova, E.G., Silaev, I., and Shiriaev, V.M. (1981). Comparative study of the radiation oxidation and X-ray chemiluminescence of globular proteins. *Biofizika*, **26**, 581–586.

Sappey, C., Legrand, P.S., Best, B.M., Favier, A., Rentier, B., and Piette, J. (1994). Stimulation of glutathione peroxidase activity decreases HIV type 1 activation after oxidative stress. *Aids Research and Human Retroviruses*, **10**, 1451–1461.

Sappey, C., Boelaert, J.R., Legrand, P.S., Forceille, C., Favier, A., and Piette, J. (1995). Iron chelation decreases NF-kappa B and HIV type 1 activation due to oxidative stress. *Aids Research and Human Retroviruses*, **11**, 1049–1061.

Sarkar, A., Bishayee, A., and Chatterjee, M. (1995). Beta-carotene prevents lipid peroxidation and red blood cell membrane protein damage in experimental hepatocarcinogenesis. *Cancer Biochemistry and Biophysics*, **15**, 111–125.

Sarnesto, A., Linder, N., and Raivio, K.O. (1996). Organ distribution and molecular forms of human xanthine dehydrogenase/xanthine oxidase protein. *Laboratory Investigations*, **74**, 48–56.

Sastry, M.S., Gupta, S.S., and Singh, A.J. (1995). Effects of imidazole and zinc on the interaction of some amino acid compounds of copper(II) with hydrogen peroxide. *BioMetals*, **8**, 174–178.

Sato, H., Takenaka, Y., Fujiwara, K., Yamaguchi, M., Abe, K., and Bannai, S. (1995). Increase in cystine transport activity and glutathione level in mouse peritoneal macrophages exposed to oxidized low-density lipoprotein. *Biochemical and Biophysical Research Communications*, **215**, 154–159.

Sattler, W., and Stocker, R. (1993). Greater selective uptake by Hep G2 cells of high-density lipoprotein cholesteryl ester hydroperoxides than of unoxidized cholesteryl esters. *Biochemical Journal*, **294**, 771–778.

Sattler, W., Mohr, D., and Stocker, R. (1994a). Rapid isolation of lipoproteins and assessment of their peroxidation by high-performance liquid chromatography postcolumn chemiluminescence. *Methods in Enzymology*, **233**, 469–489.

Sattler, W., Maiorino, M., and Stocker, R. (1994b). Reduction of HDL- and LDL-associated cholesterylester and phospholipid hydroperoxides by phospholipid hydroperoxide glutathione peroxidase and Ebselen (PZ 51). *Archives of Biochemistry and Biophysics*, **309**, 214–221.

Savenkova, M.L., Mueller, D.M., and Heinecke, J.W. (1994). Tyrosyl radical generated by myeloperoxidase is a physiological catalyst for the initiation of lipid peroxidation in low density lipoprotein. *Journal of Biological Chemistry*, **269**, 20394–20400.

Savolainen, K.M., Loikkanen, J., and Naarala, J. (1995). Amplification of glutamate-induced oxidative stress. *Toxicology Letters*, **83**, 399–405.

Sawyer, D.T., Sobkowiak, A., Matsushita, T. (1996). Metal $[ML_x; M = Fe, Cu, Co, Mn]$/hydroperoxide-induced activation ofdioxygen for the oxygenation of hydrocarbons: oxygenated Fenton chemistry. *Accounts of Chemical Research*, **29**, 409–416.

Saxton, J.M., Donnelly, A.E., and Roper, H.P. (1994). Indices of free-radical-mediated damage following maximum voluntary eccentric and concentric muscular work. *European Journal of Applied Physiology*, **68**, 189–193.

Schackelford, R.E., Misra, U.K., Florine, C.K., Thai, S.F., Pizzo, S.V., and Adams, D.O. (1995). Oxidized low density lipoprotein suppresses activation of NF kappa B in macrophages via a pertussis toxin-sensitive signaling mechanism. *Journal of Biological Chemistry*, **270**, 3475–3478.

Schacter, E., Williams, J.A., Lim, M., and Levine, R.L. (1994). Differential susceptibility of plasma proteins to oxidative modification: examination by western blot immunoassay. *Free Radical Biology and Medicine*, **17**, 429–437.

Schaich, K.M. (1980*a*). Free radical initiation in proteins and amino acids by ionizing and ultraviolet radiations and lipid oxidation—part III: free radical transfer from oxidizing lipids. *Critical Reviews of Food Science and Nutrition*, **13**, 189–244.

Schaich, K.M. (1980*b*). Free radical initiation in proteins and amino acids by ionizing and ultraviolet radiations and lipid oxidation—Part I: ionizing radiation. *Critical Reviews of Food Science and Nutrition,*, **13**, 89–129.

Schaich, K.M. (1980*c*). Free radical initiation in proteins and amino acids by ionizing and ultraviolet radiations and lipid oxidation—Part II: ultraviolet radiation and photolysis. *Critical Reviews of Food Science and Nutrition*, **13**, 131–159.

Schaich, K.M., and Karel, M. (1975). Free radicals in lysozyme reacted with peroxidizing methyl linoleate. *Journal of Food Science*, **40**, 456–459.

Schaich, K.M., and Karel, M. (1976). Free radical reactions of peroxidizing lipids with amino acids and proteins: an ESR study. *Lipids*, **11**, 392–400.

Scheuner, G., and Gabler, W. (1967). On the histochemical effect of some oxidizing agents on protein-bound amino acids. *Acta Histochemistry*, **26**, 107–121.

Schilling, B., and Lerch, K. (1995). Amine oxidases from *Aspergillus niger*: identification of a novel flavin-dependent enzyme. *Biochimica et Biophysica Acta*, **1243**, 529–537.

Schinina, M.E., Carlini, P., Polticelli, F., Zappacosta, F., Bossa, F., and Calabrese, L. (1996). Amino acid sequence of chicken Cu, Zn-containing superoxide dismutase and identification of glutathionyl adducts at exposed cysteine residues. *European Journal of Biochemistry*, **237**, 433–439.

Schlatter, D., Waldvogel, S., Zulli, F., Suter, F., Portmann, W., and Zuber, H. (1985). Purification, amino-acid sequence and some properties of the ferredoxin isolated from *Bacillus acidocaldarius*. *Biological Chemistry, Hoppe-Seyler*, **366**, 223–231.

Schmidt, R.E., Dorsey, D.A., Beaudet, L.N., Reiser, K.M., Williamson, J.R., and Tilton, R.G. (1996). Effect of aminoguanidine on the frequency of neuroaxonal dystrophy in the superior mesenteric sympathetic autonomic ganglia of rats with streptozocin-induced diabetes. *Diabetes*, **45**, 284–290.

Schmitz, S., Thomas, P.D., Allen, T.M., Poznansky, M.J., and Jimbow, K. (1995). Dual role of melanins and melanin precursors as photoprotective and phototoxic agents: inhibition of ultraviolet radiation-induced lipid peroxidation. *Photochemistry and Photobiology*, **61**, 650–655.

Schneider, J.J., Phillips, J.R., Pye, Q., Maidt, M.L., Price, S., and Floyd, R.A. (1993). Methylene blue and Rose Bengal photoinactivation of RNA bacteriophages: comparative studies of 8-oxoguanine formation in isolated RNA. *Archives of Biochemistry and Biophysics*, **301**, 91–97.

Schoneich, C. (1995). Kinetics of thiol reactions. *Methods in Enzymology*, **251**, 45–55.

Schoneich, C., and Asmus, K.D. (1990). Reaction of thiyl radicals with alcohols, ethers and polyunsaturated fatty acids: a possible role of thiyl free radicals in thiol mutagenesis? *Radiation and Environmental Biophysics*, **29**, 263–271.

Schoneich, C., and Asmus, K.-D. (1995). Determination of absolute rate constants for the reversible hydrogen-atom transfer between thiyl radicals and alcohols or ethers. *Journal of Chemical Society Faraday Transactions*, **91**, 1923–1930.

Schoneich, C., Asmus, K.D., Dillinger, U., and von Bruchhausen, F. (1989a). Thiyl radical attack on polyunsaturated fatty acids: a possible route to lipid peroxidation. *Biochemical and Biophysical Research Communications*, **161**, 113–120.

Schoneich, C., Bonifacic, M., and Asmus, K.D. (1989b). Reversible H-atom abstraction from alcohols by thiyl radicals: determination of absolute rate constants by pulse radiolysis. *Free Radical Research Communications*, **6**, 393–405.

Schoneich, C., Bonifacic, M., Dillinger, U., and Asmus, K.-D. (1990). Hydrogen abstraction by thiyl radicals from activated C–H-bonds of alcohols, ethers and polyunsaturated fatty acids. In *Sulfur-Centered Reactive Intermediates in Chemistry and Biology*, (ed. C. Chatgilialoglu, and K.D. Asmus), pp. 367–376. Plenum Press, New York.

Schoneich, C., Dillinger, U., von Bruchhausen, F., and Asmus, K.D. (1992). Oxidation of polyunsaturated fatty acids and lipids through thiyl and sulfonyl radicals: reaction kinetics, and influence of oxygen and structure of thiyl radicals. *Archives of Biochemistry and Biophysics*, **292**, 456–467.

Schoneich, C., Zhao, F., Wilson, G.S., and Borchardt, R.T. (1993). Iron-thiolate induced oxidation of methionine to methionine sulfoxide in small model peptides. Intramolecular catalysis by histidine. *Biochimica et Biophysica Acta*, **1158**, 307–322.

Schoneich, C., Zhao, F., Madden, K.P., and Bobrowski, K. (1994). Side chain fragmentation of N-terminal threonine or serine residue induced through intramolecular proton transfer to hydroxy sulfuranyl radical formed at neighboring methionine in dipeptides. *Journal of the American Chemical Society*, **116**, 4641–4652.

Schraufstatter, I.U., Browne, K., Harris, A., Hyslop, P.A., Jackson, J.H., Quehenberger, O., et al. (1990). Mechanisms of hypochlorite injury of target cells. *Journal of Clinical Investigation*, **85**, 554–562.

Schreck, R., Albermann, K., and Baeuerle, P.A. (1992). Nuclear factor kappa B: an oxidative stress-responsive transcription factor of eukaryotic cells (a review). *Free Radical Research Communications*, **17**, 221–237.

Schrover, J.M., Frank, J., van Wielink, J.E., and Duine, J.A. (1993). Quaternary structure of quinoprotein ethanol dehydrogenase from *Pseudomonas aeruginosa* and its reoxidation with a novel cytochrome *c* from this organism. *Biochemical Journal*, **290**, 123–127.

Schubert, D., and Chevion, M. (1995). The role of iron in beta amyloid toxicity. *Biochemical and Biophysical Research Communications*, **216**, 702–707.

Schuchmann, M.N., and von Sonntag, C. (1979). Hydroxyl radical-induced oxidation of 2-methyl-2-propanol in oxygenated aqueous solution. A product and pulse radiolysis study. *Journal of Physical Chemistry*, **83**, 780–784.

Schuchmann, M.N., and von Sonntag, C. (1981). Photolysis at 185 nm of dimethyl ether in aqueous solution: Involvement of the hydroxymethyl radical. *Journal of Photochemistry*, **16**, 289–295.

Schuchmann, M.N., and von Sonntag, C. (1988). The rapid hydration of the acetyl radical. A pulse radiolysis study of acetaldehyde in aqueous solution. *Journal of the American Chemical Society*, **110**, 5698–5701.

Schuchmann, M.N., Schuchmann, H.-P., and von Sonntag, C. (1989). The pK_a value of the $\cdot O_2CH_2CO_2H$ radical: The Taft σ^* constant of the $-CH_2O_2\cdot$ group. *Journal of Physical Chemistry*, **93**, 5320–5323.

Schuessler, H. (1973). X-ray inactivation of ribonuclease in the presence of EDTA. *International Journal of Radiation Biology and Related Studies in Physics, Chemistry and Medicine*, **23**, 175–182.

Schuessler, H. (1975). Effect of ethanol on the radiolysis of ribonuclease. *International Journal of Radiation Biology and Related Studies in Physics, Chemistry and Medicine*, **27**, 171–180.

Schuessler, H. (1981). Reactions of ethanol and formate radicals with ribonuclease A and bovine serum albumin in radiolysis. *International Journal of Radiation Biology and Related Studies in Physics, Chemistry and Medicine*, **40**, 483–492.

Schuessler, H., and Davies, J.V. (1983). Radiation-induced reduction reactions with bovine serum albumin. *International Journal of Radiation Biology and Related Studies in Physics, Chemistry and Medicine*, **43**, 291–301.

Schuessler, H., and Denkl, P. (1972). X-ray inactivation of lactate dehydrogenase in dilute solution. *International Journal of Radiation Biology and Related Studies in Physics, Chemistry and Medicine*, **21**, 435–443.

Schuessler, H., and Freundl, K. (1983). Reactions of formate and ethanol radicals with bovine serum albumin studied by electrophoresis. *International Journal of Radiation Biology and Related Studies in Physics, Chemistry and Medicine*, **44**, 17–29.

Schuessler, H., and Hartmann, H. (1987). The effect of a protein on the radiolysis of DNA studied by HPLC and pulse radiolysis. *International Journal of Radiation Biology and Related Studies in Physics, Chemistry and Medicine*, **52**, 269–279.

Schuessler, H., and Herget, A. (1980). Oxygen effect in the radiolysis of proteins. I. Lactate dehydrogenase. *International Journal of Radiation Biology and Related Studies in Physics, Chemistry and Medicine*, **37**, 71–80.

Schuessler, H., and Jung, E. (1989a). Protein-DNA crosslinks induced by primary and secondary radicals. *International Journal of Radiation Biology*, **56**, 423–435.

Schuessler, H., and Jung, E. (1989b). Protein-DNA-crosslinks induced by primary and secondary radicals. *Free Radical Research Communications*, **6**, 161.

Schuessler, H., and Schilling, K. (1984). Oxygen effect in the radiolysis of proteins. Part 2. Bovine serum albumin. *International Journal of Radiation Biology and Related Studies in Physics, Chemistry and Medicine*, **45**, 267–281.

Schuessler, H., Niemczyk, P., Eichhorn, M., and Pauly, H. (1975). On the radiation-induced aggregates of lactate dehydrogenase. *International Journal of Radiation Biology and Related Studies in Physics, Chemistry and Medicine*, **28**, 401–408.

Schuessler, H., Mee, L.K., and Adelstein, S.J. (1976). Reaction of ethanol radicals with ribonuclease. *International Journal of Radiation Biology and Related Studies in Physics, Chemistry and Medicine*, **30**, 467–472.

Schuessler, H., Ebert, M., and Davies, J.V. (1977). The reaction rates of electrons with native and irradiated ribonuclease. *International Journal of Radiation Biology and Related Studies in Physics, Chemistry and Medicine*, **32**, 391–396.

Schuessler, H., Davies, J.V., Scherbaum, W., and Jung, E. (1986). Reactions of reducing radicals with ribonuclease. *International Journal of Radiation Biology and Related Studies in Physics, Chemistry and Medicine*, **50**, 825–839.

Schuessler, H., Geiger, A., Hartmann, H., and Steinheber, J. (1987). The effect of a protein on the radiolysis of DNA studied by gel filtration. *International Journal of Radiation Biology and Related Studies in Physics, Chemistry and Medicine*, **51**, 455–466.

Schuessler, H., Schmerler, D.G., Danzer, J., and Jung, K.E. (1992). Ethanol radical-induced protein-DNA crosslinking. A radiolysis study. *International Journal of Radiation Biology and Related Studies in Physics, Chemistry and Medicine*, **62**, 517–526.

Schuh, J., Fairclough, G.J., and Haschemeyer, R.H. (1978). Oxygen-mediated heterogeneity of apo-low-density lipoprotein. *Proceedings of the National Academy of Science of the United States of America*, **75**, 3173–3177.

Schuler, R.H. (1977). Oxidation of ascorbate anion by electron transfer to phenoxyl radicals. *Radiation Research*, **69**, 417–433.

Schulz, J.B., Matthews, R.T., Jenkins, B.G., Ferrante, R.J., Siwek, D., Henshaw, D.R., *et al.* (1995*a*). Blockade of neuronal nitric oxide synthase protects against excitotoxicity *in vivo*. *Journal of Neuroscience*, **15**, 8419–8429.

Schulz, J.B., Matthews, R.T., Muqit, M.M., Browne, S.E., and Beal, M.F. (1995*b*). Inhibition of neuronal nitric oxide synthase by 7-nitroindazole protects against MPTP-induced neurotoxicity in mice. *Journal of Neurochemistry*, **64**, 936–939.

Schulz, J.B., Huang, P.L., Matthews, R.T., Passov, D., Fishman, M.C., and Beal, M.F. (1996). Striatal malonate lesions are attenuated in neuronal nitric oxide synthase knockout mice. *Journal of Neurochemistry*, **67**, 430–433.

Schulze, O.K., Los, M., and Baeuerle, P.A. (1995). Redox signalling by transcription factors NF-kappa B and AP-1 in lymphocytes. *Biochemical Pharmacology*, **50**, 735–741.

Schuppe, I., Moldeus, P., and Cotgreave, I.A. (1992). Protein-specific S-thiolation in human endothelial cells during oxidative stress. *Biochemical Pharmacology*, **44**, 1757–1764.

Schuppe, K.I., Moldeus, P., Bergman, T., and Cotgreave, I.A. (1994*a*). S-thiolation of human endothelial cell glyceraldehyde-3-phosphate dehydrogenase after hydrogen peroxide treatment. *European Journal of Biochemistry*, **221**, 1033–1037.

Schuppe, K.I., Gerdes, R., Moldeus, P., and Cotgreave, I.A. (1994*b*). Studies on the reversibility of protein S-thiolation in human endothelial cells. *Archives of Biochemistry and Biophysics*, **315**, 226–234.

Schwartz, C.J., Valente, A.J., and Sprague, E.A. (1993). A modern view of atherogenesis. *American Journal of Cardiology*, **71**, 9B-14B.

Schwartz, R.S., Rybicki, A.C., Heath, R.H., and Lubin, B.H. (1987). Protein 4.1 in sickle erythrocytes. Evidence for oxidative damage. *Journal of Biological Chemistry*, **262**, 15666–15672.

Schwartz, T.W. (1988). Effect of amino acid analogs on the processing of the pancreatic polypeptide precursor in primary cell cultures. *Journal of Biological Chemistry*, **263**, 11504–11510.

Schwarzberg, M., Sperling, J., and Elad, D. (1973). Photoalkylation of peptides. Visible light-induced conversion of glycine residues into branched α-amino acids. *Journal of the American Chemical Society*, **95**, 6418–6426.

Schweizer, M., and Richter, C. (1996). Peroxynitrite stimulates the pyridine nucleotide-linked Ca^{2+} release from intact rat liver mitochondria. *Biochemistry*, **35**, 4524–4528.

Scrofani, S.D., Brereton, P.S., Hamer, A.M., Lavery, M.J., McDowall, S.G., Vincent, G.A., *et al.* (1994). Comparison of native and mutant proteins provides a sequence-specific assignment of the cysteinyl ligand proton NMR resonances in the 2[Fe4S4] ferredoxin from *Clostridium pasteurianum*. *Biochemistry*, **33**, 14486–14495.

Searle, M.S., Hall, J.G., and Wakelin, P.G. (1988). ^{1}H- and ^{13}C-n.m.r. studies of the antitumour antibiotic luzopeptin. Resonance assignments, conformation and flexibility in solution. *Biochemical Journal*, **256**, 271–278.

Searle, M.S., Hall, J.G., Denny, W.A., and Wakelin, L.P. (1989). Interaction of the antitumour antibiotic luzopeptin with the hexanucleotide duplex d(5'-GCATGC)$_2$. One-dimensional and two-dimensional n.m.r. studies. *Biochemical Journal*, **259**, 433–441.

Seccia, M., Brossa, O., Gravela, E., Slater, T.F., and Cheeseman, K.H. (1991). Exposure of beta L-crystallin to oxidizing free radicals enhances its susceptibility to transglutaminase activity. *Biochemical Journal*, **274**, 869–873.

Sedee, A.G., Beijersbergen, v.H.G., Lusthof, K.J., and Lodder, G. (1984). Photosensitized irreversible binding of estrone to protein via a hydroperoxide intermediate: an explanation of (photo-) allergic side-effects of estrogens. *Biochemical and Biophysical Research Communications*, **125**, 675–681.

Segrest, J.P., Jones, M.K., Mishra, V.K., Anantharamaiah, G.M., and Garber, D.W. (1994). apoB-100 has a pentapartite structure composed of three amphipathic alpha-helical domains alternating with two amphipathic beta-strand domains. Detection by the computer program LOCATE. *Arteriosclerosis and Thrombosis*, **14**, 1674–1685.

Seitz, W. (1938). The effect of X-rays on dehyrogenases. *Radiologica*, **2**, 4–15.

Sell, D.R., and Monnier, V.M. (1989). Structure elucidation of a senescence cross-link from human extracellular matrix: implication of pentoses in the aging process. *Journal of Biological Chemistry*, **24**, 21597–21602.

Selvaraj, R.J., Paul, B.B., Strauss, R.R., Jacobs, A.A., and Sbarra, A.J. (1974). Oxidative peptide cleavage and decarboxylation by the $MPO-H_2O_2-Cl-$ anti-microbial system. *Infection and Immunity*, **9**, 255–260.

Sen, C.K., and Packer, L. (1996). Antioxidant and redox regulation of gene transcription. *FASEB Journal*, **10**, 709–720.

Seppi, C., Castellana, M.A., Minetti, G., Piccinini, G., Balduini, C., and Brovelli, A. (1991). Evidence for membrane protein oxidation during *in vivo* aging of human erythrocytes. *Mechanisms of Ageing and Development*, **57**, 247–258.

Seres, T., Ravichandran, V., Moriguchi, T., Rokutan, K., Thomas, J.A., and Johnston, R.J. (1996). Protein S-thiolation and dethiolation during the respiratory burst in human monocytes. A reversible post-translational modification with potential for buffering the effects of oxidant stress. *Journal of Immunology*, **156**, 1973–1980.

Setlow, P. (1995). Mechanisms for the prevention of damage to DNA in spores of *Bacillus* species. *Annual Reviews of Microbiology*, **49**, 29–54.

Seto, Y. (1995). Oxidative conversion of thiocyanate to cyanide by oxyhemoglobin during acid denaturation. *Archives of Biochemistry and Biophysics*, **321**, 245–254.

Sevanian, A., Davies, K.J., and Hochstein, P. (1985). Conservation of vitamin C by uric acid in blood. *Journal of Free Radical Biology and Medicine*, **1**, 117–124.

Sevanian, A., Davies, K.J., and Hochstein, P. (1991). Serum urate as an antioxidant for ascorbic acid. *American Journal of Clinical Nutrition*, **54 (Supplement 6)**, 1129S–1134S.

Sevilla, M.D. (1970). Radicals formed by electron attachment to peptides. *Journal of Physical Chemistry*, **74**, 3366–3372.

Sevilla, M.D., and Brooks, V.L. (1973). Radicals formed by the reaction of electrons with amino acids and peptides in a neutral aqueous glass. *Journal of Physical Chemistry*, **77**, 2954–2959.

Shacter, E., Stadtman, E.R., Jurgensen, S.R., and Chock, P.B. (1988). Role of cAMP in cyclic cascade regulation. *Methods in Enzymology*, **159**, 3–19.

Shacter, E., Lopez, R.L., Beecham, E.J., and Janz, S. (1990). DNA damage induced by phorbol ester-stimulated neutrophils is augmented by extracellular cofactors. Role of histidine and metals. *Journal of Biological Chemistry*, **265**, 6693–6699.

Shacter, E., Williams, J.A., and Levine, R.L. (1995). Oxidative modification of fibrinogen inhibits thrombin-catalyzed clot formation. *Free Radical Biology and Medicine*, **18**, 815–821.

Shah, G., Pinnas, J.L., Lung, C.C., Mahmoud, S., and Mooradian, A.D. (1994). Tissue-specific distribution of malondialdehyde modified proteins in diabetes mellitus. *Life Science*, **55**, 1343–1349.

Shah, M.A., Bergethon, P.R., Boak, A.M., Gallop, P.M., and Kagan, H.M. (1992). Oxidation of peptidyl lysine by copper complexes of pyrroloquinoline quinone and other quinones. A model for oxidative pathochemistry. *Biochimica et Biophysica Acta*, **1159**, 311–318.

Shaheen, A.A., and el Fattah, A.A. (1995). Effect of dietary zinc on lipid peroxidation, glutathione, protein thiol levels and superoxide dismutase activity in rat tissues. *International Journal of Biochemistry and Cellular Biology*, **27**, 89–95.

Shaish, A., Daugherty, A., O'Sullivan, F., Schonfeld, G., and Heinecke, J.W. (1995). Beta-carotene inhibits atherosclerosis in hypercholesterolemic rabbits. *Journal of Clinical Investigation*, **96**, 2075–2082.

Shang, F., and Taylor, A. (1995). Oxidative stress and recovery from oxidative stress are associated with altered ubiquitin conjugating and proteolytic activities in bovine lens epithelial cells. *Biochemical Journal*, **307**, 297–303.

Shang, F., Huang, L., and Taylor, A. (1994). Degradation of native and oxidized beta- and gamma-crystallin using bovine lens epithelial cell and rabbit reticulocyte extracts. *Current Eye Research*, **13**, 423–431.

Shao, H. (1991). [Effect of lipoperoxide on catabolism of protein in burns in rats]. *Chung Hua Wai Ko Tsa Chih*, **29**, 581–583.

Shapiro, B.N. (1991). The control of oxidant stress at fertilization. *Science*, **252**, 533–536.

Sharonov, B.P., Govorova, N., and Lyzlova, S.N. (1988). Antioxidative properties and degradation of serum proteins by active oxygen forms ($O_2^-\cdot$, OCl^-) generated by stimulated neutrophils. *Biokhimiia*, **53**, 816–825.

Sharpless, N.E., Blair, A.E., and Maxwell, C.R. (1955). Effect of ionising radiation on amino acids. II. Effect of X-rays on aqueous solutions of alanine. *Radiation Research*, **2**, 135–144.

Shatkay, A. (1973). Simultaneous growth and decay of free radicals in irradiated proteins. *Photochemistry and Photobiology*, **17**, 91–102.

Shatkay, A., and Michaeli, I. (1972). Decay kinetics of free radicals in irradiated proteins. *Photochemistry and Photobiology*, **15**, 421–442.

Shattock, M.J., Matsuura, H., and Hearse, D.J. (1991). Functional and electrophysiological effects of oxidant stress on isolated ventricular muscle: a role for oscillatory calcium release from sarcoplasmic reticulum in arrhythmogenesis? *Cardiovascular Research*, **25**, 645–651.

Shaughnessy, S.G., Whaley, M., Lafrenie, R.M., and Orr, F.W. (1993). Walker 256 tumor cell degradation of extracellular matrices involves a latent gelatinase activated by reactive oxygen species. *Archives of Biochemistry and Biophysics*, **304**, 314–321.

Shaw, E., and Dean, R.T. (1980). The inhibition of macrophage protein turnover by a selective inhibitor of thiol proteinases. *Biochemical Journal*, **186**, 385–390.

Shaw, P.J., Ince, P.G., Falkous, G., and Mantle, D. (1995). Oxidative damage to protein in sporadic motor neuron disease spinal cord. *Annals of Neurology*, **38**, 691–695.

Shechter, Y., Burstein, Y., and Patchornik, A. (1975). Selective oxidation of methionine residues in proteins. *Biochemistry*, **14**, 4497–4503.

Shechter, Y., Patchornik, A., and Burstein, Y. (1976). Selective chemical cleavage of tryptophanyl peptide bonds by oxidative chlorination with *N*-chlorosuccinimide. *Biochemistry*, **15**, 5071–5075.

Sheldahl, J.A., and Tappel, A.L. (1974). Fluorescent products from aging *Drosophila melanogaster*: an indicator of free radical lipid peroxidation damage. *Experimental Gerontology*, **9**, 33–41.

Shelton, J.R., and Kopczewski, R.F. (1967). Nitric oxide induced free-radical reactions. *Journal of the American Chemical Society*, **32**, 2908–2910.

Shen, J., Kuhn, H., Petho, S.A., and Chan, L. (1995). Transgenic rabbits with the integrated human 15-lipoxygenase gene driven by a lysozyme promoter: macrophage-specific expression and variable positional specificity of the transgenic enzyme. *FASEB Journal*, **9**, 1623–1631.

Shen, X.M., and Dryhurst, G. (1996). Oxidation chemistry of (-)-norepinephrine in the presence of L-cysteine. *Journal of Medicinal Chemistry*, **39**, 2018–2029.

Sherman, M.P., Aeberhard, E.E., Wong, V.Z., Griscavage, J.M., and Ignarro, L.J. (1993). Pyrrolidine dithiocarbamate inhibits induction of nitric oxide synthase activity in rat alveolar macrophages. *Biochemical and Biophysical Research Communications*, **191**, 1301–1308.

Shertzer, H.G., Bannenberg, G.L., Zhu, H., Liu, R.M., and Moldeus, P. (1994). The role of thiols in mitochondrial susceptibility to iron and *tert*-butyl hydroperoxide-mediated toxicity in cultured mouse hepatocytes. *Chemical Research Toxicology*, **7**, 358–366.

Shetlar, M.D., Christensen, J., and Hom, K. (1984). Photochemical addition of amino acids and peptides to DNA. *Photochemistry and Photobiology*, **39**, 125–133.

Shields, H., Haven, Y., Hamrick, P.J., and Ma, Y. (1988). An ESR study of the radicals in X-irradiated L-alpha-amino-*n*-butyric acid HCl containing 1.5% L-cysteine HCl. *Radiation Research*, **116**, 373–378.

Shiga, T., and Imaizumi, K. (1975). Electron spin resonance study on peroxidase- and oxidase-reactions of horse radish peroxidase and methemoglobin. *Archives of Biochemistry and Biophysics*, **167**, 469–479.

Shigenaga, M.K., and Ames, B.N. (1991). Assays for 8-hydroxy-2'-deoxyguanosine: a biomarker of *in vivo* oxidative DNA damage. *Free Radical Biology and Medicine*, **10**, 211–216.

Shigenaga, M.K., Gimeno, C.J., and Ames, B.N. (1989). Urinary 8-hydroxy-2'-deoxyguanosine as a biological marker of *in vivo* oxidative DNA damage. *Proceedings of the National Academy of Science of the United States of America*, **86**, 9697–9701.

Shigenaga, M.K., Park, J.W., Cundy, K.C., Gimeno, C.J., and Ames, B.N. (1990). In vivo oxidative DNA damage: measurement of 8-hydroxy-2'-deoxyguanosine in DNA and urine by high-performance liquid chromatography with electrochemical detection. *Methods in Enzymology*, **186**, 521–530.

Shigenaga, M.K., Aboujaoude, E.N., Chen, Q., and Ames, B.N. (1994*a*). Assays of oxidative DNA damage biomarkers 8-oxo-2'-deoxyguanosine and 8-oxoguanine in nuclear DNA and biological fluids by high-performance liquid chromatography with electrochemical detection. *Methods in Enzymology*, **234**, 16–33.

Shigenaga, M.K., Hagen, T.M., and Ames, B.N. (1994*b*). Oxidative damage and mitochondrial decay in aging. *Proceedings of the National Academy of Science of the United States of America*, **91**, 10771–10778.

Shimazu, F., and Tappel, A.L. (1964*a*). Selenoamino acids: decrease of radiation damage to amino acids and proteins. *Science*, **143**, 369–371.

Shimazu, F., and Tappel, A.L. (1964*b*). Comparative radiolability of amino acids of proteins and free amino acids. *Radiation Research*, **23**, 203–209.

Shimazu, F., Kumta, U.S., and Tappel, A.L. (1964). Radiation damage to methionine and its derivatives. *Radiation Research*, **22**, 276–287.

Shimomura, O., and Johnson, F.H. (1978). Peroxidized coelenterazine, the active group in the photoprotein aequorin. *Proceedings of the National Academy of Science of the United States of America*, **75**, 2611–2615.

Shinagawa, E., Matsushita, K., Adachi, O., and Ameyama, M. (1990). Evidence for electron transfer via ubiquinone between quinoproteins D-glucose dehydrogenase and alcohol dehydrogenase of *Gluconobacter suboxydans*. *Journal of Biochemistry Tokyo*, **107**, 863–867.

Shinar, E., Navok, T., and Chevion, M. (1983). The analogous mechanisms of enzymatic inactivation induced by ascorbate and superoxide in the presence of copper. *Journal of Biological Chemistry*, **258**, 14778–14783.

Shiriaev, V.M., and Sapezhinskii, I.I. (1980). Photochemiluminescence arising during sensitized photooxidation of trypsin solutions. *Biofizika*, **25**, 208–212.

Shivakumar, B.R., and Ravindranath, V. (1992). Oxidative stress induced by administration of the neuroleptic drug haloperidol is attenuated by higher doses of haloperidol. *Brain Research*, **595**, 256–262.

Shuker, D.E., Prevost, V., Friesen, M.D., Lin, D., Ohshima, H., and Bartsch, H. (1993). Urinary markers for measuring exposure to endogenous and exogenous alkylating agents and precursors. *Environmental Health Perspectives*, **99**, 33–37.

Shuter, S.L., Bernier, M., Davies, M.J., Kusama, Y., Takahashi, A., Slater, T.F., *et al.* (1989). Manipulation of myocardial alpha-tocopherol levels fails to affect reperfusion arrhythmias or functional recovery following ischemic challenge in the rat heart. *Basic Research in Cardiology*, **84**, 421–430.

Shuter, S.L., Davies, M.J., Garlick, P.B., Hearse, D.J., and Slater, T.F. (1990*a*). Studies on the effects of antioxidants and inhibitors of radical generation on free radical production in the reperfused rat heart using electron spin resonance spectroscopy. *Free Radical Research Communications*, **9**, 223–232.

Shuter, S.L., Davies, M.J., Garlick, P.B., Hearse, D.J., and Slater, T.F. (1990*b*). Myocardial tissue preparation for ESR spectroscopy: some methods may cause artifactual generation of signals. *Free Radical Research Communications*, **9**, 55–63.

Siedler, F., Quarzago, D., Rudolph, B.S., and Moroder, L. (1994). Redox-active bis-cysteinyl peptides. II. Comparative study on the sequence-dependent tendency for disulfide loop formation. *Biopolymers*, **34**, 1563–1572.

Siesjo, B.K., Katsura, K., Zhao, Q., Folbergrova, J., Pahlmark, K., Siesjo, P., *et al.* (1995*a*). Mechanisms of secondary brain damage in global and focal ischemia: a speculative synthesis. *Journal of Neurotrauma*, **12**, 943–956.

Siesjo, B.K., Zhao, Q., Pahlmark, K., Siesjo, P., Katsura, K., and Folbergrova, J. (1995*b*). Glutamate, calcium, and free radicals as mediators of ischemic brain damage. *Annals of Thoracic Surgery*, **59**, 1316–1320.

Signorini, C., Ferrali, M., Ciccoli, L., Sugherini, L., Magnani, A., and Comporti, M. (1995). Iron release, membrane protein oxidation and erythrocyte ageing. *Federation of the European Biochemical Societies Letters*, **362**, 165–170.

Sikorska, M., Kwast, W.J., Youdale, T., Richards, R., Whitfield, J.F., and Walker, P.R. (1992). The M1 subunit of rat liver ribonucleotide reductase appears to be modified by ubiquitination. *Biochemical and Cellular Biology*, **70**, 215–223.

Silverstein, R.M., and Hager, L.P. (1974). The chloroperoxidase-catalyzed oxidation of thiols and disulfides to sulfenyl chlorides. *Biochemistry*, **13**, 5069–5073.

Silvester, J.A., Timmins, G.S., and Davies, M.J. (1995). Detection of protein radicals formed by the photodynamic action of porphyrin sensitizers. *Biochemistry Society Transactions*, **23**, 261S.

Simic, M.G. (1978). Radiation chemistry of amino acids and peptides in aqueous solutions. *Journal of Agricultural and Food Chemistry*, **26**, 6–14.

Simic, M.G., and Dizdaroglu, M. (1985). Formation of radiation-induced cross-links between thymine and tyrosine: possible model for cross-linking of DNA and proteins by ionizing radiation. *Biochemistry*, **24**, 233–236.

Simic, M.G., and Taub, I.A. (1978). Fast electron transfer processes in cytochrome *c* and related metalloproteins. *Biophysics Journal*, **24**, 285–294.

Simic, M.G., Gajewski, E., Dizdaroglu, M. (1985). Kinetics and mechanisms of hydroxyl radical-induced crosslinks between phenylalanine peptides. *Radiation and Physical Chemistry*, **24**, 465–473.

Simpson, J.A., and Dean, R.T. (1990). Stimulatory and inhibitory actions of proteins and amino acids on copper-catalysed free radical generation in the bulk phase. *Free Radical Research Communications*, **10**, 303–312.

Simpson, J.A., Cheeseman, K.H., Smith, S.E., and Dean, R.T. (1988). Free-radical generation by copper ions and hydrogen peroxide. Stimulation by Hepes buffer. *Biochemical Journal*, **254**, 519–523.

Simpson, J.A., Narita, S., Gieseg, S., Gebicki, S., Gebicki, J.M., and Dean, R.T. (1992). Long-lived reactive species on free-radical-damaged proteins. *Biochemical Journal*, **282**, 621–624.

Simpson, J.A., Gieseg, S.P., and Dean, R.T. (1993). Free radical and enzymatic mechanisms for the generation of protein bound reducing moieties. *Biochimica et Biophysica Acta*, **1156**, 190–196.

Singh, B.B., and Ormerod, M.G. (1965). The effect of sulphur compounds on free radical reactions and formation in irradiated dry protein. *Biochimica et Biophysica Acta*, **109**, 204–213.

Sips, H.J., and Hamers, M.N. (1981). Mechanism of the bactericidal action of myeloperoxidase: increased permeability of the *Escherichia coli* cell envelope. *Infection and Immunity*, **31**, 11–16.

Sivaraja, M., Goodin, D.B., Smith, M., and Hoffman, B.M. (1989). Identification by ENDOR of Trp191 as the free-radical site in cytochrome *c* peroxidase compound ES. *Science*, **245**, 738–740.

Sjoberg, B.M., Graslund, A., and Eckstein, F. (1983). A substrate radical intermediate in the reaction between ribonucleotide reductase from *Escherichia coli* and 2′-azido-2′-deoxynucleoside diphosphates. *Journal of Biological Chemistry*, **258**, 8060–8067.

Sjoberg, L.B., and Bostrom, S.L. (1977). Studies in rats on the nutritional value of hydrogen peroxide-treated fish protein and the utilization of oxidized sulphur-amino acids. *British Journal of Nutrition*, **38**, 189–205.

Skaper, S.D., Facci, L., Schiavo, N., Vantini, G., Moroni, F., Dal, T.R., *et al.* (1992). Characterization of 2,4,5-trihydroxyphenylalanine neurotoxicity *in vitro* and protective effects of ganglioside GM1: implications for Parkinson's disease. *Journal of Pharmacology and Experimental Therapies*, **263**, 1440–1446.

Skaper, S.D., Negro, A., Facci, L., and Dal, T.R. (1993a). Brain-derived neurotrophic factor selectively rescues mesencephalic dopaminergic neurons from 2,4,5-trihydroxyphenylalanine-induced injury. *Journal of Neuroscience Research*, **34**, 478–487.

Skaper, S.D., Fadda, E., Facci, L., and Manev, H. (1993b). A semisynthetic glycosphingolipid (LIGA20) reduces 2,4, 5-trihydroxyphenylalanine neurotoxicity in primary neuronal cultures. *European Journal of Pharmacology*, **243**, 91–93.

Skjeldal, L., Westler, W.M., Oh, B.H., Krezel, A.M., Holden, H.M., Jacobson, B.L., *et al.* (1991). Two-dimensional magnetization exchange spectroscopy of

Anabaena 7120 ferredoxin. Nuclear Overhauser effect and electron self-exchange cross peaks from amino acid residues surrounding the 2Fe-2S* cluster. *Biochemistry*, **30**, 7363–7368.

Slagle, I.R., Ratajczak, E., Heaven, M.C., Gutman, D., and Wagner, A.F. (1985). Kinetics of polyatomic free radicals produced by laser photolysis. 4. Study of the equilibria i–C_3H_7 + O_2 $\longleftrightarrow$ i–$C_3H_7O_2$ between 592 and 692 K. *Journal of the American Chemical Society*, **107**, 1834–1845.

Slagle, I.R., Ratajczak, E., and Gutman, D. (1986). Study of the thermochemsitry of the C_2H_5 + O_2 $\longleftrightarrow$ $C_2H_5O_2$ and t–C_4H_9 + O_2 $\longleftrightarrow$ t–$C_4H_9O_2$ reactions and of the trend of alkylperoxy bond strengths. *Journal of Physical Chemistry*, **90**, 402–407.

Slater, A.F., Stefan, C., Nobel, I., van, d.D.D., and Orrenius, S. (1995). Signalling mechanisms and oxidative stress in apoptosis. *Toxicology Letters*, **83**, 149–153.

Slates, H.L., Taub, D., Kuo, C.H., and Wendler, N.L. (1963). Degradation of α-methyl-3,4-dihydroxyphenylalanine (α-methylDOPA). *Journal of Organic Chemistry*, **29**, 1424–1429.

Slyshenkov, V.S., Rakowska, M., Moiseenok, A.G., and Wojtczak, L. (1995). Pantothenic acid and its derivatives protect Ehrlich ascites tumor cells against lipid peroxidation. *Free Radical Biology and Medicine*, **19**, 767–772.

Smith, C.D., Carney, J.M., Starke, R.P., Oliver, C.N., Stadtman, E.R., Floyd, R.A., et al. (1991). Excess brain protein oxidation and enzyme dysfunction in normal aging and in Alzheimer disease. *Proceedings of the National Academy of Science of the United States of America*, **88**, 10540–10543.

Smith, C.D., Carney, J.M., Tatsumo, T., Stadtman, E.R., Floyd, R.A., and Markesbery, W.R. (1992a). Protein oxidation in aging brain. *Annals of the New York Academy of Science*, **663**, 110–119.

Smith, C.D., Carson, M., van, d.W.M., Chen, J., Ischiropoulos, H., and Beckman, J.S. (1992b). Crystal structure of peroxynitrite-modified bovine Cu,Zn superoxide dismutase. *Archives of Biochemistry and Biophysics*, **299**, 350–355.

Smith, C.E., Stack, M.S., and Johnson, D.A. (1987). Ozone effects on inhibitors of human neutrophil proteinases. *Archives of Biochemistry and Biophysics*, **253**, 146–155.

Smith, M.A., Richey, P.L., Taneda, S., Kutty, R.K., Sayre, L.M., Monnier, V.M., et al. (1994). Advanced Maillard reaction end products, free radicals, and protein oxidation in Alzheimer's disease. *Annals of the New York Academy of Science*, **738**, 447–454.

Smith, M.A., Perry, G., Richey, P.L., Sayre, L.M., Anderson, V.E., Beal, M.F., et al. (1996). Oxidative damage in Alzheimer's. *Nature*, **382**, 120–121.

Smith, P., Fox, W.M., McGinty, D.J., and Stevens, R.D. (1970). Electron paramagnetic resonance spectroscopic study of radicals derived from glycine, DL-α-alanine, and β-alanine in aqueous solution. *Canadian Journal of Chemistry*, **48**, 480–491.

Smith, W.L., and Marnett, L.J. (1991). Prostaglandin endoperoxide synthase: structure and catalysis. *Biochimica et Biophysica Acta*, **1083**, 1–17.

Smith, W.L., DeWitt, D.L., Kraemer, S.A., Andrews, M.J., Hla, T., Maciag, T., et al. (1990). Structure-function relationships in sheep, mouse, and human prostaglandin endoperoxide G/H synthases. *Advances in Prostaglandin Thromboxane and Leukotriene Research*, **20**, 14–21.

Smith, W.L., Eling, T.E., Kulmacz, R.J., Marnett, L.J., and Tsai, A. (1992). Tyrosyl radicals and their role in hydroperoxide-dependent activation and inactivation of prostaglandin endoperoxide synthase. *Biochemistry*, **31**, 3–7.

Snyder, L.M., Fortier, N.L., Trainor, J., Jacobs, J., Leb, L., Lubin, B., et al. (1985). Effect of hydrogen peroxide exposure on normal human erythrocyte deformability, morphology, surface characteristics, and spectrin-hemoglobin cross-linking. *Journal of Clinical Investigation*, **76**, 1971–1977.

Soares, F.A., Shaughnessy, S.G., MacLarkey, W.R., and Orr, F.W. (1994). Quantification and morphologic demonstration of reactive oxygen species produced by Walker 256 tumor cells *in vitro* and during metastasis *in vivo*. *Laboratory Investigations*, **71**, 480–489.

Sohal, R.S. (1991). Hydrogen peroxide production by mitochondria may be a biomarker of aging. *Mechanisms of Ageing Development*, **60**, 189–198.

Sohal, R.S. (1993). Aging, cytochrome oxidase activity, and hydrogen peroxide release by mitochondria. *Free Radical Biology and Medicine*, **14**, 583–588.

Sohal, R.S., and Brunk, U.T. (1989). Lipofuscin as an indicator of oxidative stress and aging. *Advances in Experimental Medicine and Biology*, **266**, 17–26.

Sohal, R.S., and Brunk, U.T. (1992). Mitochondrial production of pro-oxidants and cellular senescence. *Mutation Research*, **275**, 295–304.

Sohal, R.S., and Dubey, A. (1994). Mitochondrial oxidative damage, hydrogen peroxide release, and aging. *Free Radical Biology and Medicine*, **16**, 621–626.

Sohal, R.S., and Orr, W.C. (1992). Relationship between antioxidants, pro-oxidants, and the aging process. *Annals of the New York Academy of Science*, **663**, 74–84.

Sohal, R.S., and Sohal, B.H. (1991). Hydrogen peroxide release by mitochondria increases during aging. *Mechanisms of Ageing Development*, **57**, 187–202.

Sohal, R.S., and Weindruch, R. (1996). Oxidative stress, caloric restriction, and aging. *Science*, **273**, 59–63.

Sohal, R.S., Allen, R.G., and Nations, C. (1986). Oxygen free radicals play a role in cellular differentiation: an hypothesis. *Journal of Free Radical Biology and Medicine*, **2**, 175–181.

Sohal, R.S., Svensson, I., Sohal, B.H., and Brunk, U.T. (1989). Superoxide anion radical production in different animal species. *Mechanisms of Ageing Development*, **49**, 129–135.

Sohal, R.S., Marzabadi, M.R., and Brunk, U.T. (1989). Effect of ethanol on lipofuscin accumulation in cultured rat cardiac myocytes. *Free Radical Biology and Medicine*, **7**, 611–616.

Sohal, R.S., Arnold, L., and Orr, W.C. (1990a). Effect of age on superoxide dismutase, catalase, glutathione reductase, inorganic peroxides, TBA-reactive material, GSH/GSSG, NADPH/NADP$^+$ and NADH/NAD$^+$ in *Drosophila melanogaster*. *Mechanisms of Ageing Development*, **56**, 223–235.

Sohal, R.S., Arnold, L.A., and Sohal, B.H. (1990b). Age-related changes in antioxidant enzymes and prooxidant generation in tissues of the rat with special reference to parameters in two insect species. *Free Radical Biology and Medicine*, **9**, 495–500.

Sohal, R.S., Svensson, I., and Brunk, U.T. (1990c). Hydrogen peroxide production by liver mitochondria in different species. *Mechanisms of Ageing Development*, **53**, 209–215.

Sohal, R.S., Sohal, B.H., and Brunk, U.T. (1990d). Relationship between antioxidant defenses and longevity in different mammalian species. *Mechanisms of Ageing Development*, **53**, 217–227.

Sohal, R.S., Ku, H.H., and Agarwal, S. (1993a). Biochemical correlates of longevity in two closely related rodent species. *Biochemical and Biophysical Research Communications*, **196**, 7–11.

Sohal, R.S., Agarwal, S., Dubey, A., and Orr, W.C. (1993*b*). Protein oxidative damage is associated with life expectancy of houseflies. *Proceedings of the National Academy of Science of the United States of America*, **90**, 7255–7259.

Sohal, R.S., Ku, H.H., Agarwal, S., Forster, M.J., and Lal, H. (1994). Oxidative damage, mitochondrial oxidant generation and antioxidant defenses during aging and in response to food restriction in the mouse. *Mechanisms of Ageing Development*, **74**, 121–133.

Sohal, R.S., Agarwal, S., and Sohal, B.H. (1995*a*). Oxidative stress and aging in the Mongolian gerbil (*Meriones unguiculatus*). *Mechanisms of Ageing Development*, **81**, 15–25.

Sohal, R.S., Sohal, B.H., and Orr, W.C. (1995*b*). Mitochondrial superoxide and hydrogen peroxide generation, protein oxidative damage, and longevity in different species of flies. *Free Radical Biology and Medicine*, **19**, 499–504.

Sohal, R.S., Agarwal, A., Agarwal, S., and Orr, W.C. (1995*c*). Simultaneous overexpression of copper- and zinc-containing superoxide dismutase and catalase retards age-related oxidative damage and increases metabolic potential in Drosophila melanogaster. *Journal of Biological Chemistry*, **270**, 15671–15674.

Sokol, H.A., Bennett-Corniea, W., and Garrison, W.M. (1965). A marked effect of conformation in the radiolysis of poly-α-L-glutamic acid in aqueous solution. *Journal of the American Chemical Society*, **87**, 1391–1392.

Sokolovsky, M., Riordan, J.F., and Vallee, B.L. (1966). Tetranitromethane. A reagent for the nitration of tyrosyl residues in proteins. *Biochemistry*, **5**, 3582–3589.

Sokolovsky, M., Riordan, J.F., and Vallee, B.L. (1967). Conversion of 3-nitro-tyrosine to 3-aminotyrosine in peptides and proteins. *Biochemical and Biophysical Research Communications*, **27**, 20–25.

Solar, S. (1985). Reaction of hydroxyl radicals with phenylalanine in neutral aqueous solution. *Radiation and Physical Chemistry*, **26**, 103–108.

Sommer, J.H., O'Hara, P.B., Jonah, C.D., and Bershoh, R. (1982). Relative reducibilities of complexes of Fe(III), Co(III), Nm(III) and Cu(II) with apotransferrin using e^-_{aq} and $CO_2 \cdot^-$. *Biochimica et Biophysica Acta.*, **703**, 62–68.

Sonaye, B., Naik, A.A., Yadav, S.D., and Chakrabarti, S. (1995). Protein cross-linking during oxidative denaturation of methaemoglobin. *Indian Journal of Medical Research*, **101**, 75–80.

Sosnovsky, G., and Rawlinson, D.J. (1972). Free radical reactions in the presence of metal ions–reactions of nitrogen compounds. In *Advances in Free Radical Chemistry*, (ed. G.H. Williams), pp. 203–284. Logos Press, London.

Soszynski, M., and Schuessler, H. (1991). Effect of X-irradiation on erythrocyte membrane proteins. Primary radicals. *International Journal of Radiation Biology*, **60**, 859–875.

Soszynski, M., Skalski, Z., Pulaski, L., and Bartosz, G. (1995). Peroxides inhibit the glutathione S-conjugate pump. *Biochemical and Molecular Biology International*, **37**, 537–545.

Soszynski, M., Filipiak, A., Bartosz, G., and Gebicki, J.M. (1996). Effect of amino acid peroxides on the erythrocyte. *Free Radical Biology and Medicine*, **20**, 45–51.

Soulis, L.T., Cooper, M.E., Dunlop, M., and Jerums, G. (1995). The relative roles of advanced glycation, oxidation and aldose reductase inhibition in the development of experimental diabetic nephropathy in the Sprague-Dawley rat. *Diabetologia*, **38**, 387–394.

Spagnuolo, C., De Martino, F., Boffi, A., Rousseau, D.L., and Chiancone, E. (1994). Coordination and spin state equilibria as a function of pH, ionic strength, and protein concentration in oxidized dimeric *Scapharca inaequivalvis* hemoglobin. *Journal of Biological Chemistry*, **269**, 20441–20445.

Spencer, J.P.E., Jenner, A., Aruoma, O.I., Evans, P.J., Kaur, H., Dexter, D.T., *et al.* (1994). Intense oxidative DNA damage promoted by L-DOPA and its metabolites. Implications for neurodegenerative disease. *FEBS Letters*, **353**, 246–250.

Sperling, J., and Elad, D. (1971*a*). Photochemical modification of glycine containing polypeptides. *Journal of the American Chemical Society*, **93**, 967–971.

Sperling, J., and Elad, D. (1971*b*). Photoalklylation of proteins. *Journal of the American Chemical Society*, **93**, 3839–3840.

Spiegel-Adolf, M. (1931). Effects of UV rays, radium and X-rays on proteins. *Archives of Pathology*, **12**, 533–542.

Spiegel-Adolf, M., and Krumpel, O. (1927). Absorption spectra of irradiated and non-irradiated proteins. *Biochemistry Zeitschrift*, **190**, 28–41.

Spitz, D.R., Kinter, M.T., and Roberts, R.J. (1995). Contribution of increased glutathione content to mechanisms of oxidative stress resistance in hydrogen peroxide resistant hamster fibroblasts. *Journal of Cellular Physiology*, **165**, 600–609.

Splittgerber, A.G., and Tappel, A.L. (1979). Steady state and pre-steady state kinetic properties of rat liver selenium-glutathione peroxidase. *Journal of Biological Chemistry*, **254**, 9807–9813.

Spyrou, G., Bjornstedt, M., Kumar, S., and Holmgren, A. (1995). AP-1 DNA-binding activity is inhibited by selenite and selenodiglutathione. *Federation of the European Biochemist Society Letters*, **368**, 59–63.

Staal, F.J., Anderson, M.T., and Herzenberg, L.A. (1995). Redox regulation of activation of NF-kappa B transcription factor complex: effects of *N*-acetylcysteine. *Methods in Enzymology*, **252**, 168–174.

Stadtman, E.R. (1988*a*). Biochemical markers of aging. *Experimental Gerontology*, **23**, 327–347.

Stadtman, E.R. (1988*b*). Protein modification in aging. *Journal of Gerontology*, **43**, B112–B120.

Stadtman, E.R. (1990*a*). Metal ion-catalyzed oxidation of proteins: biochemical mechanism and biological consequences [published erratum appears in *Free Radical Biology and Medicine* (1991), **10**, 249]. *Free Radical Biology and Medicine*, **9**, 315–325.

Stadtman, E.R. (1990*b*). Discovery of glutamine synthetase cascade. *Methods in Enzymology*, **182**, 793–809.

Stadtman, E.R. (1990*c*). Covalent modification reactions are marking steps in protein turnover. *Biochemistry*, **29**, 6323–6331.

Stadtman, E.R. (1991). Ascorbic acid and oxidative inactivation of proteins. *American Journal of Clinical Nutrition*, **54 (Supplement 6)**, 1125S–1128S.

Stadtman, E.R. (1992). Protein oxidation and aging. *Science*, **257**, 1220–1224.

Stadtman, E.R. (1993). Oxidation of free amino acids and amino acid residues in proteins by radiolysis and by metal-catalyzed reactions. *Annual Reviews of Biochemistry*, **62**, 797–821.

Stadtman, E.R., and Berlett, B.S. (1988). Fenton chemistry revisited: amino acid oxidation. *Basic Life Science*, **49**, 131–136.

Stadtman, E.R., and Berlett, B.S. (1991). Fenton chemistry. Amino acid oxidation. *Journal of Biological Chemistry*, **266**, 17201–17211.

Stadtman, E.R., and Chock, P.B. (1978). Interconvertible enzyme cascades in metabolic regulation. *Current Topics in Cellular Regulation*, **13**, 53–95.

Stadtman, E.R., and Oliver, C.N. (1991). Metal-catalyzed oxidation of proteins. Physiological consequences. *Journal of Biological Chemistry*, **266**, 2005–2008.

Stadtman, E.R., and Wittenberger, M.E. (1985). Inactivation of *Escherichia coli* glutamine synthetase by xanthine oxidase, nicotinate hydroxylase, horseradish peroxidase, or glucose oxidase: effects of ferredoxin, putidaredoxin, and menadione. *Archives of Biochemistry and Biophysics*, **239**, 379–387.

Stadtman, E.R., Shapiro, B.M., Kingdon, H.S., Woolfolk, C.A., and Hubbard, J.S. (1968). Cellular regulation of glutamine synthetase activity in *Escherichia coli*. *Advances in Enzyme Regulation*, **6**, 257–289.

Stadtman, E.R., Oliver, C.N., Levine, R.L., Fucci, L., and Rivett, A.J. (1988). Implication of protein oxidation in protein turnover, aging, and oxygen toxicity. *Basic Life Science*, **49**, 331–339.

Stadtman, E.R., Berlett, B.S., and Chock, P.B. (1990). Manganese-dependent disproportionation of hydrogen peroxide in bicarbonate buffer. *Proceedings of the National Academy of Science of the United States of America*, **87**, 384–388.

Stadtman, E.R., Starke-Reed, P.E., Oliver, C.N., Carney, J.M., and Floyd, R.A. (1992). Protein modification in aging. *EXS*, **62**, 64–72.

Stafford, R.E., Mak, I.T., Kramer, J.H., and Weglicki, W.B. (1993). Protein oxidation in magnesium deficient rat brains and kidneys. *Biochemical and Biophysical Research Communications*, **196**, 596–600.

Stange, E., Papenberg, J., and Agostini, B. (1977). Evaluation by electron microscopy of the integrity of iodinated plasmalipoproteins. *Histochemistry*, **52**, 145–149.

Starke, P.E., Oliver, C.N., and Stadtman, E.R. (1987). Modification of hepatic proteins in rats exposed to high oxygen concentration. *FASEB Journal*, **1**, 36–39.

Starke, R.P., and Oliver, C.N. (1988). Oxidative modification of enzymes during aging and acute oxidative stress. *Basic Life Science*, **49**, 537–540.

Starke, R.P., and Oliver, C.N. (1989). Protein oxidation and proteolysis during aging and oxidative stress. *Archives of Biochemistry and Biophysics*, **275**, 559–567.

States, D.J., Dobson, C.M., Karplus, M., and Creighton, T.E. (1980). A conformational isomer of bovine pancreatic trypsin inhibitor protein produced by refolding. *Nature*, **286**, 630–632.

Steenken, S. (1987). Addition-elimination paths in electron-transfer reactions between radicals and molecules. *Journal of the Chemical Society Faraday Transactions 1*, **83**, 113–124.

Steenken, S., and O'Neill, P. (1977). Oxidative demethoxylation of methoxylated phenols and hydroxybenzoic acids by the OH radical. An *in situ* electron spin resonance, conductometric, pulse radiolysis, and product analysis study. *Journal of Physical Chemistry*, **81**, 505–508.

Steenken, S., Davies, M.J., and Gilbert, B.C. (1986). Pulse radiolysis and e.s.r. studies of the dehydration of radicals from 1,2-diols and related compounds. *Journal of the Chemistry Society, Perkins Translation*, **2**, 1003–1010.

Steffek, R.P., and Thomas, M.J. (1991). Hydrogen peroxide modification of human oxyhemoglobin. *Free Radical Research Communications*, **12–13**, 489–497.

Steffen, L.K., Glass, R.S., Sabahi, M., Wilson, G.S., Schöneich, C., Mahling, S., *et al.* (1991). OH radical induced decarboxylation of amino acids. Decarboxylation *vs* bond formation in radical intermediates. *Journal of the American Chemical Society*, **113**, 2141–2145.

Stein, G., and Weiss, J. (1949). Chemical actions of ionizing radiations on aqueous solutions. IV. The actions of X-rays on some amino acids. *Journal of the Chemical Society*, 3256–3263.

Steinebach, V., de Vries, S., and Duine, J.A. (1996). Intermediates in the catalytic cycle of copper-quinoprotein amine oxidase from *Escherichia coli*. *Journal of Biological Chemistry*, **271**, 5580–5588.

Steinhart, H. (1991). Stability of tryptophan in peptides against oxidation and irradiation. *Advances in Experimental Medical Biology*, **294**, 29–40.

Stella, L. (1983). Homolytic cyclizations of N-chloroalkenylamines. *Angewandte Chemie International, Edition in English*, **22**, 337–422.

Stelmaszynska, T., and Zgliczynski, J.M. (1978). N-(2-Oxoacyl)amino acids and nitriles as final products of dipeptide chlorination mediated by the myeloperoxidase/H_2O_2/Cl^- system. *European Journal of Biochemistry*, **92**, 301–308.

Stezowski, J.J., Gorisch, H., Dauter, Z., Rupp, M., Hoh, A., Englmaier, R., *et al.* (1989). Preliminary X-ray crystallographic study of quinoprotein ethanol dehydrogenase from *Pseudomonas aeruginosa* [letter]. *Journal of Molecular Biology*, **205**, 617–618.

Stief, T.W., Stief, M.H., Ehrenthal, W., Darius, H., and Martin, E. (1991). Nonradical oxidants of the phagocyte type induce the activation of plasmatic single chain urokinase. *Thrombosis Research*, **64**, 597–610.

Stitt, A.W., Chakravarthy, U., Archer, D.B., and Gardiner, T.A. (1995). Increased endocytosis in retinal vascular endothelial cells grown in high glucose medium is modulated by inhibitors of nonenzymatic glycosylation. *Diabetologia*, **38**, 1271–1275.

Stocker, R. (1990). Induction of haem oxygenase as a defence against oxidative stress. *Free Radical Research Communications*, **9**, 101–112.

Stocker, R. (1994). Lipoprotein oxidation: mechanistic aspects, methodological approaches and clinical relevance. *Current Opinion in Lipidology*, **5**, 422–433.

Stocker, R., and Ames, B.N. (1987). Potential role of conjugated bilirubin and copper in the metabolism of lipid peroxides in bile. *Proceedings of the National Academy of Science of the United States of America*, **84**, 8130–8134.

Stocker, R., and Peterhans, E. (1989). Antioxidant properties of conjugated bilirubin and biliverdin: biologically relevant scavenging of hypochlorous acid. *Free Radical Research Communications*, **6**, 57–66.

Stocker, R., and Peterhans, E. (1989). Synergistic interaction between vitamin E and the bile pigments bilirubin and biliverdin. *Biochimica et Biophysica Acta*, **1002**, 238–244.

Stocker, R., and Suarna, C. (1993). Extracellular reduction of ubiquinone-1 and -10 by human Hep G2 and blood cells. *Biochimica et Biophysica Acta*, **1158**, 15–22.

Stocker, R., Hunt, N.H., Weidemann, M.J., and Clark, I.A. (1986a). Protection of vitamin E from oxidation by increased ascorbic acid content within *Plasmodium vinckei*-infected erythrocytes. *Biochimica et Biophysica Acta*, **876**, 294–299.

Stocker, R., Hunt, N.H., and Weidemann, M.J. (1986b). Antioxidants in plasma from mice infected with *Plasmodium vinckei*. *Biochemical and Biophysical Research Communications*, **134**, 152–158.

Stocker, R., Yamamoto, Y., McDonagh, A.F., Glazer, A.N., and Ames, B.N. (1987a). Bilirubin is an antioxidant of possible physiological importance. *Science*, **235**, 1043–1046.

Stocker, R., Glazer, A.N., and Ames, B.N. (1987b). Antioxidant activity of albumin-bound bilirubin. *Proceedings of the National Academy of Science of the United States of America*, **84**, 5918–5922.

Stocker, R., Cowden, W.B., Tellam, R.L., Weidemann, M.J., and Hunt, N.H. (1987c). Lipids from Plasmodium vinckei-infected erythrocytes and their susceptibility to oxidative damage. *Lipids*, **22**, 51–57.

Stocker, R., McDonagh, A.F., Glazer, A.N., and Ames, B.N. (1990). Antioxidant activities of bile pigments: biliverdin and bilirubin. *Methods in Enzymology*, **186**, 301–309.

Stocker, R., Bowry, V.W., and Frei, B. (1991). Ubiquinol-10 protects human low density lipoprotein more efficiently against lipid peroxidation than does alphatocopherol. *Proceedings of the National Academy of Science of the United States of America*, **88**, 1646–1650.

Stolze, K., and Nohl., H. (1989). Detection of free radicals as intermediates in the methemoglobin formation from oxyhemoglobin induced by hydroxylamine. *Biochemical Pharmacology*, **38**, 3055–3059.

Stone, J.R., Sands, R.H., Dunham, W.R., and Marletta, M.A. (1996). Spectral and ligand-binding properties of an unusual hemoprotein, the ferric form of soluble guanylate cyclase. *Biochemistry*, **35**, 3258–3262.

Storz, G., and Tartaglia, L.A. (1992). OxyR: a regulator of antioxidant genes. *Journal of Nutrition*, **122 (Supplement 3)**, 627–630.

Storz, G., Tartaglia, L.A., and Ames, B.N. (1990a). Transcriptional regulator of oxidative stress-inducible genes: direct activation by oxidation. *Science*, **248**, 189–194.

Storz, G., Tartaglia, L.A., and Ames, B.N. (1990b). The OxyR regulon. *Antonie Van Leeuwenhoek*, **58**, 157–161.

Strack, P.R., Waxman, L., and Fagan, J.M. (1996a). Activation of the multicatalytic endopeptidase by oxidants. Effects on enzyme structure. *Biochemistry*, **35**, 7142–7149.

Strack, P.R., Waxman, L., and Fagan, J.M. (1996b). ATP-stimulated degradation of oxidatively modified superoxide dismutase by cathepsin D in cardiac tissue extracts. *Biochemical and Biophysical Research Communications*, **219**, 348–353.

Strauss, R.R., Paul, B.B., Jacobs, A.A., and Sbaraa, A.J. (1970). The role of the phagocyte in host-parasite interactions. XXVII. Myeloperoxidase-hydrogen peroxide-chloride mediated aldehyde formation and its relationship to antimicrobial activity. *Infection and Immunity*, **3**, 595–602.

Strehler, B.L., Schmid, P., Li, M.P., Martin, K., and Fliss, H. (1982). Oxidative peptide (and amide) formation from Schiff base complexes. *Journal of Molecular Evolution*, **19**, 1–8.

Stubbe, J.A. (1989). Protein radical involvement in biological catalysis? *Annual Reviews of Biochemistry*, **58**, 257–285.

Stults, N.L., Asta, L.M., and Lee, Y.C. (1989). Immobilization of proteins on oxidized crosslinked Sepharose preparations by reductive amination. *Analytical Biochemistry*, **180**, 114–119.

Stutchbury, G.M., and Truscott, R.J. (1993). The modification of proteins by 3-hydroxykynurenine. *Experimental Eye Research*, **57**, 149–155.

Stuurman, N., Floore, A., Colen, A., de Jong, L., and van Driel, R. (1992). Stabilization of the nuclear matrix by disulfide bridges: identification of matrix polypeptides that form disulfides. *Experimental Cell Research*, **200**, 285–294.

Suarna, C., Hood, R.L., Dean, R.T., and Stocker, R. (1993). Comparative antioxidant activity of tocotrienols and other natural lipid-soluble antioxidants in a homogeneous system, and in rat and human lipoproteins. *Biochimica et Biophysica Acta*, **1166**, 163–170.

Suarna, C., Dean, R.T., May, J., and Stocker, R. (1995). Human atherosclerotic plaque contains both oxidized lipids and relatively large amounts of alphatocopherol and ascorbate. *Arteriosclerosis Thrombosis and Vascular Biology*, **15**, 1616–1624.

Sud'bina, E.N., Azizova, O.A., and Kaiushin, L.P. (1973). Phototransformation of free radicals in polycrystalline proteins due to UV-radiation. Formation of peptide group radicals. *Biofizika*, **18**, 611–617.

Sugano, T., Nitta, M., Ohmori, H., and Yamaizumi, M. (1995). Nuclear accumulation of p53 in normal human fibroblasts is induced by various cellular stresses which evoke the heat shock response, independently of the cell cycle. *Journal of Cancer Research, Japan*, **86**, 415–418.

Sugumaran, M. (1991). Molecular mechanisms for mammalian melanogenesis. Comparison with insect cuticular sclerotization. *Federation of the European Biochemical Societies Letters*, **293**, 4–10.

Sugumaran, M., and Ricketts, D. (1995). Model sclerotization studies. 3. Cuticular enzyme catalyzed oxidation of peptidyl model tyrosine and dopa derivatives. *Archives of Insect Biochemistry and Physiology*, **28**, 17–32.

Sugumaran, M., Tan, S., and Sun, H.L. (1996). Tyrosinase-catalyzed oxidation of 3,4-dihydroxyphenylglycine. *Archives of Biochemistry and Biophysics*, **329**, 175–180.

Suits, A.G., Chait, A., Aviram, M., and Heinecke, J.W. (1989). Phagocytosis of aggregated lipoprotein by macrophages: low density lipoprotein receptor-dependent foam-cell formation. *Proceedings of the National Academy of Science of the United States of America*, **86**, 2713–2717.

Sukhov, N.L., Akinshin, M.A., and Ershov, B.G. (1986). Pulse radiolysis of aqueous solutions of monovalent copper. *High Energy Chemistry*, **20**, 303–306.

Sullivan, S.G., and Stern, A. (1984). Membrane protein changes induced by *tert*-butyl hydroperoxide in red blood cells. *Biochimica et Biophysica Acta*, **774**, 215–220.

Summerfield, F.W., and Tappel, A.L. (1978). Enzymatic synthesis of malonaldehyde. *Biochemical and Biophysical Research Communications*, **82**, 547–552.

Summerfield, F.W., and Tappel, A.L. (1981). Determination of malondialdehyde-DNA crosslinks by fluorescence and incorporation of tritium. *Analytical Biochemistry*, **111**, 77–82.

Summerfield, F.W., and Tappel, A.L. (1983). Determination by fluorescence quenching of the environment of DNA crosslinks made by malondialdehyde. *Biochimica et Biophysica Acta*, **740**, 185–189.

Summerfield, F.W., and Tappel, A.L. (1984*a*). Detection and measurement by high-performance liquid chromatography of malondialdehyde crosslinks in DNA. *Analytical Biochemistry*, **143**, 265–271.

Summerfield, F.W., and Tappel, A.L. (1984*b*). Vitamin E protects against methyl ethyl ketone peroxide-induced peroxidative damage to rat brain DNA. *Mutation Research*, **126**, 113–120.

Summerfield, F.W., and Tappel, A.L. (1984*c*). Cross-linking of DNA in liver and testes of rats fed 1,3-propanediol. *Chemico-Biological Interactions*, **50**, 87–96.

Summers, F.E., and Erman, J.E. (1988). Reduction of cytochrome *c* peroxidase compounds I and II by ferrocytochrome *c*. A stopped-flow kinetic investigation. *Journal of Biological Chemistry*, **263**, 14267–14275.

Sun, X., Ollagnier, S., Schmidt, P.P., Atta, M., Mulliez, E., Lepape, L., *et al.* (1996). The free radical of the anaerobic ribonucleotide reductase from *Escherichia coli* is at glycine 681. *Journal of Biological Chemistry*, **271**, 6827–6831.

Sutton, H.C. (1956). Effects of radiations on catalase solutions. I. Kinetic studies of inactivation. *Biochemical Journal*, **64**, 447–455.

Suzuki, Y.J., and Packer, L. (1995). Redox regulation of DNA-protein interactions by biothiols. *Methods in Enzymology*, **252**, 175–180.

Suzuki, Y.J., Mizuno, M., Tritschler, H.J., and Packer, L. (1995). Redox regulation of NF-kappa B DNA binding activity by dihydrolipoate. *Biochemistry and Molecular Biology International*, **36**, 241–246.

Swallow, A.J. (1960). *Radiation Chemistry of Organic Compounds*. Pergamon Press, Oxford.

Swallow, A.J. (1973). *Radiation Chemistry: An Introduction.* Longman, London.

Swamy, M.S., Tsai, C., Abraham, A., and Abraham, E.C. (1993). Glycation mediated lens crystallin aggregation and cross-linking by various sugars and sugar phosphates *in vitro. Experimental Eye Research,* **56,** 177–185.

Swartz, H.M., Bolton, J.R., and Borg, D.C. (1972). *Biological Applications of Electron Spin Resonance.* Wiley, New York.

Symons, M.C., and Petersen, R.L. (1978). The relative electron affinities of the alpha and beta chains of oxyhaemoglobin as a function of pH and added inositol hexaphosphate. An electron spin resonance study. *Biochimica et Biophysica Acta,* **537,** 70–76.

Symons, M.C.R. (1978). *Chemical and Biochemical Aspects of Electron Spin Resonance Spectroscopy.* Wiley, London.

Symons, M.C.R. (1995). Electron spin resonance studies of radiation damage to DNA and to proteins. *Radiation and Physical Chemistry,* **45,** 837–845.

Szabo, C., Salzman, A.L., and Ischiropoulos, H. (1995a). Endotoxin triggers the expression of an inducible isoform of nitric oxide synthase and the formation of peroxynitrite in the rat aorta *in vivo. Federation of the European Biochemical Societies Letters,* **363,** 235–238.

Szabo, C., Salzman, A.L., and Ischiropoulos, H. (1995b). Peroxynitrite-mediated oxidation of dihydrorhodamine 123 occurs in early stages of endotoxic and hemorrhagic shock and ischemia-reperfusion injury. *Federation of the European Biochemical Societies Letters,* **372,** 229–232.

Szalai, V.A., and Brudvig, G.W. (1996). Formation and decay of the S3 EPR signal species in acetate-inhibited photosystem II. *Biochemistry,* **35,** 1946–1953.

Szebeni, J., and Tollin, G. (1988). Some relationships between ultraviolet light and heme-protein-induced peroxidative lipid breakdown in liposomes, as reflected by fluorescence changes: the effect of negative surface charge. *Photochemistry and Photobiology,* **47,** 475–479.

Szweda, L.I., and Stadtman, E.R. (1992). Iron-catalyzed oxidative modification of glucose-6-phosphate dehydrogenase from *Leuconostoc mesenteroides.* Structural and functional changes. *Journal of Biological Chemistry,* **267,** 3096–3100.

Szweda, L.I., and Stadtman, E.R. (1993). Oxidative modification of glucose-6-phosphate dehydrogenase from *Leuconostoc mesenteroides* by an iron(II)-citrate complex. *Archives of Biochemistry and Biophysics,* **301,** 391–395.

Szweda, L.I., Uchida, K., Tsai, L., and Stadtman, E.R. (1993). Inactivation of glucose-6-phosphate dehydrogenase by 4-hydroxy-2-nonenal. Selective modification of an active-site lysine. *Journal of Biological Chemistry,* **268,** 3342–3347.

Tabira, T. (1985). Electron microscopic demonstration of polysaccharides in central and peripheral myelin by thiosemicarbazide-protein-silver staining. *Journal of Neurocytology,* **14,** 781–794.

Taborsky, G. (1973). Oxidative modification of proteins in the presence of ferrous ion and air. Effect of ionic constituents of the reaction medium on the nature of the oxidation products. *Biochemistry,* **12,** 1341–1348.

Tacchini, L., Pogliaghi, G., Radice, L., Anzon, E., and Bernelli, Z.A. (1995). Differential activation of heat-shock and oxidation-specific stress genes in chemically induced oxidative stress. *Biochemical Journal,* **309,** 453–459.

Takagi, Y., Kashiwagi, A., Tanaka, Y., Asahina, T., Kikkawa, R., and Shigeta, Y. (1995). Significance of fructose-induced protein oxidation and formation of advanced glycation end product. *Journal of Diabetes Complications,* **9,** 87–91.

Takenaka, Y., Miki, M., Yasuda, H., and Mino, M. (1991). The effect of alpha-tocopherol as an antioxidant on the oxidation of membrane protein thiols induced by free radicals generated in different sites. *Archives of Biochemistry and Biophysics*, **285**, 344–350.

Tamba, M., and Badiello, R. (1985). Reactions of selenium dioxide free radicals with amino acids and enzymes. *International Journal of Radiation Biology and Related Studies in Physics, Chemistry and Medicine*, **48**, 259–270.

Tanfani, F., Carloni, P., Damiani, E., Greci, L., Wozniak, M., Kulawiak, D., *et al.* (1994). Quinolinic aminoxyl protects albumin against peroxyl radical mediated damage. *Free Radical Research*, **21**, 309–315.

Taniguchi, H., Fuchi, K., Ohnishi, S., and Hatano, H. (1968). Free-radical intermediates in the reaction of the hydroxyl radical with amino acids. *Journal of Physical Chemistry*, **72**, 1926–1931.

Taniguchi, H., Hatano, H., Hasegawa, H., and Maruyama, T. (1970). Free-radical intermediates in the reaction of the hydroxyl radical with amino acid derivatives and related compounds. *Journal of Physical Chemistry*, **74**, 3063–3065.

Taniguchi, H., Hasumi, H., and Hatano, H. (1972). Electron spin resonance study of the amino acid radicals produced by Fenton's reagent. *Bulletin of the Chemical Society of Japan*, **45**, 3380–3383.

Tanizawa, K. (1995). Biogenesis of novel quinone coenzymes. *Journal of Biochemistry Tokyo*, **118**, 671–678.

Tanizawa, K., Matsuzaki, R., Shimizu, E., Yorifuji, T., and Fukui, T. (1994). Cloning and sequencing of phenylethylamine oxidase from *Arthrobacter globiformis* and implication of Tyr-382 as the precursor to its covalently bound quinone cofactor. *Biochemical and Biophysical Research Communications*, **199**, 1096–1102.

Tappel, A.L. (1968). Will antioxidant nutrients slow aging processes? *Geriatrics*, **23**, 97–105.

Tappel, A.L. (1970). Biological antioxidant protection against lipid peroxidation damage. *American Journal of Clinical Nutrition*, **23**, 1137–1139.

Tappel, A.L. (1972). Vitamin E and free radical peroxidation of lipids. *Annals of the New York Academy of Science*, **203**, 12–28.

Tappel, A.L. (1973). Lipid peroxidation damage to cell components. *Proceedings of the National Academy of Science of the United States of America*, **32**, 1870–1874.

Tappel, A.L. (1974). Selenium-glutathione peroxidase and vitamin E. *American Journal of Clinical Nutrition*, **27**, 960–965.

Tappel, A.L. (1975). Lipid peroxidation and fluorescent molecular damage to membranes. In *Pathology of Cell Membranes*, (ed. B.F. Trump and A.U. Arstila), pp. 145–170. Academic Press, New York.

Tappel, A.L. (1978a). Protection against free radical lipid peroxidation reactions. *Advances in Experimental Medicine and Biology*, **97**, 111–131.

Tappel, A.L. (1978b). Glutathione peroxidase and hydroperoxides. *Methods in Enzymology*, **52**, 506–513.

Tappel, A.L. (1980). Vitamin E and selenium protection from *in vivo* lipid peroxidation. *Annals of the New York Academy of Science*, **355**, 18–31.

Tappel, A.L., and Dillard, C.J. (1981). In vivo lipid peroxidation: measurement via exhaled pentane and protection by vitamin E. *Proceedings of the National Academy of Science of the United States of America*, **40**, 174–178.

Tartaglia, L.A., Storz, G., and Ames, B.N. (1989). Identification and molecular analysis of oxyR-regulated promoters important for the bacterial adaptation to oxidative stress. *Journal of Molecular Biology*, **210**, 709–719.

Tavares, P., Ravi, N., Moura, J.J., LeGall, J., Huang, Y.H., Crouse, B.R., *et al.* (1994). Spectroscopic properties of desulfoferrodoxin from *Desulfovibrio desulfuricans (ATCC 27774)*. *Journal of Biological Chemistry*, **269**, 10504–10510.

Taylor, A., and Davies, K.J. (1987). Protein oxidation and loss of protease activity may lead to cataract formation in the aged lens. *Free Radical Biology and Medicine*, **3**, 371–377.

Taylor, A., Zuliani, A.M., Hopkins, R.E., Dallal, G.E., Treglia, P., Kuck, J.F., *et al.* (1989). Moderate caloric restriction delays cataract formation in the Emory mouse. *FASEB Journal*, **3**, 1741–1746.

Taylor, S.L., and Tappel, A.L. (1976). Effect of dietary antioxidants and phenobarbital pretreatment on microsomal lipid peroxidation and activation by carbon tetrachloride. *Life Science*, **19**, 1151–1160.

Taylor, S.W., Molinski, T.F., Rzepecki, L.M., and Waite, J.H. (1991). Oxidation of peptidyl 3,4-dihydroxyphenylalanine analogues: implications for the biosynthesis of tunichromes and related oligopeptides. *Journal of Natural Products*, **54**, 918–922.

Taylor, S.W., Ross, M.M., and Waite, J.H. (1995). Novel 3,4-di- and 3,4,5-trihydroxyphenylalanine-containing polypeptides from the blood cells of the ascidians *Ascidia ceratodes* and *Molgula manhattensis*. *Archives of Biochemistry and Biophysics*, **324**, 228–240.

Tedro, S.M., Meyer, T.E., and Kamen, M.D. (1979). Primary structure of a high potential, four-iron-sulfur ferredoxin from the photosynthetic bacterium *Rhodospirillum tenue*. *Journal of Biological Chemistry*, **254**, 1495–1500.

Terato, H., and Yamamoto, O. (1994). Hydrated electron-induced inactivation of tyrosinase in aqueous solution by exposure to cobalt-60 gamma-rays. I. Cresolase activity. *Biochemistry and Molecular Biology International*, **34**, 295–300.

Tertov, V.V., Kaplun, V.V., Dvoryantsev, S.N., and Orekhov, A.N. (1995). Apolipoprotein B-bound lipids as a marker for evaluation of low density lipoprotein oxidation *in vivo*. *Biochemical and Biophysical Research Communications*, **214**, 608–613.

Teshima, S., Rokutan, K., Takahashi, M., Nikawa, T., and Kishi, K. (1996). Induction of heat shock proteins and their possible roles in macrophages during activation by macrophage colony-stimulating factor. *Biochemical Journal*, **315**, 497–504.

Tesoriere, L., Ciaccio, M., Valenza, M., Bongiorno, A., Maresi, E., Albiero, R., *et al.* (1994). Effect of vitamin A administration on resistance of rat heart against doxorubicin-induced cardiotoxicity and lethality. *Journal of Pharmacology and Experimental Therapies*, **269**, 430–436.

Test, S.T., Lampert, M.B., Ossanna, P.J., Thoene, J.G., and Weiss, S.J. (1984). Generation of nitrogen-chlorine oxidants by human phagocytes. *Journal of Clinical Investigation*, **74**, 1341–1349.

Tew, D., and Ortiz de Montellano, P.R. (1988). The myoglobin protein radical. Coupling of Tyr-103 to Tyr-151 in the H_2O_2-mediated cross-linking of sperm whale myoglobin. *Journal of Biological Chemistry*, **263**, 17880–17886.

Thanabal, V., La Mar, G.N., and de Ropp, J.S. (1988). A nuclear Overhauser effect study of the heme crevice in the resting state and compound I of horseradish peroxidase: evidence for cation radical delocalization to the proximal histidine. *Biochemistry*, **27**, 5400–5407.

Theil, E.C., Sayers, D.E., and Brown, M.A. (1979). Similarity of the structure of ferritin and iron dextran (imferon) determined by extended X-ray absorption fine structure analysis. *Journal of Biological Chemistry*, **254**, 8132–8134.

Thelander, M., Graslund, A., and Thelander, L. (1985). Subunit M2 of mammalian ribonucleotide reductase. Characterization of a homogeneous protein isolated from M2-overproducing mouse cells. *Journal of Biological Chemistry*, **260**, 2737–2741.

Thomas, E.L. (1979*a*). Myeloperoxidase-hydrogen peroxide-chloride antimicrobial system: effect of exogenous amines on antibacterial action against *Escherichia coli*. *Infection and Immunity*, **25**, 110–116.

Thomas, E.L. (1979*b*). Myeloperoxidase, hydrogen peroxide, chloride antimicrobial system: nitrogen-chlorine derivatives of bacterial components in bactericidal action against *Escherichia coli*. *Infection and Immunity*, **23**,522–531.

Thomas, E.L., and Aune, T.M. (1977). Peroxidase-catalyzed oxidation of protein sulfydryls mediated by iodine. *Biochemistry*, **16**, 3581–3586.

Thomas, E.L., and Aune, T.M. (1978*a*). Oxidation of *Escherichia coli* sulfydryl components by the peroxidase-hydrogen peroxide-iodide antimicrobial system. *Antimicrobial Agents and Chemotherapy*, **13**, 1006–1010.

Thomas, E.L., and Aune, T.M. (1978*b*). Lactoperoxidase, peroxide, thiocyanate antimicrobial system: correlation of sulfydryl oxidation with antimicrobial action. *Infection and Immunity*, **20**, 456–463.

Thomas, E.L., and Aune, T.M. (1978*c*). Susceptibility of *Escherichia coli* to bactericidal action of lactoperoxidase, peroxide, and iodide or thiocyanate. *Antimicrobial Agents and Chemotherapy*, **13**, 261–265.

Thomas, E.L., Jefferson, M.M., and Grisham, M.B. (1982). Myeloperoxidase-catalyzed incorporation of amines into proteins: role of hypochlorous acid and dichloramines. *Biochemistry*, **21**, 6299–6308.

Thomas, J.A., Chai, Y.C., and Jung, C.H. (1994). Protein S-thiolation and dethiolation. *Methods in Enzymology*, **233**, 385–395.

Thomas, E.L., Bozeman, P.M., Jefferson, M.M., and King, C.C. (1995). Oxidation of bromide by the human leukocyte enzymes myeloperoxidase and eosinophil peroxidase. Formation of bromamines. *Journal of Biological Chemistry*, **270**, 2906–2913.

Thomas, J.A., Zhao, W., Hendrich, S., and Haddock, P. (1995*a*). Analysis of cells and tissues for S-thiolation of specific proteins. *Methods in Enzymology*, **251**, 423–429.

Thomas, J.A., Poland, B., and Honzatko, R. (1995*b*). Protein sulfydryls and their role in the antioxidant function of protein S-thiolation. *Archives of Biochemistry and Biophysics*, **319**, 1–9.

Thomas, P.D., and Pozansky, M.J. (1990). Lipid peroxidation inactivates rat liver microsomal glycerol-3-phosphate acyl transferase. *Journal of Biological Chemistry*, **265**, 2684–2691.

Thomas, R.M., Nauseef, W.M., Iyer, S.S., Peterson, M.W., Stone, P.J., and Clark, R.A. (1991). A cytosolic inhibitor of human neutrophil elastase and cathepsin G. *Journal of Leukocyte Biology*, **50**, 568–579.

Thomas, S.M., Gebicki, J.M., and Dean, R.T. (1989*a*). Radical initiated alpha-tocopherol depletion and lipid peroxidation in mitochondrial membranes. *Biochimica et Biophysica Acta*, **1002**, 189–197.

Thomas, S.M., Jessup, W., Gebicki, J.M., and Dean, R.T. (1989*b*). A continuous-flow automated assay for iodometric estimation of hydroperoxides. *Analytical Biochemistry*, **176**, 353–359.

Thomas, S.R., Mohr, D., and Stocker, R. (1994). Nitric oxide inhibits indoleamine 2,3-dioxygenase activity in interferon-gamma primed mononuclear phagocytes. *Journal of Biological Chemistry*, **269**, 14457–14464.

Thomas, S.R., Neuzil, J., Mohr, D., and Stocker, R. (1995). Co-antioxidants make α-tocopherol an efficient antioxidant for LDL. *American Journal of Clinical Nutrition*, **62**, 1357S–1364S.

Thomas, T., Thomas, G., McLendon, C., Sutton, T., and Mullan, M. (1996). Beta-amyloid-mediated vasoactivity and vascular endothelial damage. *Nature*, **380**, 168–171.

Thomson, A.J., Robinson, A.E., Johnson, M.K., Moura, J.J., Moura, I., Xavier, A.V., *et al.* (1981). The three-iron cluster in a ferredoxin from *Desulphovibrio gigas*. A low-temperature magnetic circular dichroism study. *Biochimica et Biophysica Acta*, **670**, 93–100.

Thorburn, D.R., and Beutler, E. (1989). Decay of hexokinase during reticulocyte maturation: is oxidative damage a signal for destruction? *Biochemical and Biophysical Research Communications*, **162**, 612–618.

Thornalley, P.J., Wolff, S.P., Crabbe, M.J., and Stern, A. (1984). The oxidation of oxyhaemoglobin by glyceraldehyde and other simple monosaccharides. *Biochemical Journal*, **217**, 615–622.

Thorneley, R.N. (1975). Nitrogenase of *Klebsiella pneumoniae*. A stopped-flow study of magnesium-adenosine triphosphate-induced electron transfer between the compeonent proteins. *Biochemical Journal*, **145**, 391–396.

Thorpe, S., and Baynes, J.W. (1996). Role of the Maillard reaction in diabetes mellitus and disease of aging. *Drugs and Aging*, **9**, 69–77.

Thurlow, S. (1925). XXV. Studies on xanthine oxidase. IV. Relation of xanthine oxidase and similar oxidising systems to Bach's oxygenase. *Biochemical Journal*, **19**, 175–187.

Tian, L., Cai, Q., Bowen, R., and Wei, H. (1995). Effects of caloric restriction on age-related oxidative modifications of macromolecules and lymphocyte proliferation in rats. *Free Radical Biology and Medicine*, **19**, 859–865.

Till, G.O., Lutz, M.J., and Ward, P.A. (1987). Hydroxy radical as autotoxin in chemotactically activated neutrophils. *Biomedical Pharmacotherapy*, **41**, 349–354.

Timmins, G.S., and Davies, M.J. (1993*a*). An EPR spin trapping study of albumin protein radicals formed by the photodynamic action of haematoporphyrin. *Journal of Photochemistry and Photobiology B*, **21**, 167–173.

Timmins, G.S., and Davies, M.J. (1993*b*). Free radical formation in isolated murine keratinocytes treated with organic peroxides and its modulation by antioxidants. *Carcinogenesis*, **14**, 1615–1620.

Timmins, G.S., and Davies, M.J. (1993*c*). Free radical formation in murine skin treated with tumour promoting organic peroxides. *Carcinogenesis*, **14**, 1499–1503.

Timmins, G.S., and Davies, M.J. (1994). Conformational changes induced in bovine serum albumin by the photodynamic action of haematoporphyrin. *Journal of Photochemistry and Photobiology B*, **24**, 117–122.

Timmins, G.S., Davies, M.J., Song, D.X., and Muller, E.U. (1995*a*). EPR studies on the effects of complexation of heme by hemopexin upon its reactions with organic peroxides. *Free Radical Research*, **23**, 559–569.

Timmins, G.S., Davies, M.J., and Muller, E.U. (1995*b*). A study of the effects of complexation of heme by hemopexin upon its reactions with organic peroxides. *Biochemical Society Transactions*, **23**, 244S.

Tinker, D.H., and Tappel, A.L. (1983). A partial characterization of the major fluorophore of bovine ligamentum elastin. *Connective Tissue Research*, **11**, 309–319.

Tinker, D.H., Rucker, R.B., and Tappel, A.L. (1983). Variation of elastin fluorescence with method of preparation: determination of the major fluorophore of fibrillar elastin. *Connective Tissue Research*, **11**, 299–308.

Toledano, M.B., Ghosh, D., Trinh, F., and Leonard, W.J. (1993). N-terminal DNA-binding domains contribute to differential DNA-binding specificities of NF-kappa B p50 and p65. *Molecular and Cellular Biology*, **13**, 852–860.

Toledo, I., and Hansberg, W. (1990). Protein oxidation related to morphogenesis in *Neurospora crassa*. *Experimental Mycology*, **14**, 184–189.

Toledo, I., Noronha-Dutra, A.A., and Hansberg, W. (1991). Loss of NAD(P)-reducing power and glutathione disulfide excretion at the start of the inducation of aerial growth in *Neurospora crassa*. *Journal of Bacteriology*, **173**, 3243–3249.

Toledo, I., Aguirre, J., and Hansberg, W. (1994). Enzyme inactivation related to a hyperoxidant state during conidiation of *Neurospora crassa*. *Microbiology*, **140**, 2391–2397.

Toledo, I., Rangel, P., and Hansberg, W. (1995). Redox imbalance at the start of each morphogenetic step of *Neurospora crassa* conidiation. *Archives of Biochemistry and Biophysics*, **319**, 519–524.

Tomimoto, H., Akiguchi, I., Wakita, H., Kimura, J., Hori, K., and Yodoi, J. (1993). Astroglial expression of ATL-derived factor, a human thioredoxin homologue, in the gerbil brain after transient global ischemia. *Brain Research*, **625**, 1–8.

Tomoda, A., Sugimoto, K., Suhara, M., Takeshita, M., and Yoneyama, Y. (1978). Haemichrome formation from haemoglobin subunits by hydrogen peroxide. *Biochemical Journal*, **171**, 329–335.

Topchieva, I.N., Volodin, V.V., Tyukavin, Y., Osipova, S.V., Kulakov, V.N., and Banatskaya, M.I. (1991). The interaction of block copolymers of ethylene oxide and propylene oxide and their polymer-protein conjugates with lipids. *Biomedical Science*, **2**, 562–568.

Toyama, H., Fujii, A., Matsushita, K., Shinagawa, E., Ameyama, M., and Adachi, O. (1995). Three distinct quinoprotein alcohol dehydrogenases are expressed when *Pseudomonas putida* is grown on different alcohols. *Journal of Bacteriology*, **177**, 2442–2450.

Toyama, R., Mizumoto, K., Nakahara, Y., Tatsuno, T., and Kaziro, Y. (1983). Mechanism of the mRNA guanylyltransferase reaction: isolation of N epsilon-phospholysine and GMP (5' leads to N epsilon) lysine from the guanylyl-enzyme intermediate. *EMBO Journal*, **2**, 2195–2201.

Toyokuni, S., Uchida, K., Okamoto, K., Hattori, N.Y., Hiai, H., and Stadtman, E.R. (1994). Formation of 4-hydroxy-2-nonenal-modified proteins in the renal proximal tubules of rats treated with a renal carcinogen, ferric nitrilotriacetate. *Proceedings of the National Academy of Science of the United States of America*, **91**, 2616–2620.

Toyokuni, S., Mori, T., Hiai, H., and Dizdaroglu, M. (1995). Treatment of Wistar rats with a renal carcinogen, ferric nitrilotriacetate, causes DNA-protein cross-linking between thymine and tyrosine in their renal chromatin. *International Journal of Cancer*, **62**, 309–313.

Traber, J., Suter, M., Walter, P., and Richter, C. (1992). *In vivo* modulation of total and mitochondrial glutathione in rat liver. Depletion by phorone and rescue by *N*-acetylcysteine. *Biochemical Pharmacology*, **43**, 961–964.

Traber, R., Kramer, H.E., and Hemmerich, P. (1982). Mechanism of light-induced reduction of biological redox centers by amino acids. A flash photolysis study of flavin photoreduction by ethylenediaminetetraacetate and nitrilotriacetate. *Biochemistry*, **21**, 1687–1693.

Trad, C.H., and Butterfield, D.A. (1994). Menadione-induced cytotoxicity effects on human erythrocyte membranes studied by electron paramagnetic resonance. *Toxicology Letters*, **73**, 145–155.

Trad, C.H., James, W., Bhardwaj, A., and Butterfield, D.A. (1995). Selective labeling of membrane protein sulfydryl groups with methanethiosulfonate spin label. *Journal of Biochemical and Biophysical Methods*, **30**, 287–299.

Traverso, N., Pronzato, M.A., Menini, S., Odetti, P., Cottalasso, D., and Marinari, U.M. (1996). Protein peroxide generation and decay by non-enzymatic modifications. In *Abstracts of VII Biennial Meeting International Society for Free Radical Research*, p. 59, Barcelona.

Trelstad, R.L., Lawley, K.R., and Holmes, L.B. (1981). Nonenzymatic hydroxylations of proline and lysine by reduced oxygen derivatives. *Nature*, **289**, 310–322.

Trinder, P. (1980). A new method for the determination of plasma phenylalanine. *Annals of Clinical Biochemistry*, **17**, 26–30.

Trombly, R., Tappel, A.L., Coniglio, J.G., Grogan, W.J., and Rhamy, R.K. (1975). Fluorescent products and polyunsaturated fatty acids of human testes. *Lipids*, **10**, 591–596.

Troy, C.M., Stefanis, L., Prochiantz, A., Greene, L.A., and Shelanski, M.L. (1996a). The contrasting roles of ICE family proteases and interleukin-1beta in apoptosis induced by trophic factor withdrawal and by copper/zinc superoxide dismutase down-regulation. *Proceedings of the National Academy of Science of the United States of America*, **93**, 5635–5640.

Troy, C.M., Derossi, D., Prochiantz, A., Greene, L.A., and Shelanski, M.L. (1996b). Downregulation of Cu/Zn superoxide dismutase leads to cell death via the nitric oxide-peroxynitrite pathway. *Journal of Neuroscience*, **16**, 253–261.

Truscott, R.J., and Augusteyn, R.C. (1977a). Changes in human lens proteins during senile nuclear cataract formation. *Experimental Eye Research*, **24**, 159–170.

Truscott, R.J., and Augusteyn, R.C. (1977b). Oxidative changes in human lens proteins during senile nuclear cataract formation. *Biochimica et Biophysica Acta*, **492**, 43–52.

Truscott, R.J., and Augusteyn, R.C. (1977c). The state of sulphydryl groups in normal and cataractous human lenses. *Experimental Eye Research*, **25**, 139–148.

Truscott, R.J., and Elderfield, A.J. (1995). Relationship between serum tryptophan and tryptophan metabolite levels after tryptophan ingestion in normal subjects and age-related cataract patients. *Clinical Science*, **89**, 591–599.

Tsai, A.L., Palmer, G., and Kulmacz, R.J. (1992). Prostaglandin H synthase. Kinetics of tyrosyl radical formation and of cyclooxygenase catalysis. *Journal of Biological Chemistry*, **267**, 17753–17759.

Tsen, C.C., and Tappel, A.L. (1958). Oxygen lability of cysteine in haemoglobin. *Archives of Biochemistry and Biophysics*, **75**, 243–250.

Tso, J., Petrouleas, V., and Dismukes, G.C. (1990). A new mechanism-based inhibitor of photosynthetic water oxidation: acetone hydrazone. 1. Equilibrium reactions. *Biochemistry*, **29**, 7759–7767.

Tullius, T.D. (1987). Chemical 'snapshots' of DNA: using the hydroxyl radical to study the structure of DNA and DNA-protein complexes. *Trends in Biochemical Science*, **12**, 297–300.

Tullius, T.D., and Dombroski, B.A. (1985). Iron(II) EDTA used to measure the helical twist along any DNA molecule. *Science*, **230**, 679–681.

Tullius, T.D., and Dombroski, B.A. (1986). Hydroxyl radical 'footprinting': high-resolution information about DNA-protein contacts and application to lambda repressor and Cro protein. *Proceedings of the National Academy of Science of the United States of America*, **83**, 5469–5473.

Tung, T.L., Welch, G.P., Sokol, H.A., Bennett, C.W., and Garrison, W.M. (1976). Letter: Heavy-ion radiolysis of solid glycine. *Journal of the American Chemical Society*, **98**, 4341–4342.

Turnbough, C.L., and Switzer, R.L. (1975*a*). Oxygen-dependent inactivation of glutamine phosphoribosyl-pyrophosphate amidotransferase in stationary-phase cultures of B. subtilis. *Journal of Bacteriology*, **121**, 108–114.

Turnbough, C.L., and Switzer, R.L. (1975*b*). Oxygen-dependent inactivation of glutamine phosphoribosyl-pyrophosphate amidotransferase *in vitro*: model for *in vivo* inactivation. *Journal of Bacteriology*, **121**, 115–120.

Turner, J.J., Rice-Evans, C., Davies, M.J., and Newman, E.S. (1990). Free radicals, myocytes and reperfusion injury. *Biochemical Society Transactions*, **18**, 1056–1059.

Turner, J.J., Rice-Evans, C., Davies, M.J., and Newman, E.S. (1991). The formation of free radicals by cardiac myocytes under oxidative stress and the effects of electron-donating drugs. *Biochemical Journal*, **277**, 833–837.

Turowski, P.N., McGuirl, M.A., and Dooley, D.M. (1993). Intramolecular electron transfer rate between active-site copper and topa quinone in pea seedling amine oxidase. *Journal of Biological Chemistry*, **268**, 17680–17682.

Uchida, K., and Kawakishi, S. (1986). Selective oxidation of imidazole ring in histidine residues by the ascorbic acid-copper ion system. *Biochemical and Biophysical Research Communications*, **138**, 659–665.

Uchida, K., and Kawakishi, S. (1993). 2-Oxo-histidine as a novel biological marker for oxidatively modified proteins. *FEBS Letters*, **332**, 208–210.

Uchida, K., and Kawakishi, S. (1994). Identification of oxidized histidine generated at the active site of Cu,Zn-superoxide dismutase exposed to H_2O_2. Selective generation of 2-oxo-histidine at the histidine 118. *Journal of Biological Chemistry*, **269**, 2405–2410.

Uchida, K., and Stadtman, E.R. (1992*a*). Selective cleavage of thioether linkage in proteins modified with 4-hydroxynonenal. *Proceedings of the National Academy of Science of the United States of America*, **89**, 5611–5615.

Uchida, K., and Stadtman, E.R. (1992*b*). Modification of histidine residues in proteins by reaction with 4-hydroxynonenal. *Proceedings of the National Academy of Science of the United States of America*, **89**, 4544–4548.

Uchida, K., and Stadtman, E.R. (1993). Covalent attachment of 4-hydroxynonenal to glyceraldehyde-3-phosphate dehydrogenase. A possible involvement of intra- and intermolecular cross-linking reaction. *Journal of Biological Chemistry*, **268**, 6388–6393.

Uchida, K., and Stadtman, E.R. (1994). Quantitation of 4-hydroxynonenal protein adducts. *Methods in Enzymology*, **233**, 371–380.

Uchida, K., Kato, Y., and Kawakishi, S. (1990). A novel mechanism for oxidative cleavage of prolyl peptides induced by the hydroxyl radical. *Biochemical and Biophysical Research Communications*, **169**, 265–271.

Uchida, K., Szweda, L.I., Chae, H.Z., and Stadtman, E.R. (1993). Immunochemical detection of 4-hydroxynonenal protein adducts in oxidized hepatocytes. *Proceedings of the National Academy of Science of the United States of America*, **90**, 8742–8746.

Uchida, K., Toyokuni, S., Nishikawa, K., Kawakishi, S., Oda, H., Hiai, H., *et al.* (1994). Michael addition-type 4-hydroxy-2-nonenal adducts in modified low-density lipoproteins: markers for atherosclerosis. *Biochemistry*, **33**, 12487–12494.

Uchida, K., Itakura, K., Kawakishi, S., Hiai, H., Toyokuni, S., and Stadtman, E.R. (1995). Characterization of epitopes recognized by 4-hydroxy-2-nonenal specific antibodies. *Archives of Biochemistry and Biophysics*, **324**, 241–248.

Uchiumi, T., Kikuchi, M., Terao, K., and Ogata, K. (1985). Cross-linking study on protein topography of rat liver 60 S ribosomal subunits with 2-iminothiolane. *Journal of Biological Chemistry*, **260**, 5675–5682.

Ueda, J., Saito, N., and Ozawa, T. (1996). ESR Spin trapping studies on the reactions of hydroperoxides with Cu(II) comples. *Journal of Inorganic Biochemistry*, **64**, 197–206.

Ueda, K., Morita, J., Yamashita, K., and Komano, T. (1980). Inactivation of bacteriophage phi X174 by mitomycin C in the presence of sodium hydrosulfite and cupric ions. *Chemico-Biological Interactions*, **29**, 145–158.

Ueda, K., Morita, J., and Komano, T. (1982). Phage inactivation and DNA strand scission activities of 7-N-(p-hydroxyphenyl) mitomycin C. *Journal of Antibiotics Tokyo*, **35**, 1380–1386.

Ueland, P.M., Mansoor, M.A., Guttormsen, A.B., Muller, F., Aukrust, P., Refsum, H., *et al.* (1996). Reduced, oxidized and protein-bound forms of homocysteine and other aminothiols in plasma comprise the redox thiol status—a possible element of the extracellular antioxidant defense system. *Journal of Nutrition*, **126 (Supplement 4)**, 1281S-1284S.

Ukab, W.A., Sato, J., Wang, Y.M., and van Eys, J. (1981). Xylitol mediated amelioration of acetylphenylhydrazine-induced hemolysis in rabbits. *Metabolism*, **30**, 1053–1059.

Um, H.D., Orenstein, J.M., and Wahl, S.M. (1996). Fas mediates apoptosis in human monocytes by a reactive oxygen intermediate dependent pathway. *Journal of Immunology*, **156**, 3469–3477.

Unkrig, V., Neugebauer, F.A., and Knappe, J. (1989). The free radical of pyruvate formate-lyase. Characterization by EPR spectroscopy and involvement in catalysis as studied with the substrate-analogue hypophosphite. *European Journal of Biochemistry*, **184**, 723–728.

Ursini, F., Maiorino, M., Valente, M., Ferri, L., and Gregolin, C. (1982). Purification from pig liver of a protein which protects liposomes and bio-membranes from peroxidative degradation and exhibits glutathione peroxidase activity on phosphatidylcholine hydroperoxides. *Biochimica et Biophysica Acta*, **710**, 197–211.

Uyeda, M., and Peisach, J. (1981). Ultraviolet difference spectroscopy of myoglobin: assignment of pK values of tyrosyl phenolic groups and the stability of the ferryl derivatives. *Biochemistry*, **20**, 2028–2035.

Van Buskirk, J.J., Kirsch, W.M., Kleyer, D.L., Darklen, R.M., and Koch, T.H. (1984). Aminomalonic acid: identification in *E. coli* and atherosclerotic plaque. *Proceedings of the National Academy of Science of the United States of America*, **81**, 722–725.

van den Berg, J.J., Op den Kamp, J.A., Lubin, B.H., and Kuypers, F.A. (1993). Conformational changes in oxidized phospholipids and their preferential hydrolysis by phospholipase A2: a monolayer study. *Biochemistry*, **32**, 4962–4967.

van der Deen, H., and Hoving, H. (1977). Nitrite and nitric oxide treatment of Helix pomatia hemocyanin: single and double oxidation of the active site. *Biochemistry*, **16**, 3519–3525.

van der Meer, R.A., Groen, B.W., Jongejan, J.A., and Duine, J.A. (1990). The redox-cycling assay is not suited for the detection of pyrroloquinoline quinone in biological samples [see comments]. *FEBS Letters*, **261**, 131–134.

van der Vliet, A., O'Neill, C.A., Halliwell, B., Cross, C.E., and Kaur, H. (1994*a*). Aromatic hydroxylation and nitration of phenylalanine and tyrosine by peroxynitrite. Evidence for hydroxyl radical production from peroxynitrite. *FEBS Letters*, **339**, 89–92.

van der Vliet, A., Smith, D., O'Neill, C.A., Kaur, H., Darley-Usmar, V., Cross, C.E., *et al.* (1994*b*). Interactions of peroxynitrite with human plasma and its constituents; oxidative damage and antioxidant depletion. *Biochemical Journal*, **303**, 295–301.

van der Vliet, A., Eiserich, J.P., O'Neill, C.A., Halliwell, B., and Cross, C.E. (1995). Tyrosine modification by reactive nitrogen species: a closer look. *Archives of Biochemistry and Biophysics*, **319**, 341–349.

Van der Zee, J., Eling, T.E., and Mason, R.P. (1989). Formation of free radical metabolites in the reaction between soybean lipoxygenase and its inhibitors. An ESR study. *Biochemistry*, **28**, 8363–8367.

Van der Zee, J., Krootjes, B.B., Chignell, C.F., Dubbelman, T.M., and Van Steveninck, J. (1993). Hydroxyl radical generation by a light-dependent Fenton reaction. *Free Radical Biology and Medicine*, **14**, 105–113.

Van Heyningen, R. (1973). Photo-oxidation of lens proteins by sunlight in the presence of fluorescent derivatives of kynurenine, isolated from the human lens. *Experimental Eye Research*, **17**, 137–147.

van Kleef, M.A., Jongejan, J.A., and Duine, J.A. (1989). Factors relevant in the reaction of pyrroloquinoline quinone with amino acids. Analytical and mechanistic implications. *European Journal of Biochemistry*, **183**, 41–47.

Van Reyk, D.M., Brown, A.J., Jessup, W., and Dean, R.T. (1995). Batch-to-batch variation of Chelex-100 confounds metal-catalysed oxidation. Leaching of inhibitory compounds from a batch of Chelex-100 and their removal by a pre-washing procedure. *Free Radical Research*, **23**, 533–535.

Van Tamelen, E.E., Haarstad, V.B., and Orvis, R.L. (1968). Hypohalite-induced oxidative decarboxylation of α-amino acids. *Tetrahedron*, **24**, 687–704.

Vandeplassche, G., Bernier, M., Thone, F., Borgers, M., Kusama, Y., and Hearse, D.J. (1990). Singlet oxygen and myocardial injury: ultrastructural, cytochemical and electrocardiographic consequences of photoactivation of rose bengal. *Journal of Molecular and Cellular Cardiology*, **22**, 287–301.

Vanderkooi, J.M., Wright, W.W., and Erecinska, M. (1994). Nitric oxide diffusion coefficients in solutions, proteins and membranes determined by phosphorescence. *Biochimica et Biophysica Acta*, **1207**, 249–254.

Varma, S.D., and Devamanoharan, P.S. (1995). Oxidative denaturation of lens protein: prevention by pyruvate. *Ophthalmic Research*, **27**, 18–22.

Varma, S.D., Devamanoharan, P.S., Mansour, S., and Teter, B. (1994). Studies on Emory mouse cataracts: oxidative factors. *Ophthalmic Research*, **26**, 141–148.

Varma, S.D., Ramachandran, S., Devamanoharan, P.S., Morris, S.M., and Ali, A.H. (1995). Prevention of oxidative damage to rat lens by pyruvate *in vitro*: possible attenuation *in vivo*. *Current Eye Research*, **14**, 643–649.

Varsila, E., Pesonen, E., and Andersson, S. (1995). Early protein oxidation in the neonatal lung is related to development of chronic lung disease. *Acta Paediatrics*, **84**, 1296–1299.

Vecli, A., Crippa, P.R., and Santamaria, L. (1971). Light induced free radicals in hematoporphyrin-serum protein systems. *Bolletino Chimica Farmacologia*, **110**, 91–99.

Veldink, G.A., Boelens, H., Maccarrone, M., van, d.L.F., Vliegenthart, J.F., Paz, M.A., *et al.* (1990). Soybean lipoxygenase-1 is not a quinoprotein. *FEBS Letters*, **270**, 135–138.

Velez, P.C., Jimenez, D.R.M., Ebinger, G., and Vauquelin, G. (1996). Redox cycling activity of monoamine-serotonin binding protein conjugates. *Biochemical Pharmacology*, **51**, 1521–1525.

Vellieux, F.M., Frank, J., Swarte, M.B., Groendijk, H., Duine, J.A., Drenth, J., *et al.* (1986). Purification, crystallization and preliminary X-ray investigation of quinoprotein methylamine dehydrogenase from *Thiobacillus versutus*. *European Journal of Biochemistry*, **154**, 383–386.

Vellieux, F.M., Kalk, K.H., Drenth, J., and Hol, W.G. (1990). Structure determination of quinoprotein methylamine dehydrogenase from *Thiobacillus versutus*. *Acta Crystallographica B*, **46**, 806–823.

Vermeil, C., and Lefort, M. (1957). Production of tyrosine by the action of X-rays on aqueous solutions of phenylalanine. *Compote Rendus Academy Science*, **244**, 889–891.

Vertongen, F., Heyder, B.C., Fondu, P., and Mandelbaum, I. (1981). Oxidative haemolysis in protein malnutrition. *Clinica Chimica Acta*, **116**, 217–222.

Viehe, H.G., Janousek, Z., Merenyi, R., and Stella, L. (1985). The captodative effect. *Accounts of Chemical Research*, **18**, 148–154.

Viguie, C.A., Frei, B., Shigenaga, M.K., Ames, B.N., Packer, L., and Brooks, G.A. (1993). Antioxidant status and indexes of oxidative stress during consecutive days of exercise. *Journal of Applied Physiology*, **75**, 566–572.

Vilaseca, L.A., Rose, K., Werlen, R., Meunier, A., Offord, R.E., Nichols, C.L., *et al.* (1993). Protein conjugates of defined structure: synthesis and use of a new carrier molecule. *Bioconjugate Chemistry*, **4**, 515–520.

Viljoen, A.J., and Tappel, A.L. (1988a). Interactions of selenium and cadmium with metallothionein-like and other cytosolic proteins of rat kidney and liver. *Journal of Inorganic Biochemistry*, **34**, 277–290.

Viljoen, A.J., and Tappel, A.L. (1988b). Selenium-containing proteins of rat kidney. *Journal of Inorganic Biochemistry*, **33**, 263–275.

Vince, G.S., and Dean, R.T. (1987). Is enhanced free radical flux associated with increased intracellular proteolysis? *FEBS Letters*, **216**, 253–256.

Vincent, S.H. (1989). Oxidative effects of heme and porphyrins on proteins and lipids. *Seminars in Hematology*, **26**, 105–113.

Vincent, S.H., and Muller, E.U. (1987). Effects of porphyrins on proteins of cytosol and plasma. *In vitro* photo-oxidation and cross-linking of proteins by naturally occurring and synthetic porphyrins. *Journal of Laboratory and Clinical Medicine*, **110**, 475–482.

Viner, R.I., Ferrington, D.A., Huhmer, A.F., Bigelow, D.J., and Schoneich, C. (1996). Accumulation of nitrotyrosine on the SERCA2a isoform of SR Ca-ATPase of rat skeletal muscle during aging: a peroxynitrite-mediated process? *FEBS Letters*, **379**, 286–290.

Visick, J.E., and Clarke, S. (1995). Repair, refold, recycle: how bacteria can deal with spontaneous and environmental damage to proteins. *Molecular Microbiology*, **16**, 835–845.

Vissers, M.C.M., and Winterbourn, C.C. (1986). The effect of oxidants on neutrophil-mediated degradation of glomerular basement membrane collagen. *Biochimica et Biophysica Acta*, **889**, 277–286.

Vitello, L.B., Erman, J.E., Mauro, J.M., and Kraut, J. (1990). Characterization of the hydrogen peroxide-enzyme reaction for two cytochrome *c* peroxidase mutants. *Biochimica et Biophysica Acta*, **1038**, 90–97.

Vivoli, G., Bergomi, M., Rovesti, S., Pinotti, M., and Caselgrandi, E. (1995). Zinc, copper, and zinc- or copper-dependent enzymes in human hypertension. *Biological Trace Elements Resesarch*, **49**, 97–106.

Vladimirov, Y.A., Roshchupkin, D.I., and Fesenko, E.E. (1970). Photochemical reactions in amino acid residues and inactivation of enzymes during UV-irradiation. A review. *Photochemistry and Photobiology*, **11**, 227–246.

Vlessis, A.A., Muller, P., Bartos, D., and Trunkey, D. (1991). Mechanism of peroxide-induced cellular injury in cultured adult cardiac myocytes. *FASEB Journal*, **5**, 2600–2605.

Vogt, W. (1995). Oxidation of methionyl residues in proteins: tools, targets, and reversal. *Free Radical Biology and Medicine*, **18**, 93–105.

von, H.M., and Holzer, H. (1985). Oxidative inactivation of yeast fructose-1, 6-bisphosphatase. *Progress in Clinical Biological Research*, **180**, 329–340.

von, S.C. (1991). The chemistry of free-radical-mediated DNA damage. *Basic Life Science*, **58**, 287–317.

von Arx, E., and Neher, R. (1963). Eine Multidimensionale Technik Zur Chromatoagraphischen Identifizierung von Aminosäuren. *Journal of Chromatography*, **12**, 329–341.

von Sonntag, C. (1987). *The Chemical Basis of Radiation Biology*. Taylor and Francis, London.

von Sonntag, C. (1990). Free-radical reactions involving thiols and disulphides. In *Sulfur-Centered Reactive Intermediates in Chemistry and Biology*, (ed. C. Chatgilialoglu and K.D. Asmus), pp. 359–366. Plenum Press, New York.

Wade, R.S., and Castro, C.E. (1973). Oxidation of heme proteins by alkyl halides. *Journal of the American Chemical Society*, **95**, 231–234.

Wagner, A.F., Frey, M., Neugebauer, F.A., Schafer, W., and Knappe, J. (1992). The free radical in pyruvate formate-lyase is located on glycine-734. *Proceedings of the National Academy of Science of the United States of America*, **89**, 996–1000.

Wagner, J.R., Motchnik, P.A., Stocker, R., Sies, H., and Ames, B.N. (1993). The oxidation of blood plasma and low density lipoprotein components by chemically generated singlet oxygen. *Journal of Biological Chemistry*, **268**, 18502–18506.

Wagner, R.M., and Fraser, B.A. (1987). Analysis of peptides containing oxidized methionine and/or tryptophan by fast atom bombardment mass spectrometry. *Biomedical and Environmental Mass Spectrometry*, **14**, 69–72.

Waldeck, A.R., and Stocker, R. (1996). Lipid peroxidation of radical-mediated low density lipoproteins: insights obtained from kinetic modelling. *Chemical Research in Toxicology*, **9**, 954–964.

Walker, K.W., Lyles, M.M., and Gilbert, H.F. (1996). Catalysis of oxidative protein folding by mutants of protein disulfide isomerase with a single active-site cysteine. *Biochemistry*, **35**, 1972–1980.

Walling, C., and Wagner, P.J. (1964). Positive halogen compounds. X. Solvent effects in the reaction of *t*-butoxy radicals. *Journal of the American Chemical Society*, **86**, 3368–3375.

Walsh, M., Stevens, F.C., Oikawa, K., and Kay, C.M. (1978). Circular dichroism studies on Ca^{2+}-dependent protein modulator oxidized with N-chlorosuccinimide. *Biochemistry*, **17**, 3928–3930.

Wang, K., and Spector, A. (1995). Alpha-crystallin can act as a chaperone under conditions of oxidative stress. *Investigative Ophthalmology and Vision Science*, **36**, 311–321.

Wang, K., Ma, W., and Spector, A. (1995). Phosphorylation of alpha-crystallin in rat lenses is stimulated by H_2O_2 but phosphorylation has no effect on chaperone activity. *Experimental Eye Research*, **61**, 115–124.

Wang, W., and Sevilla, M.D. (1994). Reaction of cysteamine with individual DNA base radicals in gamma-irradiated nucleotides at low temperature. *International*

Journal of Radiation and Biology and Related Studies in Physical Chemistry and Medicine, **66**, 683–695.

Warburg, O., and Sakuma, S. (1923). The so-called autoxidation of cysteine. *Archives Ges Physiology (Pfluger's)*, **200**, 203–206.

Ward, W.W., and Cormier, M.J. (1975). Extraction of *Renilla*-type luciferin from the calcium-activated photoproteins aequorin, mnemiopsin, and berovin. *Proceedings of the National Academy of Science of the United States of America*, **72**, 2530–2534.

Wardman, P. (1989). Reduction potentials on one-electron couples involving free radicals in aqueous solution. *Journal of Physical Chemistry Reference Data*, **18**, 1637–1755.

Wardman, P., and Candeias, L.P. (1996). Fenton chemistry: an introduction. *Radiation Research*, **145**, 523–531.

Wardman, P., and von Sonntag, C. (1995). Kinetic factors that control the fate of thiyl radicals in cells. *Methods in Enzymology*, **251**, 31–45.

Watabe, S., Hasegawa, H., Takimoto, K., Yamamoto, Y., and Takahashi, S.Y. (1995). Possible function of SP-22, a substrate of mitochondrial ATP-dependent protease, as a radical scavenger. *Biochemical and Biophysical Research Communications*, **213**, 1010–1016.

Watt, G.D., Burns, A., Lough, S., and Tennent, D.L. (1980). Redox and spectroscopic properties of oxidized MoFe protein from *Azotobacter vinelandii*. *Biochemistry*, **19**, 4926–4932.

Watts, B.J., Barnard, M., and Turrens, J.F. (1995). Peroxynitrite-dependent chemiluminescence of amino acids, proteins, and intact cells. *Archives of Biochemistry and Biophysics*, **317**, 324–330.

Wautier, J.L., Zoukourian, C., Chappey, O., Wautier, M.P., Guillausseau, P.J., Cao, R., et al. (1996). Receptor-mediated endothelial cell dysfunction in diabetic vasculopathy. Soluble receptor for advanced glycation end products blocks hyperpermeability in diabetic rats. *Journal of Clinical Investigation*, **97**, 238–243.

Weber, T., and Bach, T.J. (1994). Conversion of acetyl-coenzyme A into 3-hydroxy-3-methylglutaryl-coenzyme A in radish seedlings. Evidence of a single monomeric protein catalyzing a FeII/quinone-stimulated double condensation reaction. *Biochimica et Biophysica Acta*, **1211**, 85–96.

Weeks, B.M., and Garrison, W.M. (1958). Radiolysis of aqueous solutions of glycine. *Radiation Research*, **9**, 291–304.

Weeks, B.M., Cole, S.A., and Garrison, W.M. (1965). Reactions of alanine with the reducing species formed in water radiolysis. *Journal of Physical Chemistry*, **69**, 4131–4137.

Weil, J.A., Bolton, J.R., and Wertz, J.E. (1994). *Electron Paramagnetic Resonance: Elementary Theory and Practical Applications*. Wiley, New York.

Weiner, L., Kreimer, D., Roth, E., and Silman, I. (1994). Oxidative stress transforms acetylcholinesterase to a molten-globule-like state. *Biochemical and Biophysical Research Communications*, **198**, 915–922.

Weiss, S.J., Lampert, M.B., and Test, S.T. (1983). Long-lived oxidants generated by human neutrophils: characterization and bioactivity. *Science*, **222**, 625–628.

Weiss, S.J., Curnutte, J.T., and Regiani, S. (1986). Neutrophil-mediated solubilization of the subendothelial matrix: oxidative and nonoxidative mechanisms of proteolysis used by normal and chronic granulomatous disease phagocytes. *Journal of Immunology*, **136**, 636–641.

Wells-Knecht, K.J., Lyons, T.J., McCance, D.R., Thorpe, S.R., Feather, M.S., and Baynes, J.W. (1994). 3-deoxyfructose concentrations are increased in human plasma and urine in diabetes. *Diabetes*, **43**, 1152–1156.

Wells-Knecht, K.J., Zyzak, D.V., Litchfield, J.E., Thorpe, S.R., and Baynes, J.W. (1995). Mechanism of autoxidative glycosylation: identification of glyoxal and arabinose as intermediates in the autoxidative modification of proteins by glucose. *Biochemistry*, **34**, 3702–3709.

Wells-Knecht, M.C., Huggins, T.G., Dyer, D.G., Thorpe, S.R., and Baynes, J.W. (1993). Oxidized amino acids in lens protein with age. Measurement of *o*-tyrosine and dityrosine in the aging human lens. *Journal of Biological Chemistry*, **268**, 12348–12352.

Wells-Knecht, M.C., Thorpe, S.R., and Baynes, J.W. (1995). Pathways of formation of glycoxidation products during glycation of collagen. *Biochemistry*, **34**, 15134–15141.

Wels, P. (1923). Effect of Rontgen rays on proteins. *Archives Ges Physiology (Pfluger's)*, **199**, 226–236.

Wels, P., and Thiele, A. (1925). Effects of Rontgen rays on proteins. II. *Archives Ges Physiology (Pfluger's)*, **209**, 49–64.

Wenger, R.H., Marti, H.H., Schuerer, M.C., Kvietikova, I., Bauer, C., Gassmann, M., *et al.* (1996). Hypoxic induction of gene expression in chronic granulomatous disease-derived B-cell lines: oxygen sensing is independent of the cytochrome *b*558-containing nicotinamide adenine dinucleotide phosphate oxidase. *Blood*, **87**, 756–761.

Werns, S.W., and Lucchesi, B.R. (1990). Free radicals and ischemic tissue injury. *Trends in Pharmacological Science*, **11**, 161–166.

Westendorp, M.O., Shatrov, V.A., Schulze, O.K., Frank, R., Kraft, M., Los, M., *et al.* (1995). HIV-1 Tat potentiates TNF-induced NF-kappa B activation and cytotoxicity by altering the cellular redox state. *EMBO Journal*, **14**, 546–554.

Westhof, E., Flossmann, W., and Muller, A. (1975). The action of ionizing radiation on protein: radical formation in L-histidine crystals. *International Journal of Radiation Biology and Related Studies in Physics, Chemistry and Medicine*, **27**, 51–62.

Wetlaufer, D.B., Branca, P.A., and Chen, G.X. (1987). The oxidative folding of proteins by disulfide plus thiol does not correlate with redox potential. *Protein Engineering*, **1**, 141–146.

Wettern, M., Parag, H.A., Pollmann, L., Ohad, I., and Kulka, R.G. (1990). Ubiquitin in *Chlamydomonas reinhardii*. Distribution in the cell and effect of heat shock and photoinhibition on its conjugate pattern. *European Journal of Biochemistry*, **191**, 571–576.

Wheelan, P., Kirsch, W.M., and Koch, T.H. (1989). Free-radical carboxylation of peptide- and protein-bound glycine to form peptide- and protein-bound aminomalonic acid (Ama). *Journal of Organic Chemistry*, **54**, 4360–4364.

Wheeler, O.H., and Montalvo, R. (1969). Radiolysis of phenylalanine and tyrosine and aqueous solution. *Radiation Research*, **40**, 1–10.

Whitaker, J.R., and Feeney, R.E. (1983). Chemical and physical modification of proteins by the hydroxide ion. *Critical Reviews of Food Science and Nutrition*, **19**, 173–212.

Whitburn, K.D. (1987). The interaction of oxymyoglobin with hydrogen peroxide: the formation of ferrylmyoglobin at moderate excesses of hydrogen peroxide. *Archives of Biochemistry and Biophysics*, **253**, 419–430.

Whitburn, K.D. (1988). The interaction of oxymyoglobin with hydrogen peroxide: a kinetic anomaly at large excesses of hydrogen peroxide. *Archives of Biochemistry and Biophysics*, **267**, 614–622.

Whitburn, K.D., Shieh, J.J., Sellers, R.M., Hoffman, M.Z., and Taub, I.A. (1989). Redox transformations in ferrimyoglobin induced by radiation-generated free radicals in aqueous solution. *Journal of Biological Chemistry*, **257**, 1860–1869.

White, F.J., Hauck, B., Kon, H., and Riesz, P. (1969). Tritium labeling of proteins by the free-radical interceptor method with the aid of electrical discharge. *Analytical Biochemistry*, **30**, 295–299.

White, F.J., Kon, H., and Riesz, P. (1971). Camparison of electrical discharge with gamma-radiation for the production of free radicals in lyophilized proteins. *Radiation Research*, **45**, 8–24.

White, S., Boyd, G., Mathews, F.S., Xia, Z.X., Dai, W.W., Zhang, Y.F., *et al.* (1993). The active site structure of the calcium-containing quinoprotein methanol dehydrogenase. *Biochemistry*, **32**, 12955–12958.

Whiteman, M., Tritschler, H., and Halliwell, B. (1996). Protection against peroxynitrite-dependent tyrosine nitration and alpha-1–antiproteinase by oxidised and reduced lipoic acid. *FEBS Letters*, **379**, 74–76.

Wickens, D.G., Li, M.K., Atkins, G., Fuller, B.J., Hobbs, K.E., and Dormandy, T.L. (1987). Free radicals in hypothermic rat heart preservation—prevention of damage by mannitol and desferrioxamine. *Free Radical Research Communications*, **4**, 189–195.

Wickens, D.G., Davies, M.J., Fairbank, J., Tay, S.K., Slater, T.F., and Dormandy, T.L. (1990). Studies on cervical intraepithelial neoplasia: the level of octadeca-9,11-dienoic acid and measurement of free radical content by electron spin resonance spectroscopy. *American Journal of Obstetrics and Gynecology*, **162**, 854–858.

Wieland, E., Schutz, E., Armstrong, V.W., Kuthe, F., Heller, C., and Oellerich, M. (1995). Idebenone protects hepatic microsomes against oxygen radical-mediated damage in organ preservation solutions. *Transplantation*, **60**, 444–451.

Wiertz, E.J.H.J., Tortorella, D., Bogyo, M., Yu, J., Mothes, W., Jones, T.R., *et al.* (1996). Sec61-mediated transfer of a membrane protein from the endoplasmic reticulum to the proteasome for destruction. *Nature*, **384**, 432–438.

Wiese, A.G., Pacifici, R.E., and Davies, K.J. (1995). Transient adaptation of oxidative stress in mammalian cells. *Archives of Biochemistry and Biophysics*, **318**, 231–240.

Wilkinson, F., and Brummer, J.G. (1981). Rate constants for the deacy and reactions of the lowest electronically excited singlet state of molecular oxygen in solution. *Journal of Physical Chemistry Reference Data*, **10**, 809–1000.

Wilks, A., and Ortiz de Montellano, P.R. (1992). Intramolecular translocation of the protein radical formed in the reaction of recombinant sperm whale myoglobin with H_2O_2. *Journal of Biological Chemistry*, **267**, 8827–8833.

Wilks, A., and Ortiz de Montellano, P.R. (1993). Rat liver heme oxygenase. High level expression of a truncated soluble form and nature of the meso-hydroxylating species. *Journal of Biological Chemistry*, **268**, 22357–22362.

Wilks, A., Torpey, J., and Ortiz de Montellano, P.R. (1994). Heme oxygenase (HO-1). Evidence for electrophilic oxygen addition to the porphyrin ring in the formation of alpha-meso-hydroxyheme. *Journal of Biological Chemistry*, **269**, 29553–29556.

Williams, M., Lagerberg, J.W., Van Steveninck, J., and Van der Zee, J. (1995). The effect of protoporphyrin on the susceptibility of human erythrocytes to oxidative stress: exposure to hydrogen peroxide. *Biochimica et Biophysica Acta*, **1236**, 81–88.

Willix, R.L., and Garrison, W.M. (1967). Chemistry of the hydrated electron in oxygen-free solutions of amino acids, peptides, and related compounds. *Radiation Research*, **32**, 452–462.

Willson, R.L. (1970). Pulse radiolysis of electron transfer in aqueous disulphide solutions. *Journal of the Chemical Society, Chemical Communications*, 1425–1426.

Willson, R.L., Dunster, C.A., Forni, L.G., Gee, C.A., and Kittridge, K.J. (1985). Organic free radicals and proteins in biochemical injury: electron- or hydrogen-transfer reactions? *Philosophical Transactions of the Royal Society of London. B Biological Sciences*, **311**, 545–563.

Wilson, J.B., Brennan, S.O., Allen, J., Shaw, J.G., Gu, L.H., and Huisman, T.H. (1993). The M gamma chain of human fetal hemoglobin is an A gamma chain with an *in vitro* modification of gamma 141 leucine to hydroxyleucine. *Journal of Chromatography*, **617**, 37–42.

Wilson, M.B., and Nakane, P.K. (1976). The covalent coupling of proteins to periodate-oxidized sephadex: a new approach to immunoadsorbent preparation. *Journal of Immunology Methods*, **12**, 171–181.

Wilson, M.T., Jensen, P., Aasa, R., Malmstrom, B.G., and Vanngard, T. (1982). An investigation by e.p.r. and optical spectroscopy of cytochrome oxidase during turnover. *Biochemical Journal*, **203**, 483–492.

Winchester, R.V., and Lynn, K.R. (1970). X and gamma radiolysis of some tryptophan dipeptides. *International Journal of Radiation Biology and Related Studies in Physics, Chemistry and Medicine*, **17**, 541–548.

Wing, S.S., Chiang, H.L., Goldberg, A.L., and Dice, J.F. (1991). Proteins containing peptide sequences related to Lys-Phe-Glu-Arg-Gln are selectively depleted in liver and heart, but not skeletal muscle, of fasted rats. *Biochemical Journal*, **275**, 165–169.

Winter, G.E.M., and Butler, A. (1996). Inactivation of vanadium bromoperoxidase: formation of 2-oxohistidine. *Biochemistry*, **35**, 11805–11811.

Winterbourn, C.C. (1985). Comparative reactivities of various biological compounds with myeloperoxidase-hydrogen peroxide-chloride, and similarity of the oxidant to hypochlorite. *Biochimica et Biophysica Acta*, **840**, 204–210.

Winterbourn, C.C., and Carrell, R.W. (1976). Oxidation of human hemoglobin by copper. Mechanism and suggested role of the thiol group of residue beta-93. *Biochemical Journal*, **165**, 141–148.

Wishnok, J.S., Tannenbaum, S.R., Stillwell, W.G., Glogowski, J.A., and Leaf, C.D. (1993). Urinary markers for exposures to alkylating or nitrosating agents. *Environmental Health Perspectives*, **99**, 155–159.

Witt, E.H., Reznick, A.Z., Viguie, C.A., Starke, R.P., and Packer, L. (1992). Exercise, oxidative damage and effects of antioxidant manipulation. *Journal of Nutrition*, **122 (Supplement 3)**, 766, 773.

Wittenberg, B.A., Kampa, L., Wittenberg, J.B., Blumberg, W.E., and Peisach, J. (1968). The electronic structure of protoheme proteins. II. An electron paramagnetic resonance and optical study of cytochrome *c* peroxidase and its derivatives. *Journal of Biological Chemistry*, **243**, 1863–1870.

Witting, P.K., Bowry, V.W., and Stocker, R. (1995). Inverse deuterium kinetic isotope effect for peroxidation in human low-density lipoprotein (LDL): a simple test for tocopherol-mediated peroxidation of LDL lipids. *FEBS Letters*, **375**, 45–49.

Wizemann, T.M., Gardner, C.R., Laskin, J.D., Quinones, S., Durham, S.K., Goller, N.L., *et al.* (1994). Production of nitric oxide and peroxynitrite in the lung during acute endotoxemia. *Journal of Leukocyte Biology*, **56**, 759–768.

Wogan, G.N. (1989). Markers of exposure to carcinogens. *Environmental Health Perspectives*, **81**, 9–17.

Wolff, S.P., and Dean, R.T. (1986). Fragmentation of proteins by free radicals and its effect on their susceptibility to enzymic hydrolysis. *Biochemical Journal*, **234**, 399–403.

Wolff, S.P., and Dean, R.T. (1987a). Glucose autoxidation and protein modification. The potential role of 'autoxidative glycosylation' in diabetes. *Biochemical Journal*, **245**, 243–250.

Wolff, S.P., and Dean, R.T. (1987b). Monosaccharide autoxidation: a potential source of oxidative stress in diabetes? Formation and reactions of peroxides in biological systems. *Bioelectrochemistry and Bioenergetics*, **18**, 283–293.

Wolff, S.P., and Dean, R.T. (1988). Aldehydes and dicarbonyls in non-enzymic glycosylation of proteins. *Biochemical Journal*, **249**, 618–619.

Wolff, S.P., Garner, A., and Dean, R.T. (1986). Free radicals, lipids and protein breakdown. *Trends in Biochemical Science*, **11**, 27–31.

Wolff, S.P., Bascal, Z.A., and Hunt, J.V. (1989). 'Autoxidative glycosylation': free radicals and glycation theory. *Progress in Clinical Biology Research*, **304**, 259–275.

Wolff, S.P., Jiang, Z.Y., and Hunt, J.V. (1991). Protein glycation and oxidative stress in diabetes mellitus and ageing. *Free Radical Biology and Medicine*, **10**, 339–352.

Wolfgang, G.H., Jolly, R.A., and Petry, T.W. (1991). Diquat-induced oxidative damage in hepatic microsomes: effects of antioxidants. *Free Radical Biology and Medicine*, **10**, 403–411.

Wondrak, G., Pier, T., and Tressl, R. (1995). Light from Maillard reaction: photon counting, emission spectrum, photography and visual perception. *Journal of Bioluminesence and Chemiluminesence*, **10**, 277–284.

Wong, C.G., Bonakdar, M., Mautz, W.J., and Kleinman, M.T. (1996). Chronic inhalation exposure to ozone and nitric acid elevates stress-inducible heat shock protein 70 in the rat lung. *Toxicology*, **107**, 111–119.

Wong, K.K., Murray, B.W., Lewisch, S.A., Baxter, M.K., Ridky, T.W., Ulissi, D.L., *et al.* (1993). Molecular properties of pyruvate formate-lyase activating enzyme. *Biochemistry*, **32**, 14102–14110.

Wood, H.N., and Balls, A.K. (1955). Enzymatic oxidation of alpha-chymotrypsin. *Journal of Biological Chemistry*, **213**, 297–305.

Wood, K.A., and Youle, R.J. (1995). The role of free radicals and p53 in neuron apoptosis *in vivo*. *Journal of Neuroscience*, **15**, 5851–5857.

Woodland, M.P., and Dalton, H. (1984). Purification and characterization of component A of the methane monooxygenase from Methylococcus capsulatus (Bath). *Journal of Biological Chemistry*, **259**, 53–59.

Woodward, H.Q. (1932). The effect of X-radiation on the viscosity of gelatin. *Journal of Physical Chemistry*, **36**, 2543–2553.

Wratten, M.L., van Ginkel, G., van't Veld, A.A., Bekker, A., van Faasen, E.E., and Sevanian, A. (1992). Structural and dynamic effects of oxidatively modified phospholipids in unsaturated lipid membranes. *Biochemistry*, **31**, 10901–10907.

Wright, N.C. (1926). Action of hypochlorites on amino acids and proteins. *Biochemical Journal*, **20**, 524–532.

Wright, N.C. (1936). The action of hypochlorites on amino acids and proteins. The effect of acidity and alkalinity. *Biochemical Journal*, **30**, 1661–1667.

Wu, X.B., Brune, B., von Appen, F., and Ullrich, V. (1992). Reversible activation of soluble guanylate cyclase by oxidizing agents. *Archives of Biochemistry and Biophysics*, **294**, 75–82.

Wurzel, H., Yeh, C.C., Gairola, C., and Chow, C.K. (1995). Oxidative damage and antioxidant status in the lungs and bronchoalveolar lavage fluid of rats exposed chronically to cigarette smoke. *Journal of Biochemical Toxicology*, **10**, 11–17.

Xanthoudakis, S., Miao, G., Wang, F., Pan, Y.C., and Curran, T. (1992*a*). Redox activation of Fos-Jun DNA binding activity is mediated by a DNA repair enzyme. *EMBO Journal*, **11**, 3323–3335.

Xanthoudakis, S., and Curran, T. (1992*b*). Identification and characterization of Ref-1, a nuclear protein that facilitates AP-1 DNA-binding activity. *EMBO Journal*, **11**, 653–665.

Xanthoudakis, S., Miao, G.G., and Curran, T. (1994). The redox and DNA-repair activities of Ref-1 are encoded by nonoverlapping domains. *Proceedings of the National Academy of Science of the United States of America*, **91**, 23–27.

Xia, C., Hu, J., Ketterer, B., and Taylor, J.B. (1996). The organization of the human GSTP1-1 gene promoter and its response to retinoic acid and cellular redox status. *Biochemical Journal*, **313**, 155–161.

Xia, Y., Dawson, V.L., Dawson, T.M., Snyder, S.H., and Zweier, J.L. (1996). Nitric oxide synthase generates superoxide and nitric oxide in arginine-depleted cells leading to peroxynitrite-mediated cellular injury. *Proceedings of the National Academy of Science of the United States of America*, **93**, 6770–6774.

Xia, Z.X., Hao, Z.P., Mathews, F.S., and Davidson, V.L. (1989). Crystallization and preliminary X-ray crystallographic study of the quinoprotein methanol dehydrogenase from bacterium W3A1. *FEBS Letters*, **258**, 175–176.

Xu, F., DeFilippi, L.J., Ballou, D.P., and Hultquist, D.E. (1993). Hydrogen peroxide-dependent formation and bleaching of the higher oxidation states of bovine erythrocyte green hemeprotein. *Archives of Biochemistry and Biophysics*, **301**, 184–189.

Xu, Y., Asghar, A., Gray, J.I., Pearson, A.M., Haug, A., and Grulke, E.A. (1990). ESR spin-trapping studies of free radicals generatred by hydrogen peroxide activation of metmyoglobin. *Journal of Agricultural and Food Chemistry*, **38**, 1494–1497.

Yablonski, M.J., and Theil, E.C. (1992). A possible role for the conserved trimer interface of ferritin in iron incorporation. *Biochemistry*, **31**, 9680–9684.

Yalcin, A.S., Sabuncu, N., and Emerk, K. (1992). Cumene hydroperoxide-induced chemiluminescence in human erythrocytes: effect of antioxidants and sulfydryl compounds. *International Journal of Biochemistry*, **24**, 499–502.

Yamada, H., Yamashita, T., Domoto, H., and Imoto, T. (1990). Reaction of hen egg-white lysozyme with tetranitromethane: a new side reaction, oxidative bond cleavage at glycine 104, and sequential nitration of three tyrosine residues. *Journal of Biochemistry, Tokyo,*, **108**, 432–440.

Yamada, M., Hearse, D.J., and Curtis, M.J. (1990). Reperfusion and readmission of oxygen. Pathophysiological relevance of oxygen-derived free radicals to arrhythmogenesis. *Circulation Research*, **67**, 1211–1224.

Yamada, M., Momose, K., Richelson, E., and Yamada, M. (1996). Sodium nitroprusside-induced apoptotic cellular death via production of hydrogen peroxide in murine neuroblastoma N1E-115 cells. *Journal of Pharmacological and Toxicological Methods*, **35**, 11–17.

Yamagata, K., Furuta, H., Oda, N., Kaisaki, P.J., Menzel, S., Cox, N.J., *et al.* (1996). Mutations in the hepatocyte nuclear factor-4alpha gene in maturity-onset diabetes of the young (MODY1). *Nature*, **384**, 458–460.

Yamaguchi, T., Nagatoshi, A., and Kimoto, E. (1985). Oxidation of nitroxide radicals by an iron-hydrogen peroxide-amino acid system. *FEBS Letters*, **192**, 259–262.

Yamamoto, O. (1973). Radiation-induced binding of phenylalanine, tryptophan and histidine mutually and with albumin. *Radiation Research*, **54**, 398–410.

Yamashita, Y., Shimokata, K., Mizuno, S., Daikoku, T., Tsurumi, T., and Nishiyama, Y. (1996). Calnexin acts as a molecular chaperone during the folding of glycoprotein B of human cytomegalovirus. *Journal of Virology*, **70**, 2237–2246.

Yamazaki, I. (1971). One-electron and two-electron transfer mechanisms in enzymic oxidation-reduction reactions. *Advances in Biophysics,*, **2**, 33–76.

Yamazaki, I., and Harada, K. (1987). Free radicals in proteins and enzymes. *Tanpakushitsu Kakusan Koso*, **32**, 1141–1150.

Yan, L.J., Traber, M.G., and Packer, L. (1995). Spectrophotometric method for determination of carbonyls in oxidatively modified apolipoprotein B of human low density lipoproteins. *Analytical Biochemistry*, **228**, 349–351.

Yan, L.J., Traber, M.G., Kobuchi, H., Matsugo, S., Tritschler, H.J., and Packer, L. (1996). Efficacy of hypochlorous acid scavengers in the prevention of protein carbonyl formation. *Archives of Biochemistry and Biophysics*, **327**, 330–334.

Yan, S.D., Yan, S.F., Chen, X., Fu, J., Chen, M., Kuppusamy, P., *et al.* (1995). Non-enzymatically glycated tau in Alzheimer's disease induces neuronal oxidant stress resulting in cytokine gene expression and release of amyloid beta-peptide. *Nature (Medicine)*, **1**, 693–699.

Yang, J.P., Merin, J.P., Nakano, T., Kato, T., Kitade, Y., and Okamoto, T. (1995). Inhibition of the DNA-binding activity of NF-kappa B by gold compounds *in vitro*. *FEBS Letters*, **361**, 89–96.

Yang, S.F. (1973). Destruction of tryptophan during the aerobic oxidation of sulfite ions. *Environmental Research*, **6**, 395–402.

Yang, X., Galeano, N.F., Szabolcs, M., Sciacca, R.R., and Cannon, P.J. (1996). Oxidized low density lipoproteins alter macrophage lipid uptake, apoptosis, viability and nitric oxide synthesis. *Journal of Nutrition*, **126 (Supplement 4)**, 1072S–1075S.

Yao, K.S., Xanthoudakis, S., Curran, T., and O'Dwyer, P.J. (1994). Activation of AP-1 and of a nuclear redox factor, Ref-1, in the response of HT29 colon cancer cells to hypoxia. *Molecular and Cellular Biology*, **14**, 5997–6003.

Yao, Y., Yin, D., Jas, G.S., Kuczer, K., Williams, T.D., Schoneich, C., *et al.* (1996). Oxidative modification of a carboxyl-terminal vicinal methionine in calmodulin by hydrogen peroxide inhibits calmodulin-dependent activation of the plasma membrane Ca-ATPase. *Biochemistry*, **35**, 2767–2787.

Yasutake, M., Ibuki, C., Hearse, D.J., and Avkiran, M. (1994). Na^+/H^+ exchange and reperfusion arrhythmias: protection by intracoronary infusion of a novel inhibitor. *American Journal of Physiology*, **267**, H2430-H2440.

Yazdanparast, R., Andrews, P., Smith, D.L., and Dixon, J.E. (1986). A new approach for detection and assignment of disulfide bonds in peptides. *Analytical Biochemistry*, **153**, 348–353.

Yelinova, V., Glazachev, Y., Khramtsov, V., Kudryashova, L., Rykova, V., and Salganik, R. (1996). Studies of human and rat blood under oxidative stress: changes in plasma thiol level, antioxidant enzyme activity, protein carbonyl content, and fluidity of erythrocyte membrane. *Biochemical and Biophysical Research Communications*, **221**, 300–303.

Yen, S.H., Liu, W.K., Hall, F.L., Yan, S.D., Stern, D., and Dickson, D.W. (1995). Alzheimer neurofibrillary lesions: molecular nature and potential roles of different components. *Neurobiological Aging*, **16**, 381–387.

Yen, Y.C., Yang, M.C., Kenny, A.D., and Pang, P.K. (1983). Parathyroid hormone (PTH) fragments relax the guinea-pig trachea *in vitro*. *Canadian Journal of Physiology and Pharmacology*, **61**, 1324–1328.

Yeo, H.C., Helbock, H.J., Chyu, D.W., and Ames, B.N. (1994). Assay of malondialdehyde in biological fluids by gas chromatography-mass spectrometry. *Analytical Biochemistry*, **220**, 391–396.

Yim, H.S., Kang, S.O., Hah, Y.C., Chock, P.B., and Yim, M.B. (1995). Free radicals generated during the glycation reaction of amino acids by methylglyoxal. A model study of protein-cross-linked free radicals. *Journal of Biological Chemistry*, **270**, 28228–28233.

Yim, M.B., Chock, P.B., and Stadtman, E.R. (1990a). Copper, zinc superoxide dismutase catalyzes hydroxyl radical production from hydrogen peroxide. *Proceedings of the National Academy of Science of the United States of America*, **87**, 5006–5010.

Yim, M.B., Berlett, B.S., Chock, P.B., and Stadtman, E.R. (1990b). Manganese(II)-bicarbonate-mediated catalytic activity for hydrogen peroxide dismutation and amino acid oxidation: detection of free radical intermediates. *Proceedings of the National Academy of Science of the United States of America*, **87**, 394–398.

Yim, M.B., Chock, P.B., and Stadtman, E.R. (1993). Enzyme function of copper, zinc superoxide dismutase as a free radical generator. *Journal of Biological Chemistry*, **268**, 4099–4105.

Yim, M.B., Chae, H.Z., Rhee, S.G., Chock, P.B., and Stadtman, E.R. (1994). On the protective mechanism of the thiol-specific antioxidant enzyme against the oxidative damage of biomacromolecules. *Journal of Biological Chemistry*, **269**, 1621–1626.

Yin, D.Z., and Brunk, U.T. (1991). Microfluorometric and fluorometric lipofuscin spectral discrepancies: a concentration-dependent metachromatic effect? *Mechanisms of Ageing and Development*, **59**, 95–109.

Yin, D., Yuan, X., and Brunk, U.T. (1995). Test-tube simulated lipofuscinogenesis. Effect of oxidative stress on autophagocytotic degradation. *Mechanisms of Ageing and Development*, **81**, 37–50.

Yin, D.Z. (1992). Lipofuscin-like fluorophores can result from reactions between oxidized ascorbic acid and glutamine. Carbonyl-protein cross-linking may represent a common reaction in oxygen radical and glycosylation-related ageing processes. *Mechanisms of Ageing and Development*, **62**, 35–45.

Yla-Herttuala, S., Lipton, B.A., Rosenfeld, M.E., Sarkioja, T., Yoshimura, T., Leonard, E.J., et al. (1991). Expression of monocyte chemoattractant protein 1 in macrophage-rich areas of human and rabbit atherosclerotic lesions. *Proceedings of the National Academy of Science of the United States of America*, **88**, 5252–5256.

Yla-Herttuala, S., Luoma, J., Viita, H., Hiltunen, T., Sisto, T., and Nikkari, T. (1995). Transfer of 15-lipoxygenase gene into rabbit iliac arteries results in the appearance of oxidation-specific lipid-protein adducts characteristic of oxidized low density lipoprotein. *Journal of Clinical Investigation*, **95**, 2692–2698.

Yonetani, T., and Schleyer, H. (1967). Studies on cytochrome *c* peroxidase. IX. The reaction of ferrimyoglobin with hydroperoxides and a comparison of peroxide-induced compounds of ferrimyoglobin and cytochrome *c* peroxidase. *Journal of Biological Chemistry*, **242**, 1974–1979.

Yoshida, H., Turner, J.E., Bolch, W.E., Jacobson, K.B., and Garrison, W.M. (1992). Measurement of products from X-irradiated glycylglycine in oxygen-free aqueous solutions. *Radiation Research*, **129**, 258–264.

Yoshioka, K., Deng, T., Cavigelli, M., and Karin, M. (1995). Antitumor promotion by phenolic antioxidants: inhibition of AP-1 activity through induction of Fra expression. *Proceedings of the National Academy of Science of the United States of America*, **92**, 4972–4976.

Young, P., Andersson, J., Sahlin, M., and Sjoberg, B.-M. (1996). Bacteriophage T4 anaerobic ribonucleotide reductase contains a stable glycyl radical at position 580. *Journal of Biological Chemistry*, **271**, 20770–20775.

Young, R.G., and Tappel, A.L. (1978). Fluorescent pigment and pentane production by lipid peroxidation in honey bees, *Apis mellifera*. *Experimental Gerontology*, **13**, 457–459.

Youngman, L.D., Park, J.Y., and Ames, B.N. (1992). Protein oxidation associated with aging is reduced by dietary restriction of protein or calories [published erratum appears in *Proceedings of the National Academy of Science of the United States of America* (1992), **15**, 11107]. *Proceedings of the National Academy of Science of the United States of America*, **89**, 9112–9116.

Yuan, X.M., Li, W., Olsson, A.G., and U.T., B. (1996). Iron in human atheroma and LDL oxidation by macrophages following erythrophagocytosis. *Atherosclerosis*, **124**, 61–73.

Zakowski, J.J., Forstrom, J.W., Condell, R.A., and Tappel, A.L. (1978). Attachment of selenocysteine in the catalytic site of glutathione peroxidase. *Biochemical and Biophysical Research Communications*, **84**, 248–253.

Zamora, R., Hidalgo, F.J., and Tappel, A.L. (1990). Oxidant-increased proteolysis in rat liver slices: effect of bromotrichloromethane, antioxidants and effectors of proteolysis. *Chemico-Biological Interactions*, **76**, 293–305.

Zamora, R., Hidalgo, F.J., and Tappel, A.L. (1991). Comparative antioxidant effectiveness of dietary beta-carotene, vitamin E, selenium and coenzyme Q10 in rat erythrocytes and plasma. *Journal of Nutrition*, **121**, 50–56.

Zavoisky, E. (1944). Paramagnetic absorption of a solution in parallel fields. *Journal of Physics USSR*, **8**, 377–380.

Zavoisky, E. (1945a). Paramagnetic relaxation of liquid solutions for perpendicular fields. *Journal of Physics USSR*, **9**, 211–216.

Zavoisky, E. (1945b). Spin-magnetic resonance in paramagnetic substances. *Journal of Physics USSR*, **9**, 245.

Zavoisky, E. (1946). Paramagnetic absorption in some salts in perpendicular magnetic fields. *Journal of Physics USSR*, **10**, 170–173.

Zemel, H., and Fessenden, R.W. (1975). Electron spin resonance studies of phenyl and pyridyl radicals in aqueous solution. *Journal of Physical Chemistry*, **79**, 1419–1427.

Zer, H., and Ohad, I. (1995). Photoinactivation of photosystem II induces changes in the photochemical reaction center II abolishing the regulatory role of the QB site in the D1 protein degradation. *European Journal of Biochemistry*, **231**, 448–453.

Zer, H., Prasil, O., and Ohad, I. (1994). Role of plastoquinol oxidoreduction in regulation of photochemical reaction center IID1 protein turnover *in vivo*. *Journal of Biological Chemistry*, **269**, 17670–17676.

Zgliczynski, J.M., and Stelmaszynska, T. (1975). Chlorinating ability of human phagocytosing leucocytes. *European Journal of Biochemistry*, **56**, 157–162.*

Zgliczynski, J.M., Stelmaszynska, T., Ostrowski, W., Naskalski, J., and Sznajd, J. (1968). Myeloperoxidase of human leukaemic leucocytes. Oxidation of amino acids in the presence of hydrogen peroxide. *European Journal of Biochemistry*, **4**, 540–547.

Zgliczynski, J.M., Stelmaszynska, T., Domanski, J., and Ostrowski, W. (1971). Chloramines as intermediates of oxidation reaction of amino acids by myeloperoxidase. *Biochimica et Biophysica Acta.*, **235**, 419–424.

Zhai, X., Lawson, C.S., Cave, A.C., and Hearse, D.J. (1993). Preconditioning and post-ischaemic contractile dysfunction: the role of impaired oxygen delivery vs extracellular metabolite accumulation. *Journal of Molecular and Cellular Cardiology*, **25**, 847–857.

Zhang, J., and Snyder, S.H. (1993). Purification of a nitric oxide-stimulated ADP-ribosylated protein using biotinylated beta-nicotinamide adenine dinucleotide. *Biochemistry*, **32**, 2228–2233.

Zhang, J., Pieper, A., and Snyder, S.H. (1995). Poly(ADP-ribose) synthetase activation: an early indicator of neurotoxic DNA damage. *Journal of Neurochemistry*, **65**, 1411–1414.

Zhang, X., Fuller, J.H., and McIntire, W.S. (1993). Cloning, sequencing, expression, and regulation of the structural gene for the copper/topa quinone-containing methylamine oxidase from *Arthrobacter strain P1*, a gram-positive facultative methylotroph. *Journal of Bacteriology*, **175**, 5617–5627.

Zhang, Y., Marcillat, O., Giulivi, C., Ernster, L., and Davies, K.J. (1990). The oxidative inactivation of mitochondrial electron transport chain components and ATPase. *Journal of Biological Chemistry*, **265**, 16330–16336.

Zhao, R., Lind, J., Merényi, G., and Eriksen, T.E. (1994). Kinetics of one-electron oxidation of thiols and hydrogen abstraction by thiyl radicals from α-amino C–H bonds. *Journal of the American Chemical Society*, **116**, 12010–12015.

Zhao, R., Lind, J., Merenyi, G., and Eriksen, T.E. (1996). The fate of glutathione thiyl radicals in oxygenated solution. In *Abstracts of VIII Biennial Meeting International Society for Free Radical Research*. p. 249, Barcelona.

Zhou, J.Q., and Gafni, A. (1991). Exposure of rat muscle phosphoglycerate kinase to a nonenzymatic MFO system generates the old form of the enzyme. *Journal of Gerontology*, **46**, B217–221.

Zhu, L., and Crouch, R.K. (1992). Albumin in the cornea is oxidized by hydrogen peroxide. *Cornea*, **11**, 567–572.

Zhu, S., Haddad, I.Y., and Matalon, S. (1996). Nitration of surfactant protein A (SP-A) tyrosine residues results in decreased mannose binding ability. *Archives of Biochemistry and Biophysics*, **333**, 282–290.

Zhuang, Z., Huang, X., and Costa, M. (1994). Protein oxidation and amino acid-DNA crosslinking by nickel compounds in intact cultured cells. *Toxicology and Applied Pharmacology*, **126**, 319–325.

Zhukov, I.I., and Unkovskaya, V.A. (1930). Influence of radon on the viscosity of gelatin solutions. *Journal of the Russian Physical Chemistry Society*, **62**, 581–600.

Zidek, L., Machala, M., and Skursky, L. (1991). Interactions of organic hydroperoxides with heme proteins. *Drug Metabolism and Drug Interaction*, **9**, 209–224.

Ziedler, U., Barth, C., and G., S. (1995). Radiation-induced and free radical-mediated inactivation of ion channels formed by the polyene antibiotic amphotericin B in lipid membranes: effect of radical scavengers and single-channel analysis. *International Journal of Radiation Biology and Related Studies in Physics, Chemistry and Medicine*, **67**, 127–134.

Zimmermann, R., Munck, E., Brill, W.J., Shah, V.K., Henzl, M.T., Rawlings, J., et al. (1978). Nitrogenase X: Mossbauer and EPR studies on reversibly oxidized MoFe protein from *Azotobacter vinelandii OP*. Nature of the iron centers. *Biochimica et Biophysica Acta*, **537**, 185–207.

Zirlin, A., and Karel, M. (1969). Oxidation effects in freeze-dried gelatin-methyl linoleate system. *Journal of Food Science*, **34**, 160–164.

Zu, J., Morita, J., Nishikawa, S., and Kashimura, N. (1996). Generation of active oxygen species by some low-molecular weight Amadori rearrangement products under physiological conditions. *Carbohydrate Letters*, **1**, 457–464.

Zweier, J.L. (1988). Measurement of superoxide-derived free radicals in the reperfused heart. *Journal of Biological Chemistry*, **263**, 1353–1357.

Zweier, J.L., Flaherty, J.T., and Weisfeldt, M.L. (1987). Direct measurement of free radical generation following reperfusion of ischemic myocardium. *Proceedings of the National Academy of Science of the United States of America*, **84**, 1404–1407.

Zwizinski, C.W., and Schmid, H.H. (1992). Peroxidative damage to cardiac mitochondria: identification and purification of modified adenine nucleotide translocase. *Archives of Biochemistry and Biophysics*, **294**, 178–183.

Index

Printed in the United Kingdom
by Lightning Source UK Ltd.
101771UKS00001B/146